Vascular Disease, Alzheimer's Disease, and Mild Cognitive Impairment

Vascular Disease, Alzheimer's Disease, and Mild Cognitive Impairment

Advancing an Integrated Approach

Edited by

DAVID J. LIBON, MELISSA LAMAR,
RODNEY A. SWENSON, AND
KENNETH M. HEILMAN

OXFORD
UNIVERSITY PRESS

OXFORD
UNIVERSITY PRESS

Oxford University Press is a department of the University of Oxford. It furthers the University's objective of excellence in research, scholarship, and education by publishing worldwide. Oxford is a registered trade mark of Oxford University Press in the UK and certain other countries.

Published in the United States of America by Oxford University Press
198 Madison Avenue, New York, NY 10016, United States of America.

Library of Congress Cataloging-in-Publication Data
Names: Libon, David J., editor. | Lamar, Melissa, editor. |
Swenson, Rodney A., editor. | Heilman, Kenneth M., 1938– editor.
Title: Vascular disease, Alzheimer's Disease, and mild cognitive impairment :
advancing an integrated approach / edited by David J. Libon, Melissa
Lamar, Rodney A. Swenson, Kenneth M. Heilman.
Description: New York : Oxford University Press, 2020. |
Includes bibliographical references and index. |
Identifiers: LCCN 2019044905 (print) | LCCN 2019044906 (ebook) |
ISBN 9780190634230 (hardback) | ISBN 9780190668556 (epub) | ISBN 9780190634254 (online)
Subjects: LCSH: Cognition disorders—Patients—Rehabilitation. |
Cerebrovascular disease—Patients—Rehabilitation. | Alzheimer's diseases—Treatment.
Classification: LCC RC553.C64 V37 2020 (print) | LCC RC553.C64 (ebook) |
DDC 616.8—dc23
LC record available at https://lccn.loc.gov/2019044905
LC ebook record available at https://lccn.loc.gov/2019044906

Contents

Preface ix
Vladimir Hachinski
Contributors xi
Introduction xv
David J. Libon, Melissa Lamar, Rodney A. Swenson, and Kenneth M. Heilman

PART 1 EPIDEMIOLOGY AND NEUROPSYCHOLOGY

1. Vascular Risk Factors and Their Relationship to Brain Aging: Findings from the Framingham Heart Study 3
Ting Fang Alvin Ang, Prajakta Joshi, and Rhoda Au
2. Heterogeneity in Alzheimer's/Vascular Spectrum Dementia 30
Sheina Emrani, Melissa Lamar, Catherine C. Price, Victor Wasserman, Emily Matusz, Rodney A. Swenson, Kenneth M. Heilman, and David J. Libon
3. Neuropsychological Contributions to the Diagnosis of Mild Cognitive Impairment Associated With Alzheimer's Disease 52
Joel Eppig, Madeleine Werhane, Emily C. Edmonds, Lisa-Delano Wood, Katherine J. Bangen, Amy Jak, Kelsey R. Thomas, Christina Wong, Alexandra Weigand, and Mark W. Bondi
4. Vascular Cognitive Impairment 83
Victor Wasserman, Sheina Emrani, Emily Matusz, Catherine C. Price, Melissa Lamar, Rodney A. Swenson, Kenneth M. Heilman, and David J. Libon
5. Decline in Everyday Functioning in MCI and Dementia: A Neuropsychological Perspective 102
Rachel Mis and Tania Giovannetti
6. Heterogeneity in Dementia and Mild Cognitive Impairment: Using Statistical Modeling Techniques 129
Deborah A. G. Drabick and Jill Rabinowitz
7. Apraxic and Action-Intentional Disorders Associated With Vascular and Degenerative Dementing Diseases 146
Kenneth M. Heilman

PART 2 NEUROIMAGING

8. Cerebral Small Vessel Disease and the Risk of Dementia and Cognition Decline 187
Emilia Salvadori, Fabio Fierini, and Leonardo Pantoni

9. Structural MRI in Alzheimer's Disease: Are We Measuring the Right Stuff? 208
Briana S. Last, Batool Rizvi, and Adam M. Brickman

10. Brain Structural Alterations Common to Cardiovascular Disease Risk Factors and Alzheimer's Dementia: Implications for Connectomics and Cognition 241
Melissa Lamar, Elizabeth A. Boots, Konstantinos Arfanakis, Lisa L. Barnes, and Julie A. Schneider

PART 3 BLOOD–BRAIN BARRIER AND CARDIOGENIC MECHANISMS

11. The Blood–Brain Barrier in Cognitive Decline and Alzheimer's Disease 261
Daniel A. Nation and Elissa McIntosh

12. Arterial Stiffening and Cerebrovascular Resistance in Cognitive Decline and Alzheimer's Disease 274
Belinda Yew, Anna Blanken, and Daniel A. Nation

13. Hemodynamics in Alzheimer's Disease and Vascular Cognitive Impairment and Dementia 302
Francis Cambronero and Angela L. Jefferson

PART 4 NEUROPATHOLOGICAL AND NEUROPHYSIOLOGICAL MECHANISMS

14. Neuropathology of Alzheimer's Disease and Vascular Dementia 333
Alifiya Kapasi and Julia A. Schneider

15. Potential of Blood- and CSF-Based Biomarkers for Alzheimer's Disease Diagnostics 375
Eric L. Goldwaser and Robert G. Nagele

16. Unraveling the Role of Mitochondria in Alzheimer's Disease: Toward Assembling the Puzzle 407
Sónia C. Correia, Paula I. Moreira, and George Perry

PART 5 TREATMENT AND INTERVENTION

17. Cognitive Change and Elective Surgeries With Anesthesia: Considerations for Neuropsychologists and the Growing Field of Perioperative Cognitive Medicine 433
Margaret E. Wiggins, Carlos Hernaiz, Brenda G. Fahy, and Catherine C. Price

18. Management of Mild Cognitive Impairment 458
Ramit Ravona-Springer and Amos D. Korczyn

Index 469

Preface

Cerebrovascular and Alzheimer disease often occur together but are usually studied apart. This book offers a timely integrated approach to both diseases. Beginning with a section on epidemiology and neuropsychology, this volume goes on to discuss and explore the neuropathological and neurophysiological mechanisms of these disorders. This book then develops a novel concept of an Alzheimer disease/vascular dementia spectrum. Sections on neuroimaging, as well as treatments and interventions, follow.

The editors have succeeded in gathering an impressive group of clinicians and scientists, who are well qualified by their achievements and leadership to make important contributions to this new integrated approach to dementing disorders.

This important book should have broad appeal to anyone studying or caring for patients with dementing disorders, as it is comprehensive, yet focused on a unitary, complementary and pragmatic approach.

Vladimir Hachinski, CM, MD, FRCPC, DSc
Professor of Neurology and Epidemiology
University of Western Ontario

Contributors

Ting Fang Alvin Ang, MD
Department of Anatomy and Neurobiology, Boston University School of Medicine
Department of Epidemiology, Boston University School of Public Health
The Framingham Heart Study, Boston University School of Medicine

Konstantinos Arfanakis, PhD
Professor
Rush Alzheimer's Disease Center, Department of Diagnostic Radiology and Nuclear Medicine, Rush University Medical Center
Department of Biomedical Engineering, Illinois Institute of Technology

Rhoda Au, PhD
Department of Anatomy and Neurobiology, Boston University School of Medicine
Department of Epidemiology, Boston University School of Public Health
The Framingham Heart Study, Boston University School of Medicine
Department of Neurology, Boston University School of Medicine
Boston University Alzheimer's Disease Center and Boston University CTE Center, Boston University School of Medicine

Katherine J. Bangen, PhD, ABPP-CN
Department of Psychiatry, University of California San Diego, School of Medicine
Veterans Affairs San Diego Healthcare System

Lisa L. Barnes, PhD
Alla V. and Solomon Jesmer Professor of Gerontology and Geriatric Medicine
Rush Alzheimer's Disease Center
Department of Neurological Sciences

Anna Blanken, MS
Department of Psychology
University of Southern California

Mark W. Bondi, PhD, ABPP-CN
Department of Psychiatry, University of California San Diego, School of Medicine
Veterans Affairs San Diego Healthcare System

Elizabeth A. Boots, MA
Department of Psychology, University of Illinois at Chicago
Rush Alzheimer's Disease Center, Rush University Medical Center

Adam M. Brickman, PhD
Professor of Neuropsychology
Taub Institute for Research on Alzheimer's Disease and the Aging Brain
Department of Neurology
College of Physicians and Surgeons, Columbia University

Francis Cambronero, AB
Neuroscience PhD Candidate
Vanderbilt Memory and Alzheimer's Center, Vanderbilt University Medical Center
Vanderbilt Brain Institute, Vanderbilt University

Sónia C. Correia, PhD
Center for Neuroscience and Cell Biology
University of Coimbra, Coimbra, Portugal

Deborah A. G. Drabick, PhD
Associate Professor
Department of Psychology, Temple University

Emily C. Edmonds, PhD
Department of Psychiatry, University of California San Diego, School of Medicine
Veterans Affairs San Diego Healthcare System

Sheina Emrani, MA
Department of Psychology
Rowan University

Joel S. Eppig, PhD
San Diego State University/University of California, San Diego, Joint Doctoral Program in Clinical Psychology
VA Puget Sound Healthcare System, Seattle Division

Brenda G. Fahy, MD
Associate Chief, Critical Care Medicine
Program Director, Adult Combined Cardiothoracic
Critical Care Medicine Fellowship
Professor of Anesthesiology
University of Florida

Fabio Fierini, MD
Psychiatry Unit, Department of Health Sciences
University of Florence, Florence

Tania Giovannetti, PhD, ABPP-CN
Associate Professor
Psychology Department, Temple University

Eric L. Goldwaser, DO, PhD
Psychiatry Resident
Physician-Scientist Training Program
University of Maryland Medical Center/ Sheppard Pratt Health System

Kenneth M. Heilman, MD
Distinguished Professor Emeritus
Department of Neurology, University of Florida College of Medicine
and Staff Neurologist, Malcom Randall Veterans Affairs Hospital

Carlos Hernaiz, BS
Clinical and Health Psychology
University of Florida

Amy J. Jak, PhD
Department of Psychiatry, University of California San Diego, School of Medicine
Veterans Affairs San Diego Healthcare System

Angela L. Jefferson, PhD
Professor of Neurology and Director of the Vanderbilt Memory and Alzheimer's Center
Department of Neurology
Vanderbilt University Medical Center

Prajakta Joshi, BDS, MPH
Department of Anatomy and Neurobiology, Boston University School of Medicine
The Framingham Heart Study, Boston University School of Medicine
Department of General Dentistry, Boston University Henry Goldman School of Dental Medicine

Alifiya Kapasi, PhD
Assistant Professor, Department of Pathology, Rush Alzheimer's Disease Center
Rush University Medical Center

Amos D. Korczyn, MD
Professor Emeritus
Departments of Neurology, Physiology and Pharmacology
Tel Aviv University
Founder and Chairman, CONy Neurology Congress

Melissa Lamar, PhD
Associate Professor
Department of Behavioral Sciences
Rush Alzheimer's Disease Center, Rush University Medical Center

Briana S. Last, MA
PhD Candidate in Clinical Psychology
Psychology Department, University of Pennsylvania

David J. Libon, PhD, ABN, FACPN
Professor
Department of Geriatrics and Gerontology and Department of Psychology
New Jersey Institute for Successful Aging
School of Osteopathic Medicine, Rowan University

Emily Matusz, MA
Research Assistant
New Jersey Institute for Successful Aging, School of Osteopathic Medicine, Rowan University

Elissa McIntosh, MA
Department of Psychology
University of Southern California

Rachel Mis, MA
Psychology Department
Temple University

Paula I. Moreira, PhD
Center for Neuroscience and Cell Biology
Laboratory of Physiology, Faculty of Medicine
University of Coimbra

Robert G. Nagele, PhD
Director, Biomarker Discovery Center
Professor of Geriatrics and Gerontology
New Jersey Institute for Successful Aging
School of Osteopathic Medicine, Rowan University

Daniel A. Nation, PhD
Department of Psychological Science
Institute for Memory Disorders and Neurological Impairments
University of California Irvine

Leonardo Pantoni, MD, PhD
Luigi Sacco Department of Biomedical and Clinical Sciences
University of Milan

George Perry, PhD
Department of Biology, College of Sciences
University of Texas

Catherine C. Price, PhD, ABPP
Paul Satz Term Professor/University of Florida Preeminent Term Professor
Director, Perioperative Cognitive Anesthesia Network Department of Clinical and Health Psychology and Department of Anesthesiology
University of Florida

Jill Rabinowitz, PhD
Assistant Research Scientist
Johns Hopkins University
Bloomberg School of Public Health and the Department of Mental Health

Ramit Ravona-Springer, MD
Memory Clinic, Division of Psychiatry, Sheba Medical Center, Ramat Gan
Sackler School of Medicine, Tel Aviv University

Batool Rizvi, MS
Research Analyst
Taub Institute for Research on Alzheimer's Disease and the Aging Brain
Department of Neurology
College of Physicians and Surgeons, Columbia University

Emilia Salvadori, PhD
NEUROFARBA Department,
Neuroscience Section
University of Florence, Italy
and IRCCS Don Carlo Gnocchi,
Florence

Julia A. Schneider, MD, MS
Professor, Department of Pathology and
Neurological Sciences
Rush Alzheimer's Disease Center, Rush
University Medical Center

Rodney A. Swenson, PhD, ABN, FACPN
Clinical Professor
Department of Psychiatry and Behavioral
Science
University of North Dakota
School of Medicine and Health
Sciences

Kelsey R. Thomas, PhD
Department of Psychiatry,
University of California San Diego,
School of Medicine
Veterans Affairs San Diego
Healthcare System

Victor Wasserman, MA
Department of Psychology
Rowan University

Alexandra J. Weigand, BA
San Diego State University/University
of California, San Diego, Joint Doctoral
Program in Clinical Psychology

Madeleine L. Werhane, MS, MPH
San Diego State University/University
of California, San Diego, Joint Doctoral
Program in Clinical Psychology

Margaret E. Wiggins, MS
Clinical and Health Psychology
University of Florida

Lisa-Delano Wood, PhD
Department of Psychiatry, University of
California San Diego, School of Medicine
Veterans Affairs San Diego
Healthcare System

Christina G. Wong, PhD
Department of Psychiatry, University of
California San Diego, School of Medicine
Veterans Affairs San Diego
Healthcare System
Lou Ruvo Center for Brain Health,
Cleveland Clinic

Belinda Yew, MS
Department of Psychology
University of Southern California

Introduction

David J. Libon, Melissa Lamar, Rodney A. Swenson, and Kenneth M. Heilman

Correlation does not necessarily provide evidence for *causation*. Understanding the etiology and developing treatments for insidious onset dementia, such as Alzheimer's disease and vascular dementia, constitute one of our most intractable public health problems. Over the last three decades, the lens through which many clinicians and investigators have tended to view the biological or etiologic basis for Alzheimer's disease has focused on the amyloid cascade hypothesis, that is, that insoluble forms of β-amyloid constitute an initial and necessary event that eventually leads to both a clinical and neuropathological diagnosis of Alzheimer's disease. Unfortunately, efforts to treat and/or modify clinically diagnosed Alzheimer's disease by targeting aggregated forms of β-amyloid have not been successful. Nonetheless, β-amyloid, in addition to other proteins, is certainly present in the brains of many patients meeting diagnostic criteria for Alzheimer's disease. However, perhaps it is worth repeating that *correlation* (i.e., measurable amounts of β-amyloid obtained either in life or quantified after death) does not necessarily provide evidence for *causation* (i.e., that insoluble β-amyloid is *the causative agent* of Alzheimer's disease).

The purpose of this volume is to present evidence that there is considerable heterogeneity in Alzheimer's disease, vascular dementia (Boyle et al., 2017, 2018) and mild cognitive impairment (MCI). Further, we maintain that because of the heterogeneity associated with Alzheimer's disease, vascular dementia, and MCI, it is more valuable to view these disorders as a *spectrum phenomenon*. To operationally define heterogeneity in Alzheimer/vascular spectrum dementia, it is valuable to pose the question, "What proportion of a patient's clinical or phenotypic presentation is associated with what proportion of underlying biological substrate?" There is now compelling evidence that statistical methods can be used to operationally define neuropsychological subtypes presenting with subtle cognitive impairment (Edmonds et al., 2016), mild cognitive impairment (Edmonds et al., 2018; Jak et al., 2016), and dementia (Libon et al., 2014). Moreover, statistical methods can be used to quantify neuropsychological patterns of behavior as related to putative biological/neuroanatomical alterations as measured with magnetic resonance imaging and other technologies (see Brickman et al.,

David J. Libon, Melissa Lamar, Rodney A. Swenson, and Kenneth M. Heilman. *Introduction*, In: *Vascular Disease, Alzheimer's Disease, and Mild Cognitive Impairment*. Edited by: David J. Libon, Melissa Lamar, Rodney A. Swenson, Kenneth M. Heilman, Oxford University Press (2020). © Oxford University Press.
DOI: 10.1093/oso/9780190634230.003.0001

2018). This methodology attempts to make the best use of all available data to *classify* patients along a neuropsychological/neurobiological continuum. On the basis of considerable evidence as described in this book, we feel that the time of *splendid isolation* is past—that is, the zeitgeist that views insidious onset dementia narrowly, as the province of one or two proteinopathies, must give way to an ecumenical approach where the variety of proteinopathies, vasculopathy, and other neuropathological disorders emerge contemporaneously, interact, and may be synergistic. Using this approach, it is our hope that new ideas will be developed that may result in successful treatment of Alzheimer/vascular spectrum dementia. Clearly, the status quo cannot continue.

The current volume is organized into five sections. In Section 1, chapters are devoted to epidemiological and neuropsychological research in MCI and Alzheimer/vascular spectrum dementia. Section 2 contains chapters describing a wide variety of neuroimaging alterations and neuroimaging technology. Section 3 explores alterations in the brain, heart, the blood–brain barrier that appear to contribute to a diagnosis of Alzheimer/vascular spectrum dementia. In Section 4, autopsy and underlying neuropathological mechanisms are discussed. Finally, Section 5 contains chapters on treatment and intervention. It is our hope that this volume will stimulate new ideas that will allow for better identification, classification, and treatment of Alzheimer/vascular spectrum dementia.

References

Boyle, P.A., Yang, J., Yu, L., Leurgans, S.E., Capuano, A.W., Schneider, J.A., Wilson, R.S., and Bennett D.A. (2017). Varied effects of age-related neuropathologies on the trajectory of late life cognitive decline. *Brain*, 140, 804–812.

Boyle, P.A., Yu, L., Wilson, R.S., Leurgans, S.E., Schneider, J.A., and Bennett D.A. (2018). Person-specific contribution of neuropathologies to cognitive loss in old age. *Annuals of Neurology*, 83, 74–83.

Brickman, A.M., Tosto, G., Gutierrez, J., Andrews, H., Gu, Y., Narkhede, A., Rizvi, B., Guzman, V., Manly, J.J., Vonsattel, J.P., and Schupf, N. (2018). An MRI measure of degenerative and cerebrovascular pathology in Alzheimer disease. *Neurology*, 91, e1402–e1412.

Jak, A.J., Preis, S.R., Beiser, A.S., Seshadri, S., Wolf, P.A., Bondi, M.W., and Au, R. (2016). Neuropsychological criteria for mild cognitive impairment and dementia risk in the Framingham Heart Study. *Journal of the International Neuropsychological Society*, 22, 937–943.

Edmonds, E.C., Delano-Wood, L., Galasko, D.R., Salmon, D.P., and Bondi, M.W., for the Alzheimer's Disease Neuroimaging Initiative. (2015). Subtle cognitive decline and biomarker staging in preclinical Alzheimer's disease. *Journal of Alzheimer's disease*, 47, 231–242.

Edmonds, E. C., Ard, M. C., Edland, S. D., Galasko, D. R., Salmon, D. P., & Bondi, M. W. (2018). Unmasking the benefits of donepezil via psychometrically precise identification of mild cognitive impairment: A secondary analysis of the ADCS vitamin E and donepezil in MCI study. *Alzheimer's & Dementia: Translational Research & Clinical Interventions*, 4, 11–18.

Libon, D.J., Drabick, D.A.G., Giovannetti, T., Price, C.C., Bondi, M.W., Eppig, J., Nieves, C., Lamar, M., Delano-Wood, L., Nation, D.A., Brennan, L., Au, R., Swenson, R. (2014). Neuropsychological syndromes associated with Alzheimer's/ Vascular spectrum dementia: A Latent Class Analysis. *Journal of Alzheimer's Disease*, 42, 999–1014.

PART 1
EPIDEMIOLOGY AND NEUROPSYCHOLOGY

1

Vascular Risk Factors and Their Relationship to Brain Aging

Findings from the Framingham Heart Study

Ting Fang Alvin Ang, Prajakta Joshi, and Rhoda Au

1. Introduction

As the aging population continues to increase rapidly, there has been a marked escalation in the incidence of neurodegenerative disorders, including dementias such as Alzheimer's disease (AD; United Nations Population Division, 2007). AD, believed to be the most common type of dementia, has been estimated to affect 9 million Americans by the year 2050 (Alzheimer's Association, 2008). Despite the overwhelming disease burden, current treatments have little to no impact on slowing down disease progression after the onset of clinical symptoms (Dash, 2011; Saxena, 2010). These present-day lackluster therapies have resulted in a paradigm shift to identify prodromal or preclinical dementia, often referred to as mild cognitive impairment (MCI), as early as possible (Petersen et al., 1999). The term *mild cognitive impairment* generally refers to a prodromal state of relatively intact functional status with some evidence of neuropsychological impairment (Petersen & Morris, 2004). Several postmortem studies have reported significant AD brain pathology in deceased individuals with MCI, indicating progression of disease from MCI to AD (Bennett, Schneider, Bienias, Evans, & Wilson, 2005; Guillozet, Weintraub, Mash, & Mesulam, 2003; Markesbery et al., 2006). In fact, some argue that MCI is not preclinical AD but a manifestation of AD in its incipient stage (Morris, 2005). Owing to these studies, the concept of a prolonged preclinical phase, extending beyond the currently defined MCI stage, is gaining much popularity (Sperling et al., 2011). One may thus theorize that AD is a life-course disease (Seshadri et al., 2006), with an insidious onset that may arise decades before overt clinical symptoms become apparent (Dubois et al., 2010; M. F. Elias et al., 2000; Rowe et al., 2010); hence, numerous investigational tests have been developed over the last decade in an attempt to pinpoint the disease onset.

Ting Fang Alvin Ang, Prajakta Joshi, and Rhoda Au, *Vascular Risk Factors and Their Relationship to Brain Aging* In: *Vascular Disease, Alzheimer's Disease, and Mild Cognitive Impairment*. Edited by: David J. Libon, Melissa Lamar, Rodney A. Swenson, Kenneth M. Heilman, Oxford University Press (2020).
DOI: 10.1093/oso/9780190634230.003.0002

The Framingham Heart Study (FHS), established in 1948, has been the longest ongoing prospective cohort study with cardiovascular diseases and stroke as initial outcomes of interest. The term *risk factors* had not been coined at the commencement of the study, and collecting data on such variables was deemed as a novel approach. The FHS adopted a presumptive multicausal approach, challenging the long-standing notion of a single-cause disease model. Additionally, the design was robust, with the application of various diagnostic procedures and regular follow-up to accurately capture the sequence of events leading to heart disease and stroke and thereby providing data on their prevalence and incidence (Dawber, Meadors, & Moore, 1951).

At its inception, 10,000 participants between the ages of 30 and 60 years who were randomly selected through a stratified sampling of families and precinct of residence were invited to participate in the study (Kannel, Feinleib, McNamara, Garrison, & Castelli, 1979). Among them, 5,209 volunteered to participate and constituted the Gen 1 cohort. An in-person interview was conducted along with a thorough physical examination and a multitude of laboratory investigations, including X-rays, electrocardiogram, and blood and urine assays. These tests were performed biennially on each participant. To assess the potential familial disease patterns, children of the Gen 1 cohort and their spouses were enrolled in 1971, constituting the Gen 2 cohort (n = 5,124), and in 2002, grandchildren of the Gen 1 cohort were also recruited, establishing the Gen 3 cohort (Gen 3; n = 4,209). Furthermore, to ensure that the study population of FHS was representative of the United States, two additional cohorts with ethnically diverse participants were recruited: the Omni Generation 1 (OmniGen 1; 1990, n = 500) and Omni Generation 2 (OmniGen 2; 2002, n = 410) cohorts. Finally, from 2003 to 2005, parents of Gen 3 who were not originally enrolled in 1971, were recruited into the New Offspring Spouses (NOS) cohort (n = 103) to maximize genetically related research. Recruitment details of FHS cohorts have been previously reported (Tsao & Vasan, 2015).

The initial intent of the FHS was to study the causal pathway of cardiovascular diseases and stroke but has been extended over recent decades to include other chronic diseases including neurodegenerative disorders. Over the past several decades, it has become apparent that there are links between cardiovascular and nervous systems illness. The FHS has capitalized on its decades of data to relate how cardiovascular risk and neurodegeneration may be related.

Neuropsychological assessment of the Gen 1 cohort participants was introduced in 1976 with the administration of a 20-minute neuropsychological protocol designed by Edith Kaplan and Martin Albert to establish a dementia-free cohort (henceforth referenced as the Kaplan–Albert test battery). Later, in 1981, the Mini-Mental Status Examination (MMSE) was introduced to objectively monitor the cognitive status of the participants in this cohort (Folstein, Folstein,

& McHugh, 1975). When participants' MMSE performance dropped 3 or more points compared to the previous exam, or dropped 5 points across all exams, they were invited for an in-depth neuropsychological test protocol and, when possible, a neurological exam. If a participant was suspected of having dementia following either or both examinations, a consensus panel determined dementia status and, if warranted, dementia subtype. Details on the FHS dementia diagnostic protocol have been specified in previous publications (Seshadri et al., 2011). Cognitive status monitoring was extended to the Gen 2 and Omni cohorts in 1991 and in 2008 to the Gen 3 and Omni 2 cohorts. Because of the younger age of the Gen 2, Gen 3, and Omni 2 cohorts, as well as their higher levels of educational attainment, the Consortium to Establish a Registry of Alzheimer's Disease (CERAD) List Learning and Victoria Stroop tests were used for cognitive screening in lieu of the MMSE.

Since 1999 administration of the in-depth neuropsychological protocol has undergone several iterations. The current neuropsychological protocol has adopted the Boston process approach (Kaplan 1988, 1990), which scores both correct and incorrect responses to neuropsychological test questions (Rhoda Au, Piers, & Devine, 2017). Additionally, beginning in 1999, participants were invited for brain magnetic resonance imaging (MRI) scans, with more than 90% of MRI scans done on the same day as the cognitive assessment (Au & Devine, 2013). The extensive cognitive data and brain MRI studies, coupled with the FHS's rich cardiovascular repository, have enabled numerous studies relating neuropsychological decline and dementia risk to various cardiovascular risk factors (Massaro et al., 2004).

Owing to its longitudinal, multi-generational nature, the FHS has become a treasure trove of data on major cardiovascular risk factors (Tsao & Vasan, 2015) and its potential impact on brain aging. For many FHS participants, cardiovascular risk data have been collected across much of the adult lifespan, enabling researchers to establish a clear longitudinal relationship with different brain aging outcomes across a wide range of age groups (Massaro et al., 2004).

In this chapter, we will highlight some of the major FHS findings regarding the associations between major cardiovascular risk factors, neuropsychological performance, brain MRI metrics, and diagnosis of clinical dementia, including AD. These major factors include hypertension, diabetes, smoking, alcohol consumption, body mass index (BMI), cholesterol and the Framingham Stroke Risk Profile score (FSRP)—a composite score of cardiovascular risk factors that predicts a person's 10-year probability of a stroke. Effects of advancing age on cognition, structural brain changes, and risk of neurocognitive outcomes have been well documented in numerous published studies (Marchant et al., 2013; Matthews et al., 2016; Ritchie, Artero, & Touchon, 2001; Schmand, Jonker,

Hooijer, & Lindeboom, 1996). Distinct gender differences have also been observed (Matthews et al., 2016; Satizabal, Beiser, & Seshadri, 2016).

2. Neuropsychological Performance

Between January 1976 and March 1978, 2,123 participants from FHS Gen 1 Cohort, aged 55 to 89 years, underwent neuropsychological testing. A protocol of eight tests assessed cognitive functions such as language, memory, learning, reproduction of designs, arousal, attention, mental control, and abstract thinking (Satizabal et al., 2016). The central aim of this neuropsychological protocol was to establish a dementia-free cohort for incident follow up. This initial assessment allowed for the FHS's first series of studies relating cardiovascular risk to cognition.

2.1. Hypertension

The FHS is credited as generating the first research describing blood pressure levels that define hypertension (Farmer, White, Abbott et al., 1987). In the United States, one out of three adults are hypertensive and the prevalence increases significantly with age, affecting 63% of adults aged 60 to 79 years and 70% among those aged 80 years or older. There is growing evidence suggesting that vascular risk factors such as hypertension increase risk for and progression of cognitive decline (M. F. Elias, Wolf, D'Agostino, Cobb, & White, 1993; Farmer et al., 1990).

Farmer et al. (1987a) pioneered one of the earliest studies to investigate the relationship between blood pressure and cognitive performance in middle-aged and elderly persons while controlling for several co-factors such as education, smoking, alcohol use, and antihypertensive treatment. In a sample of 2,032 FHS Gen 1 cohort participants aged 55 years and above, no significant association was found between blood pressure and antihypertensive treatment with cognition. When blood pressure measurements were stratified into normotensive, borderline hypertensive, and definite hypertensive categories, participants in the borderline and definite hypertension categories were found to be poorer performers on test of attention ($p < 0.05$), while those in the definite hypertension category scored lower in immediate verbal recall ($p < 0.05$). In a follow-up study on the same population, Farmer et al. (1990) found that blood pressure was inversely associated with cognitive decline in participants who were not on antihypertensive medication. By contrast, this association was not observed among those on treatment. Instead, they noted a highly significant graded relation between cognitive impairment and the probability of being off medication among the latter group at earlier testing cycles. Although the two studies yielded inconclusive results, Farmer and his colleagues paved the way for subsequent studies relating blood pressure to cognitively related outcomes.

Five years after Farmer's first study, M. F. Elias et al. (1993) examined the cognitive performance of 1,702 stroke-free Gen 1 cohort participants, focusing on three distinct blood pressure parameters: systolic blood pressure (SBP), diastolic blood pressure, and chronicity of blood pressure. Distinguishing their work from Farmer's studies, they were interested in *untreated* blood pressure and its impact on cognition. This methodological approach is of great importance, because it is technically impossible in this day and age to observe the effects of untreated hypertension, given the long-standing widespread practice of early high blood pressure intervention. Similar to the findings of Farmer's second study, they found an inverse relationship between cognitive functions and average systolic and diastolic blood pressures in participants with untreated hypertension. In a subsequent study, they further demonstrated an inverse association between visual and verbal memory tests from the Kaplan–Albert protocol and blood pressure and chronicity of hypertension (M. F. Elias, D'Agostino, Elias, & Wolf, 1995). M. F. Elias extended the research efforts to the Gen 2 cohort and found that left ventricular dilatation after adjusting for covariates, was inversely associated with Wechsler Adult Intelligence Scale (WAIS) Similarities test performance ($p < 0.05$) and visuospatial memory and organization ($p < 0.01$; M. F. Elias et al., 2007).

In addition to being an independent risk factor, hypertension seems to interact with other co-factors in affecting cognitive performance. The apolipoprotein ε4 allele (ApoE4) is a well-documented genetic risk factor for AD (Caselli et al., 2007; Knopman, Mosley, Catellier, & Coker, 2009), and it accelerates cognitive decline in ApoE4 carriers (Whitehair et al., 2010). In stratified analyses, Nishtala et al. (2014) suggested that the relationship between hypertension and cognition was exacerbated for those who were ApoE4+, as compared to those who were ApoE4–, demonstrating reduced verbal output on letter fluency (letters FAS) tests. Significant inverse associations were also observed between hypertension and output on both letter and semantic (animals) fluency among ApoE4+ participants, with no statistically significant association among the ApoE4– group. Overall, early and recent FHS studies indicated that elevated blood pressure and/or presence of hypertension might adversely influence cognition, especially executive functions, language, and memory.

2.2. Diabetes

Diabetes is a chronic disease affecting about 422 million people globally, and about 20% of individuals aged 65 years and above suffer from it (Roglic, 2016). Miles and Root (1922) first conceptualized the association between diabetes and cognition more than 85 years ago when they observed poorer performance in memory, psychomotor efficiency, and mental arithmetic tests among patients with diabetes. Following in their footsteps, several FHS researchers found a complex relationship between several risk factors, including diabetes, high blood pressure, and cognitive performance (P. K. Elias et al., 1997).

Using data from the Gen 1 Cohort participants, P. K. Elias and colleagues (1997) were the first from the FHS to examine the association between diabetes and cognition. They stratified individuals aged 55 to 88 by diabetic status to consider the impact of the onset and duration of diabetes and of hypertension, and their combination. Aligned with previous studies, the presence of diabetes and higher blood pressure were independently associated with poorer cognitive performance. In addition, longer duration of noninsulin-dependent diabetes mellitus (NIDDM) was associated with worse performance on verbal memory and verbal concept formation tests with these effects amplified in participants suffering with both hypertension and NIDDM. These findings were later reproduced by Knopman and colleagues (2001) in another large-scale community-based cohort study (Atherosclerosis Risk in Communities [ARIC]). Several years later, Akomolafe et al. (2006) re-examined these Gen 1 cohort participants and reported a relative risk of 1.15 (95% confidence interval [CI] 0.65–2.05) for AD among diabetic participants who were dementia-free (mean age = 70 years) as compared to their nondiabetic counterparts. This risk increased to 2.98 (95% CI = 1.06–8.39, $p = 0.03$) for participants without ApoE4 allele or elevated plasma homocysteine levels. This effect of diabetes was further amplified among participants who were above 75 years of age.

Tan and his team (2011) went on to evaluate the relationship among FHS Gen 2 Cohort participants and showed that diabetic status, serum hemoglobin A1c, homeostatic model assessment of insulin resistance (HOMA-IR), and fasting insulin were related to poorer executive function. Interestingly, an apparent association between diabetes and better performance in verbal memory tasks was observed, although this effect was reduced after adjusting for all covariates. More recently, Bangen et al. (2010) studied risk factors of stroke, such as diabetes and hypertension, in cognitively normal individuals, participants with AD without depression, and participants with AD and depression, using the FSRP. Although the three groups differed in terms of frequency of cardiovascular disease, there were no significant between-group differences with respect to diabetes mellitus. Nishtala et al. (2014) followed up with a subsequent study that assessed the FSRP score collected between 2005 and 2009 in the Gen 2 Cohort population. In their individual component analysis, these researchers reported that an 8-year history of diabetes was associated with poorer performance on fluency tests. Gupta et al. (2015) studied error response along with traditional measures of episodic memory to examine the association between mid-life cardiovascular risk factor and later-life cognitive function in the Gen 2 cohort. They found that participants with diabetes were 56% more likely to produce greater errors on the Logical Memory immediate free recall test condition than those without diabetes.

2.3. Smoking, Serum Cholesterol, Obesity, and Alcohol Consumption

Smoking, serum cholesterol, and obesity are well-known risk factors for cardiovascular diseases, which have been established in several landmark studies (Damen et al., 2016; P. K. Elias, Elias, D'Agostino, Sullivan, & Wolf, 2005; Garcia, McNamara, Gordon, & Kannel, 1974; Ott et al., 2004; Razani, Boone, Lesser, & Weiss, 2004; van Vliet, van de Water, de Craen, & Westendorp, 2009). In fact, due to their strong associations, several cardiovascular risk predictive models have incorporated them as part of the algorithms (Damen et al., 2016; Ott et al., 2004). Despite the overwhelming amount of research demonstrating a significant relationship between cardiovascular health and brain health, the connection between these variables and cognition remains ambiguous due to inconsistent results across studies. In the case of smoking, some researchers have reported an association with cognitive function (Razani et al., 2004); however, others have demonstrated little to no association (Akomolafe et al., 2006). For instance, Razani et al. (2004) suggested that even though there was no difference in cognition between nonsmokers and light/moderate smokers, heavy smokers seemed to suffer from executive function deficits. Similar poor outcomes regarding executive function have since been reported (Debette et al., 2011; Gupta et al., 2015; Nishtala et al., 2014). Debette et al. (2011) examined 1,352 nondemented FHS Gen 2 Study participants and concluded that smoking status increased the rate of progression of vascular brain injury, global and hippocampal atrophy, and a decline in executive function a decade later. Nishtala et al. (2014) analyzed the association between FSRP and cognition and reported that current smoking status, as an individual component, negatively influenced cognition, such that smokers performed slower in the Trails B test. Gupta et al. (2015) studied error response along with traditional measures of episodic memory to examine the association between midlife cardiovascular risk factors and later-life cognitive function, in the Gen 2 cohort. Their study found that participants who smoked were 60%

more likely to produce a high number of errors on the Wechsler Memory Scale (WMS) Visual Reproduction delay-free recall test condition than those who did not smoke.

The relationship between serum cholesterol and cognition is complex. Participants from the FHS Gen 1 Cohort underwent biannual total cholesterol determinations over a period of 16 to 18 years. Those who were free from dementia and stroke were invited for detailed neuropsychological testing. Low serum total cholesterol levels, which may be secondary to poor nutrition and chronic medical illness, were found to correlate with poorer cognitive performance for abstract reasoning, attention/concentration, verbal fluency, and executive functioning (P. K. Elias et al., 2005). In contrast, individuals with higher total cholesterol levels in midlife have been shown to be at a greater risk of late-life cognitive impairment (van Vliet et al., 2009). Taken together, these studies suggest that both low and high levels of total cholesterol can negatively impact cognition and thus maintaining normal cholesterol levels is warranted to best preserve brain health.

Obesity has been shown to be an important independent risk factor for cardiovascular diseases and diabetes in both genders (Garcia et al., 1974; Hubert, Feinleib, McNamara, & Castelli, 1983). M. F. Elias et al. (2003) reported that the combined effects of obesity and hypertension were associated with poorer verbal (WMS Logical Memory–Immediate Recall) as well as visual memory (WMS Visual Reproduction and Logical Memory-Delayed Recall) in late middle-aged and elderly men, but not in women. In the same vein, a follow-up with the same FHS population demonstrated that obesity was associated with a decline in cognitive performance in men but not women (M. F. Elias, Elias, Sullivan, Wolf, & D'Agostino, 2005). For men, this decrease was observed for every cognitive test measure except WMA Paired Associates learning. In a later study, Wolf et al. (2007) found that indices of obesity (BMI and Waist–Hip Ratio) were each significantly related to poorer performance on tests measuring executive function and visual episodic memory (i.e., Trails B, WMS Visual Reproductions–Immediate and Delayed Recall).

2.4. Alcohol Consumption

Previously, the common belief associated alcohol consumption at any level with poorer cognitive performance (P. K. Elias et al., 1995; P. K. Elias, Elias, D'Agostino, Silbershatz, & Wolf, 1999). However, in one of the earliest cognition-related studies on the FHS Gen 1 Cohort, Farmer, White, Kittner et al. (1987b) demonstrated that alcohol consumption was associated with better verbal episodic memory (WMS Logical Memory–Immediate and Delayed Free Recall) and executive abilities (letter fluency). In another study, M. F. Elias et al. (1993) examining the relationship between blood pressure and cognition in the Gen 1 cohort, moderate alcohol consumption was positively associated with better performance on cognitive test. Some gender differences have been reported. Studies that examined older participants indicated that the relationship between alcohol consumption and cognitive performance might be best described as a U- or J-shaped curve (P. K. Elias et al., 1995; Parker, Parker, Brody, & Schoenberg, 1983). For example, P. K. Elias et al. (1999) found that moderate drinking (2–4 drinks/day) had a beneficial effect on verbal and visual memory for woman. In contrast to the protective effects of moderate alcohol consumption demonstrated by previous research, this study found that moderate alcohol consumption was not protective against normal age-related differences in total brain volume (TBV). Gender-specific analyses showed that adjusted mean total cerebral brain volume (TCBV) was higher for women than men in every category of alcohol consumption and the linear regression curve for the association between alcohol consumption and TCBV was steeper for women. Unlike hypertension and diabetes, the relationship between smoking, serum cholesterol, obesity, and alcohol consumption seems to be less definitive, suggesting the need for more research.

2.5. Arterial Stiffness and Pressure Pulsatility

Beyond conventional cardiovascular risk factors, researchers are discovering new connections between cognition and novel cardiovascular metrics including arterial stiffness and pressure pulsatility, two important risk factors with well-documented correlation with atherosclerotic burden. Not surprisingly arterial stiffness and pressure pulsatility have been shown to be strongly associated with cardiovascular endpoints (Knopman et al., 2001). Tsao et al. (2016) reported that elevated arterial stiffness and pressure pulsatility might lead to faster rate of neurocognitive decline. In their study, Gen 2 cohort participants with higher baseline inverse-transformed carotid-femoral pulse wave velocity (CFPWV) and central pulse pressure demonstrated a greater drop in executive function and verbal abstraction test performance over time. Putting these results in a temporal perspective, one standard deviation increase in CFPWV is associated with nearly 1 year of brain aging.

Pulse pressure, an index of vascular aging, has been associated with neurodegenerative changes before the onset of clinically diagnosed dementia across a broad age range. Among very old participants, higher pulse pressure was also associated with cerebral amyloidosis in the presence of neurodegeneration and accelerated progression to dementia. Furthermore, diastolic contributions were limited to relatively younger participants in the study, while systolic contributions were found only in very old participants (Maillard et al., 2012). This topic is described in greater detail by Yew and colleagues (Chapter 12, this volume).

2.6. Cumulative Vascular Risk Factors/FSRP

In an attempt to calculate the conditional probability of a health outcome, several composite risk scores have been developed over the past few decades. The FHS published its first risk score in 1988, commonly known as the Framingham Risk Score (FRS). This index takes into consideration an array of risk factors (e.g., age, gender, smoking status, SBP, presence of hypertension, and cholesterol profile) to estimate the 10-year cardiovascular risk of an individual. FRS is now widely used in the medical community to manage moderate- to high-risk patients. Following in the footsteps of FRS, FHS constructed the FSRP, a predictive model for the probability of stroke within an individual in the next 10 years (Wolf, D'Agostino, Belanger, & Kannel, 1991). Unlike individual risk factors, composite risk scores like FRS and FRSP avoid the dependence of a single predictor variable and hence minimize overreacting and allow more logical risk classification of patients at risk.

There is an apparent inverse relationship between FSRP and memory function. Using the WMS Visual Reproductions subtest, Gupta et al. (2015) found that a higher FSRP score during midlife was associated with poorer visual memory test performance. This is especially so among participants who were smokers, as they performed poorer compared to their nonsmoker counterparts in both WMS Visual Reproduction Immediate and Delayed free recall test conditions ($p < 0.02$ and $p < 0.04$, respectively). In addition to visual memory deficits, M. F. Elias et al. (2004) demonstrated that a 10% increment in 10-year risk for stroke correlated with poorer performance in other cognitive domains including reasoning, visual organization, attention, and visual scanning and motor speed.

In conclusion, lifetime exposure to major cardiovascular risk factors, specifically hypertension, diabetes mellitus, arterial stiffness, and pressure pulsatility adversely impact cognitive function in various domains, particularly in older individuals. Hence, prevention and appropriate management of cardiovascular risk factors are crucial to minimize the risk of cognitive decline later in life (Table 1.1).

3. Brain MRI

MRI is very useful in identifying a wide number of anatomic biomarker associated with both normal and pathological aging including lower brain volume,

Table 1.1 Midlife Cardiovascular Risk Factors Associations with Cognition in FHS Gen 1 Cohort and FHS Gen 2 Cohort

	Cognitive Functions	Blood Pressure	Diabetes	Serum Total Cholesterol	Alcohol Consumption	Cigarette Smoking	Obesity	FSRP
40–54 years old	L							
	VM							
	Vis. M							–
	A/C							–
	EF	–				NS		–
	LA	–	–			NS		
	VO							–
55–64 years old	L	NS		NS				
	VM	–	+	NS		NS	NS	
	Vis. M	–	U	NS	+	NS	–	–
	A/C	U	–					–
	EF	–	–	–		–	U	–
	LA		–					
	VO	–						–

(Continued)

Table 1.1 (Continued)

	Cognitive Functions	Blood Pressure	Diabetes	Serum Total Cholesterol	Alcohol Consumption	Cigarette Smoking	Obesity	FSRP
65–74 years old	L	U	–	NS	U	NS	NS	
	VM	–	–	NS	U	NS	U	
	Vis. M	–	–	NS	U	NS	–	–
	A/C	+	NS	–	U	NS	NS	–
	EF	–	–	–	U	–	U	–
	LA	U	–	–	U	NS	–	
	VO							–
>75 years old	L	NS	–	NS				
	VM	–	U					
	Vis. M	–	–				–	–
	A/C	+						–
	EF	–		–				
	LA	NS						

Notes: Empty fields mean no study performed. FHS, Framingham Heart Study; FSRP, Framingham Stroke Risk Profile; NS, not significant; U, unclear relationship; +, direct relationship; –, inverse relationship; L, learning; VM, verbal memory; Vis. M, visual memory; A/C, attention/concentration; EF, executive functioning; LA, language; VO, visuoperceptual organization; CVRF, cardiovascular risk factor.

asymptomatic cerebral infarcts, and white matter hyperintensity (WMH) lesions. A number of neuroradiological markers have been associated with impaired neuropsychological test performance in AD and MCI (Au et al., 2006). In 1999, the FHS started collecting MRI brain data of its Gen 1 and Gen 2 cohort participants, and a decade later, Gen 3 participants were included (DeCarli, 2016). To facilitate the investigation of structural brain changes in normal aging and different stages of cognitive decline, extensive data were collected on numerous MRI measures including TCBV, white WMH volume (WMHV) and silent cerebral infarcts (SCI).

3.1. Hypertension, Blood Pressure, and Atrial Fibrillation

Clinically relevant and modifiable vascular events such as midlife SBP has been associated with clinically asymptomatic infarcts, brain atrophy, gray matter atrophy, and white matter injury, including WMH lesions (Maillard et al., 2012). Abnormal white matter signals have been linked with brain atrophy, focal neurologic signs, reduced cerebral blood flow, and worse performance on neuropsychological tests (DeCarli et al., 1995). For example, among 1,352 nondemented FHS Gen 2 participants, Debette et al. (2011) showed that hypertension and increased SBP were significant predictors of WMHV progression and worse performance on executive tests. Similar results were subsequently reproduced by Maillard et al. (2016) who examined 579 younger adults (mean age = 39.2 ± 8.4) from the FHS Gen 3 cohort and reported that increasing SBP was associated with reduced gray matter volume as well as injury to white matter microstructure. On the contrary, WMHV was not associated with SBP. Thus, more longitudinal studies are needed to investigate whether prolonged elevated SBP during early adulthood has cumulative deleterious effects on white matter integrity.

SCIs are parenchymal lesions that have the MRI characteristics of previous infarcts but are not necessarily associated with clinical signs or symptoms corresponding to a stroke (Masuda, Nabika, & Notsu, 2001). These lesions may be seen in both healthy individuals as well as those with hypertension, stroke, and cognitive decline (Vermeer et al., 2003). In 2,040 participants from the FHS Gen 2 Cohort, hypertension and SBP were independently associated with an increased risk of SCIs. Furthermore, the presence of SCIs was associated with a twofold increase in the risk of atrial fibrillation (Das et al., 2008), suggesting that early and timely treatment of hypertension and atrial fibrillation may help to reduce the occurrence of SCIs. Overall, these findings suggest the insidious effects of elevated blood pressure and atrial fibrillation on brain structure leading to apparent vascular injury and subsequent cognitive decline even in young adults and thus further underscore the need for early diagnosis and appropriate treatment.

3.2. Diabetes

Data from the FHS has link diabetes with a number of neuroradiological alternations well-known to be associated with cognitive compromise. For example, Debette et al. (2011) showed that increasing annual temporal horn volume (THV) of lateral ventricles, a surrogate marker of accelerated hippocampal atrophy, was significantly related to midlife diabetes in FHS Gen 2 Cohort. Tan and colleagues (2011) observed a strong correlation between duration of diabetes and TCBV as well as a 1.24% difference in TCBV between those with and without diabetes, an equivalent to the effect of 6 years of chronological aging. By contrast, no association has been found between diabetes and other MRI measures such as SCIs in the FHS Gen 2 cohort (Das et al., 2008; Jeerakathil et al., 2004).

3.3. Diet, BMI, Cholesterol, Alcohol, and Smoking

There is a growing interest in assessing dietary, nutrition, and lifestyle patterns as potentially modifiable factors in the delay or prevention of cognitive dysfunction (Otaegui-Arrazola, Amiano, Elbusto, Urdaneta, & Martinez-Lage, 2014). Choline is a precursor to the neurotransmitter acetylcholine, which plays an important role in cognition and the loss of cholinergic neurons have been associated with cognitive decline and AD (Davies, 1999; Muir, 1997). Higher intake of choline among 1,391 FHS Gen 2 participants resulted in better performance on verbal memory tests.

Numerous lifestyle habits such as smoking and alcohol consumption have been known to play direct or indirect roles in the etiopathogenic mechanisms of neurodegeneration and cardiovascular comorbidities, such as hypercholesterolemia and obesity. Among midlife smokers from FHS Gen 2 cohort, there was a marked reduction in TBV and an increased risk of greater THV and WMHV. Investigators also showed that an increasing waist to hip ratio was associated with a marked reduction in TBV (Wolf et al., 2007). However, like diabetes, these factors were not associated with the presence of SCIs (Das et al., 2008; Jeerakathil et al., 2004).

3.4. Arterial Stiffness and Pressure Pulsatility

As previously mentioned, the increase in arterial stiffness and pressure pulsatility are age-related changes that cause aortic remodeling, which progressively negatively affect arterial hemodynamics, leading to neurovascular injury and impaired neuropsychological functioning (Maillard et al., 2012; Tsao et al., 2016). Tsao et al. (2016) reported that Gen 2 cohort participants with higher baseline inverse-transformed CFPWV experienced greater degree of cognitive decline. These findings were complemented by Maillard et al. (2012) in Gen 3 participants, where higher CFPWV was continued to be associated with lower fractional anisotropy within voxels that covered 25.5 cc of white matter and lower gray matter density in voxels that covered 0.93 cc of gray matter. This study also identified a significant negative relation between CFPWV with fractional anisotropy measures with increasing age.

Based on these results, we can conclude that CFPWV may be superior predictor for white matter integrity as compared to other novel hemodynamic measures even among younger individuals. Still, additional research is needed before definitive conclusions can be drawn due to the cross-sectional design and difference in age in these studies.

3.5. Cumulative Vascular Risk Factors/FSRP

Seshadri et al. (2004) evaluated 909 stroke and dementia-free FHS Gen 2 participants and found a strong inverse association between TCBV and FSRP score. This association was partly attributed to age, since TCBV was reduced by 1.9% and stroke risk increased with each decade in age. This relationship remained robust even after adjusting WMHV, SCIs, and ApoE4 status. These researchers were found also found that increased TCBV was associated with poorer performance on tests measuring attention and visuospatial and executive functioning. Das et al. (2008) examined the correlation between FSRP and SCI and found that two were significantly related. Among the individual components of FSRP, hypertension, atrial fibrillation, and SBP were significantly related to SCIs. The results of these studies not only highlight the potential benefits of early detection and management of stroke risk factors during midlife, but also emphasize the need for physicians to actively intervene at young adulthood for high-risk patients to minimize irreversible brain injury that may lead to eventual cognitive decline.

In summary, the compendium of findings across FHS studies suggest that healthy lifestyle practices that include regular blood pressure monitoring, not smoking, and eating a choline-rich diet appear to minimize adverse structural brain changes. Indeed, exposures to cumulative effects of various cardiovascular risk factors are likely associated with negative structural brain alterations, which, in turn, can result in neuropsychological dysfunction (Table 1.2).

Table 1.2 Midlife Cardiovascular Risk Factors Associations with Brain MRI in FHS Gen 1 and Gen 2 Cohorts

		Blood Pressure	Diabetes	Hypercholesterolemia	Alcohol Consumption	Cigarette Smoking	Obesity	FSRP
55–64 years old	WMH	+	NS	NS		+	U	–
	TCBV	NS	U	NS		–		
	THV	NS	+	NS		+	U	
	HV		NS					
	SCI	+	NS	NS		NS	U	+
	CM	+	NS	NS		NS		
65–74 years old	WMH	+						–
	TCBV					–		
	THV		+			+		
	HV							
	SCI							+
	CM							

>75 years old	WMH	U
	TCBV	
	THV	
	HV	
	SCI	
	CM	

Notes: Empty fields indicate no study performed. MRI, magnetic resonance imaging; FHS, Framingham Heart Study; NS: not significant; U, unclear relationship; +, direct relationship; –, inverse relationship; WMH, white matter hyperintensity; TCBV, total cranial brain volume; THV, temporal horn volume; HV, hippocampal volume; SCI, silent cerebral infarcts; CM, cerebral microbleeds; CVRF, cardiovascular risk factor.

4. MCI, Dementia, and Alzheimer's Disease

At its inception, the FHS primarily focused on cardiovascular diseases. This has expanded over time to include a multitude of outcomes including stroke, cancer and other common chronic diseases. The Epidemiology of Dementia Study was established in 1974 with the principal objective of identifying incident cases of dementia among its participants. Those who were free of stroke and dementia were followed from 1976 to 1978 and their baseline cognitive assessment was measured using the Kaplan–Albert protocol (Seshadri et al., 2011).

With the increase in the average lifespan of individuals, there was a marked rise in the incidence of AD and other types of neurodegenerative diseases. Thus, the pursuit for an early and accurate diagnosis of these diseases has become critical. Wolf et al. (2012), through the vast body of their work, recognized that atherosclerosis, cardiovascular disease, and cardiovascular risk factors contribute to the development of cognitive decline, dementia, vascular cognitive impairment and AD. In the last decade, increasingly non-FHS studies also reported associations between vascular risk factors and neurodegenerative outcomes.

Pase and colleagues (Pase, Beiser, Aparicio et al., 2016; Pase, Beiser, Enserro et al., 2016; Pase, Beiser, Himali et al., 2016) have published a series of papers demonstrating an association between several cardiovascular markers and the outcome of dementia later in life. Individuals with higher continuous aortic stiffness were at a higher risk of developing MCI, all-cause dementia, and AD (Pase, Beiser, Himali et al., 2016). This association was increased in nondiabetic individuals who were in the top two quintiles of aortic stiffness. In tandem to the results on aortic stiffness, they found that both Gen 1 and Gen 2 individuals, who had high interarm differences in SBP (≥10 mm Hg) *and* were carriers of an ApoE4 allele, were predisposed to dementia such as AD (Pase, Beiser, Aparicio et al., 2016). Further, Gen 2 participants who obtained a better Ideal Cardiovascular Health score were less likely to develop dementia (Pase, Beiser, Enserro et al., 2016). Jefferson et al. (2015) reinforced these findings showing that lower cardiac output relative to their body surface area was nearly three times more likely to develop dementia and AD as compared to their counterparts with normal cardiac output.

FHS researchers have also discovered multiple biomarkers that are associated with cardiovascular risk and dementia. For example, elevated plasma homocysteine concentration is linked to new onset of stroke (Bostom et al., 1999). Plasma homocysteine concentration is also associated the eventual emergence of AD (Seshadri, 2006; Seshadri et al., 2002). Serum brain derived neurotrophic factor (BDNF) is a biomarker of physical activity, which in turn has been widely documented as linked to cardiovascular risk factors and disease. Although BDNF was not associated with elevated risk for AD or all-cause dementia among

Table 1.3 Midlife Cardiovascular Risk Factors Associations with AD and Other Types of Dementia in FHS Gen 1 and Gen 2 Cohorts

		ApoE4	Diabetes	WMH	Serum Brain-Derived Neurotrophic Factor	Brain Injury	Serum Thryoid-Stimulating Hormone (TSH)	Biomarkers of Insulin Resistance	Interarm Difference in Systolic Blood Pressure
55 to 64 years old	MCI	+		+		+			
	AD	+			NS	+			+
	A-C. D	+		+	NS	+			+
65 to 74 years old	MCI					+			
	AD		+		+	+	+	+	+
	A-C. D		+		+	+	+	+	+
>75 years old	MCI								
	AD				+				
	A-C. D				+				

Notes: Empty fields mean no study performed. AD, Alzheimer's disease; FHS, Framingham Heart Study; NS, not significant; +, direct relationship; MCI, mild cognitive impairment; A-C. D, all-cause dementia; ApoE4, apolipoprotein 4; WMH, white matter hyperintensity.

participants aged 55 to 64, it is a risk factor for participants above 65 years of age (Weinstein et al., 2014). Schaefer et al. (2006) examined another serum biomarker that has also been linked to cardiovascular risk, phosphatidylcholine docosahexaenoic acid (PC DHA), which appears to have a protective effect against AD, such that higher serum level demonstrated a 47% reduction in the risk of developing all-cause dementia. Other serum biomarkers that have previously been linked to cardiovascular risk and disease have been founded to be associated to all-cause dementia and/or AD, such as thyroid stimulating hormone (Tan et al., 2008), biomarkers of insulin resistance (van Himbergen et al., 2012), plasma leptin (Lieb et al., 2009), bone mineral density (Tan et al., 2005), and inflammatory markers (Tan et al., 2007; Table 1.3).

5. Conclusion

As one of the longest ongoing community-based epidemiological studies, the FHS has championed the research on cardiovascular diseases and its associated risk factors for close to than 70 years. With the subsequent introduction of neuropsychological protocols and brain MRI scans, investigators have been able to capitalize on its robust infrastructure and rich data repository to establish associations between cardiovascular diseases and its risk factors with cognition and neurodegenerative outcomes. In this chapter, we highlighted the effects of cardiovascular risk factors on cognition, brain structure, and risk of all-cause dementia or AD. The FHS studies suggest a complex synergistic relationship between cardiovascular risk factors, cognition, and changes in brain structures. Means to accurately diagnose AD and other dementia syndromes continues to be vexing. The solution to this problem will require a multidisciplinary approach, looking beyond the conventional neuropsychological and MRI metrics and taking into consideration the individual's cardiovascular health status and genetic profile. The FHS findings provided in this chapter suggest that consideration of vascular pathways is a major contributing factor to dementia such as AD.

References

Akomolafe, A., Beiser, A., Meigs, J. B., Au, R., Green, R. C., Farrer, L. A., . . . Seshadri, S. (2006). Diabetes mellitus and risk of developing Alzheimer disease: Results from the Framingham Study. *Archives of Neurology*, *63*(11), 1551–1555. https://doi.org/10.1001/archneur.63.11.1551

Alzheimer's Association. (2008). 2008 Alzheimer's disease facts and figures. *Alzheimer's Dement*, *4*(2), 110–33.

Au, R., & Devine, S. (2013). Implementing the Boston process approach in the Framingham Heart Study: It is possible. In L. Ashendorf, R. Swenson, & D. J. Libon (Eds.), *The Boston process approach to neuropsychological assessment: A practitioner's guide*. New York, NY: Oxford University Press.

Au, R., Massaro, J. M., Wolf, P. A., Young, M. E., Beiser, A., Seshadri, S., . . . DeCarli, C. (2006). Association of white matter hyperintensity volume with decreased cognitive functioning: The Framingham Heart Study. *Archives of Neurology*, *63*(2), 246–250. http://doi.org/10.1001/archneur.63.2.246

Au, R., Piers, R. J., & Devine, S. (2017). How technology is reshaping cognitive assessment: Lessons from the Framingham Heart Study. *Neuropsychology*, *31*(8), 846–861. http://doi.org/10.1037/neu0000411

Bangen, K. J., Delano-Wood, L., Wierenga, C. E., McCauley, A., Jeste, D. V, Salmon, D. P., & Bondi, M. W. (2010). Associations between stroke risk and cognition in normal aging and Alzheimer's disease with and without depression. *International Journal of Geriatric Psychiatry*, *25*(2), 175–182. http://doi.org/10.1002/gps.2317

Bennett, D. A., Schneider, J. A., Bienias, J. L., Evans, D. A., & Wilson, R. S. (2005). Mild cognitive impairment is related to Alzheimer disease pathology and cerebral infarctions. *Neurology*, *64*(5), 834–41.

Bostom, A. G., Rosenberg, I. H., Silbershatz, H., Jacques, P. F., Selhub, J., D'Agostino, R. B., . . . Wolf, P. A. (1999). Nonfasting plasma total homocysteine levels and stroke incidence in elderly persons: The Framingham Study. *Annals of Internal Medicine*, *131*(5), 352–355.

Caselli, R. J., Reiman, E. M., Locke, D. E. C., Hutton, M. L., Hentz, J. G., Hoffman-Snyder, C., . . . Osborne, D. (2007). Cognitive domain decline in healthy apolipoprotein E epsilon4 homozygotes before the diagnosis of mild cognitive impairment. *Archives of Neurology*, *64*(9), 1306–1311. http://doi.org/10.1001/archneur.64.9.1306

Damen, J. A. A. G., Hooft, L., Schuit, E., Debray, T. P. A., Collins, G. S., Tzoulaki, I., . . . Moons, K. G. M. (2016). Prediction models for cardiovascular disease risk in the general population: Systematic review. *BMJ (Clinical Research Ed.)*, *353*, i2416.

Das, R. R., Seshadri, S., Beiser, A. S., Kelly-Hayes, M., Au, R., Himali, J. J., . . . Wolf, P. A. (2008). Prevalence and correlates of silent cerebral infarcts in the Framingham offspring study. *Stroke*, *39*(11), 2929–2935. http://doi.org/10.1161/STROKEAHA.108.516575

Dash, S. K. (2011). Future targeted disease modifying drugs for Alzheimer's disease. *Recent Patents on CNS Drug Discovery*, *6*(1), 65–76.

Davies, P. (1999, April). Challenging the cholinergic hypothesis in Alzheimer disease. *JAMA*, *281*(15), 1433–1434.

Dawber, T. R., Meadors, G. F., & Moore, F. E. (1951). Epidemiological approaches to heart disease: The Framingham Study. *American Journal of Public Health*, *41*(3), 279–281. http://doi.org/10.2105/AJPH.41.3.279

Debette, S., Seshadri, S., Beiser, A., Au, R., Himali, J. J., Palumbo, C., . . . DeCarli, C. (2011). Midlife vascular risk factor exposure accelerates structural brain aging and cognitive decline. *Neurology*, *77*(5), 461–468. http://doi.org/10.1212/WNL.0b013e318227b227

DeCarli, C. (2016). Prevalence of MRI Abnormalities in the Framingham Study. *Alzheimer's & Dementia: The Journal of the Alzheimer's Association*, *12*(7), P267. http://doi.org/10.1016/j.jalz.2016.06.483

DeCarli, C., Murphy, D. G., Tranh, M., Grady, C. L., Haxby, J. V, Gillette, J. A., . . . Rapoport, S. I. (1995). The effect of white matter hyperintensity volume on brain structure, cognitive performance, and cerebral metabolism of glucose in 51 healthy adults. *Neurology*, *45*(11), 2077–2084.

Dubois, B., Feldman, H. H., Jacova, C., Cummings, J. L., DeKosky, S. T., Barberger-Gateau, P., . . . Scheltens, P. (2010). Revising the definition of Alzheimer's disease: A new lexicon. *The Lancet Neurology*, *9*(11), 1118–1127. http://doi.org/10.1016/S1474-4422(10)70223-4

Elias, M. F., Beiser, A., Wolf, P. A., Au, R., White, R. F., & D'Agostino, R. B. (2000). The preclinical phase of Alzheimer disease. *Archives of Neurology*, *57*(6), 808. http://doi.org/10.1001/archneur.57.6.808

Elias, M. F., D'Agostino, R. B., Elias, P. K., & Wolf, P. A. (1995). Neuropsychological test performance, cognitive functioning, blood pressure, and age: The Framingham Heart Study. *Experimental Aging Research*, *21*(4), 369–391. http://doi.org/10.1080/03610739508253991

Elias, M. F., Elias, P. K., Sullivan, L. M., Wolf, P. A., & D'Agostino, R. B. (2003). Lower cognitive function in the presence of obesity and hypertension: The Framingham heart study. *International Journal of Obesity and Related Metabolic Disorders*, *27*(2), 260–268. http://doi.org/10.1038/sj.ijo.802225

Elias, M. F., Elias, P. K., Sullivan, L. M., Wolf, P. A., & D'Agostino, R. B. (2005). Obesity, diabetes and cognitive deficit: The Framingham Heart Study. *Neurobiology of Aging*, *26*(Suppl 1), 11–16. http://doi.org/10.1016/j.neurobiolaging.2005.08.019

Elias, M. F., Sullivan, L. M., D'Agostino, R. B., Elias, P. K., Beiser, A., Au, R., . . . Wolf, P. A. (2004). Framingham stroke risk profile and lowered cognitive performance. *Stroke*, *35*(2), 404–409. http://doi.org/10.1161/01.STR.0000103141.82869.77

Elias, M. F., Sullivan, L. M., Elias, P. K., D'Agostino, R. B. S., Wolf, P. A., Seshadri, S., . . . Vasan, R. S. (2007). Left ventricular mass, blood pressure, and lowered cognitive performance in the Framingham offspring. *Hypertension*, *49*(3), 439–445. http://doi.org/10.1161/01.HYP.0000256361.68158.24

Elias, M. F., Wolf, P. A., D'Agostino, R. B., Cobb, J., & White, L. R. (1993). Untreated blood pressure level is inversely related to cognitive functioning: The Framingham Study. *American Journal of Epidemiology*, *138*(6), 353–364.

Elias, P. K., D'Agostino, R. B., Elias, M. F., & Wolf, P. A. (1995). Blood pressure, hypertension, and age as risk factors for poor cognitive performance. *Experimental Aging Research*, *21*(4), 393–417. http://doi.org/10.1080/03610739508253992

Elias, P. K., Elias, M. F., D'Agostino, R. B., Cupples, L. A., Wilson, P. W., Silbershatz, H., & Wolf, P. A. (1997). NIDDM and blood pressure as risk factors for poor cognitive performance: The Framingham Study. *Diabetes Care*, *20*(9), 1388–1395.

Elias, P. K., Elias, M. F., D'Agostino, R. B., Silbershatz, H., & Wolf, P. A. (1999). Alcohol consumption and cognitive performance in the Framingham Heart Study. *American Journal of Epidemiology*, *150*(6), 580–589.

Elias, P. K., Elias, M. F., D'Agostino, R. B., Sullivan, L. M., & Wolf, P. A. (2005). Serum cholesterol and cognitive performance in the Framingham Heart Study. *Psychosomatic Medicine*, *67*(1), 24–30. http://doi.org/10.1097/01.psy.0000151745.67285.c2

Farmer, M. E., Kittner, S. J., Abbott, R. D., Wolz, M. M., Wolf, P. A., & White, L. R. (1990). Longitudinally measured blood pressure, antihypertensive medication use, and cognitive performance: The Framingham Study. *Journal of Clinical Epidemiology*, *43*(5), 475–480.

Farmer, M. E., White, L. R., Abbott, R. D., Kittner, S. J., Kaplan, E., Wolz, M. M., . . . Wolf, P. A. (1987a). Blood pressure and cognitive performance: The Framingham Study. *American Journal of Epidemiology*, *126*(6), 1103–1114.

Farmer, M. E., White, L. R., Kittner, S. J., Kaplan, E., Moes, E., McNamara, P., . . . Feinleib, M. (1987b). Neuropsychological test performance in Framingham: A descriptive study. *Psychological Reports*, *60*(3 Pt 2), 1023–1040. http://doi.org/10.2466/pr0.1987.60.3c.1023

Folstein, M. F., Folstein, S. E., & McHugh, P. R. (1975). "Mini-mental state": A practical method for grading the cognitive state of patients for the clinician. *Journal of Psychiatric Research*, *12*(3), 189–198. http://doi.org/10.1016/0022-3956(75)90026-6

Garcia, M. J., McNamara, P. M., Gordon, T., & Kannel, W. B. (1974). Morbidity and mortality in diabetics in the Framingham population: Sixteen year follow-up study. *Diabetes*, *23*(2), 105–111.

Guillozet, A. L., Weintraub, S., Mash, D. C., & Mesulam, M. M. (2003). Neurofibrillary tangles, amyloid, and memory in aging and mild cognitive impairment. *Archives of Neurology*, *60*(5), 729–736.

Gupta, A., Preis, S. R., Beiser, A., Devine, S., Hankee, L., Seshadri, S., . . . Au, R. (2015). Mid-life cardiovascular risk impacts memory function: The Framingham Offspring Study. *Alzheimer Disease and Associated Disorders*, *29*(2), 117–123. http://doi.org/10.1097/WAD.0000000000000059

Hubert, H. B., Feinleib, M., McNamara, P. M., & Castelli, W. P. (1983). Obesity as an independent risk factor for cardiovascular disease: A 26-year follow-up of participants in the Framingham Heart Study. *Circulation*, *67*(5), 968–977.

Jeerakathil, T., Wolf, P. A., Beiser, A., Hald, J. K., Au, R., Kase, C. S., . . . DeCarli, C. (2004). Cerebral microbleeds: Prevalence and associations with cardiovascular risk factors in the Framingham Study. *Stroke*, *35*(8), 1831–1835. http://doi.org/10.1161/01.STR.0000131809.35202.1b

Jefferson, A. L., Beiser, A. S., Himali, J. J., Seshadri, S., O'Donnell, C. J., Manning, W. J., . . . Benjamin, E. J. (2015). Low cardiac index is associated with incident dementia and Alzheimer disease: The Framingham Heart Study. *Circulation*, *131*(15), 1333–1339. http://doi.org/10.1161/CIRCULATIONAHA.114.012438

Kannel, W. B., Feinleib, M., McNamara, P. M., Garrison, R. J., & Castelli, W. P. (1979). An investigation of coronary heart disease in families: The Framingham offspring study. *American Journal of Epidemiology*, *110*(3), 281–290.

Kaplan, E. (1988). A process approach to neuropsychological assessment. In T. Boll & B. R. Bryant (Eds.), *Clinical neuropsychology and brain function: Research, measurement, and practice: Master lectures*. Washington, DC: American Psychological Association.

Kaplan, E. (1990). The process approach to neuropsychological assessment of psychiatric patients. *Journal of Neuropsychiatry and the Clinical Neurosciences*, *2*, 72–87.

Knopman, D., Boland, L. L., Mosley, T., Howard, G., Liao, D., Szklo, M., . . . Folsom, A. R. (2001). Cardiovascular risk factors and cognitive decline in middle-aged adults. *Neurology*, *56*(1), 42–48.

Knopman, D. S., Mosley, T. H., Catellier, D. J., & Coker, L. H. (2009). Fourteen-year longitudinal study of vascular risk factors, APOE genotype, and cognition: The ARIC MRI Study. *Alzheimer's & Dementia: The Journal of the Alzheimer's Association*, *5*(3), 207–214. http://doi.org/10.1016/j.jalz.2009.01.027

Lieb, W., Beiser, A. S., Vasan, R. S., Tan, Z. S., Au, R., Harris, T. B., . . . Seshadri, S. (2009). Association of plasma leptin levels with incident Alzheimer disease and MRI measures of brain aging. *JAMA*, *302*(23), 2565–2572. http://doi.org/10.1001/jama.2009.1836

Maillard, P., Mitchell, G. F., Himali, J. J., Beiser, A., Tsao, C. W., Pase, M. P., . . . DeCarli, C. (2016). Effects of arterial stiffness on brain integrity in young adults from the Framingham Heart Study. *Stroke*, *47*(4), 1030–1036. http://doi.org/10.1161/STROKEAHA.116.012949

Maillard, P., Seshadri, S., Beiser, A., Himali, J. J., Au, R., Fletcher, E., . . . DeCarli, C. (2012). Effects of systolic blood pressure on white-matter integrity in young adults in the Framingham Heart Study: A cross-sectional study. *The Lancet Neurology*, *11*(12), 1039–1047. http://doi.org/10.1016/S1474-4422(12)70241-7

Marchant, N. L., Reed, B. R., Sanossian, N., Madison, C. M., Kriger, S., Dhada, R., . . . Jagust, W. J. (2013). The aging brain and cognition: Contribution of vascular injury and aβ to mild cognitive dysfunction. *JAMA Neurology*, *70*(4), 488–495. http://doi.org/10.1001/2013.jamaneurol.405

Markesbery, W. R., Schmitt, F. A., Kryscio, R. J., Davis, D. G., Smith, C. D., & Wekstein, D. R. (2006). Neuropathologic substrate of mild cognitive impairment. *Archives of Neurology*, *63*(1), 38–46.

Massaro, J. M., D'Agostino, R. B. S., Sullivan, L. M., Beiser, A., DeCarli, C., Au, R., . . . Wolf, P. A. (2004). Managing and analysing data from a large-scale study on Framingham Offspring relating brain structure to cognitive function. *Statistics in Medicine*, *23*(2), 351–367. http://doi.org/10.1002/sim.1743

Masuda, J., Nabika, T., & Notsu, Y. (2001). Silent stroke: Pathogenesis, genetic factors and clinical implications as a risk factor. *Current Opinion in Neurology*, *14*(1), 77–82.

Matthews, F. E., Stephan, B. C. M., Robinson, L., Jagger, C., Barnes, L. E., Arthur, A., & Brayne, C. (2016). A two decade dementia incidence comparison from the Cognitive Function and Ageing Studies I and II. *Nature Communications*, *7*, 11398. http://doi.org/10.1038/ncomms11398

Miles, W. R., & Root, H. F. (1922). Psychological tests applied to diabetic patients. *Archives of Internal Medicine*, *30*(6), 767–777.

Morris, J. C. (2005). Early-stage and preclinical Alzheimer disease. *Alzheimer Disease and Associated Disorders*, *19*(3), 163.

Muir, J. L. (1997). Acetylcholine, aging, and Alzheimer's disease. *Pharmacology Biochemistry and Behavior*, *56*(4), 687–696. http://doi.org/10.1016/S0091-3057(96)00431-5

Nishtala, A., Preis, S. R., Beiser, A., Devine, S., Hankee, L., Seshadri, S., . . . Au, R. (2014). Midlife cardiovascular risk impacts executive function: Framingham offspring study. *Alzheimer Disease and Associated Disorders*, *28*(1), 16–22. http://doi.org/10.1097/WAD.0b013e3182a715bc

Otaegui-Arrazola, A., Amiano, P., Elbusto, A., Urdaneta, E., & Martinez-Lage, P. (2014). Diet, cognition, and Alzheimer's disease: Food for thought. *European Journal of Nutrition*, *53*(1), 1–23. http://doi.org/10.1007/s00394-013-0561-3

Ott, A., Andersen, K., Dewey, M. E., Letenneur, L., Brayne, C., Copeland, J. R. M., . . . Launer, L. J. (2004). Effect of smoking on global cognitive function in nondemented elderly. *Neurology*, *62*(6), 920–924.

Parker, D. A., Parker, E. S., Brody, J. A., & Schoenberg, R. (1983). Alcohol use and cognitive loss among employed men and women. *American Journal of Public Health*, *73*(5), 521–526.

Pase, M. P., Beiser, A., Aparicio, H., DeCarli, C., Vasan, R. S., Murabito, J., & Seshadri, S. (2016). Interarm differences in systolic blood pressure and the risk of dementia and subclinical brain injury. *Alzheimer's & Dementia: The Journal of the Alzheimer's Association*, *12*(4), 438–445. http://doi.org/10.1016/j.jalz.2015.09.006

Pase, M. P., Beiser, A., Enserro, D., Xanthakis, V., Aparicio, H., Satizabal, C. L., . . . Seshadri, S. (2016). Association of ideal cardiovascular health with vascular brain injury and incident dementia. *Stroke, 47*(5), 1201–1206. http://doi.org/10.1161/STROKEAHA.115.012608

Pase, M. P., Beiser, A., Himali, J. J., Tsao, C., Satizabal, C. L., Vasan, R. S., . . . Mitchell, G. F. (2016). Aortic stiffness and the risk of incident mild cognitive impairment and dementia. *Stroke, 47*(9), 2256–2261. http://doi.org/10.1161/STROKEAHA.116.013508

Petersen, R. C., & Morris, J. C. (2004). Mild cognitive impairment as a clinical entity and treatment target. *Archives of Neurology, 62*(7), 1160–1163; discussion 1167. http://doi.org/10.1001/archneur.62.7.1160

Petersen, R. C., Smith, G. E., Waring, S. C., Vnik, R. J., Tangalos, E. G., & Kokmen, E. (1999). Mild cognitive impairment: Clinical characterization and outcome. *Archives of Neurology, 56*(3), 303–8.

Razani, J., Boone, K., Lesser, I., & Weiss, D. (2004). Effects of cigarette smoking history on cognitive functioning in healthy older adults. *American Journal of Geriatric Psychiatry, 12*(4), 404–411. http://doi.org/10.1176/appi.ajgp.12.4.404

Ritchie, K., Artero, S., & Touchon, J. (2001). Classification criteria for mild cognitive impairment: A population-based validation study. *Neurology, 56*(1), 37–42.

Roglic, G. (2016). WHO Global report on diabetes: A summary. *International Journal of Noncommunicable Diseases, 1*(1), 3.

Rowe, C. C., Ellis, K. A., Rimajova, M., Bourgeat, P., Pike, K. E., Jones, G., . . . Villemagne, V. L. (2010). Amyloid imaging results from the Australian Imaging, Biomarkers and Lifestyle (AIBL) study of aging. *Neurobiology of Aging, 31*(8), 1275–1283. http://doi.org/10.1016/j.neurobiolaging.2010.04.007

Satizabal, C., Beiser, A. S., & Seshadri, S. (2016). Incidence of dementia over three decades in the Framingham Heart Study. *New England Journal of* Medicine, *375*, 92–94. http://doi.org/10.1056/NEJMc1604823

Saxena, U. (2010). Alzheimer's disease amyloid hypothesis at crossroads: Where do we go from here? *Expert Opinion on Therapeutic Targets, 14*(12), 1273–7.

Schaefer, E. J., Bongard, V., Beiser, A. S., Lamon-Fava, S., Robins, S. J., Au, R., . . . Wolf, P. A. (2006). Plasma phosphatidylcholine docosahexaenoic acid content and risk of dementia and Alzheimer disease: The Framingham Heart Study. *Archives of Neurology, 63*(11), 1545–1550. http://doi.org/10.1001/archneur.63.11.1545

Schmand, B., Jonker, C., Hooijer, C., & Lindeboom, J. (1996). Subjective memory complaints may announce dementia. *Neurology, 46*(1), 121–125.

Seshadri, S. (2006). Elevated plasma homocysteine levels: Risk factor or risk marker for the development of dementia and Alzheimer's disease? *Journal of Alzheimer's Disease, 9*(4), 393–398.

Seshadri, S., Beiser, A., Au, R., Wolf, P. A., Evans, D. A., Wilson, R. S., . . . Chui, H. C. (2011). Operationalizing diagnostic criteria for Alzheimer's disease and other age-related cognitive impairment-Part 2. *Alzheimer's & Dementia: The Journal of the Alzheimer's Association, 7*(1), 35–52. http://doi.org/10.1016/j.jalz.2010.12.002

Seshadri, S., Beiser, A., Kelly-Hayes, M., Kase, C. S., Au, R., Kannel, W. B., & Wolf, P. A. (2006). The lifetime risk of stroke: Estimates from the Framingham Study. *Stroke, 37*(2), 345–350. http://doi.org/10.1161/01.STR.0000199613.38911.b2

Seshadri, S., Beiser, A., Selhub, J., Jacques, P. F., Rosenberg, I. H., D'Agostino, R. B., . . . Wolf, P. A. (2002). Plasma homocysteine as a risk factor for dementia and Alzheimer's disease. *New England Journal of Medicine, 346*(7), 476–483. http://doi.org/10.1056/NEJMoa011613

Seshadri, S., Wolf, P. A., Beiser, A., Elias, M. F., Au, R., Kase, C. S., . . . DeCarli, C. (2004). Stroke risk profile, brain volume, and cognitive function: The Framingham Offspring Study. *Neurology, 63*(9), 1591–1599.

Sperling, R. A., Aisen, P. S., Beckett, L. A., Bennett, D. A., Craft, S., Fagan, A. M., . . . Phelps, C. H. (2011). Toward defining the preclinical stages of Alzheimer's disease: Recommendations from the National Institute on Aging-Alzheimer's Association workgroups on diagnostic guidelines for Alzheimer's disease. *Alzheimers Dement, 7*(3), 280–92.

Tan, Z. S., Beiser, A. S., Fox, C. S., Au, R., Himali, J. J., Debette, S., . . . Seshadri, S. (2011). Association of metabolic dysregulation with volumetric brain magnetic resonance imaging and cognitive markers of subclinical brain aging in middle-aged adults: The Framingham Offspring Study. *Diabetes Care, 34*(8), 1766–1770. http://doi.org/10.2337/dc11-0308

Tan, Z. S., Beiser, A. S., Vasan, R. S., Roubenoff, R., Dinarello, C. A., Harris, T. B., . . . Seshadri, S. (2007). Inflammatory markers and the risk of Alzheimer disease: The Framingham Study. *Neurology, 68*(22), 1902–1908. http://doi.org/10.1212/01.wnl.0000263217.36439.da

Tan, Z. S., Beiser, A., Vasan, R. S., Au, R., Auerbach, S., Kiel, D. P., . . . Seshadri, S. (2008). Thyroid function and the risk of Alzheimer disease: The Framingham Study. *Archives of Internal Medicine, 168*(14), 1514–1520. http://doi.org/10.1001/archinte.168.14.1514

Tan, Z. S., Seshadri, S., Beiser, A., Zhang, Y., Felson, D., Hannan, M. T., . . . Kiel, D. P. (2005). Bone mineral density and the risk of Alzheimer disease. *Archives of Neurology, 62*(1), 107–111. http://doi.org/10.1001/archneur.62.1.107

Tsao, C. W., Himali, J. J., Beiser, A. S., Larson, M. G., DeCarli, C., Vasan, R. S., . . . Seshadri, S. (2016). Association of arterial stiffness with progression of subclinical brain and cognitive disease. *Neurology, 86*(7), 619–626. http://doi.org/10.1212/WNL.0000000000002368

Tsao, C. W., & Vasan, R. S. (2015). Cohort profile: The Framingham Heart Study (FHS): Overview of milestones in cardiovascular epidemiology. *International Journal of Epidemiology, 44*(6), 1800–1813. http://doi.org/10.1093/ije/dyv337

United Nations Population Division. (2007). *World population aging 2007*. New York, NY: United Nations.

van Himbergen, T. M., Beiser, A. S., Ai, M., Seshadri, S., Otokozawa, S., Au, R., . . . Schaefer, E. J. (2012). Biomarkers for insulin resistance and inflammation and the risk for all-cause dementia and Alzheimer disease: Results from the Framingham Heart Study. *Archives of Neurology, 69*(5), 594–600. http://doi.org/10.1001/archneurol.2011.670

van Vliet, P., van de Water, W., de Craen, A. J. M., & Westendorp, R. G. J. (2009). The influence of age on the association between cholesterol and cognitive function. *Experimental Gerontology, 44*(1–2), 112–122. http://doi.org/10.1016/j.exger.2008.05.004

Vermeer, S. E., Hollander, M., van Dijk, E. J., Hofman, A., Koudstaal, P. J., & Breteler, M. M. B. (2003). Silent brain infarcts and white matter lesions increase stroke risk in the general population: The Rotterdam Scan Study. *Stroke, 34*(5), 1126–1129. http://doi.org/10.1161/01.STR.0000068408.82115.D2

Weinstein, G., Beiser, A. S., Choi, S. H., Preis, S. R., Chen, T. C., Vorgas, D., . . . Seshadri, S. (2014). Serum brain-derived neurotrophic factor and the risk for dementia: The Framingham Heart Study. *JAMA Neurology, 71*(1), 55–61. http://doi.org/10.1001/jamaneurol.2013.4781

Whitehair, D. C., Sherzai, A., Emond, J., Raman, R., Aisen, P. S., Petersen, R. C., & Fleisher, A. S. (2010). Influence of apolipoprotein E varepsilon4 on rates of cognitive and functional decline in mild cognitive impairment. *Alzheimer's & Dementia: The Journal of the Alzheimer's Association*, *6*(5), 412–419. http://doi.org/10.1016/j.jalz.2009.12.003

Wolf, P. A. (2012). Contributions of the Framingham Heart Study to stroke and dementia epidemiologic research at 60 years. *Archives of Neurology*, *69*(5), 567–571. http://doi.org/10.1001/archneurol.2011.977

Wolf, P. A., Beiser, A., Elias, M. F., Au, R., Vasan, R. S., & Seshadri, S. (2007). Relation of obesity to cognitive function: Importance of central obesity and synergistic influence of concomitant hypertension: The Framingham Heart Study. *Current Alzheimer Research*, *4*(2), 111–116.

Wolf, P. A., D'Agostino, R. B., Belanger, A. J., & Kannel, W. B. (1991). Probability of stroke: A risk profile from the Framingham Study. *Stroke*, *22*(3), 312–318.

2
Heterogeneity in Alzheimer's/Vascular Spectrum Dementia

Sheina Emrani, Melissa Lamar, Catherine C. Price, Victor Wasserman, Emily Matusz, Rodney A. Swenson, Kenneth M. Heilman, and David J. Libon

1. Introduction

The prevailing point of view suggests that Alzheimer's disease (AD) and vascular dementia (VaD) are independent forms of dementia. However, over the last decade a robust and emerging body of research has shown that many patients diagnosed with either AD or VaD present with biological substrates associated with both dementia syndromes to suggest considerable pathological and clinical heterogeneity. The notion that the pathological changes associated with these two disorders are additive, synergistic, or directly related to each other is the subject of lively debate (Esiri et al., 1999; Sweeney et al., 2019). An emerging challenge regarding the classification of these disorders is not necessarily the diagnosis of a specific clinical/pathological syndrome; rather, determining *how much* or *what proportion* of a patient's clinical or phenotypic presentation is associated with *what type* of underlying neuropathology. The determination of *how much* or *what proportion* requires an inclusive algorithm that defines meaningful neuropsychological phenotypes along with biological indicators of dementia obtained from imaging and fluid biomarkers. This type of algorithm for classifying AD/VaD spectrum dementia is very different from current dementia diagnostic schemes where the presence of a single fluid biomarker or a positive finding from an imaging study determines the diagnosis (Jack et al., 2018). We would submit that models associating phenotypic features—largely defined using neuropsychological tests—coupled with the quantification of underlying biological substrate would be a more heuristically meaningful method for AD/VaD classification. This type of algorithm, gaining traction in the literature (Bondi et al., 2014; Edmonds et al., 2015, 2019; Eppig et al., 2012; Libon et al., 2010, 2011; 2014; Wong et al., 2018), is particularly relevant for selecting patients and formulating expected outcomes for clinical trials designed to treat dementia (Edmonds et al., 2018).

Sheina Emrani, Melissa Lamar, Catherine Price, Victor Wasserman, Emily Matusz, Rodney Swenson, Kenneth M. Heilman, and David J. Libon, *Heterogeneity in Alzheimer's/Vascular Spectrum Dementia* In: *Vascular Disease, Alzheimer's Disease, and Mild Cognitive Impairment*. Edited by: David J. Libon, Melissa Lamar, Rodney A. Swenson, Kenneth M. Heilman, Oxford University Press (2020).
DOI: 10.1093/oso/9780190634230.003.0003

1.1. The Amyloid Cascade Hypothesis

The amyloid cascade hypothesis (Hardy & Higgins 1992; Hardy et al., 2014) continues to be the dominant biological model attempting to explain the mechanistic sequence of events that precipitate and ultimately lead to a clinical/pathological diagnosis of AD (Hardy & Selkoe, 2002; Selkoe, 2000). According to this model (Hardy & Higgins; 1992), abnormal aggregation of beta-amyloid (Aβ) induces a cascade of events that result in pathological changes and subsequent neurodegeneration. The nexus of the amyloid cascade hypothesis revolves around aberrant cleavage of the amyloid precursor protein (APP). APP has been implicated in the migration of neurons during early development and has been linked to synaptic formation; nonetheless, the principal function(s) of APP are not well understood. Under usual circumstances, APP is cleaved by α-secretase (alpha-secretase) followed by γ-secretase (gamma-secretase) resulting in extracellular fragment (sAPPα). The events associated with the α-secretase are thought to be relatively benign. Problems arise with the occurrence of APP cleavage made by β-secretase (beta-secretase), again followed by γ-secretase resulting in the accumulation of insoluble Aβ peptides. Insoluble Aβ peptides aggregate to form plaques thus constituting one of the major hallmarks features of AD pathology (Hardy, 2014). These events appear to suggest a complex, but nonetheless linear, relationship linking derailed APP cleavage with clinically diagnosed AD.

There are growing criticisms of the amyloid cascade hypothesis as *the* causative model for clinical diagnosed AD (Drachman, 2014; Herrup 2015). First, the presence of significant amyloid should result in AD; however, research shows that the presence of amyloid does not necessarily result in the emergence of clinical signs of AD. Indeed, past research shows that many individuals with high amyloid burden do not necessarily present with clinical signs of dementia. Another problem with the amyloid cascade hypothesis is that clinical improvement should occur when amyloid is removed from patients' brains. Prior clinical trials show that there are agents may be able to reduce the amyloid burden; however, these agents have little or no effect subsequent performance on neuropsychological tests (Holmes et al., 2008). These observations have led some researchers to suggest that amyloid burden could be *necessary but not sufficient* for the development of AD. Clearly, biologic markers measuring Aβ levels are clearly necessary for any proposed diagnostic or classification model of dementia. While we acknowledge that, the criticisms of the amyloid cascade hypothesis do not obviate the putative role of insoluble Aβ in the genesis of dementia such as AD, the prevailing evidence suggests that for the majority of patient clinical vascular alterations and AD-type pathology co-exist and are important to eventual emergence of AD/VaD spectrum dementia.

1.2. Vascular Disease and Dementia

There is no single theory'\ that links vascular disease with dementia. Rather, the evidence that vascular disease is associated with dementia, such as AD comes from a variety of sources. First, perfusion deficits due to compromised cardiac functioning and cerebral arterial disease are associated with the eventual emergence of dementia such as AD (Cermakova et al., 2015; Jefferson et al., 2018). Second, research has associated a number of vascular risk factors including midlife hypertension (Kalaria, 2012; Reitz et al., 2007), hypercholesterolemia (Craft, 2009; Hughes & Craft, 2016), diabetes mellitus (DM; Craft, 2009; Jayaraman & Pike, 2014), midlife obesity (Kalaria, 2010), smoking (Barnes & Yaffe, 2011), and physical inactivity (Barnes & Yaffe, 2011) with AD/VaD dementia. Third, epidemiological research including data from the Framingham Heart Study (Farmer et al., 1990) and the Rotterdam Study (De Leeuw et al., 2001; Ott et al., 1998, 1999) also link clinical vascular risk factors to reduced performance on neuropsychological tests, as well as the emergence of clinical syndromes such as mild cognitive impairment (MCI) and dementia including AD. Fourth, all of the previously listed vascular risk factors are easily identifiable and potentially treatable. Managing medical illnesses associated with cardiovascular risk including diet and other modifiable life style factors like cardiovascular fitness (DeFina et al., 2013) are powerful tools in either delaying or preventing the onset of dementia (Serrano-Pozo & Growdon, 2019).

There is also emerging research demonstrating complex interrelationships between vascular risk factors and traditional AD pathology. For example, Clark and colleagues (2019) studied a group of community volunteers with and without vascular risk such as hypertension and obesity and concurrent elevated β-amyloid. Patients with both vascular risk and elevated β-amyloid performed worse on immediate and delay free recall on a serial list-learning test. Clark and colleagues (2019) also found that elevated β-amyloid and subsequent reduced performance on memory tests appeared to be moderated by the presence of vascular risk factors. Iturria-Medina and colleagues (2016) sought to characterize the temporal ordering of factors related to the eventual emergence of AD including amyloid-β deposition, glucose metabolism, cerebral blood flow, resting functional magnetic resonance imaging (MRI) neuronal activity (structural MRI), neuropsychological abilities, and peripheral protein levels (cerebrospinal fluid [CSF] and plasma). This study found that vascular dysregulation within the brain was, in fact, an early marker for pathological events related to the emergence of AD.

Animal models have also demonstrated the intricate relationship between AD-type pathology and vascular factors. Sadowski et al. (2004) looked at double transgenic AD mouse model expressing both APP and PSEN1 and found that ischemia resulted in long-term disturbances of Aβ homeostasis. Additionally, Aβ deposition combined with vascular pathology had a synergistic effect on the emergence of cognitive deficits. The authors proposed that in homeostatic conditions, the blood–brain barrier (BBB) is able to modulate soluble Aβ peptides via receptor-specific mechanisms. However, ischemic damage and/or the presence of vessel amyloid may override homeostatic functions and have negative consequences on the BBB. Further, other studies have shown that Aβ appears to render the brain more vulnerable to ischemic injury (Attems & Jellinger, 2014) including hypoxia with ischemia that promote Aβ cleavage from APP by upregulating β-secretase expression (Iadecola, 2010). As such, it is important to consider vascular contributions in tandem with traditional markers of AD neuropathology as adverse influencers on memory and other neurocognitive domains.

As described in the previous discussion, there are complex interrelationships between vascular risk factors and traditional AD pathology. Many patients seen for dementia evaluation present with a long history of cardiovascular risk (hypertension, diabetes, compromised cardiac functioning), and measurable evidence of vascular compromise as seen on MRI scans such as subcortical infarcts, dilatation of perivascular space, microbleeds, and white matter hyperintensities. In these patients, an analysis of biomarkers and brain scans may also be positive for changes that are associated with AD; however, the presence of vascular disease is often ignored or minimized in comparison to laboratory signs of AD. From a clinical perspective, overlooking or underestimating the contribution of vascular risk and their concomitant medical conditions increase the probability of emergent dementia. Together, the previously discussed data support the notion that AD/VaD dementia may be best understood as a spectrum illness.

2. Neuropathology Heterogeneity in AD/VaD Spectrum Dementia

There is now a growing body of research demonstrating considerable heterogeneity with respect to the neuropathology underlying insidious onset AD/VaD spectrum dementia (Chui & Ramirez-Gomez, 2015; Sachdev et al., 2014). Recent epidemiological and community-based research clearly show the presence of *mixed neuropathology* in many if not the majority of patients diagnosed with dementia (Brayne et al., 2009; Brenowitz et al., 2017; James, Bennett, Boyle, Leurgans, & Schneider, 2012; Schneider, Arvanitakis, Bang, & Bennett, 2007; Schneider, Aggarwal, Barnes, Boyle, & Bennett, 2009). For example, Wharton and colleagues (2011) and Schneider and colleagues (2009) found mixed AD/VaD pathology to be quite common, if not the norm, in their samples. White et al. (2002) studied participants from the Honolulu Aging Study and found numerous microinfarcts in their sample of patients with dementia. These researchers concluded that vascular disease might be as plausible a cause for dementia as AD pathology. More recently, Boyle and colleagues (2019) examined over 1,000 participants. Eight types of neuropathology (i.e., macroscopic infarct, Lewy bodies, hippocampal sclerosis, TDP-43, cerebral amyloid angiopathy [CAA], atherosclerosis, and arteriosclerosis) including neuropathology traditionally associated with AD (i.e., neuritic plaques/neurofibrillary tangles) were quantified. They found that approximately 67.5% of cases with dementia could be attributable to some combination of all eight neuropathologic indices.

Considerable heterogeneity of brain pathology has also been described in clinic-based samples. Post mortem examinations described by Wang et al. (2012) found that actual cases of so-called pure AD (i.e., plaques and tangles) were less common than those with mixed AD/VaD. Azarpazhooh et al. (2018) identified 10 studies describing approximately 3,000 where neuropathology data were available. An overwhelming number of patients (77%–86%) had evidence of vascular and/or mixed neuropathology whereas only 45% of patients displayed relatively circumscribed AD pathology. These researchers observed that many cases of dementia might have been delayed or prevented with better management of vascular risk factors.

Recent evidence suggests that upon autopsy, approximately one third of patients diagnosed with VaD showed evidence of basal forebrain, cholinergic deficits. A similar phenomenon has been described in patients diagnosed with AD. Impaired cholinergic transmission in VaD include a reduction in cholinergic nerve terminals, decreased activity of choline acetyltransferace (enzyme for acetylcholine synthesis) in the cortex, hippocampus, and striatum, and degeneration of nicotinic cholinergic neurotransmission and receptors (Kalaria, 2002). In subsequent research Kalaria et al. (2012) also noted that mixed AD/VaD is far more prevalent than either "pure" AD or VaD dementia syndromes. In sum, neuropathological heterogeneity is not just present but is likely present for the majorly of AD/VaD patients. The lack of appreciation of these relationships may have contributed to the failure of clinical trials designed to treat dementia such as AD.

3. Vascular Dysfunction as Both a Mediator and Moderator of AD/VaD Dementia Spectrum

Risk factors for both VaD and AD include a wide range of cardiovascular illness including atrial fibrillation, atherosclerosis, CAA, coronary artery disease, MRI defined microvascular changes, metabolic syndromes (i.e., DM, hypertension, and dyslipidemia), APOE4 allele, smoking, among other factors (Kalaria, 2002; Attems & Jellinger, 2014). Proposed mechanisms and derivative neuropathology as related to AD for some of these risk factors are described in the following text.

3.1. Alterations in the Blood–Brain Barrier

There is now keen interest in understanding the mechanism underlying breach in the BBB as related to the eventual emergence of AD and other dementia syndromes (Kalaria, 1998; Sweeney et al., 2018, 2019). The neurovascular unit is composed of endothelial cells, pericytes, vascular smooth muscle cells, glia, and neurons, which together act to control BBB permeability and blood flow. Research suggests that impaired BBB functioning can result in the accumulation of toxic molecules within the brain. Alterations in the BBB likely contribute to neuronal degeneration and the emergence of AD pathology (Sweeney et al., 2018, 2019; Zlokovic, 2011). For example, pericytes help regulate BBB permeability. Pericyte injury has been shown to be present in both postmortem analyses of patients with AD and in CSF of living MCI patients (Nelson et al., 2016). The microstructural changes found in pericytes (e.g., intracellular inclusions, large lipid granules) correlate with capillary reduction, dilation of vessels, and the appearance of tortuous vessels (Hughes & Craft, 2016; Sweeney et al., 2015; Nelson et al., 2016).

3.2. The Two-Hit Vascular Hypothesis

According to the two-hit hypothesis, vascular risk factors and cerebrovascular damage (hit 1) is the primary, causal insult promoting BBB dysfunction and reduction in cerebral blood flow, and ultimately lead to accumulation of Aβ and other neuropathology in the brain (hit 2; Zlokovic, 2011). This model has two arms—a non-Aβ pathway and an amyloidogenic Aβ pathway. In the non-Aβ pathway, circulating neurotoxic molecules (e.g., thrombin, plasminogen, fibrinogen) and hypoperfusion induce early neuronal dysfunction. In the amyloidogenic Aβ pathway, Aβ clearance is derailed by BBB dysfunction. In turn, this leads to overexpression and enhanced processing of APP that promote Aβ accumulation. The increase in Aβ (hit 2) amplifies neuronal dysfunction and accelerates the neurodegenerative processes of AD. Furthermore, Aβ is known to be a potent vasoconstrictor, thus impairing the mechanisms regulating the cerebral circulation and perpetuating vascular dysfunction and neuropathology.

3.3. Type 2 Diabetes Mellitus

In normal brain function insulin is readily transported across the BBB through a receptor-mediated process (Li et al., 2007; Sadowski et al., 2004; Sweeney et al., 2019; Talbot et al., 2012). Insulin receptors within the central nervous system are found in astrocytes and neuronal synapses and are highly concentrated in the olfactory bulb, cerebral cortex, hippocampus, hypothalamus, amygdala, and septum. Insulin influences vasoreactivity, capillary recruitment, vasodilation, and regional blood flow. As such, insulin resistance can result in vasoconstriction and reduction of capillary recruitment. Endothelial dysfunction due to insulin resistance reduces insulin transport and ultimately capillary recruitment and microvascular blood flow (Craft, 2009; Hughes & Craft, 2016). The ramifications of endothelial dysfunction secondary to insulin resistance is downstream neurovascular unit dysfunction and derailed coordinated interaction between astrocytes, neuron, and endothelium that augment vasoconstriction and inflammation.

Growing evidence supports the notion that type 2 DM is a major vascular risk factor and contributes to the development of AD. In a mouse model of diabetes, reduced brain insulin signaling was associated with increased tau phosphorylation, while raising plasma insulin levels through intravenous infusion in human AD patients increased CSF levels of $A\beta_{42}$ (Craft, 2009). Vascular alterations and increased BBB permeability have also been shown in DM patients (Hughes & Craft, 2016; Nelson et al., 2016). The mechanistic underpinnings of linking diabetes and dementia-related changes in the brain include increased levels of receptor for advanced glycation end-products (RAGE and AGEs), vascular inflammation, reduced insulin transport across the BBB, insulin resistance, and impaired insulin signaling (Jayaraman & Pike, 2014).

3.4. Hypertension

Hypertension impairs functional hyperemia, or the way in which brain activity and blood flow are synchronized (Craft, 2009; Kalaria, 2010). Functional hyperemia is induced by structural alterations of blood vessels (i.e., dysregulation of vasoactive mediators) and inadequate cerebral autoregulation. Animal models show that Aβ accumulation increases hypertension and induces vascular dysfunction that weakens functional hyperemia (Craft, 2009; Hughes & Craft, 2016). Indeed, postmortem analyses found greater AD pathology in hypertensive older adults (Hughes and Craft, 2016).

3.5. Hyperlipidemia

Hyperlipidemia has been shown to contribute to VaD, small vessel disease, and AD (Kalaria, 2010; Kivipelto et al., 2005). A meta-analytic study found that midlife total cholesterol levels were associated with increased risk for all dementias (Craft, 2009; Hughes & Craft, 2016). Dyslipidemia has also been linked to insulin-resistant syndrome, as insulin is a primary regulator of lipid metabolism. Further, lipids and lipoproteins play a critical role in Aβ production and clearance. For example, a rodent model found that increased peripheral, very low-density lipoprotein (LDL) secretion precedes Aβ accumulation in the brain suggesting that high-fat diet increases amyloid burden (Craft, 2009). Further, highly lipidated APOE increases Aβ brain efflux and reduces Aβ deposition whereas poorly lipidated APOE increases amyloid burden.

3.6. APOE Epsilon 4 Allele

The presence of the APOE epsilon4 allele has traditionally been viewed as a risk factor for AD. APOE is known to function as a lipid transport protein and ligand for LDL receptors and plays a role in cholesterol metabolism (Huang & Mahley, 2014; Mahley, 2016). Yip and colleagues (2005) autopsied the brains of patients with confirmed AD to assess the relationship between the APOE allele and the presence of cerebrovascular lesions. Brains positive for the E4 allele also had a greater amount of small vessel arteriolosclerosis. Specifically, the E4 allele was associated with greater thickness in the walls of blood vessels. The E4 allele was also associated with micro infarcts in the deep gray matter nuclei. APOE4 is also known to increase BBB damage (e.g., astrocytes, tight junctions), CAA, and fibrinogen deposits, and negatively affects clearance of Aβ (Zlokovic, 2011; Sweeney et al., 2015; Nelson, 2016). The interaction between APOE4, Aβ, and BBB are known and hypothesized to cause dysfunction via an upregulation of RAGE and downregulation of LDL receptor-related protein 1 (LRP-1; Donahue & Johanson, 2008).

The accumulated results suggests that decreased regional blood flow, reduction of glucose transport and use, loss of vascular innervation, damage to neurovascular regulation, Aβ deposition found in capillaries and basement membrane breakdown, and BBB impairment of amyloid clearance are all implicated in AD and VaD (Attems & Jellinger, 2014). Final end products of these changes include structural alteration as seen on MRI scans (i.e., lacunes, infarct, white matter alterations [WMAs]); compromised neuronal metabolism (e.g., reduction in glucose), and the formation of neuritic lesions (i.e., neurofibrillary tangles).

In sum, the research just described shows complex interrelationships between vascular dysfunction and reduced capacity for Aβ clearance suggesting a dual-direction relationship and a negative feedback loop. The intimate connections between vascular risk factors and AD pathology provide further justification for the notion that AD/VaD dementia should be viewed as a spectrum illness.

4. Neuropsychological Heterogeneity in Alzheimer's/ Vascular Spectrum Dementia

4.1. Statistically Modeling of AD/VaD Spectrum Neuropsychological Phenotypes

Past research analyzing neuropsychological test performance using statistical modeling techniques reveal the presence of clinical or phenotypic heterogeneity. Research conducted by both Price et al. (2005, 2015) and Libon et al. (2008) are emblematic. Both studies used a simple visual rating scale (Junque et al., 1990) that measured the severity of MRI WMAs to reclassify patients diagnosed clinically with either AD or VaD into three group: patients with mild, moderate, and severe MRI WMA. Price and colleagues (2005) constructed two neuropsychological indices measuring executive control/visuoconstruction abilities versus episodic memory/language abilities. At least four key findings emerged from this research. First, there was a double dissociation between patients reclassified as presenting with mild versus severe MRI WMAs. Patients with mild WMA clearly performed worse on the episodic memory/language index. On the other hand, patients with severe WMA were particularly impaired on the executive control/visuoconstruction index. Thus, based on severity of MRI-determined WMAs, two distinct *single-domain* neuropsychological syndromes were observed. Second, reclassified patients who presented with moderate WMA were equally impaired when executive control/visuoconstruction abilities versus episodic memory/language abilities were compared. In this sense, these patients can be viewed as presenting with a *multidomain* neuropsychological syndrome. Third, of the three MRI-determined WMA groups, the mixed or multidomain group contained the largest number of patients suggesting that clinical heterogeneity is quite common. Fourth, when each neuropsychological index was analyzed, the mixed/multidomain patients tended to produce scores that were less impaired than their single domain counterparts. Libon et al. (2008) largely replicated these findings of Price et al. (2005).

The significance of this research begs the question—Can neuropsychological phenotypes in AD/VaD spectrum dementia as previously defined provide information about the *type and penetrance* of neuropathology underlying these single domain and multidomain syndromes? For example, the amnestic/language deficits that were predominant in patients with mild WMA could suggest relative circumscribed gray matter pathology located in temporal brain regions, perhaps revolving around the presence of AD-related pathology. By contrast, the dysexecutive/visuoconstruction impairment seen in patients with severe WMA is most likely due to vascular disease that serves to disconnect or disrupt connectivity with the frontal lobes with the frontal lobes (Lamar et al., 2008). The multidomain neuropsychological presentation seen in the patients with moderate WMAs could suggest dementia associated with multiple neuropathological alterations that are widely distributed throughout the brain but, perhaps, are not as penetrant as seen in the two single domain groups.

4.2. AD/VaD Neuropsychological Phenotypes Using Latent Class Analysis

To gain more knowledge regarding the presence of distinct phenotypic syndromes in patients diagnosed clinically with either AD or VaD, Libon et al. (2014) used latent class analysis (LCA) to examine a corpus of six neuropsychological test scores measuring executive control/working memory; naming/lexical retrieval. LCA found evidence for four distinct groups or classes. This included two *single domain* groups typified by executive impairment and amnesia, respectively. In addition, two *mixed/multidomain* neuropsychological groups were found where neuropsychological impairment tended to be equally distributed across the three neuropsychological domains that were entered into the statistical model. However, the two mixed groups were distinguished by the fact that one group presented with moderate impairment across neuropsychological tests while the other mixed group presented with relatively mild neuropsychological impairment. Consistent with data reported by Price et al. (2005) and Libon et al. (2008) the majority of patients presented with the mixed domain-nonspecific profiles. In sum, all three experiments provide evidence that phenotypic heterogeneity is the norm rather than the exception in AD/VaD spectrum dementia, and that the neuropsychological profiles seen in AD/VaD spectrum dementia patients can be quite nuanced.

4.3. Statistically Modeling of Neuropsychological Phenotypes: Implication for Treatment

Edmonds et al. (2018) use statistical model procedures as previously described in their reanalysis of the original donepezil/vitamin E trial designed to treat

MCI (Petersen et al., 2005). The original trial defined MCI using Petersen criteria (2004, 2005) and reported only modest treatment effects. Edmonds et al. (2018) used cluster analysis to reclassify participants into groups presenting with amnestic MCI, mixed MCI, and cognitively normal participants. Subsequent analyses of the effect of drug on neurocognition after removing a statistically determined cognitively normal group revealed substantially lower rate of progression to dementia and better performance on memory tests. Thus, overall results described by Edmonds et al. (2018) found better treatment effect as compared to the original research findings. These data underscore the efficacy of statistical modeling techniques to characterize neuropsychological test performance. The results reported by Edmonds et al. (2018) clearly have important implications for all clinical trial designed to treat dementia.

5. Heterogeneity in AD/VaD Spectrum Dementia Patient: Context Independent Versus Context Dependent Neuropsychological Profiles

The neuropsychology of the insidious onset AD/VaD spectrum dementia often involves two broad types of neuropsychological impairments: dysexecutive impairment including working memory, information processing speed, and visuoconstruction and the presence of clinical of amnesia along with impaired access and/or degraded semantic knowledge (see Lamar et al., 2010; Libon et al., 2004, 2017, for a review). Certainly, circumscribed neuropsychological disabilities involving language and visuospatial impairment such as posterior cortical atrophy are well-known (Benson, 1988; da Silva et al., 2017; Suárez-González et al., 2015). Nonetheless, we maintain that, broadly speaking, dysexecutive and amnestic/language impairment tend to be the dominant patterns of impairment seen in patients with the AD/VaD spectrum dementia.

The traditional means by which neuropsychological heterogeneity in AD/VaD spectrum dementia is assessed has been to calculate relative impairment as expressed with simple test scores (Libon et al., 2008, 2014; Price et al., 2005). However, another potentially informative means to assess for heterogeneity in AD/VaD spectrum dementia is through an analysis of the hypothetical constructs (Cronbach & Meehl, 1955) underlying executive and amnestic/language impairment are expressed across neurocognitive domains. In past research, we have used constructs suggested by A. R. Luria (1980) and Joaquin Fuster (2008) as heuristics to place empirical or clinical evidence of dysexecutive and amnestic/language impairment into a theoretical framework.

Luria's construct of *pathological inertia* suggests that dysregulated frontal systems operations are due to the presence of actual frontal lobe lesions and/

or significant disturbance between frontal lobe regions and other areas of the brain. Indeed, the overall significance of MRI evidence of subcortical WMA (leukoaraiosis) in AD/VaD spectrum dementia is the extent to which these vascular lesions essentially disrupt or disconnect the capacity of frontal regions to regulate and direct behavior. Significant disconnections between frontal regions and other areas of brain in AD/VaD spectrum dementia often translate into severe executive impairment. Luria's construct of pathological inertia was originally applied narrowly to describe the variety of *motor perseverations* produced by patients with frontal lobe lesions. As described in the following text, we have expanded upon Luria's term *pathological inertia* to illustrate how dysexecutive behavior is seen not just on tests traditionally thought to measure executive abilities but also on tests that assess language and episodic memory abilities.

5.1. Context Independence Versus Context Dependence:

When conducting clinical evaluation for the diagnosis of dementia or MCI, it is important to note when executive impairment is *ubiquitous*, that is, seen across virtually many neuropsychological domains including tests that assess language and episodic memory. These neuropsychological syndromes can be described as *context independent*, that is, not necessarily linked or confined to a single neuropsychological domain. By contrast, other AD/VaD spectrum dementia patients can present with circumscribed or relatively narrow neuropsychological deficits. In these dementia patients, the neuropsychological profile can be described as *context dependent*, suggesting that significant neuropsychological impairment is more or less confined to a comparatively narrow array of neuropsychological abilities.

The distinction between context independent and context dependent neuropsychological AD/VaD dementia syndromes is not just a question of semantics. These distinctions could form the basis of a more heuristically meaningful scheme to classify AD/VaD spectrum dementia that maximizes the use of neuropsychological assessment as a grouping variable. Described in the following discussion is some of our prior research describing *context-independent* versus *context-dependent* neuropsychological syndromes in AD/VaD spectrum dementia.

5.2. Executive Dysregulation and Perseveration

Lamar et al. (1997) studied the severity and nature of graphomotor perseveration in patients thought to have either AD or VaD. The patients with VaD demonstrated extensive WMA on MRI scans. Not surprisingly, these patients produced more total perseverations compared to AD patients where MRI scans showed minimal to mild WMAs. Perhaps more interesting were the *types* of perseverations produced by the patients with VaD and AD. The perseverations produced by VaD patients were consistent with motor impersistence (Kim et al., 2016) such that these patients demonstrated an inability to desist from a motor act when their behavior was no longer productive. In addition, these graphomotor perseverations were correlated with poor performance on other executive and motor tests. In this sense, the pattern of perseveration obtained with these patients is an example of *context independence.*

By contrast, patients with AD who had minimal to mild WMAs primarily made errors in their *mode of output* such as producing a written response in words when asked to draw geometric figures. Impaired access and/or degraded lexical/semantic representations could account for this behavior. Indeed, these errors were highly correlated with impaired performance on language tests such as the Boston Naming Test and the animal fluency test. Thus, the errors produced by patients with AD can be viewed as *context dependent*, perhaps subordinate to impaired lexical/semantic processing, a common neuropsychological deficit in patients with AD. The importance of this data is that different neurocognitive constructs likely underlie executive impairment in both groups.

5.3. Verbal Concept Formation

Additional evidence supporting the heuristic value of the distinction between context independent versus context dependent neuropsychological impairment in AD/VaD spectrum dementia is provided by an analysis of errors made on tests assessing verbal concept formation. Giovannetti et al. (2001) coded errors produced by AD/VaD dementia spectrum patients from the Wechsler Adult Intelligence Scale–Revised Similarities subtest. In this research, only errors or zero-point responses was examined. Some errors were coded as *out-of-set* (e.g., *dog–lion*—"one barks and the other growls") such that the patient demonstrated that he or she was not operating within the parameters of the test (i.e., how are the word pairs alike). Juxtaposed to this type of error are *in-set* (e.g., *dog–lion*—"They're alive) where patients demonstrated an ability to respond as requested (i.e., provide the superordinate relationship between test stimuli). However, their response is obviously superficial. Principal component analysis found that *out-of-set* errors were clearly associated with measures of executive impairment. By contrast, *in-set* errors were associated with neuropsychological measures related to impairment in language and lexical access. Moreover, AD patients tended to produce a greater proportion of *in-set* errors whereas patients with

VaD produced a greater proportion of *out-of-set* errors. Consistent with analyses of graphomotor perseverations in AD/VaD spectrum described by Lamar et al. (1997), *out-of-set* errors appears to be *context independent* (i.e., a component of an overall dysexecutive syndrome). By contrast, the production of *in-set* errors appears to be *context dependent*, perhaps related to poor access to and/or degraded semantic knowledge.

5.4. Episodic Memory Test Performance

Context independent versus context dependent neuropsychological impairment is clearly present in the pattern of performance produced by AD/VaD spectrum dementia patients on verbal serial list learning tests, including the Philadelphia (repeatable) Verbal Learning Test (PrVLT). This test is a nine-word verbal serial list-learning task designed and modeled after the California Verbal Learning Test (CVLT-I; Delis et al., 1987). Price et al. (2009) examined performance on this test produced from a large group of AD/VaD spectrum patients. Patients were, again, sorted into three groups on the basis of MRI WMA (Junque et al., 1990), that is, mild, moderate, severe WMAs.

The overall pattern of performance produced by patients with severe WMA can be viewed as *context independent* in that their pattern of performance appeared to be part of their overarching executive impairment. For example, these patients obtained relatively better scores on the delayed Recognition Discriminability Index as compared to delay free recall. In addition, the delay recognition foils endorsed by this group tended to be drawn from the list B interference test condition, suggesting the presence of a source recall, retrieval-based profile.

By contrast, a very different profile was seen in patients with minimal to mild MRI WMA. First, these patients produced very low scores on both delay free recall and the delay Recognition Discriminability Index and tended to endorse numerous recognition foils. In addition, these patients generated many extra-list cued recall intrusion errors. The production of serial list learning cued recall intrusion errors have been associated with parahippocampal damage (Desgranges et al., 2002; Lekeu et al., 2003). It was also observed that the extra-list intrusion errors produced by these patients were very prototypic as related to their semantic category (e.g., "dog" for the animal category & "apple" for fruit). All of these features are consistent with the presence of clinical amnesia.

The third group, patients with moderate WMAs, tended to occupy a middle position as compared to other groups. These patients produced some, but fewer, extralist intrusion errors than patients with little WMA, but also tended to endorse the list B interference foils similar to patients with severe WMA.

In sum, this research found very different patterns of performance in AD/VaD spectrum patients and provides additional evidence supporting the heuristic value of analyzing context dependent versus context independent neuropsychological syndromes. Moreover, these data likely suggest that different patterns of neuropathology underlie the patterns of impairment seen in all three groups.

6. Impaired Temporal Gradients in AD/VaD Spectrum Dementia

Fuster (2008) suggests that significant frontal lobe recruitment is necessary when neurocognitive operations are novel, when behavior deviates from the routine, and, most important, when there is significant time between the initiation of a response to when the test is successfully brought to fruition. The construct of *temporal gradient* has been proposed by Fuster (2008) to describe the operations of frontal regions to recruit and coordinate the multitude of neurocognitive operations for successful completion of goal-directed behavior. Implicit in the construct of temporal gradients is the idea that *when* or *where* both errors and correct responses occur is as revealing as the final overall test score. In a series of experiments, we have tried to leverage this construct to place into context dysexecutive behavior seen in patients with AD/VaD spectrum dementia.

Lamar et al. (2002) undertook several experiments to test the notion that dysexecutive behavior in AD/VaD spectrum dementia can be understood in terms of Fuster's model of *temporal gradients*. In one experiment, AD/VaD spectrum dementia patients were asked to complete the Boston Revision of the Wechsler Memory Scale Mental Control subtest. Total test performance differed between groups such that VaD patients performed worse than AD patients. Subsequent analyses divided the test performance into three test epochs (i.e., the beginning third, the middle third, and the latter third). In this sense test epoch was used to operationally define Fuster's construct of temporal gradients. When performance was assessed as a function of time or test epoch, patients with VaD produced a striking negative slope such that performance worsened from test epoch 1 to test epoch 2, and from test epoch 2 to test epoch 3. AD patients produced a different profile. For these patients, performance declined from test epoch 1 to test epoch 2 with no additional decline.

In a second experiment, Lamar et al. (2002) looked at letter fluency test performance (letters FAS), measured by total output in each 15 second test epoch. In this experiment, AD/VaD spectrum dementia patients and patients with dementia due to Parkinson's disease (PD) were studied. Patients with PD often present with disproportionate executive impairment (Tröster, 2011). Thus, these patients were recruited as a control group. The a priori prediction was that patients with PD would perform in a manner similar to patients with VaD. Performance on this test was assessed as a percentage of total output for each 15-second epoch. As predicted, VaD and PD patients generated a similar pattern of performance such that maximum output was generated in the first 15 seconds of the test. By contrast, there was little difference between AD and normal control participants.

In both of these experiments, a negative slope as a function of time typified the pattern of performance produced by VaD patients. This suggests that overall test impairment seen in these experiments is likely due to an inability to recruit and coordinate the neurocognitive resources necessary to bring these tests to fruition. In this context, the striking negative slope produced by VaD patients can be interpreted as derailed temporal gradients.

7. Diagnosing Versus Classifying AD/VaD Spectrum Dementia

Over 100 years after the death of Professor Aloysius Alzheimer, there is now a renewed appreciation of the importance of vascular disease as related to insidious onset dementia syndromes. The data that have accumulated over the past several decades suggest that vascular risk factors such as hypertension, diabetes, and heart disease increases the probability of not only structural lesions seen on computer tomography or MRI scans, but also the derailing upstream biological mechanism affecting the neurovascular unit and may potentiate traditional AD pathology. The only logical conclusion is that the biological mechanisms associated with AD and VaD, once thought be independent, are, in fact, intricately related. As such heterogeneity in the form of combined clinical-pathological syndromes are quite common, with so-called *pure AD or pure VaD* syndromes being infrequent. In this chapter, we have reviewed how theoretical constructs as well as multivariate statistical analysis are able to differentiate highly nuanced *context-specific*/single domain and *context-independent*/mixed/multidomain AD/VaD spectrum syndromes. A wealth of information regarding the brain-behavior relations that underlie these syndromes is now available. This information can be used to help develop a more effective nosology or classification of AD/VaD spectrum dementia syndromes.

The use of fluid biomarker and in vivo imaging techniques are valid to the extent that these technologies can measure the presence and, perhaps, the severity of AD-related neuropathology. However, this does not tell the whole story. Vascular risk factors and imaging evidence of vascular disease must be afforded equal importance as AD fluid/imaging biomarkers to fully understand and appreciate what can only be described as a highly contextualized, multidimensional view of AD/VaD spectrum dementia.

The traditional use of neuropsychological assessment in dementia research has primarily been to assess outcome. This needs to change. As demonstrated by Edmonds et al. (2018), neuropsychological assessment can and should be used as an independent variable to classify patients for treatment. The neuropsychological research reviewed herein clearly demonstrate how one can leverage theoretical meaningful constructs to define empirically meaningful single and multidomain clinical syndromes. Additional studies are needed to better understand how single and multidomain AD/VaD spectrum neuropsychological syndromes are associated with specific panels of underlying neuropathology.

In sum, we maintain that *classification* of the neuropsychological syndromes using neuropsychological statistical methods should be integrated into current AD/VaD diagnostic schemes. This kind of paradigm explicitly jettisons the notion of syndromic or pathological "purity." Rather, this type of synthesis maximizes and puts to best use all available data to manage and treat what has become the leading public health problem of our age.

References

Attems, J., & Jellinger, K. A. (2014). The overlap between vascular disease and Alzheimer's disease-lessons from pathology. *BMC Medicine*, *12*(1), 206.

Azarpazhooh, M. R., Avan, A., Cipriano, L. E., Munoz, D. G., Sposato, L. A., & Hachinski, V. (2018). Concomitant vascular and neurodegenerative pathologies double the risk of dementia. *Alzheimer's & Dementia*, *14*(2), 148–156.

Barnes D. E., & Yaffe K. (2011). The projected effect of risk factor reduction on Alzheimer's disease prevalence. *Lancet Neurology*, *10*, 819–828.

Benson, D. F., Davis, R. J., & Snyder, B. D. (1988). Posterior cortical atrophy. *Archives of Neurology*, *45*(7), 789–793. http://doi.org/10.1001/archneur.1988.00520310107024

Bondi, M. W., Edmond, E. C., Jak, A. J., Clark, L. R., Delano-Wood, L., McDonald, C.R., . . . Salmon, D. P.; Alzheimer's Disease Neuroimaging Initiative. (2014). Neuropsychological criteria for mild cognitive impairment improves diagnostic precision, biomarker associations, and progression rates. *Journal of Alzheimer's Disease*, 42, 275–289.

Bondi, M. W., & Smith, G. E. (2014). Mild cognitive impairment: A concept and diagnostic entity in need of input from neuropsychology. *Journal of the International Neuropsychological Society*, *20*, 129–134.

Boyle, P. A., Yu, L., Leurgans, S. E., Wilson, R. S., Brookmeyer, R., Schneider, J. A., & Bennett, D. A. (2019). Attributable risk of Alzheimer's dementia attributed to age-related neuropathologies. *Annals of Neurology*, *85*(1), 114–124.

Brayne, C., Richardson, K., Matthews, F. E., Fleming, J., Hunter, S., Xuereb, J. H., . . . Dening, T. (2009). Neuropathological correlates of dementia in over-80-year-old brain donors from the population-based Cambridge City Over-75s Cohort (CC75C) study. *Journal of Alzheimer's Disease*, *18*(3), 645–658.

Brenowitz, W. D., Keene, C. D., Hawes, S. E., Hubbard, R. A., Longstreth, W. T., Jr., Woltjer, R. L., . . . Kukull, W. A. (2017). Alzheimer's disease neuropathologic change, Lewy body disease, and vascular brain injury in clinic-and community-based samples. *Neurobiology of Aging*, *53*, 83–92.

Cermakova, P., Eriksdotter, M., Lund, L. H., Winblad, B., Religa, P., & Religa, D. (2015). Heart failure and Alzheimer' s disease. *Journal of Internal Medicine*, *277*(4), 406–425.

Chui, H. C., & Ramirez-Gomez, L. (2015). Clinical and imaging features of mixed Alzheimer and vascular pathologies. *Alzheimer's Research and Therapy*, 7(1), 21. doi:10.1186/s13195-015-0104-7

Clark, L. R., Koscik, R. L., Allison, S. L., Berman, S. E., Norton, D., Carlsson, C. M., . . . Johnson, S.C. (2019). Hypertension and obesity moderate the relationship between β-amyloid and cognitive decline in midlife. *Alzheimer's & Dementia*, *15*, 418–428.

Craft, S. (2009). The role of metabolic disorders in Alzheimer disease and vascular dementia: Two roads converged. *Archives of Neurology*, *66*(3), 300–305.

Cronbach, L. J., & Meehl, P. E. (1955). Construct validity in psychological tests. *Psychological Bulletin*, *52*, 281–302.

da Silva, M. N., Millington, R. S., Bridge, H., James-Galton, M., & Plant. G. T. (2017). Visual dysfunction in posterior cortical atrophy. *Frontiers in Neurology*, *8*, 389. doi:10.3389/fneur.2017.00389S

DeFina, L. F., Willis, B. L., Radford, N. B., Gao, A., Leonard, D., Haskell, W. L., . . . Berry, J. D. (2013). The association between midlife cardiorespiratory fitness levels and later-life dementia: A cohort study. *Annals of Internal Medicine*, *158*(3), 162–168.

De Leeuw, F. E., De Groot, J. C., Achten, E., Oudkerk, M., Ramos, L. M. P., Heijboer, R., . . . Breteler, M. M. B. (2001). Prevalence of cerebral white matter lesions in elderly people: a population based magnetic resonance imaging study: The Rotterdam Scan study. *Journal of Neurology, Neurosurgery & Psychiatry*, *70*(1), 9–14.

Delis, D. C. Kramer, J. H., Kaplan, E., & Ober, B. A. (1987). *The California Verbal Learning Test*. New York, NY: Psychology Corporation.

Desgranges, B., Baron, J. C., Giffard, B., Chételat, G., Lalevée, C., Viader, F., . . . Eustache F. (2002). The neural basis of intrusions in free recall and cued recall: A PET study in Alzheimer's disease. *Neuroimage*, *17*, 1658–1664.

Donahue, J. E., & Johanson, C. E. (2008). Apolipoprotein E, amyloid-β, and blood–brain barrier permeability in Alzheimer disease. *Journal of Neuropathology & Experimental Neurology*, *67*(4), 261–270.

Drachman, D. A. (2014). The amyloid hypothesis, time to move on: Amyloid is the downstream result, not cause, of Alzheimer's disease. *Alzheimer's and Dementia*, *10*, 372–380.

Edmonds, E. C., Ard, M. C., Edland, S. D., Galasko, D. R., Salmon, D. P., & Bondi, M. W. (2018). Unmasking the benefits of donepezil via psychometrically precise identification of mild cognitive impairment: A secondary analysis of the ADCS vitamin E and donepezil in MCI study. *Alzheimer's & Dementia*, *4*, 11–18.

Edmonds, E. C., Delano-Wood, L., Galasko, D. R., Salmon, D. P., & Bondi, M. W.; Alzheimer's Disease Neuroimaging Initiative. (2015). Subtle cognitive decline and biomarker staging in preclinical Alzheimer's Disease. *Journal of Alzheimer's Disease*, *47*, 231–242.

Edmonds, E. C., McDonald, C. R., Marshall, A., Thomas, K. R., Eppig, J., Weigand, W. J., . . . Bondi, M. W.; Alzheimer's Disease Neuroimaging Initiative. (2019). Early versus late MCI: Improved MCI staging using a neuropsychological approach. *Alzheimer's and Dementia, 15*(5), 699–708. doi:10.1016/j.jalz.2018.12.009

Eppig, J., Wambach, D., Nieves, C., Price, C. C., Lamar, M., Delano-Wood, L., . . . Lippa, C. (2012). Dysexecutive functioning in mild cognitive impairment: Derailment in temporal gradients. *Journal of the International Neuropsychological Society, 18*(1), 20–28.

Esiri, M. M., Nagy, Z., Smith, M. Z., Barnetson, L., & Smith, A. D. (1999). Cerebrovascular disease and threshold for dementia in the early stages of Alzheimer's disease. *Lancet, 354*, 919–920.

Farmer, M. E., Kittner, S. J., Abbott, R. D., Wolz, M. M., Wolfs, P. A., & White, L. R. (1990). Longitudinally measured blood pressure, antihypertensive medication use, and cognitive performance: The Framingham Study. *Journal of Clinical Epidemiology, 43*(5), 475–480.

Fuster, J. M. (2008). *The prefrontal cortex: Anatomy, physiology, and neuropsychology of the executive lobe* (3nd ed.). New York, NY: Lippincott-Raven Press.

Giovannetti, T., Lamar, M., Cloud, B.S ., Swenson, R., Fein, D., Kaplan, E., & Libon, D. J. (2001). Different underlying mechanisms for deficits in concept formation in dementia. *Archives of Clinical Neuropsychology, 16*, 547–560.

Hardy, J., Bogdanovic, N., Winblad, B., Portelius, E., Andreasen, N., Cedazo-Minguez, A., & Zetterberg, H. (2014). Pathways to Alzheimer's disease. *Journal of Internal Medicine, 275*(3), 296–303.

Hardy, J. A., & Higgins, G. A. (1992). Alzheimer's disease: the amyloid cascade hypothesis. *Science*, 256(5054), 184–185.

Hardy, J., & Selkoe, D. J. (2002). The amyloid hypothesis of Alzheimer's disease: progress and problems on the road to therapeutics. *Science*, 297, 353–356.

Herrup, K. (2015). The case for rejecting the amyloid cascade hypothesis. *Nature Neuroscience, 18*(6), 794–799.

Holmes, C., Boche, D., Wilkinson, D., Yadegarfar, G., Hopkins, V., Bayer, A., . . . Nicoll, J. A. R. (2008). Long-term effects of Abeta42 immunisation in Alzheimer's disease: follow-up of a randomised, placebo-controlled phase I trial. *Lancet (London, England), 372*(9634), 216–223. http://doi.org/10.1016/S0140-6736(08)61075-2

Huang, Y., & Mahley, R. W. (2014). Apolipoprotein E: structure and function in lipid metabolism, neurobiology, and Alzheimer's diseases. *Neurobiology of Disease, 72*, 3–12.

Hughes, T. M., & Craft, S. (2016). The role of insulin in the vascular contributions to age-related dementia. *Biochimica et Biophysica Acta (BBA)–Molecular Basis of Disease, 1862*(5), 983–991.

Iadecola, C. (2010). The overlap between neurodegenerative and vascular factors in the pathogenesis of dementia. *Acta Neuropathologica, 120*(3), 287–296.

Iturria-Medina, Y., Sotero, R. C., Toussaint, P. J., Mateos-Pérez, J. M., Evans, A. C., Weiner, M. W., . . . Trojanowki, J. Q. (2016). Early role of vascular dysregulation on late-onset Alzheimer's disease based on multifactorial data-driven analysis. *Nature Communications, 7*, 11934.

Jack, C. R., Jr, Bennett, D. A., Blennow, K., Carrillo, M. C., Dunn, B., Haeberlein, S. B., . . . Contributors (2018). NIA-AA Research Framework: Toward a biological definition of Alzheimer's disease. *Alzheimer's & Dementia: The Journal of the Alzheimer's Association, 14*(4), 535–562. doi:10.1016/j.jalz.2018.02.018

James, B. D., Bennett, D. A., Boyle, P. A., Leurgans, S., & Schneider, J. A. (2012). Dementia from Alzheimer disease and mixed pathologies in the oldest old. *JAMA, 307*(17), 1798–1800.

Jayaraman, A., & Pike, C. J. (2014). Alzheimer's disease and type 2 diabetes: multiple mechanisms contribute to interactions. *Current Diabetes Reports*, *14*(4), 476.

Jefferson, A. L., Cambronero, F. E., Liu, D., Moore, E. E., Neal, J. E., Terry, J. G., Nair, S., . . . Carr, J. J. (2018). Higher aortic stiffness is related to lower cerebral blood flow and preserved cerebrovascular reactivity in older adults. *Circulation*, 138, 1951–1962.

Junque, C., J. Pujol, Vendrell, P., Bruna, O., Jódar, M., Ribas, J. C., . . . Marti-Vilalta, J. L. (1990). Leuko-araiosis on magnetic resonance imaging and speed of mental processing. *Archives of Neurology*, *47*, 151–156.

Kalaria, R. (2002). Similarities between Alzheimer's disease and vascular dementia. *Journal of the Neurological Sciences*, *203*, 29–34.

Kalaria, R. N. (2010). Vascular basis for brain degeneration: Faltering controls and risk factors for dementia. *Nutrition Reviews*, *68*(Suppl_2), S74–S87.

Kalaria, R.N., Akinyemi, R., & Ihara, M. (2012). Does vascular pathology contribute to Alzheimer changes? *Journal of the Neurological. Sciences*, *322*, 141–147.

Kalaria, R. N., Cohen, D. L., Premkumar, D. R. D., Nag, S., LaManna, J. C., & Lust, W. D. (1998). Vascular endothelial growth factor in Alzheimer's disease and experimental cerebral is chemia. *Molecular Brain Research*, *62*(1), 101–105.

Kim, G. H., Seo, S. W., Jung, K., Kwon, O. H., Kwon, H., Kim, J. H., . . . Na, D. L. (2016). The neural correlates of motor intentional disorders in patients with subcortical vascular cognitive impairment. *Journal of Neurology, 263*, 89–99. doi:10.1007/s00415-015-7946-6

Kivipelto, M., Ngandu, T., Fratiglioni, L., Viitanen, M., Kåreholt, I., Winblad, B., . . . Nissinen, A. (2005). Obesity and vascular risk factors at midlife and the risk of dementia and Alzheimer disease. *Archives of Neurology*, *62*(10), 1556–1560.

Lamar, M., Catani, M., Price, C. C., Heilman, K. M., & Libon, D. J. (2008).The impact of region specific leukoaraiosis on working memory deficits in dementia. *Neuropsychologia*, *46*, 2597–2601.

Lamar, M., & Libon, D. J. (2010). Perseveration. In J. Kreutzer, J. DeLuca, & B. Caplan (Eds.), *The encyclopedia of clinical neuropsychology* (pp. 78–83). New York, NY: Springer.

Lamar, M., K. Podell, Carew, T. G., Cloud, B. S., Resh, R., Kennedy, C., . . . Libon, D. J. (1997). Perseverative behavior in Alzheimer's disease and subcortical ischemic vascular dementia. *Neuropsychology*, *11*, 523–534.

Lamar, M., Price, C. C., Davis, K. L., Kaplan, E., & Libon, D. J. (2002). Capacity to maintain mental set in dementia. *Neuropsychologia*, *40*, 435–445.

Lamar, M., Price, C. C., Giovannetti, T., Swenson, R., & Libon, D. J. (2010). The dysexecutive syndrome associated with ischaemic vascular disease and related subcortical neuropathology: a Boston process approach. *Behavioural Neurology*, *22*(1–2), 53–62.

Lekeu, F., Van der Linden, M., Chicherio, C., Collette, F., Degueldre, C., & Fanck, G. (2003). Brain correlates of performance in a free/cued recall task with semantic encoding in Alzheimer disease. *Alzheimer Disease and Associated Disorders*, *17*, 35–45.

Li, Z. G., Zhang, W., & Sima, A. A. (2007). Alzheimer-like changes in rat models of spontaneous diabetes. *Diabetes*, *56*(7), 1817–1824.

Libon, D. J., Bondi, M. W., Price, C. C., Lamar. M., Eppig, J., Wambach, D. M., . . . Penney, D.L. (2011). Verbal serial list learning in mild cognitive impairment: A profile analysis of interference, forgetting, and errors. *Journal of the International Neuropsychological Society*, *17*, 905–914.

Libon, D. J., Drabick, D. A. G., Giovannetti, T., Price, C. C., Bondi, M. W., Eppig, J., Nieves, C., . . . Swenson, R. (2014). Neuropsychological syndromes associated with Alzheimer's/vascular spectrum dementia: A latent class analysis. *Journal of Alzheimer's Disease, 42*, 999–1014.

Libon, D. J., Price, C .C., Garrett, K. D, & Giovannetti, T. (2004). From Binswanger's disease to Leukoaraiosis: What we have learned about subcortical vascular dementia. *Clinical Neuropsychologist, 18*, 83–100.

Libon, D. J., Price, C. C., Giovannetti, T., Swenson, R., Bettcher, B. M., Heilman, K. M., & Pennisi, A. (2008). Linking MRI hyperintensities with patterns of neuropsychological impairment: evidence for a threshold effect. *Stroke, 39*(3), 806–813.

Luria, A. R. (1980). *Higher cortical functions*. New York, NY: Basic Books.

Mahley, R. W. (2016). Apolipoprotein E: From cardiovascular disease to neurodegenerative disorders. *Journal of Molecular Medicine, 94*(7), 739–746.

Nelson, A. R., Sweeney, M. D., Sagare, A. P., & Zlokovic, B. V. (2016). Neurovascular dysfunction and neurodegeneration in dementia and Alzheimer's disease. *Biochimica et Biophysica Acta (BBA)–Molecular Basis of Disease, 1862*(5), 887–900.

Ott, A., Breteler, M. M., Harskamp, F. V., Stijnen, T., & Hofman, A. (1998). Incidence and risk of dementia: The Rotterdam Study. *American Journal of Epidemiology, 147*(6), 574–580.

Ott, A., Stolk, R. P., Van Harskamp, F., Pols, H. A. P., Hofman, A., & Breteler, M. M. B. (1999). Diabetes mellitus and the risk of dementia: The Rotterdam Study. *Neurology, 53*(9), 1937–1942.

Petersen, R. C. (2004). Mild cognitive impairment as a diagnostic entity. *Journal of Internal Medicine, 256*(3), 183–194.

Petersen, R. C., & Morris, J. C. (2005). Mild cognitive impairment as a clinical entity and treatment target. *Archives of Neurology*, 62, 1160–1163.

Petersen, R. C., Thomas, R. G., Grundman, M., Bennett, D., Doody, R., Ferris, S., . . . Pfeiffer, E. (2005). Vitamin E and donepezil for the treatment of mild cognitive impairment. *New England Journal of Medicine, 352*(23), 2379–2388.

Price, C. C., Garrett, K. D., Jefferson, A. L., Cosentino, S., Tanner, J., Penney, D. L., . . . Libon, D.J. (2009).The role of leukoaraiosis severity on learning and memory in dementia: Performance differences on a 9-word list learning test. *Clinical Neuropsychologist, 23*, 1–18.

Price, C. Jefferson, A. L., Merino, J., Heilman, K., & Libon, D. J. (2005). Towards an operational definition of the Research Criteria for Subcortical Vascular Dementia: Integrating neuroradiological and neuropsychological data. *Neurology*, 65, 376–382.

Price, C. C., Tanner, J. T., Schmalfuss, I., Heilman, K. M., & Libon, D. J. (2015). Dissociating statistically determined Alzheimer/vascular dementia neuropsychological syndromes using white and gray neuroradiological parameters. *Journal of Alzheimer's Disease, 48*(3), 833–847

Reitz, C., Tang, M. X., Manly, J., Mayeux, R., & Luchsinger, J. A. (2007). Hypertension and the risk of mild cognitive impairment. *Archives of Neurology, 64*(12), 1734–1740.

Sachdev, P., Kalaria, R., O'Brien, J., Skoog, I., Alladi, S., & Black, S.E. (2014). Diagnostic criteria for vascular cognitive disorders: A VASCOG statement. *Alzheimer Disease and Associated Disorders, 28*, 206–218.

Sadowski, M., Pankiewicz, J., Scholtzova, H., Li, Y. S., Quartermain, D., Duff, K., & Wisniewski, T. (2004). Links between the pathology of Alzheimer's disease and vascular dementia. *Neurochemical Research, 29*(6), 1257–1266.

Schneider, J. A., Arvanitakis, Z., Bang, W., & Bennett, D. A. (2007). Mixed brain pathologies account for most dementia cases in community-dwelling older persons. *Neurology, 69*, 2197–2204.

Schneider, J. A., Arvanitakis, Z., Leurgans, S. E., & Bennett, D. A. (2009). The neuropathology of probable Alzheimer disease and mild cognitive impairment. *Annals of Neurology, 66*, 200–208.

Selkoe, D. J. (2000). Toward a comprehensive theory for Alzheimer's disease. Hypothesis: Alzheimer's disease is caused by the cerebral accumulation and cytotoxicity of amyloid beta-protein. *Annual of the New York Academy of Science, 924*, 17–25.

Serrano-Pozo, A., & Growdon, J. H. (2019). Is Alzheimer's disease risk modifiable? *Journal of Alzheimer's Disease, 67*, 795–819.

Suárez-González, A., Henley, S.M., Walton, J., & Crutch, S. (2015). Posterior cortical atrophy: an atypical variant of Alzheimer disease. *Psychiatric Clinics in North America, 38*, 211–220.

Sweeney, M. D., Montagne, A., Sagare, A. P., Nation, D. A., Schneider, L. S., Chui, H. C., . . . Jacobs, R. E. (2019). Vascular dysfunction: The disregarded partner of Alzheimer's disease. *Alzheimer's & Dementia, 15*(1), 158–167.

Sweeney, M. D., Sagare, A. P., & Zlokovic, B. V. (2015). Cerebrospinal fluid biomarkers of neurovascular dysfunction in mild dementia and Alzheimer's disease. *Journal of Cerebral Blood Flow & Metabolism, 35*(7), 1055–1068.

Sweeney, M. D., Sagare, A. P., & Zlokovic, B. V. (2018). Blood–brain barrier breakdown in Alzheimer disease and other neurodegenerative disorders. *Nature Reviews Neurology, 14*(3), 133–150.

Talbot, K., Wang, H. Y., Kazi, H., Han, L. Y., Bakshi, K. P., Stucky, A., . . . Arvanitakis, Z. (2012). Demonstrated brain insulin resistance in Alzheimer's disease patients is associated with IGF-1 resistance, IRS-1 dysregulation, and cognitive decline. *Journal of Clinical Investigation, 122*, 1316–1338.

Tröster, A. (2011). A précis of recent advances in the neuropsychology of mild cognitive impairment(s) in Parkinson's disease and a proposal of preliminary research criteria. *Journal of the International Neuropsychological Society*, 17, 393–406.

Wang, B. W., Lu, E., Mackenzie, I. R. A., Assaly, M., Jacova, C., Lee, P. E., . . . Hsiung, G. Y. R. (2012). Multiple pathologies are common in Alzheimer patients in clinical trials. *Canadian Journal of Neuroscience, 39*, 592–599.

White, L., Petrovitch, H., Hardman, J., Nelson, J., Davis, D. G., & Ross, G. W. (2002). Cerebrovascular pathology and dementia in autopsied Honolulu-Asia Aging Study participants. *Annual of the New York Academy of Science, 977*, 9–23.

Wharton, S. B., Brayne, C., Savva, G. M., Matthews, F. E., Forster, G., Simpson, J., . . . Ince, P. G, for the Medical Research Council Cognitive Function and Aging Study. (2011). Epidemiological neuropathology: The MRC Cognitive Function and Aging study experience. *Journal of Alzheimer's Disease, 25*, 359–372.

Wong, C. G., Thomas, K. R., Edmonds, E. C., Weigand, A. J., Bangen, K. J., Eppig, J. S., . . . Bondi, M. B. (2018). Neuropsychological criteria for mild cognitive impairment in the Framingham Heart Study's oldest-old. *Dementia and Geriatric Cognitive Disorder, 46*, 253–265.

Yip, A. G., McKee, A. C., Green, R. C., Wells, J., Young, H., Cupples, L. A., & Farrer, L. A. (2005). APOE, vascular pathology, and the AD brain. *Neurology, 65*(2), 259–265.

Zlokovic, B. V. (2011). Neurovascular pathways to neurodegeneration in Alzheimer's disease and other disorders. *Nature Reviews Neuroscience, 12*, 723–738.

3

Neuropsychological Contributions to the Diagnosis of Mild Cognitive Impairment Associated With Alzheimer's Disease

Joel Eppig, Madeleine Werhane, Emily C. Edmonds, Lisa-Delano Wood, Katherine J. Bangen, Amy Jak, Kelsey R. Thomas, Christina Wong, Alexandra Weigand, and Mark W. Bondi

1. Introduction

Mild cognitive impairment (MCI) is an intermediate stage between normal aging and, with many patients, the development of dementia such as Alzheimer's disease (AD). Patients with MCI demonstrate cognitive impairment in the presence of generally intact functional abilities (Albert et al., 2011). Over the last several decades, there has been a rapid growth in research to better understand and characterize MCI. This growth has been driven in part by the need to accurately identify individuals with an increased risk of AD, prior to the onset of frank dementia. Currently, 5.3 million older adults are estimated to have AD dementia in the United States; by 2050, that number is projected to increase to 13.8 million (Alzheimer's Association, 2017). AD has a devastating personal impact on patients and loved ones, as well as tremendous societal burden in the form of high healthcare costs and caregiving requirements. Unfortunately, the pharmaceutical trials for AD have generally failed to produce any meaningful disease modifying effects (Cummings, Morstorf, & Zhong, 2014).

In light of this history, researchers and healthcare professionals increasingly acknowledge that the best chance to avoid an impending public health crisis involving AD is to target putative neurodegenerative illness well before the development of dementia and irreversible neuronal loss (Sperling et al., 2014). Past research has demonstrated that individuals diagnosed with MCI are at a greater risk of progression to AD dementia, although specific conversion and reversion rates vary based on the sample (i.e., community versus clinic-based) and definition of MCI (Aerts et al., 2017; Canevelli et al., 2016; Marcos et al., 2016; Mitchell & Shiri-Feshki, 2009; Petersen et al., 2001; Ward, Tardiff, Dye & Arrighi, 2013). Thus, both *accurate and consistent* diagnosis of MCI is critical for improving

Joel Eppig, Madeleine Werhane, Emily C. Edmonds, Lisa-Delano Wood, Katherine J. Bangen, Amy Jak, Kelsey R. Thomas, Christina Wong, Alexandra Weigand, and Mark W. Bondi, *Neuropsychological Contributions to the Diagnosis of Mild Cognitive Impairment Associated With Alzheimer's Disease* In: *Vascular Disease, Alzheimer's Disease, and Mild Cognitive Impairment.* Edited by: David J. Libon, Melissa Lamar, Rodney A. Swenson, Kenneth M. Heilman, Oxford University Press (2020).
DOI: 10.1093/oso/9780190634230.003.0004

identification of individuals at risk for AD, treatment outcome, and clinical practice. This chapter will review the evolution of the concept of MCI as well as recent contributions from the field of neuropsychology by discussing: (a) the origins of MCI and conventional diagnostic criteria; (b) current diagnostic criteria for MCI; (c) neuropsychological heterogeneity in empirically derived MCI; (d) actuarial neuropsychological criteria in the diagnosis and subtyping of MCI; and (e) the relationship between biological and neuroimaging markers and MCI subtypes.

2. The Origins of Mild Cognitive Impairment and Conventional Diagnostic Criteria

2.1. Identifying Prodromal Dementia

The concept of MCI was introduced in the early 1980s (Reisberg et al., 2008). Two staging systems were proposed—the Clinical Dementia Rating (CDR) and the Global Deterioration Scale (GDS)—each independently developed to help clinicians evaluate cognitive and functional abilities in people who are aging and have dementia (Hughes et al., 1982; Reisberg et al., 1982). Despite differences in these scales and operationalization of stages, both systems provided a means to characterize an individual on a spectrum ranging from normal (i.e., no cognitive and functional complaints or deficits), a stage denoted prodromal dementia, to severe dementia (i.e., significant cognitive and functional impairments). On the CDR, a rating of 0.5 represents "questionable dementia" (Hughes et al., 1982). A GDS of 3—coined as "mild cognitive decline"—suggests the presence of mild but clear-cut clinical and functional deficits.

2.2. Conventional Diagnostic Criteria for Mild Cognitive Impairment

At the turn of the 21st century, Petersen et al. (2001) proposed criteria that would form the foundation for the *conventional* diagnosis of MCI. However, from a neuropsychological perspective, this early definition was focused solely on the presence of memory deficits in addition to complaints involving instrumental activities of daily living (IADLs). Nonetheless, Petersen's initial criteria for MCI overlapped with a CDR of 0.5 and GDS of 3 such that MCI was proposed to encompass (a) a memory complaint, preferably corroborated by an informant; (b) impaired memory function for age and education; (c) preserved general cognitive function; (d) intact activity of daily living; and (e) not demented (Petersen et al., 2001). The generally exclusive focus on "memory" as the predominant neuropsychological impairment in MCI was (and remains) consistent with research demonstrating that patients with MCI often perform worse on memory measures than healthy older adults, while retaining intact performance in other cognitive domains (Petersen et al., 1999).

Although Petersen et al.'s (2001) model of MCI built upon the CDR and GDS framework, critiques pointed to the overly narrow definition of impairment. Thus, Petersen (2004) and an International Working Group on Mild Cognitive Impairment (Winblad et al., 2004) recommended MCI criteria include (1) not normal, but not demented (i.e., does not meet criteria via *Diagnostic and Statistical Manual of Mental Disorders* (DSM; fourth edition) or the *International Classification of Diseases* (10th edition) for a dementia syndrome); (2a) cognitive decline by self- and/or informant-report and impairment on objective cognitive tasks; *and/or* (2b) evidence of decline over time on objective cognitive tasks; and (3) preserved basic activities of daily living/ minimal impairment in complex instrumental functions. Importantly, the authors expanded the definition of cognitive impairment to include both memory and nonmemory domains. These criteria form the basis of the four commonly used *conventional* MCI subtypes: (a) single-domain amnestic MCI, (b) single-domain nonamnestic MCI, (c) multidomain amnestic MCI, and (d) multidomain nonamnestic MCI.

Despite these improvements, the Petersen (2004) and Winblad et al. (2004) criteria for MCI tended to predominantly revolve around the presence or absence of memory impairment by anchoring MCI subtypes to "amnestic" or "nonamnestic" deficits. Thus, a limitation of these classification systems involves the grouping of potentially unique cognitive profiles together into a general "nonamnestic" label, with little empirical evidence to support this arbitrary combination. Another difficulty involved the cut-score(s) to determine the presence of cognitive impairment; Petersen (1999) initially defined an abnormal score as falling 1.5 standard deviations (SDs) below age and education matched control subjects for amnestic MCI. Subsequently, Petersen (2004) suggested that this criterion may need to be adjusted for certain factors such as low educational attainment. Finally, questions remain regarding the paradigm and specific tests used to assess for amnestic impairment (i.e., paragraph recall, serial list learning). For example, in many settings delayed recognition testing is omitted despite substantial empirical research suggesting that clinical amnesia is best diagnosed using both delayed free recall and recognition test performance (Price et al., 2009). Despite these methodological issues, *conventional diagnostic criteria* (Petersen & Morris, 2005) continues to be the method of choice in research including clinical trials targeting MCI and other large-scale studies such as the Alzheimer's Disease Neuroimaging Initiative ([ADNI]; Weiner et al., 2013).

3. Current Diagnostic Criteria for Mild Cognitive Impairment

Most recently, the National Institute on Aging-Alzheimer's Association (NIA-AA) revisited the criteria for MCI in 2011 (Albert et al., 2011). Although the framework established by Petersen (2004) and Winblad et al. (2004) is largely retained, Albert et al. (2011) proposed key distinctions between clinical and research criteria, with the latter using a staging scheme to reflect the likelihood of AD etiology based upon biomarker and neuroimaging profiles.

3.1. Core Clinical Criteria

Currently, the core clinical criteria for MCI *due to AD* include (a) concern regarding cognitive decline; (b) impairment in one or more cognitive domains; (c) preservation of independence in functional abilities (i.e., only mild problems with complex functional tasks, often with reduced efficiency); and (d) not demented (Albert et al., 2011). The authors provide clinicians a significant degree of latitude in the application of each criterion and acknowledge the inherent difficulty obtaining the information necessary to make appropriate judgments along with the adjustment of expectations based on specific individual factors (e.g., educational level). Importantly, Albert et al. (2011) recognize that while episodic memory is the most common cognitive deficit in individuals with MCI who progress to AD dementia, initial impairment can also occur in other domains such as attention, language, visuospatial skills, and executive functioning. Consistent with Petersen (2001), these authors also suggest that cognitive scores in individuals with MCI may be 1.0 to 1.5 SDs below age- and education-adjusted norms on culturally appropriate neuropsychological tests and also suggest that this range should be view as a guideline rather than a specific cut-point.

3.2. AD Staging Criteria

In addition to the core clinical MCI criteria, Albert et al. (2011) emphasize the inclusion of biomarker and neuroimaging data to stage the likelihood of AD etiology in MCI research, including (a) biomarkers of beta amyloid (Aβ); (b) biomarkers of neuronal injury (i.e., tau, hippocampal volume loss, reduced glucose metabolism or perfusion of the temporoparietal cortex); and (c) markers associated with biochemical change (i.e., inflammation, oxidative stress). Aβ and neuronal injury biomarkers with "AD-positive" or "abnormal" signatures are incorporated into the research criteria for MCI due to AD. Albert et al. goes on to propose a scheme with three levels of likelihood—high, intermediate, and unlikely, reflecting a combination of positivity on Aβ and/or neuronal injury biomarkers in addition to core clinical MCI criteria. Additionally, if Aβ and/ or neuronal injury biomarkers are untested or indeterminate, an individual otherwise meeting the core clinical MCI criteria would be deemed "uninformative." Markers associated with biochemical change—although a promising area of study—are not included in this stating scheme until further research determines their appropriate utility. Albert et al. also recognize that new biomarkers associated with AD will likely be identified in the future and will need to be integrated after their validity have been properly established. This situation is currently unfolding with the advent of positron emission tomography tau imaging (tau positron emission tomography [PET]), which was not available in 2011. As tau PET is established as a key neuroimaging marker of AD pathology (Gordon et al., 2016), MCI staging criteria will need to be revisited to incorporate this biomarker.

4. Neuropsychological Heterogeneity in Empirically Derived Mild Cognitive Impairment

Recently, increased attention has been given to the heterogeneity of MCI diagnostic subtypes, both with respect to neuropsychological performance as well as the neurobiological underpinnings of the syndrome. While the evolution of conventional MCI diagnostic criteria acknowledges the existence of MCI subtypes their characterization is largely based on clinical and/or professional opinion rather than concrete operational definitions that could be subjected to empirical examination. Given that the accurate identification of meaningful dementia prodromes depends on the use of valid diagnostic criteria, a body of neuropsychological research has emerged over the past decade that has employed sophisticated statistical methods to empirically characterize MCI subtypes (Bondi et al., 2014; Clark et al., 2013; Delano-Wood et al., 2009; Edmonds et al., 2015, 2016, 2018; Eppig et al., 2012; 2017; Hanfelt et al., 2011; Libon et al., 2010, 2011; McGuiness et al., 2015). These studies differ regarding test selection, neuropsychological domains assessed, and cut-scores used to define impairment. Nonetheless, results have robustly produced three to four unique MCI subgroups involving amnestic, dysexecutive, and language impairment. The following section provides a review of how person-centered statistical techniques, such as cluster analysis and mixture models, have been used to identify unique MCI subtypes.

4.1. Cluster Analytic Models of MCI

One of the first studies to employ statistical methods to define MCI subtypes was conducted by Delano-Wood et al. (2009). In this research, a protocol of neuropsychological tests was subjected to cluster analysis using a sample of 70 older adults diagnosed with MCI using Petersen and Morris's (2005) conventional criteria (i.e., subjective memory complaints; normal activities of daily living (ADL); absence of dementia; Mini-Mental State Examination [MMSE] ≥24; and mild quantifiable cognitive impairment). In an attempt to balance the increased sensitivity of a more liberal cutoff (i.e., 1 SD below the mean) with Petersen et al.'s (1999) criteria, the authors chose a cut-score of 1.2 SDs below the mean to signify cognitive impairment. All participants were administered a neuropsychological protocol measuring constructional praxis, learning and memory, verbal fluency, naming, executive functions, and processing speed. Using Ward's minimum variance cluster analysis, Delano-Wood et al. found three distinct neuropsychological MCI subtypes: (a) a group with impairment in memory and language (memory/language MCI: 25.7%); (b) a group with impairment in executive functions and processing speed (executive/processing speed MCI: 25.7%); and (c) a group with mild impairment only in memory (amnestic MCI: 48.6%). Furthermore, Delano-Wood et al. observed that these MCI subtypes presented with different patterns of periventricular and subcortical white matter pathology. The amnestic MCI group was also younger and had more years of education than the memory/language MCI group.

In a separate study, Libon et al. (2010) also provided evidence for three MCI subtypes using cluster analysis on a sample of memory clinic patients (*n* = 77). Participants were diagnosed with MCI using conventional Petersen criteria as previously described. A group of community dwelling, healthy normal control participants (*n* = 55) were recruited to calculate normative z-scores. Libon et al. (2010) employed a K-means cluster analysis on the neuropsychological scores, specifying a priori three clusters. Three unique neuropsychological MCI subtypes emerged: (a) a group with impairment in executive and language abilities (executive/language MCI: 27.3%); (b) a group with mixed impairment characterized by low scores on memory and verbal fluency (both animals and letter fluency; mixed MCI: 25.7%); and (c) a group with substantial impairment only in memory (amnestic MCI: 48.6%). The three MCI subtypes were not found to differ in age or years of education.

Clark et al. (2013) also performed a cluster analysis on a sample of participants (*n* = 134) diagnosed using conventional MCI diagnostic criteria. Participants with MCI received a comprehensive neuropsychological protocol comprised of 13 tests assessing five cognitive domains, with at least two measures in each domain (i.e., language, episodic memory, processing speed, attention/ executive control, visuospatial operations). Cognitively normal participants (n = 57) were used to calculate normative z-scores on these tests. Using Ward's minimum variance cluster analysis, Clark et al. (2013) also found evidence for three distinct neuropsychological phenotypes (a) mild memory and language impairment (amnestic/language MCI: 29.1%); (b) mixed impairment across all domains except attention (mixed MCI: 23.1%); and, most interestingly, (c) a large group of individuals with intact performance on all cognitive measures (i.e., cluster-derived normal: 47.8%). Demographically, the mixed MCI group was significantly older than cluster-derived normal participants and had fewer years of education than both other groups. The cluster-derived normal group was also comprised of more women than the other groups. Most important, the cluster-derived normal group was not significantly different than the normal controls (used in z-score generation) on all 13 neuropsychological measures, suggesting that conventional Petersen criteria erroneously identified these individuals with MCI (i.e., false-positives).

The finding reported by Clark et al. (2013) were followed by Edmonds et al. (2015) who examined a large group of patients from the ADNI (n = 825) where MCI was diagnosed using conventional criteria where the key memory measure of limited to delay free recall obtained from the Wechsler Memory Scale–Revised (WMS-R), Logical Memory II, Story A delayed recall. A significant strength of Edmonds et al. involved the use of a robust normal control sample (n = 284) to standardize performance. These individuals continued to be identified by ADNI as normal on longitudinal follow-up (range from 1–7 years) removing the likelihood of including individuals with incipient MCI or dementia. Edmonds et al. analyzed six age- and education-adjusted neuropsychological z-scores that were independent of diagnosis and equally distributed across the domains of attention/executive functions, language, and episodic memory. Ward's minimum variance cluster analysis produced four unique cognitive phenotypes including (a) an amnestic MCI group (amnestic, 34.9%); (b) a predominant naming/language deficit and mild memory impairment MCI group (dysnomic MCI, 18.5%); and (c) a MCI group with impairment across all three domains, although differentially in attention/executive functions (dysexecutive/mixed MCI: 12.4%).

However, consistent with Clark et al. (2013), a large fourth cluster of cluster-derived normal participants (34.2%) was found. This group performed within normal limits on all six neuropsychological measures (mean z-scores ranged from −0.26 to 0.87), despite their scores on the WMS-R Logical Memory-II Story A, MMSE, and CDR that led to an ADNI MCI diagnosis. Compared to the robust normal controls, cluster-derived normal participants performed statistically worse only on a verbal memory measure of delay free recall. However, further examination indicated that there was less than a one-word raw score difference

(7.1 vs. 7.9 words) and average performance remained within-normal limits ($z = -0.26$). The cluster-derived normal group also performed significantly better than amnestic MCI on memory measures, dysexecutive/mixed MCI on attention/ executive function measures, and dysnomic MCI on language measures (Edmonds et al., 2015).

The existence of this cluster-derived normal group—approximately one third of individuals ADNI diagnosed as MCI—provided additional evidence that conventional Petersen diagnostic criteria for MCI is susceptible to false-positive errors. The notion that individuals in this group were incorrectly assigned a diagnosis of MCI was further supported by cerebrospinal fluid (CSF) AD biomarker profiles that did not significantly differ from robust normal controls. Edmonds et al. (2015) also analyzed longitudinal data over an average of 23 months and found that the cluster-derived normal group had lower rates of progression to AD and higher rates of reversion to "cognitively normal" (both diagnoses were made using ADNI criteria) than those participants in the other three MCI groups.

4.2. Latent Mixture Models of MCI

In addition to cluster analytic techniques, researchers have also utilized latent mixture models, such as latent profile analysis (LPA) and latent class analysis (LCA), to classify cognitive subtypes in MCI (Eppig et al., 2017; Hanfelt et al., 2011; McGuinness et al., 2015). Latent mixture models offer several statistical advantages over cluster analysis including a model-driven approach (see Chapter 6 of this volume for details). Studies have used LPA or LCA to identify three to seven neuropsychological classes (Eppig et al., 2017; Hanfelt et al., 2011; McGuinness et al., 2015), with varying results based on the sample characteristics (e.g., community vs. clinic-based), and tests chosen as indicators (e.g., inclusion of cognitive and noncognitive measures).

Hanfelt et al. (2011) initially employed LCA on MCI participants ($n = 1{,}655$) from the Uniform Data Set (UDS) of 29 NIH Alzheimer's Disease Centers (ADC). Participants were recruited from both the community and clinic samples. Inclusion criteria were (a) consensus diagnosis of MCI from the clinicians at each ADC; (b) available information on age, years of education, and race; and (c) MMSE $\geq$22. Neuropsychological measures of global cognition, executive functions, language, visuomotor processing speed, and learning and memory were selected from the core cognitive UDS protocol. Standardized regression based formulas, adjusting for age, education, race, and the education*race interaction were derived from cognitively normal individuals in the UDS and subsequently applied to the MCI participants to calculate z-scores for each cognitive measure. In addition to neuropsychological assessment, the authors measured activities of daily living, psychiatric and behavioral problems, and depression via informant and self-reported inventories. Hanfelt et al. (2011) found a complex LCA solution of 7 subgroups, including (a) *minimally impaired* (12%), which were indistinguishable from the cognitively normal group on UDS variables; (b) *pure amnestic* (16%), characterized by a subtle impairment in delayed memory; (c) *amnestic with functional impairments and neuropsychiatric features* (16%), characterized by impairments in both immediate and delayed memory, difficulties performing ADLs, and neuropsychiatric disturbances; (d) *mixed multidomain* (12%), characterized by impairments across cognitive domains including episodic and semantic memory, language, and executive function; (e) *mixed multidomain with functional impairments and neuropsychiatric features* (12%), characterized by difficulties performing ADLs, the presence of neuropsychiatric disturbances, and impairments across a broader spectrum of cognitive domains including attention and visuomotor skills; (f) *functional impairments and neuropsychiatric features* (15%), a subgroup experiencing functional and behavioral impairments but with no neuropsychological impairment; and finally, (g) *executive function and language impairments* (18%), a subgroup distinguished by neuropsychological impairment in non-memory domains. Interestingly, these subgroups differed with respect to cerebrovascular disease (CVD) as measured by the Rosen Modification of the Hachinski Ischemic Score (RMHIS) such that the *amnestic multidomain with functional impairments and neuropsychiatric features* and *functional impairments and neuropsychiatric features* classes had a significantly greater likelihood (at least 3.8×) of CVD compared to the *minimally impaired* class.

Another study by McGuinness et al. (2015) examined MCI patients ($n = 139$) from a hospital memory clinic comparing conventional Petersen and Morris's (2005) criteria versus empirically derived LPA subgroups. A group of healthy, cognitively normal controls ($n = 98$) were also recruited. All participants were administered a neuropsychological protocol assessing learning/memory, attention/executive functions, language, and visuospatial ability. Age- and education-adjusted z-scores were calculated for each neuropsychological measure relative to normal control performance. Using conventional diagnostic criteria, impairment in a cognitive domain was designated as <1.5 SDs below the mean on at least one test. Also, in accordance with Petersen (2004) nosology, participants were labeled as presenting with single-domain amnestic (sd-aMCI), multidomain amnestic (md-aMCI), single-domain nonamnestic (sd-naMCI), and multidomain nonamnestic MCI (md-naMCI) or as having no impairment of clinical significance. Conventional Petersen (2004) criteria classified 9.4% as sd-aMCI, 46.8% as md-aMCI, 18.7% as sd-naMCI, and 7.2% as md-naMCI. The remaining 18.0% were identified with no impairment. A Cox proportional hazard ratio

(HR) and Kaplan–Meier analysis indicated that the md-aMCI group was at significantly increased risk of conversion to dementia within 2 years (HR = 3.7) compared to all other conventional Petersen MCI subtypes. However, using LPA, McGuinness et al. (2015) determined that a three-subgroup solution was the best-fitting model, with (a) an amnestic MCI group (36.7%); (b) a mixed or multidomain MCI group (40.3%); and (c) a LPA-derived cognitively intact group (23.0%) consistent with findings described by both Clark et al. (2013) and Edmonds et al. (2015).

Regression using proportional LPA membership indicated that the cognitively intact and amnestic MCI groups were significantly more likely to revert to normal (odds ratio [OR] = 41.33 and 14.99, respectively) and significantly less likely to progress to dementia upon follow-up (OR = 0.11 and 0.18, respectively), as compared to the mixed MCI subgroup. A Cox proportional HR indicated that the mixed subgroup was more likely to convert to dementia (HR = 3.7) compared to the other two groups. McGuinness et al. (2015) also cross-tabulated empirically derived LPA MCI classes against the conventional Petersen (2004) MCI subtypes and found substantial concordance between conventional sd-aMCI and the amnestic MCI subgroup (92.3% classification overlap) as well as significant agreement between conventional md-aMCI and the mixed MCI subgroup.

Most recently, Eppig et al. (2017) applied LPA to a sample of ADNI participants with the aim of identifying distinct neuropsychological classes among MCI participants ($n = 806$). Similar to Edmonds et al. (2015), MCI was diagnosed by ADNI using conventional Petersen (2004) criteria and a robust ADNI normal control sample ($n = 260$) was used to generate age-, education-, and sex-adjusted normative z-scores. Distinct from Edmonds et al. (2015), eight neuropsychological measures representing four cognitive (i.e., attention/executive functions, language, episodic memory, and visuoconstructional ability) were included in the LPA. Eppig et al. determined a three-class LPA solution as the best-fitting model, included an amnestic MCI group (56.5%), a mixed MCI group (13.2%), and a false-positive group with intact neuropsychological performance on all measures (LPA-derived normal: 30.4%) consistent with past work (Bondi et al., 2014; Edmonds et al., 2015, 2016; McGuinness et al., 2015).

Moreover, the amnestic and mixed MCI subgroups were more likely to be apolipoprotein E (APOE) ε4-positive on genotyping, display greater evidence for AD on the basis of CSF biomarkers and progress to dementia at a higher rate than the LPA-derived normal class. Eppig et al. (2017) also found that the percentage of conversion to dementia in the LPA-derived normal class was almost half of the proportion that converted to dementia in Edmonds et al.'s (2015) cluster-derived normal group (5.8% vs. 10.7%, respectively). As both studies used a highly overlapping sample from ADNI (97.7% concordance), this result provides support for the preferential use of LPA versus cluster analysis in future MCI classification research. Finally, Eppig et al. found disparities among the classes with regard to ADNI wave of enrollment (i.e., ADNI-1, -GO, or -2), suggesting potential methodological problems in ADNI's recruitment and characterization of MCI that may be differentially contributing to the problem of false-positive diagnoses.

4.3. Acetylcholinesterase Inhibitors in Statistically Defined MCI

Donepezil, an acetylcholinesterase inhibitor, is a common medication used to mitigate cognitive decline associated with AD (Birks & Harvey, 2018; Thomas et al., 2005). Although clinically indicated for the treatment of AD dementia, acetylcholinesterase inhibitors are not currently recommended for use in MCI due to a lack of empirical support (Petersen et al., 2018). However, as previously described, the potential for diagnostic errors using conventional Petersen MCI criteria is a serious methodological problem such that the inadvertent inclusion of false-positive participants into pharmacological trials designed to treat prodromal AD may attenuate beneficial effects.

Edmonds et al. (2018) explored this notion by reanalyzing data from the double-blind Alzheimer's Disease Cooperative Study (ADCS) vitamin E and donepezil trial for MCI (Petersen et al., 2005). The original double-blind trial randomized 769 MCI participants diagnosed using conventional Petersen criteria into control (i.e., placebo & Vitamin E) versus donepezil treatment groups (Petersen et al., 2005). The results of the original trial demonstrated that the donepezil group had a lower rate progression to dementia compared to control groups. However, these effects did not persist over the remaining 24 months of the study (Petersen et al., 2005).

Edmonds et al. (2018) re-examined these data by empirically classifying the original MCI participants ($n = 756$) on the basis of baseline neuropsychological tests of attention/executive functions, language, and episodic memory. Cluster analysis established three groups: (a) amnestic MCI (31.1%), (b) mixed MCI (39.0%), and (c) cognitively normal participants (29.9%) representing false-positive diagnostic errors. This cognitively normal group was subsequently remove from subsequent analysis. When Edmonds et al. compared the remaining treatment and control (vitamin E + placebo) groups, the authors found that the donepezil group had a lower rate progression to dementia over the entire 36 months of the study than the control group. Furthermore, the donepezil group demonstrated better overall immediate recall for verbal memory measures across the 36 months than the control group. Most impressively, the results of Edmonds et al. represented an *increase* in treatment effect relative to the original ADCS trial, despite an almost 30% reduction in sample size. This finding further highlights the critical contribution of neuropsychology to the accurate diagnosis of MCI.

4.4 Summary of Statistical Approaches to Classify MCI

Studies employing statistical techniques to classify MCI have consistently found three to four empirical subtypes despite methodological differences in definition of impairment, cognitive domains examined, neuropsychological tests administered, and type of statistical model (Table 3.1).

Additional important findings regarding research using empirical methods to define MCI subtypes are list as follows.

1. Empirical MCI subtypes have nuanced neuropsychological profiles, with unique patterns of impairment across varying cognitive domains (Libon et al., 2010, 2012; Clark et al., 2013; Delano-Wood et al., 2009; Edmonds et al., 2015; Epping, 2011; Hanfelt et al., 2011).
2. Single-domain or "pure" amnestic MCI emerges as a consistent subtype across all studies, typically representing a plurality of individuals (Delano-Wood et al., 2009; Edmonds et al., 2015, 2018; Libon et al., 2010).
3. Mixed MCI, as defined by the presence of impairment across the majority of neuropsychological domains, is also a consistent subtype across all studies. Importantly, these individuals appear to be at greatest risk for progression to dementia (Edmonds et al., 2015, 2018; McGuiness et al., 2015).
4. Conventional MCI criteria (Petersen & Morris, 2005) may be highly susceptible to false-positive diagnostic errors. Several studies employing statistical classification methods have independently identified a group of individuals originally diagnosed with MCI using conventional Petersen criteria that nonetheless demonstrate intact performance across neuropsychological tests (Clark et al., 2013; Edmonds et al., 2015, 2018; Eppig et al., 2017; Hanfelt et al., 2011; McGuinness et al., 2015). Estimates on the prevalence of these cognitively normal false-positive MCI participants ranges from 23% to 48%, an alarmingly high rate of potential diagnostic errors. This finding has obvious implications for research on the development of disease modifying medications to treat AD (Edmonds et al., 2018) as well as the quality of clinical care provided to patients and families. In response to these concerns, it is apparent a more rigorous, sophisticated, *neuropsychological* paradigm for identifying MCI subtypes may greatly benefit diagnostic accuracy.

Table 3.1 Results of Cluster Analytic and Mixture Model Approaches in Conventional MCI

Study	Statistical Model	Neuropsychological Domains	Sample Size	Number of Subgroups	MCI Subtypes (Proportion of Sample)
Clark et al. (2013)	Ward's method cluster analysis	Attention; episodic memory; executive functions; language; visuospatial ability	$n = 134$	4	Cognitively normal (47.8%) Memory/language (29.1%) Mixed/intact attention (23.1%)
Delano-Wood et al. (2009)	Ward's method cluster analysis	Constructional praxis; episodic memory; executive functions; language; processing speed	$n = 70$	3	Amnestic (48.6%) Memory/language (25.7%) Executive/processing speed (25.7%)
Edmonds et al. (2015)	Ward's method cluster analysis	Attention and executive functions; episodic memory; language	$n = 825$	4	Amnestic (34.9%) Cognitively normal (34.2%) Memory/language (18.5%) Executive/mixed (12.4%)
Edmonds et al. (2018)	Ward's method cluster analysis	Attention and executive functions; episodic memory; language	$n = 756$	3	Mixed (39.0%) Amnestic (31.1%) Cognitively normal (29.9%)
Eppig et al. (2017)	Latent profile analysis	Attention and executive functions; episodic memory; language; visuoconstructional copy	$n = 806$	3	Amnestic (56.5%) Cognitively normal (30.4%) Mixed (13.2%)

Hanfelt et al. (2011)	Latent profile analysis	Attention; depression; episodic memory; executive functions; functional ability; global cognition; processing speed; psychiatric symptoms	$n = 1{,}655$	7	Executive/language (18%) Amnestic (16%) Amnestic + functional/ psych (16%) Functional + psych (15%) Mixed (12%) Mixed + functional/ psych (12%) Cognitively normal (12%)
Libon et al. (2010)	K-means cluster analysis	Episodic memory; executive functions; language	$n = 77$	3	Amnestic (48.6%) Executive/language (27.3%) Mixed (25.7%)
McGuinness et al. (2015)	Latent profile analysis	Attention and executive functions; episodic memory; language; visuospatial ability	$n = 139$	3	Mixed (40.3%) Amnestic (36.7%) Cognitively normal (23.0%)

Note: MCI, mild cognitive impairment.

5. A Neuropsychological Approach to MCI Diagnosis: The Development and Validation of the Comprehensive Criteria

5.1. Origins of Comprehensive Diagnostic Criteria for MCI

Despite improvements over the last decade regarding the definition of MCI, there is lively debate regarding how to operationalize specific criterion. The evaluation of MCI continues to rely largely on subjective rating scales, brief cognitive screens, and/or a single impaired test score (e.g., Logical Memory delay free recall) rather than objective empirical methods as previously described (see Bondi et al., 2014, for a review). In an effort to address these issues, a new set of neuropsychological-based diagnostic criteria known as the *comprehensive criteria* have been developed for the purpose of more accurately diagnosing MCI subtypes. The following section discusses the origins, psychometric properties, and empirical validity of this approach.

Jak, Bondi, et al. (2009) introduced the term *comprehensive* diagnostic criteria for MCI by comparing the psychometric performances of five different MCI diagnostic strategies on a comprehensive neuropsychological protocol. In this community-based study, 90 nondemented and neurologically normal older adults were classified via consensus diagnosis as either normally aging or having MCI based on five different strategies (i.e., historical, typical, comprehensive, liberal, and conservative). A subset of 73 participants was evaluated 17 months later to determine the stability of the diagnosis. All five diagnostic strategies varied based on the cutoff used to determine objective cognitive impairment and the number of neuropsychological tests within a cognitive domain necessary for an MCI diagnosis (Table 3.2).

Of these five approaches, the comprehensive diagnostic criteria described in the following text were developed to address the pitfalls common to many MCI diagnostic paradigms. First, a lower cutoff for impairment of 1 SD below normative data (compared to 1.5 SDs) was adopted to improve the balance between reliability and sensitivity of the criteria to detect mild impairment (Heaton, Grant, & Matthews, 1991; Heaton, Miler, Taylor, & Grant, 2004). Second, special consideration was given to the fact that the interpretive value of an isolated impaired score is often limited. Heaton and colleagues (1991, 2004) reported that the majority of neurologically normal adults obtained *at least one* "abnormal' test score when administered the expanded Halsead–Reitan neuropsychological test battery and that the prevalence of these false-positive impaired scores is even higher in the older adult population. Critically, Palmer and colleagues (1998) found that a considerable number of healthy older adults earned one impaired score in *two* different cognitive domains, but that few (approximately 5% or less) had two or more impaired scores within the same cognitive domain. Thus, the

Table 3.2 MCI Diagnostic Schemes

Criteria	Origin	Impairment Cutoff (SD Below Age-Appropriate Norms)	Number of Tests Required to Be Impaired for MCI Diagnosis
Historical	Original Petersen (2001)	>1.5 SD	1 (WMS-R LM subtest only)
Typical (aka conventional)	Petersen and Morris (2005)	>1.5 SD	1 (within any cognitive domain)
Comprehensive	Jak et al. (2009)	> 1 SD	2 (within any cognitive domain)
Liberal	Jak et al. (2009)	> 1 SD	1 (within any cognitive domain)
Conservative	Jak et al. (2009)	> 1.5 SD	2 (within any cognitive domain)

Notes: MCI diagnostic schemes as compared in Jak et al. (2009). MCI, mild cognitive impairment; WMS-R LM, Wechsler Memory Scale–Revised–Logical Memory.

comprehensive MCI criteria required that, for a domain to be considered impaired, performance on *two or more* tests within a domain must be impaired (Jak, Bondi, et al., 2009).

5.2. Stability of the Comprehensive Criteria for MCI

Unsurprisingly, Jak, Bondi, et al. (2009) confirmed that the rate of MCI diagnosis varied widely depending on the criteria used (range = 10%–74%) such that a 2% to 30% of individuals demonstrated diagnostic instability over time (i.e., changed to MCI or cognitively normal diagnosis between baseline and follow-up). Moreover, there was considerable variability regarding the percentage of individuals within this subset that reverted from MCI back to normal cognition at follow up (range = 0%–15%). The authors noted that single domain, nonamnestic MCI was particularly unstable compared to other subtypes. These findings not only confirmed the need for a consensus on the ideal scheme for MCI diagnosis, but also quantified the discrepancies between extant and novel neuropsychological-based schemes with respect to sensitivity to impairment and stability.

In an attempt to provide insight into the most appropriate MCI diagnostic approach for research and clinical practice, Jak, Bondi, et al. (2009) further discussed the relative benefits and drawbacks of each of the diagnostic approaches. It was noted that, compared to the conventional MCI diagnostic criteria (Petersen & Morris, 2005), the comprehensive criteria offered an improved balance between sensitivity and specificity to detect *mild* impairment. Specifically, comprehensive criteria outperformed other schemes with respect to diagnostic stability over time. That is, schemes that only required an impaired score on one test within a single cognitive domain led to a relatively highly percentage (i.e., 18%–33%) of individuals who changed MCI subtype over time. Thus, it was determined that the comprehensive criteria offered the best balance between sensitivity and specificity while also maintaining a satisfactory level of diagnostic stability compared to the other potential schemes.

5.3. Validity of Comprehensive MCI Diagnostic Criteria

There is now accumulating research supporting the validity of the comprehensive MCI diagnostic criteria (Jak, Bondi, et al., 2009). Critically, statistical classification of individuals diagnosed with comprehensive MCI criteria has demonstrated that, unlike conventional Petersen criteria for MCI, a cognitively normal subgroup as described in previous research is consistently absent (e.g., Bondi et al., 2014; Clark et al., 2013; Jak et al., 2016). This finding supports the advantage of using comprehensive MCI criteria to minimize problematic false-positive diagnostic errors. These findings are further confirmed in a study that compared rates of progression to dementia between the conventional and comprehensive criteria in 1,203 participants in the Framingham Heart Study (FHS; Jak et al., 2016). The comprehensive MCI criteria had a similar—albeit slightly increased—association with dementia risk compared to the conventional criteria over an average period of 9.7 years (HR = 3.30, $p < 0.0001$, and HR = 2.64, $p < 0.0002$, respectively); however, comprehensive criteria resulted in approximately *30% fewer participants* diagnosed with MCI. The authors concluded that, again, this discrepancy in MCI diagnoses between these two criteria confirmed the susceptibility of the conventional criteria to false-positive MCI diagnoses in otherwise cognitively normal individuals.

In a follow-up FHS study among 347 "oldest-old" participants (i.e., 79 to 102 years old), Wong et al. (2018) also compared conventional and comprehensive criteria for MCI. These authors found that both diagnostic schemes were associated with increased conversion to dementia versus cognitively normal participants over an average period of 5.7 years. However, when both diagnostic schemes were included in the same model only the comprehensive MCI criteria continued to significantly predict conversion to dementia (comprehensive criteria: HR = 2.43, $p < 0.001$; conventional criteria: HR = 1.45, $p = 0.11$). Additional analysis by Wong et al. demonstrated that participants diagnosed with comprehensive MCI criteria were less likely to revert to cognitively normal (7.4%) than individuals diagnosed with conventional MCI criteria (13.6%), extending the notion that the comprehensive criteria are more sensitive and specific to the accurate identification of prodromal dementia.

Further evidence supporting the validity of comprehensive criteria for MCI comes from research examining the association between neuropathologic biomarkers of AD and disease progression. Jak, Urban, et al. (2009) examined whether the association between MCI status and bilateral hippocampal volume differed depending on diagnostic scheme (i.e., comprehensive vs. conventional) in 65 nondemented, community-dwelling older adults. The authors found that when participants were diagnosed using comprehensive criteria, hippocampal volume was significantly smaller in amnestic MCI compared to the cognitively normal or nonamnestic MCI groups. No such differences were observed between groups when the conventional MCI criteria were applied to the sample. Bondi and colleagues (2014) evaluated the diagnostic precision of both the comprehensive and conventional criteria by comparing associations with AD biomarkers and rates of dementia progression in 1,150 ADNI participants. For this study ADNI participants were diagnosed at baseline as either cognitively normal or MCI based on both the conventional criteria as operationalized by ADNI, and the comprehensive criteria by Jak, Bondi, et al. Similar to prior work (Edmonds et al., 2015), cluster and discriminant function analyses were obtained using neuropsychological measures of attention/executive functions, language, and episodic memory. Groups were compared on APOE ε4 genotype, AD-specific biomarkers in CSF including amyloid beta, total tau, and phosphorylated tau, and clinical outcome. Comprehensive diagnostic criteria demonstrated stronger associations with CSF AD biomarkers, APOE ε4 genotype, and later progression to AD. These findings challenge the empirical validity of the conventional MCI classification system in addition to providing an alternative diagnostic method that may help mitigate the rate of false-positive diagnostic errors.

6. Biological and Neuroimaging Markers Associated With MCI Subtypes

The identification of sensitive biological and neuroimaging markers for MCI has become an essential component of AD research. One approach to validate the use of operationally defined MCI subtypes involves the association of these subgroups with relevant brain regions on neuroimaging as well as sensitive AD biomarkers. Next, we review the current literature exploring both traditional (i.e., magnetic resonance imaging [MRI], CSF biomarkers) and more recent (i.e., white matter changes) measures of putative biomarkers discriminating between MCI subtypes.

6.1. Hippocampal Atrophy in MCI Subtypes

One of the most pronounced features of AD is the progressive and extensive nature atrophy involving the temporal lobe (i.e., hippocampus, entorhinal cortex, inferior temporal cortex, and uncus), and extending to parietal and frontal regions at later stages (Braak & Braak, 1995; Josephs et al., 2008). Not surprisingly, the majority of the studies have reported significantly smaller hippocampal volumes in individuals with amnestic MCI compared to nonamnestic MCI (Eliassen et al., 2017; He et al., 2009; Jak, Urban, et al., 2009). Furthermore, hippocampal volumes observed in amnestic MCI are generally intermediate between those in normal aging and AD (Mariani, Monastero, & Mecocci, 2007), although they have greater similarity to volumes observed in early AD than cognitive normal older adults (Stoub, Rogalski, Leurgans, & Bennett, 2010).

Mixed results have been reported when amnestic MCI is compared to multi-domain MCI. Becker and colleagues (2006) reported that hippocampal volumes in individuals with multi-domain MCI were not statistically different than normal controls, but were significantly larger than both the amnestic MCI and AD groups. Conversely, Eliassen, et al. (2017) reported that individuals with multidomain MCI had more extensive overall and subfield-specific atrophy of the hippocampus as compared to individuals with amnestic MCI and normal controls.

6.2. Cortical Atrophy in MCI Subtypes

Progressive involvement of cortical and subcortical gray matter regions affected by AD has been reported in longitudinal studies using voxel-based morphometry to study amnestic MCI (Goerlich et al., 2017; Whitwell et al., 2007), a pattern of atrophy that mirrors the neurofibrillary pathological staging scheme proposed by Braak and Braak (1991). However, there is preliminary evidence to suggest heterogeneity *within* the amnestic MCI subtype itself with respect to patterns of gray matter atrophy. For example, Kim et al. (2011) identified three subgroups of amnestic MCI based on impairment on either verbal, visual, or both types of memory tests. It was found that the verbal-amnestic MCI group had greater cortical thinning in the left anterior and medial temporal regions compared normal controls, while no differences were observed between visual-amnestic MCI and normal controls.

There are also a handful of studies that have attempted to explore more widespread cortical and subcortical atrophy differences across MCI subtypes. Guan et al. (2017) classified MCI subtypes in a sample of community-dwelling older adults using cross-sectional and longitudinal MRI-based biomarkers. Amnestic and nonamnestic MCI was differentiated with baseline gray matter structures including the hippocampus, amygdala and frontal pole. Additionally, Bell-McGinty and colleagues (2005) reported greater volume loss in the left entorhinal cortex and inferior parietal lobe in individuals with amnestic compared to multidomain MCI. In another study, a multidomain MCI group exhibited neuropathological changes in other brain regions including smaller right inferior frontal gyrus, right middle temporal gyrus, and bilateral superior temporal gyrus as compared to amnestic MCI (Becker et al., 2006).

In a follow-up study of Edmonds et al. (2015), Edmonds and colleagues (2016) investigated the relationship between patterns of cortical atrophy and empirically derived MCI subtypes in ADNI participants with MRI. These authors demonstrated an ordered pattern of cortical atrophy corresponding to the neuropsychological profile of each MCI subtype (i.e., amnestic MCI, dysnomic MCI, dysexecutive/mixed MCI, and cluster-derived normal), likely a reflection of increasing disease severity. Specifically, in comparison to robust normal controls, the amnestic MCI group presented with cortical thinning primarily relegated to the bilateral medial and lateral temporal lobe regions; the dysnomic MCI group exhibited cortical thinning in the bilateral medial and lateral temporal lobe regions (left > right) as well as some frontal lobe regions; and the dysexecutive/mixed MCI group demonstrated widespread bilateral cortical thinning across frontal, temporal, parietal, and cingulate regions, with relative sparing of occipital and paracentral cortices. When the cortical atrophy profiles of these three MCI subtypes were compared to each other, the authors observed that the dysexecutive/mixed MCI group displayed greater cortical thinning than the amnestic MCI group in frontal (left caudal middle frontal gyrus), lateral temporal (left superior temporal gyrus, left middle temporal gyrus, left inferior temporal gyrus), and parietal regions (left supramarginal gyrus, left and right inferior parietal cortex, and right precuneus) of the brain (Edmonds et al., 2016).

With respect to the cluster-derived normals, Edmonds et al. (2016) observed relatively intact medial and lateral temporal lobe cortical thickness compared to amnestic and dysnomic MCI groups and relatively intact cortical thickness in frontal, temporal, and parietal regions compared to dysexecutive/mixed MCI patients. Perhaps most notably, the cluster-derived normal group did not demonstrate any significant differences in regional cortical thickness from robust normal controls. Thus, the data reported by Edmonds et al. (2016) provide further support to the notion that ADNI participants have been erroneously diagnosed with MCI due to the susceptibility of conventional Petersen criteria to false positive diagnostic errors, while adding to the growing literature on cortical atrophy differences across MCI subtypes.

6.3. AD Protein Pathology in MCI

The traditional hallmark features of AD includes accumulation of Aβ peptides and hyperphosphorylated tau (p-tau). Until recently, the abnormal accumulation of these proteins in the brain of living individuals has been assessed indirectly by measuring CSF levels of Aβ and p-tau. Accordingly, studies that have aimed to identify potential differences in AD protein accumulation across MCI subtypes have largely relied on CSF measures of AD biomarkers.

Many studies have generally reported negative results with respect to AD CSF biomarker differences between MCI subtypes (Bondi et al., 2014; Edmonds et al., 2015, 2016; Eliassen et al., 2015; Eppig et al., 2017). However, Edmonds et al., 2015 noted significant differences in cluster-derived MCI subtypes when AD CSF biomarkers of p-tau$_{181p}$, Aβ$_{1\text{-}42}$, and the p-tau$_{181p}$/Aβ$_{1\text{-}42}$ ratio were assessed dichotomously. The cluster-defined dysexecutive/mixed MCI subgroup was observed to have a significantly greater proportion of AD CSF-positive individuals as compared to the amnestic and dysnomic subtypes. These differences were not observed when CSF biomarkers were analyzed as a continuous measure. The authors concluded that the dysexecutive/mixed group may represent a more pathologically advanced stage of MCI relative to the amnestic and dysnomic groups.

Recent advances in imaging methodology have allowed for the in vivo inspection of cortical Aβ in the human brain during life by employing radioactive tracers (e.g., Pittsburgh Compound B, florbetapir) and PET imaging. This technology has allowed for a more direct, sensitive assessment of amyloid burden compared the CSF measurements of Aβ. At the current time only one study to our knowledge has investigated cortical amyloid burden differences across MCI subtypes (Bangen et al., 2016). In this study, florbetapir PET imaging was used to assess cortical Aβ levels and interactions with APOE ε4 genotype status across cluster-derived MCI subgroups and cognitively normal older adults. Dysexecutive/mixed and amnestic MCI groups had significantly greater levels of cortical Aβ compared to the cluster-derived normal and normal control groups (which did not significantly differ from each other). Additionally, a group × APOE genotype interaction was observed such that APOE ε4 carriers within the amnestic MCI, cluster-derived normal, and normal groups had significantly greater cortical Aβ accumulation relative to their noncarrier counterparts, although this pattern was not found in dysexecutive/mixed MCI group. Given that the dysexecutive/mixed MCI group was also characterized by greater cognitive impairment and amyloid accumulation compared to the other participant groups, these findings further add accumulating evidence suggesting that the dysexecutive/mixed MCI group may represent a later, more progressed stage of MCI. As such, the APOE genotype findings might suggest a decreased role of the APOE ε4 allele in AD pathology in later stages of disease as compared to earlier stages (e.g., as captured by the amnestic MCI subgroup).

6.4. White Matter Pathology in MCI

Although the neurodegenerative progression of AD has been traditionally characterized by the cortical accumulation of abnormal proteins (i.e., amyloid beta, tau) and diffuse gray matter atrophy, this framework has recently been expanded to include early pathological changes in white matter macro- and microstructure (see Chapters 9 and 10 of this volume). One of the most common neuroimaging findings associated with aging is the presence of white matter macrostructural abnormalities, typically reflected by white matter hyperintensity (WMH) burden in subcortical and periventricular brain regions (Brickman et al., 2013). Importantly, WMH pathology is present in roughly 40% to 50% of older adults over age 50 (Schenk, Wuerz, & Lerner, 2013; Grueter & Schulz, 2012). Numerous studies have shown that WMH are associated with cognitive impairment (Delano-Wood et al., 2008, 2009; DeCarli et al., 1995; Au et al., 2006; Silbert, Howieson, Dodge, & Kaye, 2008; Silbert, Nelsen, Howieson, Moore, & Kaye, 2009), as well as dementia onset and progression (Brickman et al., 2015; Wolf, Ecke, Bettin, Dietrich, & Gertz, 2000). Accordingly, some have suggested that widespread white matter changes may be among the very earliest manifestations of the disease (see Brickman et al., 2013 for a review; Brickman et al., 2015).

With respect to the differences between MCI subtypes, several studies have reported no significant differences in WMH burden between individuals diagnosed with amnestic and nonamnestic MCI using the conventional criteria (Casado et al., 2015; Devine, Fonseca, & Walker, 2013; Guan et al., 2017; He et al., 2009). However, Delano-Wood et al. (2009) examined WMH burden in statistically defined MCI subtypes (amnestic MCI, memory/language MCI, executive/processing speed MCI and found regional differences in periventricular (pWML) versus deep white matter lesions (dWML). Specifically, the cluster-defined executive/processing speed group exhibited greater total WML burden than the memory/language and amnestic MCI groups, and greater dWML burden than the memory/language MCI group. Conversely, the amnestic MCI group displayed less pWML and dWML burden compared to both the memory/ language and amnestic MCI groups. The executive/processing speed group also had a higher dWML versus pWML load, yet the opposite pattern was observed in the memory/language MCI group (higher pWML vs. dWML burden). The authors interpreted these findings as consistent with past work, such that pWML along the borders of the ventricles may be related to age-associated changes in the ependymal lining, whereas dWML may reflect disrupted projection fibers of fronto-subcortical pathways via pathological small vessel disease. Delano-Wood et al. not only provide evidence supporting district subgroups within MCI based on both cognitive performance and neuropathological findings, but further emphasize the methodological and theoretical advantages of empirically-based approaches towards characterizing these subgroups.

6.5. Diffusion Tensor Imaging and MCI

The development of diffusion tensor imaging (DTI), a well-established, noninvasive MRI technique that uses patterns of water diffusion in brain tissue to describe white matter pathways and microstructure in vivo, has been particularly useful for characterizing the white matter changes that occur in various normal and pathologic aging conditions. Only a few studies have explored DTI-defined white matter microstructural differences between MCI subgroups (Haller et al., 2010, 2013; Grambaite et al., 2011; Gyebnar et al., 2018; Sali et al., 2013; Thillainades et al., 2010; Yu, Zhao, Li, & Yin, 2017; Zhuang et al., 2010), several of which are impacted by small sample sizes and underpowered statistical models. Nonetheless, there appears to be some preliminary evidence suggesting DTI-defined differences involving white matter microstructural differences between amnestic and nonamnestic MCI groups (Gyebnár et al., 2018; Haller et al., 2013, Thillainadesan et al., 2012; Zhuang et al., 2010). While the specific regions identified in white matter group-level differences vary somewhat across studies, most conclude that the pattern of white matter changes observed in the amnestic MCI is more consistent with the pathological progression of AD compared to nonamnestic MCI. There are, however, several studies that have reported no significant differences between MCI subtypes (Grambaite et al., 2011; Haller et al., 2010; Sali et al., 2013). Given the limited nature of the existing literature, combined with notable methodological variability, it is difficult to reconcile these discrepant findings at this time.

6.6. APOE Genotype

Given that the environment in which pathological mechanisms are initiated and perpetuated is influenced by genetic factors, it is necessary to understand how certain genes may influence the development and progression of MCI across different subtypes. Although there are a multitude of genetic factors that affect brain structure and function, APOE is by far the most prominent genetic risk factor for cognitive decline and AD (Corder et al., 1993; Saunders et al., 1993).

The APOE genes codes for the ApoE protein, which—in the brain—is produced primarily by astrocytes and microglia, although neurons also express ApoE in response to excitotoxicity (Huang & Mahley, 2014). With respect to the its role in the brain, ApoE appears to be involved with phospholipid and cholesterol transport between cells, as well as receptor-mediated plasma lipoprotein metabolism (Guo, LaDu, & Van Eldik, 2004). Three polymorphisms in the APOE gene code one of its three isoforms: APOE- ε2, APOE-ε3, and APOE-ε4. A loss in normal APOE function has been observed in APOE-ε4 carriers, negatively impacting synaptic plasticity, Aβ accumulation, neuronal recovery from neurodegeneration, and neuroinflammatory metabolic processes (Hayashi, Campenot, Vance, & Vance, 2004). Approximately 14% of the population has at least one copy of the APOE ε4 allele (Cedazo-Mínguez & Cowburn, 2001; Zannis et al., 1993) with each copy of the ε4 allele increasing the risk of developing AD at a younger median age (Corder et al., 1993; Farrer et al., 1997). Nonetheless, the exact mechanism(s) by which APOE genotype confers risk for AD remains elusive.

Although extensive research exists documenting differences in APOE genotype between individuals with MCI and cognitively normal older adults, there is an extremely limited number of studies that have explored differences *across* MCI subtypes. While the majority of these studies have reported no significant differences between MCI subtypes (Bondi et al., 2014; Edmonds et al., 2015; Eppig et al., 2017), one study did observe that APOE ε4 subtype was twice as prevalent in amnestic MCI as compared to nonamnestic MCI individuals (He et al., 2009). Additionally, it has been reported that the effect of the APOE ε4 allele on AD cortical pathology may differ between MCI subtypes (Bangen et al., 2016). Thus, it is clear that future research is warranted to further explore the potential role of APOE genotype, as well as other genetic biomarkers, across different MCI subtypes. Such research may inform the genetic roots of some of the heterogeneity observed within the MCI and furthermore help gauge risk for different clinical outcomes following MCI diagnosis.

7. Summary and Conclusion

Since the construct of MCI was introduced in the 1980s, there has been substantial research designed to improve both diagnostic sensitivity and specificity with the ultimate goal of improving the accurate identification of individuals at risk for developing AD. The definition of MCI has evolved over time from the early conceptual framework put forth by Petersen and colleagues (Petersen et al., 1999; Petersen, 2004; Winblad et al., 2004), to the current diagnostic criteria (Albert et al., 2011) that better reflect the cognitive and neuropathological heterogeneity that has been increasingly recognized within MCI (Bondi et al., 2014; Clark et al., 2013; Delano-Wood et al., 2009; Edmonds et al., 2015, 2016; Eppig et al., 2012, 2017; Libon et al., 2010, 2011; Hanfelt et al., 2011; McGuinness et al., 2015). Despite these improvements a growing body of neuropsychological research using statistical algorithms to classify MCI suggests conventional, Petersen diagnostic criteria for MCI result in a sizeable minority of individuals representing false-positive diagnostic errors. This is a serious problem to the extent Petersen criteria are used to in pharmacological trials to assess for potential benefits of disease modifying medication. A new set of neuropsychological-based diagnostic criteria—the "comprehensive criteria"—has been developed for the improved diagnosis of MCI. Critically, these criteria emphasize the use of comprehensive neuropsychological protocols and strategic impairment cutoffs to improve the MCI diagnosis accuracy. Not only do the comprehensive criteria demonstrate improved stability, reduced false-positive and false-negative rates, and greater correlation with biomarkers of risk relative to other approaches across a variety of aging samples, but there is also accumulating evidence to suggest that these criteria convey an advantage for describing the neuropsychological and biological heterogeneity that underlie MCI. Combined, these findings challenge the empirical validity of the conventional MCI classification system and implore the field to consider using an actuarial classification strategy to improve the accuracy of MCI diagnosis in both research and clinical settings.

References

Aerts, L., Heffernan, M., Kochan, N. A., Crawford, J. D., Draper, B., Trollor, J. N., . . . Brodaty, H. (2017). Effects of MCI subtype and reversion on progression to dementia in a community sample. *Neurology, 88*(23), 2225–2232.

Albert, M. S., DeKosky, S. T., Dickson, D., Dubois, B., Feldman, H. H., Fox, N. C., . . . Snyder, P. J. (2011). The diagnosis of mild cognitive impairment due to Alzheimer's disease: Recommendations from the National Institute on Aging-Alzheimer's Association workgroups on diagnostic guidelines for Alzheimer's disease. *Alzheimer's & Dementia, 7*(3), 270–279.

Alzheimer's Association. (2017). 2017 Alzheimer's disease facts and figures. *Alzheimer's & Dementia, 13*(4), 325–373.

Au, R., Massaro, J. M., Wolf, P. A., Young, M. E., Beiser, A., Seshadri, S., . . . DeCarli, C. (2006). Association of white matter hyperintensity volume with decreased cognitive functioning: The Framingham Heart Study. *Archives of Neurology, 63*(2), 246–250.

Bangen, K. J., Clark, A. L., Werhane, M., Edmonds, E. C., Nation, D. A., Evangelista, N., . . . Delano-Wood, L. (2016). Cortical amyloid burden differences across empirically-derived mild cognitive impairment subtypes and interaction with APOE ε4 genotype. *Journal of Alzheimer's Disease, 52*(3), 849–861.

Becker, J. T., Davis, S. W., Hayashi, K. M., Meltzer, C. C., Toga, A. W., Lopez, O. L., & Thompson, P. M. (2006). Three-dimensional patterns of hippocampal atrophy in mild cognitive impairment. *Archives of Neurology, 63*(1), 97–101.

Bell-McGinty, S., Lopez, O. L., Meltzer, C. C., Scanlon, J. M., Whyte, E. M., DeKosky, S. T., & Becker, J. T. (2005). Differential cortical atrophy in subgroups of mild cognitive impairment. *Archives of Neurology, 62*(9), 1393–1397.

Birks, J. S., & Harvey, R. J. (2018). Donepezil for dementia due to Alzheimer's disease. *Cochrane Database Systematic Review, 6*, CD001190.

Bondi, M. W., Edmonds, E. C., Jak, A. J., Clark, L. R., Delano-Wood, L., McDonald, C. R., . . . Salmon, D. P. (2014). Neuropsychological criteria for mild cognitive impairment improves diagnostic precision, biomarker associations, and progression rates. *Journal of Alzheimer's Disease, 42*(1), 275–289.

Braak, H., & Braak, E. (1991). Neuropathological staging of Alzheimer-related changes. *Acta Neuropathologica, 82*(4), 239–259.

Braak, H., & Braak, E. V. A. (1995). Staging of Alzheimer's disease-related neurofibrillary changes. *Neurobiology of Aging, 16*(3), 271–278.

Brickman, A. M. (2013). Contemplating Alzheimer's disease and the contribution of white matter hyperintensities. *Current Neurology and Neuroscience Reports, 13*(12), 415.

Brickman, A. M., Zahodne, L. B., Guzman, V. A., Narkhede, A., Meier, I. B., Griffith, E. Y., . . . Luchsinger, J. A. (2015). Reconsidering harbingers of dementia: Progression of parietal lobe white matter hyperintensities predicts Alzheimer's disease incidence. *Neurobiology of Aging, 36*(1), 27–32.

Canevelli, M., Grande, G., Lacorte, E., Quarchioni, E., Cesari, M., Mariani, C., . . . Vanacore, N. (2016). Spontaneous reversion of mild cognitive impairment to normal cognition: A systematic review of literature and meta-analysis. *Journal of the American Medical Directors Association, 17*(10), 943–948.

Casado Naranjo, I., Portilla Cuenca, J. C., Duque de San Juan, B., García, A. F., Sevilla, R. R., Serrano Cabrera, A., . . . Ramírez Moreno, J. M. (2015). Association of vascular factors and amnestic mild cognitive impairment: A comprehensive approach. *Journal of Alzheimer's Disease, 44*(2), 695–704.

Cedazo-Mínguez, A., & Cowburn, R. F. (2001). Apolipoprotein E: A major piece in the Alzheimer's disease puzzle. *Journal of Cellular and Molecular Medicine, 5*(3), 254–266.

Clark, L. R., Delano-Wood, L., Libon, D. J., McDonald, C. R., Nation, D. A., Bangen, K. J., . . . Bondi, M. W. (2013). Are empirically-derived subtypes of mild cognitive impairment consistent with conventional subtypes?. *Journal of the International Neuropsychological Society, 19*(06), 635–645.

Corder, E. H., Saunders, A. M., Strittmatter, W. J., Schmechel, D. E., Gaskell, P. C., Small, G., . . . Pericak-Vance, M. A. (1993). Gene dose of apolipoprotein E type 4 allele and the risk of Alzheimer's disease in late onset families. *Science, 261*(5123), 921–923.

Cummings, J. L., Morstorf, T., & Zhong, K. (2014). Alzheimer's disease drug-development pipeline: Few candidates, frequent failures. *Alzheimer's Research & Therapy, 6*(4), 37.

DeCarli, C., Murphy, D. G. M., Tranh, M., Grady, C. L., Haxby, J. V., Gillette, J. A., . . . Schapiro, M. B. (1995). The effect of white matter hyperintensity volume on brain structure, cognitive performance, and cerebral metabolism of glucose in 51 healthy adults. *Neurology, 45*(11), 2077–2084.

Delano-Wood, L., Abeles, N., Sacco, J. M., Wierenga, C. E., Horne, N. R., & Bozoki, A. (2008). Regional white matter pathology in mild cognitive impairment: Differential influence of lesion type on neuropsychological functioning. *Stroke, 39*(3), 794–799.

Delano-Wood, L., Bondi, M. W., Sacco, J., Abeles, N. O. R. M., Jak, A. J., Libon, D. J., & Bozoki, A. (2009). Heterogeneity in mild cognitive impairment: Differences in neuropsychological profile and associated white matter lesion pathology. *J Int Neuropsychol Soc, 15*(6), 906–914.

Devine, M. E., Fonseca, J. A. S., & Walker, Z. (2013). Do cerebral white matter lesions influence the rate of progression from mild cognitive impairment to dementia? *International Psychogeriatrics, 25*(1), 120–127.

Edmonds, E. C., Bangen, K. J., Delano-Wood, L., Nation, D. A., Furst, A. J., Salmon, D. P., & Bondi, M. W.; Alzheimer's Disease Neuroimaging Initiative. (2016). Patterns of cortical and subcortical amyloid burden across stages of preclinical Alzheimer's disease. *Journal of the International Neuropsychological Society, 22*(10), 978–990.

Edmonds, E. C., Delano-Wood, L., Clark, L. R., Jak, A. J., Nation, D. A., McDonald, C. R., . . . Bondi, M. W.; Alzheimer's Disease Neuroimaging Initiative. (2015). Susceptibility of the conventional criteria for mild cognitive impairment to false-positive diagnostic errors. *Alzheimer's & Dementia, 11*(4), 415–424.

Edmonds, E. C., Eppig, J., Bondi, M. W., Leyden, K. M., Goodwin, B., Delano-Wood, L., & McDonald, C. R.; Alzheimer's Disease Neuroimaging Initiative. (2016). Heterogeneous cortical atrophy patterns in MCI not captured by conventional diagnostic criteria. *Neurology, 87*(20), 2108–2116.

Edmonds, E. C., Ard, M. C., Edland, S. D., Galasko, D. R., Salmon, D. P., & Bondi, M. W. (2018). Unmasking the benefits of donepezil via psychometrically precise identification of mild cognitive impairment: A secondary analysis of the ADCS vitamin E and donepezil in MCI study. *Alzheimer's & Dementia, 4*, 11–18.

Eliassen, C. F., Selnes, P., Almdahl, I. S., Reinvang, I., Fladby, T., & Hessen, E. (2015). Hippocampal subfield atrophy in multi-domain but not amnestic mild cognitive impairment. *Dementia and Geriatric Cognitive Disorders, 40*(1-2), 44–53.

Eppig, J., Wambach, D., Nieves, C., Price, C. C., Lamar, M., Delano-Wood, L., . . . Libon, D. J. (2012). Dysexecutive functioning in mild cognitive impairment: Derailment in temporal gradients. *Journal of the International Neuropsychological Society, 18*(1), 20–28. http://doi.org/10.1017/S1355617711001238

Eppig, J. S., Edmonds, E. C., Campbell, L., Sanderson-Cimino, M., Delano-Wood, L., & Bondi, M. W.; Alzheimer's Disease Neuroimaging Initiative. (2017). Statistically derived subtypes and associations with cerebrospinal fluid and genetic biomarkers in mild cognitive impairment: A latent profile analysis. *Journal of the International Neuropsychological Society, 23*(7), 564–576.

Farrer, L. A., Cupples, L. A., Haines, J. L., Hyman, B., Kukull, W. A., Mayeux, R., . . . Van Duijn, C. M. (1997). Effects of age, sex, and ethnicity on the association between apolipoprotein E genotype and Alzheimer disease: A meta-analysis. *JAMA, 278*(16), 1349–1356.

Goerlich, K. S., Votinov, M., Dicks, E., Ellendt, S., Csukly, G., & Habel, U. (2017). Neuroanatomical and Neuropsychological Markers of Amnestic MCI: A Three-Year Longitudinal Study in Individuals Unaware of Cognitive Decline. *Frontiers in Aging Neuroscience*, *9*, 34.

Gordon, B. A., Friedrichsen, K., Brier, M., Blazey, T., Su, Y., Christensen, J., . . . Morris, J. C. (2016). The relationship between cerebrospinal fluid markers of Alzheimer pathology and positron emission tomography tau imaging. *Brain*, *139*(8), 2249–2260.

Grambaite, R., Reinvang, I., Selnes, P., Fjell, A. M., Walhovd, K. B., Stenset, V., & Fladby, T. (2011). Pre-dementia memory impairment is associated with white matter tract affection. *Journal of the International Neuropsychological Society*, *17*(1), 143–153.

Grueter, B. E., & Schulz, U. G. (2012). Age-related cerebral white matter disease (leukoaraiosis): A review. *Postgraduate Medical Journal*, *88*(1036), 79–87.

Guan, H., Liu, T., Jiang, J., Tao, D., Zhang, J., Niu, H., . . . Brodaty, H. (2017). Classifying MCI Subtypes in Community-Dwelling Elderly Using Cross-Sectional and Longitudinal MRI-Based Biomarkers. *Frontiers in Aging Neuroscience*, *9*, 309.

Guo, L., LaDu, M. J., & Van Eldik, L. J. (2004). A dual role for apolipoprotein E in neuroinflammation. *Journal of Molecular Neuroscience*, *23*(3), 205–212.

Gyebnár, G., Szabó, Á., Sirály, E., Fodor, Z., Sákovics, A., Salacz, P., . . . Csukly, G. (2018). What can DTI tell about early cognitive impairment?–Differentiation between MCI subtypes and healthy controls by diffusion tensor imaging. *Psychiatry Research: Neuroimaging*, *272*, 46–57.

Haller, S., Missonnier, P., Herrmann, F. R., Rodriguez, C., Deiber, M. P., Nguyen, D., . . . Giannakopoulos, P. (2013). Individual classification of mild cognitive impairment subtypes by support vector machine analysis of white matter DTI. *American Journal of Neuroradiology*, *34*(2), 283–291.

Haller, S., Nguyen, D., Rodriguez, C., Emch, J., Gold, G., Bartsch, A., . . . Giannakopoulos, P. (2010). Individual prediction of cognitive decline in mild cognitive impairment using support vector machine-based analysis of diffusion tensor imaging data. *Journal of Alzheimer's Disease*, *22*(1), 315–327.

Hanfelt, J. J., Wuu, J., Sollinger, A. B., Greenaway, M. C., Lah, J. J., Levey, A. I., & Goldstein, F. C. (2011). An exploration of subgroups of mild cognitive impairment based on cognitive, neuropsychiatric and functional features: Analysis of data from the National Alzheimer's Coordinating Center. *American Journal of Geriatric Psychiatry*, *19*(11), 940–950.

Hayashi, H., Campenot, R. B., Vance, D. E., & Vance, J. E. (2004). Glial lipoproteins stimulate axon growth of central nervous system neurons in compartmented cultures. *Journal of Biological Chemistry*, *279*(14), 14009–14015.

He, J., Farias, S., Martinez, O., Reed, B., Mungas, D., & DeCarli, C. (2009). Differences in brain volume, hippocampal volume, cerebrovascular risk factors, and apolipoprotein E4 among mild cognitive impairment subtypes. *Archives of Neurology*, *66*(11), 1393–1399.

Heaton, R. K., Grant, I., & Matthews, C. G. (1991). *Comprehensive norms for an expanded Halstead–Reitan battery: Demographic corrections, research findings, and clinical applications; with a supplement for the Wechsler Adult Intelligence Scale–Revised (WAIS-R)*. Lutz, FL: Psychological Assessment Resources.

Heaton, R. K., Miller, S. W., Taylor, M. J., & Grant, I. (2004). *Revised comprehensive norms for an expanded Halstead–Reitan battery: Demographically adjusted neuropsychological norms for African American and Caucasian adults.* Lutz, FL: Psychological Assessment Resources.

Huang, Y., & Mahley, R. W. (2014). Apolipoprotein E: structure and function in lipid metabolism, neurobiology, and Alzheimer's diseases. *Neurobiology of Disease, 72 Pt A*, 3–12. http://doi.org/10.1016/j.nbd.2014.08.025

Hughes, C. P., Berg, L., Danziger, W. L., Coben, L. A., & Martin, R. (1982). A new clinical scale for the staging of dementia. *British Journal of Psychiatry, 140*(6), 566–572.

Jak, A. J., Bondi, M. W., Delano-Wood, L., Wierenga, C., Corey-Bloom, J., Salmon, D. P., & Delis, D. C. (2009). Quantification of five neuropsychological approaches to defining mild cognitive impairment. *American Journal of Geriatric Psychiatry, 17*(5), 368–375.

Jak, A. J., Preis, S. R., Beiser, A. S., Seshadri, S., Wolf, P. A., Bondi, M. W., & Au, R. (2016). Neuropsychological criteria for mild cognitive impairment and dementia risk in the Framingham Heart Study. *Journal of the International Neuropsychological Society, 22*(9), 937–943.

Jak, A. J., Urban, S., McCauley, A., Bangen, K. J., Delano-Wood, L., Corey-Bloom, J., & Bondi, M. W. (2009). Profile of hippocampal volumes and stroke risk varies by neuropsychological definition of mild cognitive impairment. *Journal of the International Neuropsychological Society, 15*(6), 890–897.

Josephs, K. A., Whitwell, J. L., Ahmed, Z., Shiung, M. M., Weigand, S. D., Knopman, D. S., . . . Jack, C. R. (2008). β-amyloid burden is not associated with rates of brain atrophy. *Annals of Neurology, 63*(2), 204–212.

Kim, M. J., Im, K., Lee, J. M., Park, A., Chin, J., Kim, G. H., . . . Na, D. L. (2011). Cortical thinning in verbal, visual, and both memory-predominant mild cognitive impairment. *Alzheimer Disease & Associated Disorders, 25*(3), 242–249.

Libon, D. J., Xie, S. X., Eppig, J., Wicas, G., Lamar, M., Lippa, C., . . . Wambach, D. M. (2010). The heterogeneity of mild cognitive impairment: A neuropsychological analysis. *Journal of the International Neuropsychological Society, 16*(01), 84–93.

Marcos, G., Santabárbara, J., Lopez-Anton, R., De-la-Cámara, C., Gracia-García, P., Lobo, E., . . . Brayne, C. (2016). Conversion to dementia in mild cognitive impairment diagnosed with DSM-5 criteria and with Petersen's criteria. *Acta Psychiatrica Scandinavica, 133*(5), 378–385.

Mariani, E., Monastero, R., & Mecocci, P. (2007). Mild cognitive impairment: A systematic review. *Journal of Alzheimer's Disease, 12*(1), 23–35.

McGuinness, B., Barrett, S. L., McIlvenna, J., Passmore, A. P., & Shorter, G. W. (2015). Predicting conversion to dementia in a memory clinic: A standard clinical approach compared with an empirically defined clustering method (latent profile analysis) for mild cognitive impairment subtyping. *Alzheimer's & Dementia, 1*(4), 447–454.

Mitchell, A. J., & Shiri-Feshki, M. (2009). Rate of progression of mild cognitive impairment to dementia: Meta-analysis of 41 robust inception cohort studies. *Acta Psychiatrica Scandinavica, 119*(4), 252–265.

Palmer, B. W., Boone, K. B., Lesser, I. M., & Wohl, M. A. (1998). Base rates of "impaired" neuropsychological test performance among healthy older adults. *Archives of Clinical Neuropsychology, 13*(6), 503–511.

Petersen, R. C. (2004). Mild cognitive impairment as a diagnostic entity. *Journal of Internal Medicine, 256*(3), 183–194.

Petersen, R. C., & Morris, J. C. (2005). Mild cognitive impairment as a clinical entity and treatment target. *Archives of Neurology, 62*(7), 1160–1163.

Petersen, R. C., Doody, R., Kurz, A., Mohs, R. C., Morris, J. C., Rabins, P. V., . . . Winblad, B. (2001). Current concepts in mild cognitive impairment. *Archives of Neurology, 58*(12), 1985–1992.

Petersen, R. C., Lopez, O., Armstrong, M. J., Getchius, T. S. D., Ganguli, M., Gloss, D., . . . Rae-Grant, A. (2018). Practice guideline update summary: Mild cognitive impairment. *Neurology, 90*(3), 126–135.

Petersen, R. C., Smith, G. E., Waring, S. C., Ivnik, R. J., Tangalos, E. G., & Kokmen, E. (1999). Mild cognitive impairment: Clinical characterization and outcome. *Archives of Neurology, 56*(3), 303–308.

Petersen, R. C., Thomas, R. G., Grundman, M., Bennett, D., Doody, R., Ferris, S., . . . Pfeiffer, E. (2005). Vitamin E and donepezil for the treatment of mild cognitive impairment. *New England Journal of Medicine, 352*(23), 2379–2388.

Price, C. C., Garrett, K. D., Jefferson, A. L., Cosentino, S., Tanner, J. J., Penney, D. L., . . . Libon, D. J. (2009). Leukoaraiosis severity and list-learning in dementia. *Clinical Neuropsychologist, 23*(6), 944–961. http://doi.org/10.1080/13854040802681664

Reisberg, B., Ferris, S. H., de Leon, M. J., & Crook, T. (1982). The Global Deterioration Scale for assessment of primary degenerative dementia. *American Journal of Psychiatry, 139*(9), 1136–1139.

Reisberg, B., Ferris, S. H., Kluger, A., Franssen, E., Wegiel, J., & De Leon, M. J. (2008). Mild cognitive impairment (MCI): A historical perspective. *International Psychogeriatrics, 20*(1), 18–31.

Sali, D., Verganelakis, D. A., Gotsis, E., Toulas, P., Papatriantafillou, J., Karageorgiou, C., . . . Papadimitriou, A. (2013). Diffusion tensor imaging (DTI) in the detection of white matter lesions in patients with mild cognitive impairment (MCI). *Acta Neurologica Belgica, 113*(4), 441–451.

Saunders, A. M., Strittmatter, W. J., Schmechel, D., George-Hyslop, P. S., Pericak-Vance, M. A., Joo, S. H., . . . Hulette, C. (1993). Association of apolipoprotein E allele ϵ4 with late-onset familial and sporadic Alzheimer's disease. *Neurology, 43*(8), 1467–1472.

Schenk, C., Wuerz, T., & Lerner, A. J. (2013). Small vessel disease and memory loss: What the clinician needs to know to preserve patients' brain health. *Current Cardiology Reports, 15*(12), 427.

Silbert, L. C., Howieson, D. B., Dodge, H., & Kaye, J. A. (2009). Cognitive impairment risk: White matter hyperintensity progression matters. *Neurology, 73*(2), 120–125.

Silbert, L. C., Nelson, C., Howieson, D. B., Moore, M. M., & Kaye, J. A. (2008). Impact of white matter hyperintensity volume progression on rate of cognitive and motor decline. *Neurology, 71*(2), 108–113.

Sperling, R. A., Rentz, D. M., Johnson, K. A., Karlawish, J., Donohue, M., Salmon, D. P., & Aisen, P. (2014). The A4 study: Stopping AD before symptoms begin? *Science Translational Medicine, 6*(228), 228fs13–228fs13.

Stoub, T. R., Rogalski, E. J., Leurgans, S., & Bennett, D. A. (2010). Rate of entorhinal and hippocampal atrophy in incipient and mild AD: Relation to memory function. *Neurobiology of Aging, 31*(7), 1089–1098.

Thillainadesan, S., Wen, W., Zhuang, L., Crawford, J., Kochan, N., Reppermund, S., . . . Sachdev, P. (2012). Changes in mild cognitive impairment and its subtypes as seen on diffusion tensor imaging. International *Psychogeriatrics, 24*(9), 1483–1493.

Thomas, D. A., Libon, D. J., & Ledakis, G. (2005). Treating dementia patients with vascular lesions with donepezil: A preliminary analysis. *Applied Neuropsychology*, 12, 12–18.

Ward, A., Tardiff, S., Dye, C., & Arrighi, H. M. (2013). Rate of conversion from prodromal Alzheimer's disease to Alzheimer's dementia: A systematic review of the literature. *Dementia and Geriatric Cognitive Disorders Extra, 3*(1), 320–332.

Weiner, M. W., Veitch, D. P., Aisen, P. S., Beckett, L. A., Cairns, N. J., Green, R. C., . . . Morris, J. C. (2013). The Alzheimer's Disease Neuroimaging Initiative: A review of papers published since its inception. *Alzheimer's & Dementia, 9*(5), e111–e194.

Whitwell, J. L., Przybelski, S. A., Weigand, S. D., Knopman, D. S., Boeve, B. F., Petersen, R. C., & Jack, C. R., Jr. (2007). 3D maps from multiple MRI illustrate changing atrophy patterns as subjects progress from mild cognitive impairment to Alzheimer's disease. *Brain, 130*(7), 1777–1786.

Winblad, B., Palmer, K., Kivipelto, M., Jelic, V., Fratiglioni, L., Wahlund, L. O., . . . Arai, H. (2004). Mild cognitive impairment–beyond controversies, towards a consensus: Report of the International Working Group on Mild Cognitive Impairment. *Journal of Internal Medicine, 256*(3), 240–246.

Wolf, H., Ecke, G. M., Bettin, S., Dietrich, J., & Gertz, H. J. (2000). Do white matter changes contribute to the subsequent development of dementia in patients with mild cognitive impairment? A longitudinal study. *International Journal of Geriatric Psychiatry, 15*(9), 803–812.

Wong, C. G., Thomas, K. R., Edmonds, E. C., Weigand, A. J., Bangen, K. J., Eppig, J. S., . . . Edland, S. D. (2018). Neuropsychological Criteria for Mild Cognitive Impairment in the Framingham Heart Study's Old-Old. *Dementia and Geriatric Cognitive Disorders, 46*(5-6), 253–265.

Yu, Y., Zhao, W., Li, S., & Yin, C. (2017). MRI-based comparative study of different mild cognitive impairment subtypes: Protocol for an observational case–control study. *BMJ Open, 7*(3), e013432.

Zannis, V. I., Kardassis, D., & Zanni, E. E. (1993). Genetic mutations affecting human lipoproteins, their receptors, and their enzymes. In H. Harris & K. Hirschhorn (Eds.), *Advances in human genetics 21* (pp. 145–319). Boston, MA: Springer.

Zhuang, L., Wen, W., Zhu, W., Trollor, J., Kochan, N., Crawford, J., . . . Sachdev, P. (2010). White matter integrity in mild cognitive impairment: A tract-based spatial statistics study. *Neuroimage, 53*(1), 16–25.

4
Vascular Cognitive Impairment

Victor Wasserman, Sheina Emrani, Emily Matusz, Catherine C. Price, Melissa Lamar, Rodney A. Swenson, Kenneth M. Heilman, and David J. Libon

1. Introduction

Vascular cognitive impairment (VCI) is a clinical syndrome in which there is a decline in neurocognitive functions induced by cerebrovascular disease. This decline can vary in severity, ranging from mild neurocognitive decline to dementia (Moorhouse & Rockwood, 2008). The etiological processes leading to VCI are diverse. In clinical practice, an etiological perspective frequently distinguishes between cognitive change associated with cortical territory infarction and change related to subcortical infarction. These cortical territory vascular incidents can be caused by large or mid-sized vessel thrombosis in the carotid, vertebral, the middle cerebral, anterior cerebral, and posterior cerebral arteries. Subcortical causes are more heterogeneous and may involve so-called strategic stroke in subcortical locations (e.g., thalamic and basal ganglia; Zhao et al., 2018) and small vessel disease, lacunes, and leukoaraiosis (Erkinjuntti, 2003). In addition, cerebral hypoperfusion has been described as a common pathophysiological process underlying white matter changes and may contribute to neurodegeneration and cognitive decline involved in vascular dementia (VaD; Duncombe et al., 2017).

The diagnostic criteria for VCI can be variable (Skrobot et al., 2017; Smith, 2017) with several groups putting forward competing diagnostic criteria. These diagnostic criteria share similarities but differ with respect to the emphasis placed on information drawn from patient history, physical examination, diagnostic testing, neurocognitive profile, and neuroimaging (American Psychiatric Association, 2013; Gorelick et al., 2011; Sachdev et al., 2014). A fundamental issue regarding VCI is the actual pathophysiological relationship between evidence for the presence of vascular disease and accompanying neurocognitive impairments. This chapter will be divided into five parts. First, we present a short historical review of VCI. The second part of this chapter will present a brief review the epidemiological research on VCI. Third, we will review the neuropsychological literature as related to VCI and vascular mild cognitive impairment (MCI). Fourth, we will discuss recent findings associating biomarkers with VCI.

Victor Wasserman, Sheina Emrani, Emily Matusz, Catherine C. Price, Melissa Lamar, Rodney Swenson, Kenneth H. Heilman, and David J. Libon, *Vascular Cognitive Impairment* In: *Vascular Disease, Alzheimer's Disease, and Mild Cognitive Impairment.* Edited by: David J. Libon, Melissa Lamar, Rodney A. Swenson, Kenneth M. Heilman, Oxford University Press (2020). © Oxford University Press.
DOI: 10.1093/oso/9780190634230.003.0005

Finally, the last part of this chapter will address public health and treatment issues.

2. Vascular Cognitive Impairment: Historical and Modern Perspectives

The term *multi-infarct dementia* (MID) was suggested by Hachinski and colleagues (Hachinski et., 1974, 1975) to identify patients where dementia was linked to a de novo vascular event. The Hachinski Ischemic Scale lists a number of clinical characteristics associated with ischemic stroke and has been used to differentiate AD from MID. The term *vascular cognitive impairment* also dates from the work of Hachinski and colleagues (Bowler, 2004, 2005; Bowler & Hachinski, 1995; Devasenapathy & Hachinski, 2000; Hachinski, 1994). Hachinski and colleagues used the term to describe a broad continuum of neurocognitive and functional alterations, ranging from minimal/mild prodromal states to the presence of clinical dementia.

The rationale underlying the introduction of the term VCI revolves around three considerations. First, it is evident that there are diverse neuroradiological and clinical presentations of disorders where vascular disease is believed to be either the cause or a contributing factor to a decline in neurocognitive functions. Second, Hachinski and colleagues have commented that cerebrovascular and cardiovascular risk factors could, in many cases, be identified (Wardlaw et al., 2013). The identification of cerebrovascular and cardiovascular risk factors, along with treatment, may have a meaningful effect on the course of this illness. Third, Hachinski and colleagues have pointed out the tendency to view all insidious onset dementia through the lens of Alzheimer's disease (AD; i.e., the *Alzheimerization* of dementia; see Libon, Price, Heilman, & Grossman, 2006, for a review). The *Alzheimerization of dementia* also tends to view memory impairment as the most common and salient neurocognitive characteristic. This point of view has been challenged. Libon et al. (2011) noted that an *impairment on a memory test* is not always the same as the presence of *clinical amnesia*. For example, there are patients who present with low scores on both delayed free recall and recognition tests and other patients who score higher on recognition compared to delay free recall. Unfortunately, these differences have not always been appreciated.

VCI has come to mean different things to different people. For example, Román and colleagues (2004) suggested reserving the term VCI to describe situations when vascular disease is only associated with mild changes in neurocognition and do not meet criteria for dementia. This perspective was echoed by Erkinjuntti and Rockwood (2003). More recently, VCI has come to be an umbrella term describing a spectrum of neurocognitive impairments (Moorhouse & Rockwood, 2008), including what has been described as both vascular MCI and VaD.

Clinical classification criteria for VCI were published as part of the fifth edition of the *Diagnostic and Statistical Manual of Mental Disorders* (DSM-5; American Psychiatric Association, 2013; Table 4.1). In addition, the International Society of Vascular Behavioral and Cognitive Disorders (VAS-COG; Sachdev et al., 2014) and the American Heart Association (Gorelick et al., 2011) have both suggested criteria for classifying neurocognitive impairment with vascular contributions (Table 4.1).

These criteria are, for the most part, similar, requiring objective evidence of a decline in neurocognitive function, either following a vascular event or accompanied by evidence of cerebrovascular disease. While naming conventions differ, these criteria also allow for the classification of vascular MCI or VaD, depending upon the severity of symptoms. All of these criteria allow for the subclassification of possible or probable VCI depending on the availability of supporting evidence, enabling a diagnosis of VCI in the absence of neuroimaging or in the presence of evidence of another neurocognitive disorder. The DSM-5 criteria are notable for not requiring evidence of cerebrovascular disease from neuroimaging to diagnose VCI, while the VAS-COG provide additional criteria for specifying underlying cerebrovascular pathology. The Vascular Impairment of Cognition Classification Consensus Study (VICCCS; Skrobot et al., 2017) surveyed an international sample of clinicians and researchers to achieve a conceptual consensus for VCI, along with VCI subtypes such as multi-infarct dementia, mixed dementia, and poststroke dementia and have suggested areas of research that could further support the construct and subtyping of VCI. These suggestions include determining if subtypes of mild VCI are empirically supported and improving our understanding of the relative contribution of co-occurring pathology in cases of mixed dementia and dementia comorbid with psychiatric disorders or other neurodegenerative conditions.

3. Empirical Support for the Construct of VCI

Data supporting the validity of VCI as a diagnostic construct come from several sources: (a) research demonstrating differences in the rate and presentation of mild/prodromal neurocognitive impairment to the emergence of VaD versus conversion to AD; (b) research associating vascular risk factors with the eventual emergence of dementia; and (c) research demonstrating a unique neurocognitive profile associated with mild/potential predementia states with vascular underpinnings.

Table 4.1 Comparison of diagnostic criteria for VCI.

	DSM-5	American Heart Association/ American Stroke Association	VAS-COG Society
Diagnostic classification	(a) Mild vascular neurocognitive disorder (b) Major vascular neurocognitive disorder	(a) Vascular mild cognitive impairment; (b) Vascular dementia	(a) Vascular mild cognitive disorder; (b) vascular major cognitive disorder
Clinical evidence of vascular cause	Cognitive deficits are temporally related to cerebrovascular events *or* the pattern of cognitive change indicates decline in attention, processing speed and executive function	Cognitive deficits are temporally related to cerebrovascular events *or* the severity and pattern of cognitive change is related to diffuse, subcortical cerebrovascular pathology	Physical signs suggest a stroke *or* cognitive deficits are temporally related to cerebrovascular events *or* the pattern of cognitive change indicates decline in attention, processing speed, and executive function with additional changes in gait, mood lability/ personality, or urinary symptoms
Requirement for neuroimaging evidence of cerebrovascular disease	No	Yes	Yes
Requirement for a temporal relationship between vascular event and cognitive change	Yes	Yes	Yes

Criteria for "possible" VCI	Applicable when meeting criteria but without supporting neuroimaging *or* without an established temporal relationship between cerebrovascular event and cognitive changes	Applicable when there is also evidence of other neurodegenerative conditions *or* when necessary criterion such as neuroimaging or cognitive assessment are missing or incomplete.	Applicable when meeting criteria but without supporting neuroimaging
Criteria contraindicating VCI	Another disease or disorder better explains cognitive impairment	Applicable when meeting criteria but without supporting neuroimaging *or* without an established temporal relationship between cerebrovascular event and cognitive changes	Evidence of one or more non-vascular disorders sufficient to explain the cognitive impairment

Notes: Adapted from Smith (2017). DSM-5, Diagnostic and Statistical Manual of Mental Disorders (fifth edition; American Psychiatric Association, 2013); VCI, vascular cognitive impairment.

3.1. Conversion From Mild Cognitive Impairment to Dementia

Past research has attempted to identify means to distinguish individuals presenting with a prodromal VaD versus prodromal AD and to document differential rates of conversion to a dementia syndrome. In a meta-analysis, Zhang and colleagues (2012) found that among their participants, AD was more prevalent than VaD in all age groups. Likewise, Ohara and colleagues (2017) observed that AD was more prevalent in a Japanese sample than VaD. Both studies also found that the prevalence of VaD among Chinese and Japanese populations had declined or held constant since 1985, while the prevalence of AD has risen. Changes in diagnostic criteria may underlie these observed changes in prevalence (Prince et al., 2016).

Epidemiological studies of neurocognitive impairment have noted a consistent contribution of cerebrovascular events to mild impairment in the absence of additional underlying pathology. Data obtained from a community sample found that in 13% of patients with amnestic MCI and 19% of those with nonamnestic MCI, the presence of infarcts was the most prominent neuropathological alteration upon autopsy (Schneider, Arvanitakis, Leurgans, & Bennett, 2009). The overall prevalence of MCI attributable to a vascular cause without corresponding AD pathology in this sample was 16%. The Canadian Study of Health and Aging reported that 15.4% of patients with neurocognitive impairment—no dementia (CIND) was related to vascular injury alone (Graham et al., 1997).

Zanetti and colleagues (2006) conducted a population study and identified individuals with MCI who were either amnesic or had evidence of executive dysfunction. The amnesic group was characterized by poor performance on tests of memory while the dysexecutive group was characterized by slower time to completion on Trail Making Test Part B and reduced output on tests of letter fluency. Upon follow-up, most patients in the amnesic and dysexecutive groups went on to develop AD and VaD, respectively. In sum, these studies appear to suggest that the course that ultimately leads to a clinical diagnosis of either AD versus VaD differs. The pathway that ultimately leads to AD is likely more homogenous than that which leads VaD (Sachdev et al., 2004).

3.2. Mild Cognitive Impairment and Vascular Risk Factors

Several studies have attempted to evaluate the relationship between risk factors for stroke and the evolution to dementia. An and Li (2015) reported that VCI in poststroke individuals, who were without cognitive impairment prior to their stroke there was a significant association with vascular risk factors, including elevated blood pressure, homocysteine, atrial fibrillation, glycosylated hemoglobin, and tobacco and alcohol use. In a study of single and multidomain amnestic MCI patients, Villeneuve and colleagues (2009) observed that there was a greater vascular burden in patients with amnestic MCI who exhibited lower performance on tests that assessed executive functions. A significant vascular burden was also found to be common in patients with multidomain neurocognitive impairments. These findings suggests a relationship between vascular burden and greater heterogeneity of impaired functions in MCI. Takahashi and colleagues (2019) reported the ability to identify individuals with amnestic MCI within 2 weeks of an acute ischemic stroke using a magnetic resonance imaging (MRI) visual rating scales of medial temporal atrophy along with poor performance on the delayed recall on the Montreal Cognitive Assessment (MoCA). In contrast, Smith and colleagues (2018), in an exploratory study of hypertensive individuals with and without MCI, found that the volume of white matter hyperintensities, silent brain infarcts, and microbleeds were not associated with performance on neurocognitive testing. Rather, episodic memory performance as measured with the California Verbal Learning II (CVLT-II) and the Wechsler Memory Scale Logical Memory II was associated with beta-amyloid deposition, as detected by Pittsburgh Compound B positron emission tomography scan, suggests that AD pathology may be a factor in neurocognitive decline even in those people with a notable VCI risk.

3.3. Neuropsychological and Behavioral Tests Predicting Conversion of Vascular MCI to VaD

Some research investigating conversion to AD suggests that, before actual dementia develops, isolated memory impairment is present (Albert, 2002). However, more recent research regarding this relationship demonstrates variable results. For example, Rist and colleagues (2013) found that patients with stroke or a transient ischemic attack who had worse performance on the Mini-Mental State Examination (MMSE) at baseline were at a high risk of converting to dementia, even without a recurrent stroke. In contrast with these findings, Stephan and colleagues (2017) reported that patients with hypertension, peripheral vascular disease, or chronic heart disease were at an increased risk of developing dementia within 2 years, but that the development of dementia was not related to impaired cognition when initially assessed with the MMSE or Cambridge Cognition Examination (CAMCOG). Smith and colleagues (2015) obtained data from an asymptomatic, middle-aged community and found that slower gait was associated with an increase in silent brain infarcts detected on MRI. White matter hyperintensity volume in the supratentorial region was also correlated with slower gait, as well as worse performance on neuropsychological testing.

The results of these studies appear to be variable likely due to multiple factors. First, there is overreliance on using brief neurocognitive screening measures such as the MoCA and MMSE. Second, the plethora of neuropsychological tests used from study to study places some limits on the external validity of these studies. Tests that assess working memory and information processing speed have been shown to differentiate patients with AD from VaD (Lamar et al., 2007; Lamar, Price, Cynthia, Kaplan, & Libon, 2002); however, discriminating between AD and VaD on the basis of executive dysfunction at the individual level is not always reliable (Andruita et al., 2018; Ramirez-Gomez et al., 2017).

4. Neuropsychology of VCI

One consistent finding that has emerged over the last several years is the dissociation on neuropsychological testing between VaD and AD. Patients with VaD tend to reveal a greater impairment on tests of executive control, visuoconstruction, and information processing speed than AD patients. In contrast, the patients with AD often reveal worse performance on tests of episodic memory and tests assessing lexical retrieval (Desmond, 2004; Libon et al., 1998; Libon, Price, Davis Garrett, & Giovannetti, 2004; Price, Jefferson, Merino, Heilman, & Libon, 2005; Sachdev et al., 2004).

4.1. VCI and Poststroke Cognitive Disabilities

Kramer and colleagues (2002) examined a group of nondemented patients with subcortical lacunes who suffered one or more subcortical lacunes. Compared to a control group, patients with a prior stroke obtained lower scores on tests of processing speed and had impaired inhibition (Stroop Test), impairments in novel-concept formation with disengagement (California Card Sort Test), and impaired performance on the initiation-perseveration portion of the Mattis Dementia Rating Scale. No differences were noted, however, on tests of language or memory. Poor performance on these executive control measures were also positively correlated with periventricular and deep white matter signal hyperintensities. In a follow-up study, this same research group studied a group of patients with and without dementia and found that subcortical lacunes correlated with reduced activity in the dorsolateral prefrontal cortex (Reed et al., 2004). Reduced dorsolateral prefrontal activity was also selectively correlated with poorer performance on these executive tests.

Grau-Olivares and colleagues (2010) studied patients with first-ever lacunar infarct with and without vascular MCI. Vascular MCI patients presented with greater impairment upon an 18-month follow-up on testing such as verbal fluency, Stroop Interference, and the Trail Making Tests. Compared to non-MCI, the vascular MCI group also showed improvement on memory testing. Nyenhuis and colleagues (2004) used logistic regression analysis and were able to show that nondemented, poststroke patients could be classified on the basis of slower performance on tests related to information processing speed and episodic memory. Jokinen and colleagues (2006) also found that a combination of reduced performance on tests of executive control and delayed memory best characterized their sample of nondemented, poststroke patients. Finally, Nakaoku and colleagues (2018) reported reduced cerebral blood flow in regions comprising the prefrontal-subcortical circuits among stroke patients was associated with poorer executive function, attention, language, and delayed recall on MoCA.

4.2. VCI and Subcortical White Matter Disease

A variety of studies have examined patients with mild cognitive deficits associated with MRI evidence of subcortical white matter disease. Consistent with studies that have evaluated patients with dementia who have significant white matter disease, these patients are impaired on a wide number of executive function tests. For example, Garrett and colleagues (2004) studied patients characterized as presenting with vascular CIND (VaCIND) who had subcortical white matter disease and found that poor performance on tests assessing neurocognitive flexibility (Trail Making Tests–Parts A and B), letter fluency, and delayed recognition memory (California Verbal List Learning Test). Sachdev and colleagues (2004) assessed a large number of nondemented VCI patients with evidence of prior stroke or transient ischemic attacks. When compared to healthy controls, these patients obtained lower scores on tests of abstraction, mental flexibility, working memory, and information processing speed when compared to controls. There was a high correlation between impairments on executive control tests and deep white matter hyperintensities on MRI, as defined by the number or volume of infarcts. Gasparovic and colleagues (2013) measured brain metabolites in the white matter above the lateral ventricles using MR spectroscopy in patients with white matter alterations following diagnosis of ischemic vascular disease, multiple infarcts, mixed dementia, and leukoaraiosis. In this sample, total creatine and *N*-acetyl aspartyl compounds were positively associated with executive function and attention. White matter metabolite levels were also more strongly associated with neurocognitive performance than white matter hyperintensity volume from fluid-attenuated inversion recovery (FLAIR)

MRI, suggesting that white matter metabolic status may be a better predictor of cognitive changes from VCI pathology than lesion volume.

Finally, in a study of white matter damage involving the cholinergic system in individuals characterized with vascular MCI, Liu and colleagues (2017) found that lower fractional anisotropy in three pathways projecting from the nucleus basalis of Maynert may be responsible for both the specific executive dysfunction common in VCI and may partially mediate downstream difficulty seen on these assessing episodic memory, language, and processing speed. These pathways projected to the bilateral cingulum, bilateral external capsule, and bilateral claustrum, respectively. A longitudinal study of individuals with mixed VCI/AD pathology and pure VCI found that those with mixed pathology characterized by amyloid-beta depositions declined faster and to a more severe degree over the 3 years following a vascular event (W. Liu et al., 2015).

In sum, the literature on profiles of neuropsychological deficits associated with suspected VCI generally supports the notion of differential impairment on tests of executive control for patients with subcortical cerebrovascular accident and subcortical white matter disease. However, the neuropsychological tests employed in these studies are quite variable. The exact relationship between performance on executive tests and performance on neuropsychological tests measuring other domains of cognition are lacking. Finally, virtually all prior studies have been empirical in nature and have not put forward an explanation of the neurocognitive constructs or mechanisms that underlie or explain why subcortical vascular disease results in differential executive impairment. In this regard, the imaging and electrophysiological literature cited above offer some intriguing possibilities.

5. Biomarkers for Vascular Cognitive Impairment

Recently, there has been great interest in a variety of physiological biomarkers and their ability to identify individuals who may be either clinically diagnosed with VCI and/or to predict the eventual onset of dementia.

5.1. Arterial Integrity and VCI

There has been recent interest in measuring intima-media thickness to obtain a measure of carotid stenosis (Johnston et al., 2004; Talelli et al., 2004). Li and colleagues (2017) observed that, in a poststroke Chinese sample using the MMSE, the degree of carotid artery stenosis was positively correlated with VCI risk after 1 year. Carotid-femoral pulse wave velocity (PWV) is another technique used to assess arterial integrity. Several research groups have used PWV as a measure of arterial "stiffness." Hughes and colleagues (2018) reported associations between arterial stiffness detected with PWV and lower brain volume in brain regions vulnerable to AD pathology, as well as elevated white matter hyperintensity burden, particularly among MCI individuals.

Another potential arterial biomarker is increased distal resistance to blood flow, as measured by calculating a middle cerebral artery-pulsatility index (MCA-PI), obtainable via ultrasound of the M1 segment of both middle cerebral arteries. López-Olóriz and colleagues (2014) recruited an asymptomatic, community-living, middle-aged sample with a high risk for stroke and VCI, who underwent neuropsychological assessment, ultrasound, and MRI. Neuropsychological performance, MCA-PI, and white matter integrity were independently associated with one another in this sample, with elevated MCA-PI correlating with reduced performance in executive functioning, attention, verbal fluency, episodic memory, and psychomotor speed. Increased MCA-PI may be indicative of white matter lesion volume (Xiong et al., 2013) and leukoaraiosis (Webb et al., 2012) in stroke patients.

A longitudinal study of the Cardiovascular Health Study Cognition Study tracked dementia conversion of 532 older adults between 1998 and 2013 (Cui et al., 2018). PWV was significantly associated with dementia risk among older adults and weakly associated with MCI, while measures of blood pressure were not. These results aligned with those of the Framingham Heart Study, who sampled 1,101 participants and observed an increased 10-year risk for MCI, AD, and all-cause dementia associated with PWV (Pase et al., 2016). However, the association between PWV and incident dementia was only significant among non-diabetic participants in this sample, while hypertension was not associated with alternations in cognition.

These types of biomarkers are relatively inexpensive and non-invasive. Combining information derived from these techniques with comprehensive neuropsychological assessment and information derived from MRI studies could offer more insight into the interaction between vascular anatomy and cognitive functioning. These research paradigms show promise that an analysis of arterial integrity might be an effective biomarker for VCI and/VaD.

5.2. Blood Biomarkers and VCI

In connection with subcortical small vessel disease, several potential biomarkers of VCI have been identified including elevated cerebrospinal fluid (CSF)/blood albumin ratio, which is thought to indicate blood–brain barrier disruption; CSF neurofilment, a marker of axonal damage; altered CSF matrix metalloproteinases, indicating extracellular matrix breakdown; and blood inflammatory cytokines and adhesion molecules (Wallin et al., 2017). Evidence reported by Guoping and colleagues (2015) suggests a change in peripheral T cell immune response may be a marker of VCI. In a study of poststroke patients with vascular MCI, VaD, and no cognitive impairment, VCI patients demonstrated a decrease in $CD4^+$ regulatory T cells that play a role in managing inflammation and an increase in interleukin 6, a tumor necrosis factor. These markers were also associated with lower performance on the executive function subscale of the Vascular Dementia Assessment Scale cognitive subscale (VDAS-cog).

6. Treatment and Public Health Issues

Less studied, but equally important as identifying the constituent components of VCI, is research documenting the societal costs associated with VCI (Hill, Fillit, Shah, del Valle, & Futterman, 2005; Rockwood, Brown, Merry, Sketris, & Fisk, 2002; Sicras et al., 2005). Hsu and colleagues (2018) reported that aerobic training improved executive function and neuronal efficiency involving frontoparietal neuro-networks after 6 months among older adults who have had subcortical ischemic events. Pedelty and Nyenhuis (2006) suggested that anticholinesterase agents and *N*-methyl-d-aspartate (NMDA) antagonists may result in clinical improvement among patients with VCI. To treat VCI, these researchers stress the need for the early identification and prevention of risk factors associated with vascular disease.

There also has been interest in the possible beneficial role of vitamin antioxidants in the treatment of VCI. In a study conducted in southern Italy the "Mediterranean diet," which includes high-energy intake of monounsaturated fatty acids, was associated with reduction of neurocognitive impairments (Panza et al., 2004). Recent guidelines for the prevention of stroke and transient ischemic attack advocate for the use of antithrombotic, antihypertensive, and lipid-lowering drugs in conjunction with exercise and a diet high in fish, fiber, fruits, vegetables, and olive oil (Kernan et al., 2014). The Mediterranean diet also allows for modest alcohol consumption. Data from the Rotterdam Study (Ruitenberg et al., 2002) found that light to moderate drinking (one to three drinks per day) was associated with a lower risk of any dementia (hazard ratio 0.58, 95% confidence interval 0.38–0.90) including VaD. The Dietary Approach to Stop Hypertension (DASH) is a nonpharmacological method of managing high blood pressure and has been shown to be effective in reducing risk for CVD, with improved effectiveness in individuals with higher cardiometabolic risk (Siervo et al., 2015). The Mediterranean–DASH Diet Intervention for Neurodegenerative Delay (MIND) diet attempts to integrate these dietary approaches to risk factor management, and highlights the empirical support for green leafy vegetables and berries in preventing cognitive decline (Morris et al., 2015). Douiri and colleagues (2013) reported on prevention of VCI in a large sample drawn from the South London Stroke Resister. In this sample, there was a reduced risk among those with a history of ischemic stroke for developing cognitive impairment with treatments using an antihypertensive medication, statin, or a combination of aspirin and dipyridamole. A combination of antihypertensive, antithrombotic agents, and lipid-lowering agents also contribute to reduced risk for VCI. Dementia prevalence studies report that incident dementia, regardless of type, may be declining in high-income, developed countries (Langa et al., 2017; Prince et al., 2016), where medication to manage cardiovascular disease risk factors are more affordable and available (Khatib et al., 2016). The impact of this decline in prevalence has been difficult to measure and may be attenuated by longer survival with dementia (Prince et al., 2016).

7. Summary

As noted, during the late 1980s and 1990s there was tendency to view AD and VaD as separate and distinct entities. We now understand that the separation of AD from VaD is more nuanced and more complex than previously appreciated (Libon et al., 2014). Research into VCI provides an excellent platform by which to study brain–behavior relationships and is the latest chapter in the evolving study of the interaction between AD and VaD.

The population and clinic studies reviewed above suggest individuals with VCI who may be at risk for the future development of VaD can be identified. The most common methods for identifying persons with suspected VCI includes a combination of neuropsychological tests and close attention to medical risk factors for stroke. VCI appears to be associated with a relatively greater impairment on tests assessing executive functions including working memory and information processing speed. Emerging assessment techniques such as measuring carotid intima-media thickness and arterial PWV might become tools that can help identify those at risk for developing VCI. The analysis of blood biomarkers also holds promise in furthering our understanding of prodromal dementia states.

In North America, the ongoing retirement of the baby boomer generation has sharpened our interest in identifying prodromal dementia states as early as possible. However, dementia is a worldwide public health problem. The manner in which dementia presents in various parts of the world is likely quite diverse. For all of these reasons, greater sophistication is needed to operationally define VCI. Combining statistical modeling procedures using the previously discussed assessment techniques, along with the longitudinal assessment of participants drawn from both the community and memory clinics, may ultimately lead to appropriate diagnostic criteria. The development of these criteria has the potential of preventing and alleviating suffering throughout the world.

References

Albert, M. S. (2002). Memory decline: The boundary between aging and age-related disease. *Annals of Neurology*, *51*(3), 282–284. http://doi.org/10.1002/ana.10156

American Psychiatric Association. (2013). *Diagnostic and Statistical Manual of Mental Disorders* (5th ed.). Arlington, VA: American Psychiatric Association.

An, X., & Li, C. (2015). Analysis of risk factors for vascular cognitive impairment in patients with cerebral infarction. *Cell Biochemistry and Biophysics*, *71*(2), 673–677. http://doi.org/10.1007/s12013-014-0246-4

Andruita, D., Roussel, M., Barbay, M., Despretz-Wannepain, S., Godefroy, O.; GRECogVASC Study Group. (2018). Differentiating between Alzheimer's disease and vascular cognitive impairment: Is the "memory versus executive function" contrast still relevant? *Journal of Alzheimer's Disease*, *63*, 625–633.

Bowler, J. V. (2004). Vascular cognitive impairment. *Stroke*, *36*, 386–388. http://doi.org/10.1161/01.str.0000115301.12426.2b

Bowler, J. V. (2005). Vascular cognitive impairment. *Journal of Neurology, Neurosurgery, and Psychiatry*, *76*, 35–44. http://doi.org/10.1136/jnnp.2005.082313

Bowler, J. V., & Hachinski, V. C. (1995). Vascular cognitive impairment: A new approach to vascular dementia. *Bailliere's Clinical Neurology*, *4*(2), 357–376.

Cui, C., Sekikawa, A., Kuller, L. H., Lopez, O. L., Newman, A. B., Kuipers, A. L., & Mackey, R. H. (2018). Aortic stiffness is associated with increased risk of incident dementia in older adults. *Journal of Alzheimer's Disease*, *66*(1), 297–306. http://doi.org/10.3233/JAD-180449

Desmond, D. W. (2004). The neuropsychology of vascular cognitive impairment: Is there a specific cognitive deficit? *Journal of the Neurological Sciences*, *226*(1–2), 3–7. http://doi.org/10.1016/j.jns.2004.09.002

Devasenapathy, A., & Hachinski, V. C. (2000). Vascular cognitive impairment. *Current Treatment Options in Neurology*, *2*, 61–71.

Douiri, A., McKevitt, C., Emmett, E. S., Rudd, A. G., & Wolfe, C. D. A. (2013). Long-term effects of secondary prevention on cognitive function in stroke patients. *Circulation*, *128*(12), 1341–1348. http://doi.org/10.1161/CIRCULATIONAHA.113.002236

Duncombe, J., Kitamura, A., Hase, Y., Ihara, M., Kalaria, R. N., & Horsburgh, K. (2017). Chronic cerebral hypoperfusion: a key mechanism leading to vascular cognitive impairment and dementia: Closing the translational gap between rodent models and human vascular cognitive impairment and dementia. *Clinical Science*, *131*(19), 2451–2468. http://doi.org/10.1042/CS20160727

Erkinjuntti, T. (2003). Subcortical ischemic vascular disease and dementia. *International Psychogeriatrics*, *15*(Suppl. 1), 23–26.

Erkinjuntti, T., & Rockwood, K. (2003). Vascular dementia. *Seminars in Clinical Neuropsychiatry*, *8*(1), 37–45. http://doi.org/10.1053/scnp.2003.50004

Garrett, K. D., Browndyke, J. N., Whelihan, W., Paul, R. H., DiCarlo, M., Moser, D. J., . . . Ott, B. R. (2004). The neuropsychological profile of vascular cognitive impairment—no dementia: Comparisons to patients at risk for cerebrovascular disease and vascular dementia. *Archives of Clinical Neuropsychology, 19*(6), 745–757. http://doi.org/10.1016/j.acn.2003.09.008

Gasparovic, C., Prestopnik, J., Thompson, J., Taheri, S., Huisa, B., Schrader, R., . . . Rosenberg, G. A. (2013). 1H-MR spectroscopy metabolite levels correlate with executive function in vascular cognitive impairment. *Journal of Neurology, Neurosurgery and Psychiatry, 84*(7), 715–721. http://doi.org/10.1136/jnnp-2012-303878

Gorelick, P. B., Scuteri, A., Black, S. E., Decarli, C., Greenberg, S. M., Iadecola, C., . . . Seshadri, S. (2011). Vascular contributions to cognitive impairment and dementia: A statement for healthcare professionals from the American Heart Association/American Stroke Association. *Stroke, 42*(9), 2672–2713. http://doi.org/10.1161/STR.0b013e3182299496

Graham, J. E., Rockwood, K., Beattie, B. L., Eastwood, R., Gauthier, S., Tuokko, H., & McDowell, I. (1997). Prevalence and severity of cognitive impairment with and without dementia in an elderly population. *Lancet, 349*(9068), 1793–1796. http://doi.org/10.1016/S0140-6736(97)01007-6

Grau-Olivares, M., Arboix, A., Junqué, C., Arenaza-Urquijo, E. M., Rovira, M., & Bartrés-Faz, D. (2010). Progressive gray matter atrophy in lacunar patients with vascular mild cognitive impairment. *Cerebrovascular Diseases, 30*(2), 157–166. http://doi.org/10.1159/000316059

Guoping, P., Wei, W., Xiaoyan, L., Fangping, H., Zhongqin, C., & Benyan, L. (2015). Characteristics of the peripheral T cell immune response of patients at different stages of vascular cognitive impairment. *Immunology Letters, 168*(1), 120–125. http://doi.org/10.1016/j.imlet.2015.09.015

Hachinski, V. C. (1994). Vascular dementia: A radical redefinition. *Dementia (Basel, Switzerland), 5*(3–4), 130–132.

Hachinski, V. C., Iliff, L. D., Zilhka, E., Du Boulay, G. H., McAllister, V. L., Marshall, J., . . . Symon, L. (1975). Cerebral blood flow in dementia. *Archives of Neurology, 32*(9), 632–637. http://doi.org/10.1001/archneur.1975.00490510088009

Hachinski, V. C., Lassen, N. A., & Marshall, J. (1974). Multi-infarct dementia. A cause of mental deterioration in the elderly. *Lancet (London, England), 2*(7874), 207–210. http://doi.org/10.1016/s0140-6736(74)91496-2

Hill, J., Fillit, H., Shah, S. N., del Valle, M. C., & Futterman, R. (2005). Patterns of healthcare utilization costs for vascular dementia in a community-dwelling population. *Journal of Alzheimer's Disease, 8*, 43–50.

Hsu, C. L., Best, J. R., Davis, J. C., Nagamatsu, L. S., Wang, S., Boyd, L. A., . . . Liu-Ambrose, T. (2018). Aerobic exercise promotes executive functions and impacts functional neural activity among older adults with vascular cognitive impairment. *British Journal of Sports Medicine, 52*(3), 184–191. http://doi.org/10.1136/bjsports-2016-096846

Hughes, T. M., Wagenknecht, L. E., Craft, S., Mintz, A., Heiss, G., Palta, P., . . . Gottesman, R. F. (2018). Arterial stiffness and dementia pathology: Atherosclerosis Risk in Communities (ARIC)-PET Study. *Neurology, 90*(14), e1248–e1256. http://doi.org/10.1212/WNL.0000000000005259

Johnston, S. C., O'Meara, E. S., Manolio, T. A., Lefkowitz, D., O'Leary, D. H., Goldstein, S., . . . Longstreth, W. T., Jr. (2004). Cognitive impairment and decline are associated with carotid artery disease in patients without clinically evident cerebrovascular disease. *Annals of Internal Medicine, 140*, 237–247.

Jokinen, H., Kalska, H., Mantyla, R., Pohjasvaara, T., Ylikoski, R., Hietanen, M., . . . Erkinjuntti, T. (2006). Cognitive profile of subcortical ischaemic vascular disease. *Journal of Neurology, Neurosurgery, and Psychiatry*, *77*, 28–33.

Kernan, W. N., Ovbiagele, B., Black, H. R., Bravata, D. M., Chimowitz, M. I., Ezekowitz, M. D., . . . Wilson, J. A. (2014). Guidelines for the prevention of stroke in patients with stroke and transient ischemic attack: A guideline for healthcare professionals from the American Heart Association/American Stroke Association. *Stroke*, *45*, 2160–2236. http://doi.org/10.1161/STR.0000000000000024

Khatib, R., McKee, M., Shannon, H., Chow, C., Rangarajan, S., Teo, K., . . . Yusuf, S. (2016). Availability and affordability of cardiovascular disease medicines and their effect on use in high-income, middle-income, and low-income countries: An analysis of the PURE study data. *The Lancet*, *387*(10013), 61–69. http://doi.org/10.1016/S0140-6736(15)00469-9

Kramer, J. H., Reed, B. R., Mungas, D., Weiner, M. W., & Chui, H. C. (2002). Executive dysfunction in subcortical ischaemic vascular disease. *Journal of Neurology, Neurosurgery, and Psychiatry*, *72*(2), 217–220.

Lamar, M., Price, C. C., Cynthia, D., Kaplan, E., & Libon, D. J. (2002). Capacity to maintain mental set in dementia. *Neuropsychologia*, *40*(4), 435–445. http://doi.org/10.1016/s0028-3932(01)00125-7

Lamar, M., Price, C. C., Libon, D. J., Penney, D. L., Kaplan, E., Grossman, M., & Heilman, K. M. (2007). Alterations in working memory as a function of leukoaraiosis in dementia. *Neuropsychologia*, *45*(2), 245–254. http://doi.org/10.1016/j.neuropsychologia.2006.07.009

Langa, K. M., Larson, E. B., Crimmins, E. M., Faul, J. D., Levine, D. A., Kabeto, M. U., & Weir, D. R. (2017). A comparison of the prevalence of dementia in the United States in 2000 and 2012. *JAMA Internal Medicine*, *177*(1), 51. http://doi.org/10.1001/jamainternmed.2016.6807

Li, X., Ma, X., Lin, J., He, X., Tian, F., & Kong, D. (2017). Severe carotid artery stenosis evaluated by ultrasound is associated with post stroke vascular cognitive impairment. *Brain and Behavior*, *7*(1), 1–7. http://doi.org/10.1002/brb3.606

Libon, D. J., Bogdanoff, B., Cloud, B. S., Skalina, S., Carew, T. G., Gitlin, H. L., & Bonavita, J. (1998). Motor Learning and quantitative measures of the hippocampus and subcortical white alterations in Alzheimer's disease and Ischaemic Vascular Dementia. *Journal of Clinical and Experimental Neuropsychology*, *20*, 30–41.

Libon, D. J., Bondi, M. W., Price, C. C., Lamar, M., Eppig, J., Wambach, D. M., . . . Penney, D. L. (2011). Verbal serial list learning in mild cognitive impairment: A profile analysis of interference, forgetting, and errors. *Journal of the International Neuropsychological Society*, *17*(5), 905–914. http://doi.org/10.1017/S1355617711000944

Libon, D. J., Drabick, D. A. G., Giovannetti, T., Price, C. C., Bondi, M. W., Eppig, J., . . . Swenson, R. (2014). Neuropsychological syndromes associated with Alzheimer's/Vascular spectrum dementia: A latent class analysis. *Journal of Alzheimer's Disease*, *42*, 999–1014.

Libon, D. J., Price, C. C., Davis Garrett, K., & Giovannetti, T. (2004). From Binswanger's disease to leuokoaraiosis: What we have learned about subcortical vascular dementia. *Clinical Neuropsychologist*, *18*(1), 83–100. http://doi.org/10.1080/13854040490507181

Libon, D. J., Price, C. C., Heilman, K. M., & Grossman, M. (2006). Alzheimer's "other dementia." *Cognitive and Behavioral Neurology*, *19*, 112–116.

Liu, Q., Zhu, Z., Teipel, S. J., Yang, J., Xing, Y., Tang, Y., & Jia, J. (2017). White matter damage in the cholinergic system contributes to cognitive impairment in subcortical vascular cognitive impairment, no dementia. *Frontiers in Aging Neuroscience, 9*, 1–9. http://doi.org/10.3389/fnagi.2017.00047

Liu, W., Wong, A., Au, L., Yang, J., Wang, Z., Leung, E. Y. L., . . . Mok, V. C. T. (2015). Influence of amyloid-β on cognitive decline after stroke/transient ischemic attack: Three-year longitudinal study. *Stroke, 46*(11), 3074–3080. http://doi.org/10.1161/STROKEAHA.115.010449

López-Olóriz, J., López-Cancio, E., Arenillas, J. F., Hernández, M., Dorado, L., Dacosta-Aguayo, R., . . . Mataró, M. (2014). Diffusion tensor imaging, intracranial vascular resistance and cognition in middle-aged asymptomatic subjects. *Cerebrovascular Diseases, 38*(1), 24–30. http://doi.org/10.1159/000363620

Moorhouse, P., & Rockwood, K. (2008). Vascular cognitive impairment: current concepts and clinical developments. *Lancet Neurology, 7*(3), 246–255. http://doi.org/10.1016/S1474-4422(08)70040-1

Morris, M. C., Tangney, C. C., Wang, Y., Sacks, F. M., Barnes, L. L., Bennett, D. A., & Aggarwal, N. T. (2015). MIND diet slows cognitive decline with aging. *Alzheimer's & Dementia, 11*(9), 1015–1022. http://doi.org/10.1016/j.jalz.2015.04.011

Nakaoku, Y., Oishi, N., Hase, Y., Hase, M., Saito, S., Mitsueda, T., . . . Takahashi, R. (2018). Montreal Cognitive Assessment score correlates with regional cerebral blood flow in post-stroke patients. *Clinical Neurology and Neurosurgery, 174*, 68–74. http://doi.org/10.1016/j.clineuro.2018.09.004

Nyenhuis, D. L., Gorelick, P. B., Geenen, E. J., Smith, C. A., Gencheva, E., Freels, S., & deToledo-Morrell, L. (2004). The pattern of neuropsychological deficits in Vascular Cognitive Impairment-No Dementia (Vascular CIND). *Clinical Neuropsychologist, 18*(1), 41–49. http://doi.org/10.1080/13854040490507145

Ohara, T., Hata, J., Yoshida, D., Mukai, N., Nagata, M., Iwaki, T., . . . Ninomiya, T. (2017). Trends in dementia prevalence, incidence, and survival rate in a Japanese community. *Neurology, 88*(20), 1925–1932. http://doi.org/10.1212/WNL.0000000000003932

Panza, F., Solfrizzi, V., Colacicco, A. M., D'Introno, A., Capurso, C., Torres, F., . . . Capurso, A. (2004). Mediterranean diet and cognitive decline. *Public Health Nutrition, 7*(7), 959–963.

Pase, M. P., Beiser, A., Himali, J. J., Tsao, C., Satizabal, C. L., Vasan, R. S., . . . Mitchell, G. F. (2016). Aortic stiffness and the risk of incident mild cognitive impairment and dementia. *Stroke, 47*(9), 2256–2261. http://doi.org/10.1161/STROKEAHA.116.013508

Pedelty, L., & Nyenhuis, D. L. (2006). Vascular cognitive impairment. *Current Treatment Options in Cardiovascular Medicine, 8*(3), 243–250.

Price, C. C., Jefferson, A. L., Merino, J. G., Heilman, K. M., & Libon, D. J. (2005). Subcortical vascular dementia: integrating neuropsychological and neuroradiologic data. *Neurology, 65*(3), 376–382. http://doi.org/10.1212/01.wnl.0000168877.06011.15

Prince, M., Ali, G. C., Guerchet, M., Prina, A. M., Albanese, E., & Wu, Y. T. (2016). Recent global trends in the prevalence and incidence of dementia, and survival with dementia. *Alzheimer's Research and Therapy, 8*(1). http://doi.org/10.1186/s13195-016-0188-8

Ramirez-Gomez, L., Zheng, L., Reed, B. R., Kramer, J., Mungas, D., Zarow, C., . . . Chui, H. (2017). Neuropsychological profiles differentiate Alzheimer disease from subcortical ischemic vascular dementia in an autopsy-defined cohort. *Dement Geriatr Cogn Disord, 44*, 1–11. http://doi.org/10.1097/OGX.0000000000000256.Prenatal

Reed, B. R., Eberling, J. L., Mungas, D., Weiner, M., Kramer, J. H., & Jagust, W. J. (2004). Effects of white matter lesions and lacunes on cortical function. *Archives of Neurology, 61*(10), 1545–1550. http://doi.org/10.1001/archneur.61.10.1545

Rist, P. M., Chalmers, J., Arima, H., Anderson, C., MacMahon, S., Woodward, M., . . . Tzourio, C. (2013). Baseline cognitive function, recurrent stroke, and risk of dementia in patients with stroke. *Stroke, 44*(7), 1790–1795. http://doi.org/10.1161/STROKEAHA.111.680728

Rockwood, K., Brown, M., Merry, H., Sketris, I., & Fisk, J. (2002). Societal costs of vascular cognitive impairment in older adults. *Stroke, 33*(6), 1605–1609.

Román, G. C., Sachdev, P., Royall, D. R., Bullock, R. A., Orgogozo, J.-M., Lopez-Pousa, S., . . . Wallin, A. (2004). Vascular cognitive disorder: a new diagnostic category updating vascular cognitive impairment and vascular dementia. *Journal of the Neurological Sciences, 226*(1–2), 81–87. http://doi.org/10.1016/j.jns.2004.09.016

Ruitenberg, A., Van Swieten, J. C., Witteman, J. C. M., Mehta, K. M., Van Duijn, C. M., Hofman, A., & Breteler, M. M. B. (2002). Alcohol consumption and risk of dementia: The Rotterdam Study. *Lancet, 359*(9303), 281–286. http://doi.org/10.1016/S0140-6736(02)07493-7

Sachdev, P. S., Brodaty, H., Valenzuela, M., Wen, W., Ross, A., Howard, L., . . . Berman, K. (2004). The neuropsychological profile of vascular cognitive impairment in stroke patients. *International Psychogeriatrics, 15*, 72–73.

Sachdev, P. S., Kalaria, R., O'Brien, J., Skoog, I., Alladi, S., Black, S. E., . . . Scheltens, P. (2014). Diagnostic criteria for vascular cognitive disorders. *Alzheimer Disease & Associated Disorders, 28*(3), 206–218. http://doi.org/10.1097/WAD.0000000000000034

Schneider, J. A., Arvanitakis, Z., Leurgans, S. E., & Bennett, D. A. (2009). The neuropathology of probable Alzheimer's disease and mild cognitive impairment. *Annals of Neurology, 66*(2), 200–208.

Sicras, A., Rejas, J., Arco, S., Flores, E., Ortega, G., Esparcia, A., . . . Gordillo, M. J. (2005). Prevalence, resource utilization and costs of vascular dementia compared to Alzheimer's dementia in a population setting. *Dementia and Geriatric Cognitive Disorders, 19*(5–6), 305–315. http://doi.org/10.1159/000084556

Siervo, M., Lara, J., Chowdhury, S., Ashor, A., Oggioni, C., & Mathers, J. C. (2015). Effects of the dietary approach to stop hypertension (DASH) diet on cardiovascular risk factors: A systematic review and meta-analysis. *British Journal of Nutrition, 113*(1), 1–15. http://doi.org/10.1017/S0007114514003341

Skrobot, O. A., O'Brien, J. T., Black, S., Chen, C., DeCarli, C., Erkinjuntti, T., . . . Kehoe, P. G. (2017). The Vascular Impairment of Cognition Classification Consensus Study. *Alzheimer's & Dementia : The Journal of the Alzheimer's Association, 13*(6), 624–633. http://doi.org/10.1016/j.jalz.2016.10.007

Smith, E. E. (2017). Clinical presentations and epidemiology of vascular dementia. *Clinical Science, 131*(11), 1059–1068. http://doi.org/10.1042/CS20160607

Smith, E. E., Muzikansky, A., McCreary, C. R., Batool, S., Viswanathan, A., Dickerson, B. C., . . . Blacker, D. (2018). Impaired memory is more closely associated with brain beta-amyloid than leukoaraiosis in hypertensive patients with cognitive symptoms. *PLOS ONE, 13*(1), e0191345. http://doi.org/10.1371/journal.pone.0191345

Smith, E. E., O'Donnell, M., Dagenais, G., Lear, S. A., Wielgosz, A., Sharma, M., . . . Yusuf, S. (2015). Early cerebral small vessel disease and brain volume, cognition, and gait. *Annals of Neurology, 77*(2), 251–261. http://doi.org/10.1002/ana.24320

Stephan, B. C. M., Minett, T., Muniz-Terrera, G., Harrison, S. L., Matthews, F. E., & Brayne, C. (2017). Neuropsychological profiles of vascular disease and risk of dementia: Implications for defining vascular cognitive impairment no dementia (VCI-ND). *Age and Ageing*, *46*(5), 755–760. http://doi.org/10.1093/ageing/afx016

Takahashi, Y., Saito, S., Yamamoto, Y., Uehara, T., Yokota, C., Sakai, G., . . . Ihara, M. (2019). Visually-rated medial temporal lobe atrophy with lower educational history as a quick indicator of amnestic cognitive impairment after stroke. *Journal of Alzheimer's Disease*, *67*(2), 621–629. http://doi.org/10.3233/JAD-180976

Talelli, P., Ellul, J., Terzis, G., Lekka, N. P., Gioldasis, G., Chrysanthopoulou, A., & Papapetropoulos, T. (2004). Common carotid artery intima media thickness and post-stroke cognitive impairment. *Journal of the Neurological Sciences*, *223*(2), 129–134. http://doi.org/10.1016/j.jns.2004.05.013

Villeneuve, S., Belleville, S., Massoud, F., Bocti, C., & Gauthier, S. (2009). Impact of vascular risk factors and diseases on cognition in persons with mild cognitive impairment. *Dementia and Geriatric Cognitive Disorders*, *27*(4), 375–381. http://doi.org/10.1159/000209965

Wallin, A., Kapaki, E., Boban, M., Engelborghs, S., Hermann, D. M., Huisa, B., . . . Rosenberg, G. (2017). Biochemical markers in vascular cognitive impairment associated with subcortical small vessel disease: A consensus report. *BMC Neurology*, *17*(1), 1–12. http://doi.org/10.1186/s12883-017-0877-3

Wardlaw, J. M., Smith, E. E., Biessels, G. J., Cordonnier, C., Fazekas, F., Frayne, R., . . . Dichgans, M. (2013). Neuroimaging standards for research into small vessel disease and its contribution to ageing and neurodegeneration. *Lancet Neurology*, *12*(8), 822–838. http://doi.org/10.1016/S1474-4422(13)70124-8

Webb, A. J. S., Simoni, M., Mazzucco, S., Kuker, W., Schulz, U., & Rothwell, P. M. (2012). Increased cerebral arterial pulsatility in patients with leukoaraiosis: Arterial stiffness enhances transmission of aortic pulsatility. *Stroke*, *43*(10), 2631–2636. http://doi.org/10.1161/STROKEAHA.112.655837

Xiong, Y. Y., Mok, V. C. T., Wong, A., Leung, T., Chen, X. Y., Chu, W. C. W., . . . Wong, K. S. (2013). Evaluation of age-related white matter changes using transcranial Doppler ultrasonography. *Journal of Neuroimaging*, *23*(1), 53–57. http://doi.org/10.1111/j.1552-6569.2011.00649.x

Zanetti, M., Ballabio, C., Abbate, C., Cutaia, C., Vergani, C., & Bergamaschini, L. (2006). Mild cognitive impairment subtypes and vascular dementia in community-dwelling elderly people: A 3-year follow-up study. *Journal of the American Geriatrics Society*, *54*(4), 580–586. http://doi.org/10.1111/j.1532-5415.2006.00658.x

Zhang, Y., Xu, Y., Nie, H., Lei, T., Wu, Y., Zhang, L., & Zhang, M. (2012). Prevalence of dementia and major dementia subtypes in the Chinese populations: A meta-analysis of dementia prevalence surveys, 1980-2010. *Journal of Clinical Neuroscience*, *19*(10), 1333–1337. http://doi.org/10.1016/j.jocn.2012.01.029

Zhao, L., Biesbroek, J. M., Shi, L., Liu, W., Kuijf, H. J., Chu, W. W. C., . . .Wong, A. (2018). Strategic infarct location for post-stroke cognitive impairment: A multivariate lesion-symptom mapping study. *Journal of Cerebral Blood Flow and Metabolism*, *38*(8), 1299–1311. http://doi.org/10.1177/0271678X17728162

5

Decline in Everyday Functioning in MCI and Dementia

A Neuropsychological Perspective

Rachel Mis and Tania Giovannetti

1. Introduction

Everyday activities, such as grooming and meal preparation, are cognitively complex tasks that involve the coordination of multiple cognitive, perceptual, and motor operations. Consequently, it is not surprising that as cognition changes over time, older adults experience changes in their ability to smoothly and efficiently perform everyday activities. Mild difficulties in the performance of everyday tasks have been reported in people with MCI; in dementia, impairment in everyday activities is a diagnostic criterion that is associated with a wide spectrum of negative outcomes. Everyday difficulties have been linked to decreased quality of life, frustration, depression (Adam, van der Linden, Jullerat, & Salmon, 2000; Espiritu et al., 2001; Hargrave, Reed, & Mungus, 2000), and institutionalization (Knopman, Berg, & Thomas, 1999; Knopman, Kitto, Deinard, & Heiring, 1988; Newens, Forster, & Kay, 1995; Smith, Kokmen, & O'Brien, 2000) as well as caregiver burden (DeBettignies, Mahurin, & Pirozzolo, 1990) and costs of care (Albert et al., 1999; Wolinsky, Callahan, Fitzgerald, & Johnson, 1993). Neuropsychologists are often consulted to comment on patients' abilities to live independently and to make recommendations on methods of improving everyday functioning. Therefore, it is imperative to understand the association between the cognitive constructs that are precisely measured in the neuropsychological evaluation and everyday functioning.

Rachel Mis and Tania Giovannetti, *Decline in Everyday Functioning in MCI and Dementia* In: *Vascular Disease, Alzheimer's Disease, and Mild Cognitive Impairment.* Edited by: David J. Libon, Melissa Lamar, Rodney A. Swenson, Kenneth M. Heilman, Oxford University Press (2020). © Oxford University Press. DOI: 10.1093/oso/9780190634230.003.0006

2. Terminology and Methodology

2.1. Terminology

The terminology used in the literature on everyday functioning varies widely but should be precisely defined to prevent confusion. The terms "activities of daily living" (ADL) or "instrumental activities of daily living" (IADL) have been used to refer to a range of basic (ADL) and complex (IADL) activities that are necessary for successful daily functioning. ADL and IADL include ambulation and transportation, communication, toileting, meal preparation, and a range of other tasks. In our research, we prefer the term "everyday activities" to denote a subset of ADL/IADL that possess the following features: (a) multiple subtasks and steps; (b) serial order constraints on task steps; (c) require object selection and use; and (d) a practical end-goal. Everyday activities require the coordination of numerous neurocognitive functions, including object selection, tool use, serial ordering, sustained attention, working memory, performance/error monitoring, and others. Other terms have been used to denote everyday activities in the literature, including "routine activities/ action," "naturalistic activities/ action," and "pragmatic action" (Schwartz, 2006; Schwartz & Buxbaum, 1997).

An array of terms also has been used to refer to difficulties performing everyday activities, including "ideational apraxia," "conceptual apraxia," "action disorganization syndrome," "disability," and so on (Humphreys & Forde, 1998; Ochipa, Rothi, & Heilman, 1992; Rothi, Ochipa, & Heilman, 1991; Schwartz, 2006). Some of these terms denote the putative mechanisms responsible for difficulties (e.g., conceptual apraxia). We prefer the descriptive term "everyday action difficulties" to refer to subtle changes in everyday activities that are reported in healthy aging and are noted with greater frequency or severity in mild cognitive impairment (MCI). We use the term "everyday action impairment" to refer to more serious problems in everyday activities that lead to loss of independence and that are associated with dementia and disability.

2.2. Methodology

Accurate and detailed assessment of everyday actions can be challenging. Most often, clinicians and researchers use questionnaires to evaluate everyday action (Farias et al., 2008; Gitlin, Corcoran, Winter, Boyce, & Hauk, 2001; Lawton &

Brody, 1969; Marcotte & Grant, 2009; Pfeffer, Kurosaki, Harrah, Chance, & Filos, 1982). Patient self-reports have questionable validity due to a range of factors, such as limited insight, impaired memory for errors and problems, poor judgment, denial of deficit, and so on (Hoeymans, Feskens, van den Bos, & Kromhout, 1996; Kempen, Steverink, Ormel, & Deeg, 1996; Kiyak, Teri, & Borson, 1994; Ostbye, Tyas, McDowell, & Koval, 1997; Rubenstein, Schairer, Wieland, & Kane, 1984; Sands, Ferreira, Stewart, Brod, & Yaffe, 2004; Zanetti, Geroldi, Frisoni, Bianchetti, & Trabucchi, 1999). Consequently, neuropsychologists in most settings rely on informant-report questionnaires; however, empirical findings also cast doubt on the validity of informant reports. For example, there is low agreement between informant reports and both clinician reports (Loewenstein et al., 1989; Lukovits & McDaniel, 1992) and performance-based assessment of functional abilities (Loewenstein et al., 1992; Mangone et al., 1993; Martyr & Clare, 2018; Zanetti et al., 1995; Zanetti et al., 1999).

Variability across patients' current and past daily routines is another potential source of error when using questionnaire measures. A person who typically performs only a few everyday tasks throughout the day may be judged by an informant to be less impaired than a person who typically performs a wide array of diverse tasks. Direct observations of everyday action performance have consistently shown very strong effects of task demands (e.g., number of task steps required to reach a goal) and context such as the location of task objects (Bickerton, Humphreys, & Riddoch, 2007; Giovannetti et al., 2007, 2010; Humphreys & Forde, 1998; Schwartz, Fitzpatrick-DeSalme, & Carew, 1995). Even identical tasks that require completion of the very same goal will be more or less difficult depending on the presence of distractor objects or the extent of clutter and disorganization in the home. Thus, failure to control task requirements and contexts precludes the objective evaluation of everyday action impairment. Another limitation of questionnaires is that they fail to provide information regarding patients' specific everyday problems (e.g., failure to complete task steps *vs.* inaccurate execution of task steps). Most rating instruments require collateral informants simply to note whether a patient performs a task independently, with help, or not at all. Functional abilities may be overestimated on such a scale, particularly when patients are able to achieve overall task goals inefficiently or with high rates of errors (Foundas et al., 1995).

Contemporary questionnaires address some of the aforementioned limitations by including questions that target specific functional domains and by asking to report on change in functional abilities from a premorbid level. The Everyday Cognition (ECog) Scale (Farias et al., 2006, 2008) includes a patient and informant version that evaluate recent *changes* in everyday functioning across six domains: memory, visuospatial tasks, organization, language, planning, and divided attention. The ECog includes 39 questions (e.g., memory: "Remembering a few shopping items without a list") that are scored using a 4-point response option, ranging from 1 (better or no change) to 4 (consistently much worse). These scores may be calculated separately for each of the six domains. The ECog was developed following extensive piloting of test questions. It is sensitive to mild difficulties and has excellent psychometric properties (Farias et al., 2006, 2008). A short form of the ECog that includes only 12 items (ECog-12) has also been validated (Farias et al., 2011).

The structure of the ECog is a significant improvement of older questionnaires formats. However, all questionnaires are vulnerable to the limitations associated with an inaccurate or unavailable informant. Informants are rarely screened for cognitive difficulties and yet informants with cognitive limitations may be just as prone to recall or judgment error as patients. Additionally, the stress of caregiving may make informants vulnerable to cognitive failures (Vitaliano et al., 2005). A range of informant characteristics have been examined in relation to reports of everyday functioning, with depression and level of caregiver burden showing significant associations with informant reports of functioning (Arguelles, Loewenstein, Eisdorfer, & Arguelles, 2001; Loewenstein et al., 2001; Martyr & Clare, 2018; Zanetti et al., 1999). Informant ratings also are influenced by the extent of time spent with the patient; even informants who live with patients may rarely *directly* observe patients' performance of everyday tasks, particularly if functional difficulties are mild and do not disrupt independence. Some adults are not comfortable asking a relative to report on their functioning, and many do not have a knowledgeable or healthy informant. As of 2014, over a quarter (28%) of noninstitutionalized adults over age 65 live alone and the proportion of elders living alone increases with advanced age when functional difficulties may be more likely to emerge (e.g., 46% of women aged 75 and over lived alone; U.S. Department of Health and Human Services, 2014).

Performance-based measures address many of the drawbacks of questionnaires, as they (a) do not rely upon the retrospective report and judgment of the patient or an informant, (b) may be standardized for uniform administration across patients, and (c) may be scored using detailed analyses to elucidate the nature of functional deficits across patients and populations. Work from our laboratory has relied heavily on the Naturalistic Action Test (NAT), a performance-based measure (Schwartz, Buxbaum, Ferraro, Veramonti, & Segal, 2003; Schwartz, Segal, Veramonti, Ferraro, & Buxbaum, 2002). The NAT includes a comprehensive error scoring system to code a range of overt error types and characterize the nature of everyday action impairments. The NAT requires the completion of everyday tasks (e.g., prepare toast and coffee, wrap a gift, etc.) with little guidance from the examiner. All necessary objects and distractors are available on the table for each item. Object placement, instructions, cueing, and scoring procedures are standardized and detailed in the test manual (see www.ncrrn.org/assessment/nat). The NAT error taxonomy includes omissions (failure to perform a task step), various types of commissions (inaccurate execution of a task step; e.g., sequence, perseveration, etc.), and action additions (performance of an extra, off-task step). The NAT error taxonomy has been published (Buxbaum, Schwartz, & Montgomery, 1998; Schwartz, Buxbaum et al., 1998; Schwartz, Montgomery et al., 1998; Schwartz et al., 1995; Schwartz, Reed, Montgomery, Palmer, & Mayer, 1991), and other investigators have used very similar detailed schemes to characterize performance on a range of everyday tasks (Forde & Humphreys, 2002; Humphreys & Forde, 1998; Park et al., 2012; Ramsden, Kinsella, Ong, & Storey, 2008). The NAT error coding system offers the opportunity to characterize both overall level of impairment (i.e., total errors) as well as specific functional problems (i.e., error distributions). High interrater reliability and normative data (including cut scores) have been reported (Buxbaum et al., 1998; Giovannetti, Libon, & Hart, 2002; Giovannetti, Libon, Buxbaum, & Schwartz, 2002; Schwartz et al., 2003; Schwartz, Buxbaum et al., 1998; Schwartz, Montgomery et al., 1998; Sestito, Schmidt, Gallo, Giovannetti, & Libon, 2005).

Performance-based assessments have been expanded in several ways to increase the sensitivity for detecting functional changes in healthy older adults and functional difficulties in people with MCI. The error coding system of the NAT has been expanded to include a new error category, called microerrors or microslips (Bettcher, Giovannetti, Macmullen, & Libon, 2008; Giovannetti, Schwartz, & Buxbaum, 2007; Seligman, Giovannetti, Sestito, & Libon, 2014). Microerrors/microslips are inefficient behaviors and erroneous reaching to or touching target and non-target objects (Seligman et al., 2014). Microerrors/microslips are more sensitive to subtle functional difficulties than the more egregious errors (i.e., omission, commission) captured by the original NAT taxonomy (Seligman, Giovannetti, Hulswit, & Divers, 2017; Seligman et al., 2014). Another approach to increase the sensitivity of performance-based tests is to increase task complexity and to require multitasking. The day-out task requires participants to perform several tasks to prepare for a day out (e.g., pack a bag, take medication, plan bus route) in a multiple-room apartment (McAlister & Schmitter-Edgecombe, 2013; Sanders & Schmitter-Edgecombe, 2012). Results from the day-out task have shown that healthy older adults completed tasks less efficiently and accurately than healthy younger adults, and older adults with MCI required more time as well as failed to accurately complete the tasks and were less efficient than healthy older adults (Schmitter-Edgecombe, McAlister, & Weakley, 2012).

One major limitation of performance-based methods is that they require extensive time to administer and score. To address this limitation, investigators have developed nonimmersive virtual reality tasks modeled after the NAT. In older adults with dementia, performance on a virtual kitchen coffee task performed with a mouse interface significantly correlated with performance of real tasks, cognitive tests, and informant reports of functioning. However, scoring of the coffee task was done offline by human coders (Allain et al., 2014). A more recent virtual kitchen task, called the Virtual Kitchen Challenge was designed with a touch screen interface to make the task more naturalistic and enable detection of microerrors (i.e., inefficient misreaching errors). The Virtual Kitchen currently includes two tasks of comparable complexity (breakfast, lunch) selected to be appropriate for individuals with a range of cognitive abilities. The Virtual Kitchen Challenge software enables automated online scoring of detailed metrics pertaining to performance accuracy and efficiency, without the need for human error coding. Preliminary results with the Virtual Kitchen Challenge show healthy older adults perform less efficiently than healthy young adults and automated performance metrics are meaningfully and significantly associated with human error coding, real task performance, and tests of cognitive abilities (Giovannetti et al., 2019).

The benefits of control and standardization afforded by performance-based, laboratory tasks may underestimate functioning in real life where performance may be facilitated by basic drives (e.g., hunger) and the familiar home context (Giovannetti et al., 2006). Alternatively, performance-based assessment may overestimate patients' abilities, because performance is evaluated only for a short time and in a highly structured setting (e.g., with all necessary objects within view and available to the participant without searching or planning; Farias et al., 2008). Only unobtrusive, direct observations in the naturalistic context can offer an unbiased assessment of real world functioning. Home visits by clinicians are expensive and obtrusive (and may bias results); however, advances in home and action monitoring through sensors and wearable technologies are making this approach more accurate, affordable, and efficient (Cook & Schmitter-Edgecombe, 2009). Recent studies have shown differences on automated measures of daily computer use (Kaye et al., 2014) and walking trajectories (Dodge, Mattek, Austin, Hayes, & Kaye, 2012) between healthy elderly and people with MCI. Continuous monitoring yields massive amounts of data and will require advanced analyses to efficiently find meaningful patterns to decipher participants' level of functioning and reasons for functional difficulties. Many direct observation methods also do not offer any form of standardization that will allow for easy aggregation of data or comparisons across participants. For these reasons, home monitoring is generally not incorporated into the clinical evaluation and has only been used in relatively few empirical studies.

Our brief review of the challenges of everyday action assessment highlight several of the limitations of all currently available assessment methods. Because of methodological limitations, it is crucial to consider the goal of the evaluation when selecting the appropriate measure or measures. Questionnaires may be preferred when the evaluation is focused on the impact of neuropsychological deficits on an individual's everyday life, disability, and independence. The decision to use self- or informant-report may be simple (i.e., if an informant is unavailable) or more complex when the capacity of the informant is uncertain and the patient has incomplete insight. Performance-based measures may be preferred when standardized assessment is required to compare performance to a normative sample tested under the same conditions. Performance-based measures also are essential when the focus of the evaluation is to understand *how* everyday action performance is affected by neurocognitive deficits and task context. In an analogous manner, although a list-learning test is an artificial assessment of episodic memory, it is essential to determine the extent of episodic memory impairment relative to a normative sample as well as to determine the extent to which encoding is impaired relative to retrieval, whether the participant engages in organizational strategies or benefits from cues, and so on. Then, the *consequence* of the patient's specific memory difficulties on everyday functioning may be assessed via informant questionnaires or direct observation in the home. Thus, when assessing everyday action, the goal of the evaluation should inform the method for everyday action assessment, and given that all methods have some limitations, a multimodal assessment is almost always optimal.

In the following discussion, we will use the terminology described earlier to review the current literature on everyday functioning in MCI and dementia. Our review will focus on findings from questionnaires and performance-based tests, which when considered together, show meaningful associations between level and type of cognitive impairment and everyday functioning.

3. Cognitive Factors that Affect Everyday Functioning

3.1. Level of Cognitive Impairment

Everyday action impairment associated with loss of autonomy is a core criterion of Alzheimer's disease (AD; Albert et al., 2011; McKhann et al., 2011). Mild to moderate stages of AD involve a loss of independence in complex everyday tasks, such as cooking and managing finances, while the more severe stages of AD involve a loss of the ability to perform basic everyday tasks, such as feeding and bathing oneself (Green, Mohs, Schmeidler, Aryan, & Davis, 1993). Paul and colleagues (2000) reported that participants with vascular dementia (VaD) with both white matter ischemia and cortical infarcts displayed greater cognitive impairment and greater impairment in everyday activities compared to VaD participants with white matter ischemia only, although the groups did not differ on more basic everyday tasks. Although other factors such as behavioral disturbances (Lechowski et al., 2003) and apathy likely play a role (Boyle et al., 2003a), level of cognitive impairment remains one of the strongest predictors of functional ability (Lechowski et al., 2003), such that a more severe impairment in cognition results in a correspondingly more severe impairment in functional activities. Some studies examining the relation between neuropsychiatric disturbances and functional impairment have theorized that psychiatric symptoms arise from neurobiological correlates shared by the cognitive processes relevant to functional abilities (e.g., executive functioning; Tekin, Fairbanks, O'Connor, Rosenberg, & Cummings, 2001).

The extent to which everyday functioning in affected in MCI is less clearly understood (Albert et al., 2011; Brown, Devanand, Liu, Caccappolo, & Alzheimer's Disease Neuroimaging Initiative, 2011). Diagnostic criteria for MCI require that everyday action difficulties, if present, do not rise to the level where there is a loss of independence in functional activities (Albert et al., 2011; McKhann et al., 2011). Nonetheless, recent research suggests that everyday action difficulties are observed in the MCI phase (Bangen et al., 2010; Giovannetti et al., 2008a; Griffith et al., 2003; Farias et al., 2006). Farias and colleagues (2006) found that a sample of participants with MCI reported ratings that were approximately one standard deviation worse than normal controls on the everyday memory domain of the ECog and approximately one half of a standard deviation worse on the remaining domains. Similar to cognitive decline, problems with functional activities start with subtle deficits in healthy older adults and decline gradually (Tucker-Drob, 2011). Importantly, subtle functional changes have even been found to predict conversion from normal aging to MCI (Farias et al., 2013; Nowrangi, Rosenberg, & Leoutsakos, 2016).

Some studies suggest that financial abilities are some of the earliest domains of everyday functioning to decline with increasing cognitive impairment, and difficulty managing finances has been demonstrated to emerge in MCI (Han, Boyle, James, Yu, & Bennett, 2015; Bangen et al., 2010; Griffith et al., 2003; Marson, 2001). Studies examining literacy, or the ability to understand, access, and utilize domain-specific conceptual information, have supported the link between early cognitive decline and difficulties in financial matters (Yu, Wilson, Schneider, Bennett, and Boyle, 2017; Boyle et al., 2013; Han et al. 2015). Lower financial literacy, combined with health literacy, has been shown to predict incident dementia in community-dwelling older adults (Yu et al., 2017), and declines in executive functioning and memory that occur with increasing age have been associated with lowered financial and health literacy in non-demented community-dwelling older adults (Boyle et al., 2013). Other studies suggest that despite experiencing age-related cognitive decline in fluid cognitive abilities (e.g., processing speed, working memory, etc.), healthy older adults continue to make sound financial decisions and adaptive financial behaviors (Li et al., 2015;

Xiao & Chen, 2015). Thus, although difficulties in managing finances may be a sensitive behavioral marker of neurodegenerative processes, further research in this area is required.

Level of cognitive impairment has been shown to differentially influence self- and informant reports of everyday functioning. As stated earlier, informant report is typically preferred over self-report when investigating everyday function in dementia, as people with dementia often demonstrate a tendency to underreport impairments. However, results from recent studies suggest that in the earliest stage of cognitive decline, self-report may be more accurate than informant-report, which may underestimate functional difficulties (Martyr & Clare, 2018). Okonkwo and colleagues examined the relation between self- and informant-report and a performance-based measures of financial ability. In comparing self-report and performance-based measures, although participants with MCI were more likely to overestimate their abilities with increasing cognitive impairment compared to healthy controls, self-reports of financial ability by participants with MCI were more consistent with the performance-based measure than were the informant-reports (Okonkwo et al., 2008). Thus, it may be worth considering level of overall cognitive impairment when selecting the optimal method of everyday action assessment.

Significant discrepancies between self-and informant-report also have been reported in samples including people with MCI and healthy older adults. Edmonds, Delano-Wood, Galasko, Salmon, and Bondi (2014) compared self- versus informant-reports of IADL impairment on the ECog in samples of MCI participants and cognitively normal individuals with subjective cognitive complaints. Participants defined as cognitively normal overreported functional difficulties compared to their informant-reports, whereas participants with amnestic MCI significantly *underreported* functional difficulties as compared to their informant reports. Thus, the discrepancy between self- and informant-report of everyday functioning was related to level cognitive impairment even within a sample of older adults without dementia. As everyday action difficulties could be an important early indicator of risk for progression to dementia, it will be important for future research to understand and characterize the changes in everyday action functioning in healthy and dysfunctional aging as well as determining which methods are most accurate at identifying functional change.

On performance-based tasks of everyday function, level of cognitive impairment has been strongly associated with overall task accomplishment and total errors. Overt errors, particularly omissions, are infrequent in participants at the early stages of cognitive decline but become more frequent as cognitive impairment worsens (Giovannetti, et al., 2008a, 2008b). For example, Giovannetti and colleagues (2008a) found that individuals with MCI made more errors than healthy older adults on the NAT, but fewer errors than people with dementia. MCI participants were similar to controls in the distribution of error types, with approximately 70% of total errors classified as commission (i.e., disorganized sequencing of steps, inaccurate object selection, etc.). By contrast, dementia participants showed a more even distribution of omission and commission errors. Thus, mild cognitive difficulties are associated with increased inefficiency and error-prone action, but as overall level of cognitive impairment increases, individuals are less able to achieve task goals (i.e., they make more omission errors).

The resource theory is an account of everyday action impairment that emphasizes the strong association between everyday action ability and level of global cognitive ability. The resource theory was initially developed to explain the results of three studies on everyday function conducted on stroke and brain injury populations undergoing acute, inpatient rehabilitation (Schwartz, Buxbaum et al., 1998; Schwartz, Montgomery et al., 1998; Buxbaum, 1998). The resource theory posits that impairment in everyday function is best explained by overall level of cognitive functioning, irrespective of the specific cognitive abilities that are affected (e.g., executive functioning, episodic memory). According to the resource theory, everyday activities require attentional resources, which are limited in capacity. Everyday activities also are so cognitively complex that an individual may compensate for specific cognitive impairments by recruiting other intact cognitive processes. For example, a problem with episodic memory may be compensated for by relying on relatively preserved executive skills to organize the task objects before and during task performance. However, such compensation requires additional attentional resources and will make the individual vulnerable to errors at points of the everyday task that are most complex (e.g., when there are many distractors, between subtasks, etc.; Buxbaum, Schwartz, & Montgomery, 1998; Schwartz, Buxbaum et al., 1998; Schwartz, Montgomery et al., 1998; Giovannetti et al., 2002). As a result, the types of errors observed across individuals with different cognitive impairments will be similar. Giovannetti and colleagues (2002) found support for the resource theory in a study of dementia participants. Specifically, overall cognitive functioning was the best predictor of errors on the NAT, and the pattern of overt errors (e.g., omission, sequence, addition, etc.) made by dementia participants was similar to that exhibited by participants with closed head injury and right and left hemisphere stroke, disorders that differ in patterns of cognitive impairments and neuropathology. Later studies described in the following text have not fully supported the resource theory and have suggested that the pattern of everyday action impairment meaningfully differs across individuals with different types of cognitive impairments (i.e., omission–commission model).

3.2. Type of Cognitive Impairment: Episodic Memory and Executive Functioning

The large majority of studies examining the role of specific cognitive processes in everyday functioning using self- or informant-report questionnaires have shown significant associations with measures of episodic memory and executive functioning. Studies of heterogeneous samples have suggested that episodic memory impairment may be most salient in disrupting everyday functioning, particularly in early dementia and MCI (Farias et al., 2006; Kazui et al., 2005; Tuokko, Morris, & Ebert, 2005). However, Boyle and colleagues (2003b) found that measures of executive functioning, but not memory or other cognitive domains, correlated with informant-based ratings of everyday functioning in a sample of participants with VaD.

Other studies have further demonstrated that executive functioning is a strong predictor of future functional decline. Cahn-Weiner et al. (2007) examined the relation between executive functioning, episodic memory, and neuroimaging factors with baseline and follow-up everyday functioning in a sample of participants who were cognitively normal or were diagnosed with MCI, AD, VaD, or mixed dementia. While both executive functioning and episodic memory were related to level of everyday function at baseline, only executive functioning predicted rate of decline in everyday functioning over time. When both cognitive and neuroimaging variables were included in the model, memory and hippocampal volume were associated with baseline everyday functioning, but once again, only executive functioning independently predicted rate of decline in everyday functioning. In a sample of participants with VaD, Boyle, Paul, Moser, and Cohen (2004) examined the relation between baseline executive functioning abilities and subcortical hyperintensities on magnetic resonance imaging and informant report of everyday function measured at 1-year follow-up. Baseline executive functioning significantly accounted for decline in everyday function at 1-year, even after accounting for global cognitive functioning and subcortical hyperintensities.

Cahn-Weiner and colleagues (2007) posited two possible explanations for the predictive relationship of executive functioning with everyday functioning. First, the authors proposed that executive functioning itself could play an essential role in rate of functional decline. Intact executive functioning abilities may allow a person to compensate for decline in other cognitive domains, such as episodic memory, while an impairment in executive functioning would mean that an individual is impaired at organizing other, intact cognitive processes in pursuit of a goal. Cited in support of this interpretation, Royall and colleagues (2004, 2005, 2006) have found that changes in executive functioning, but not memory, account for decline in everyday functioning impairment over time. Alternatively,

Cahn-Weiner et al. (2007) proposed that decline in executive functioning may represent a later stage in the disease process where multiple cognitive abilities are also impaired, thus resulting in greater impairment of everyday functioning. Indeed, the study noted that multidomain MCI has been found to progress to dementia at a faster rate than single-domain amnestic MCI (Alexopoulos et al., 2006; Meyer, Xu, Thornby, Chowdhury, & Quach, 2002). However, Cahn-Weiner et al. (2007) commented that they found no relation between cortical volume loss at baseline and rate of functional decline, which is inconsistent with this second interpretation.

3.3. Multidimensionality of Everyday Function and the Omission–Commission Model

It is worth considering that the specific cognitive processes linked to everyday functioning may depend, at least in part, upon the complexity of the everyday activity or the particular demands of the activity. For example, Jefferson et al. (2006) found that while executive functioning predicted change in complex everyday tasks performance in participants with VaD, memory performance predicted change in more basic everyday tasks. However, when considering relations between specific cognitive abilities and everyday functioning, most studies using questionnaires have treated everyday functioning as a unitary construct, examining associations between overall level of functional ability and performance on measures of specific cognitive processes. Most everyday activities are cognitively complex and require multiple cognitive processes, and therefore most complex cognitive tasks are differentially affected by specific cognitive impairments. For example, in the domain of language, executive retrieval deficits may disrupt language expression while leaving basic language comprehension relatively spared (Hurley et al., 2012). Likewise, there is mounting evidence from performance-based tests that individuals with different types of cognitive impairment show different forms of functional impairment. Giovannetti, Schmidt, Gallo, Sestito, and Libon (2006) compared NAT performance between participants with subcortical VaD, who showed impaired executive functioning but relatively spared episodic and semantic memory, and participants with AD, who showed the reverse pattern of cognitive deficits. The two groups did not differ in overall dementia severity, and thus expectedly did not differ in the overall score obtained on the NAT. However, the groups did differ in the *pattern* of everyday performance across tasks, with the VaD group committing a higher rate of commission errors and accomplishing fewer steps in the presence of visual and semantic distractor objects.

Additionally, Giovannetti and colleagues (2008b) found that errors of omission (i.e. leaving out a step) dissociate from errors of commission (i.e. performing steps incorrectly). Even in a sample limited to participants with AD, those with comparable overall NAT scores could exhibit varying patterns of errors, characterized by mostly omission errors, mostly commission errors, or mixed errors. Furthermore, only omission errors were predicted by overall dementia severity and episodic memory, while commission errors were predicted by measures of executive functioning. These studies and others (Kessler, Giovannetti, & MacMullen, 2007; Bailey, Kurby, Giovannetti & Zacks, 2013; Giovannetti et al., 2012; Seidel et al., 2013) contributed to the development of the omission–commission model of functional impairment. This model posits that omission errors are associated with episodic memory deficits, as individuals are unable to recall the correct steps required for successful completion of the task. In contrast, commission errors result from problems with planning and attention due to executive functioning deficits.

The omission–commission model also is supported by evidence from neuroimaging. Seidel et al. (2013) examined relations between volumes of cortical gray matter, hippocampus, caudate nucleus, and intact white matter in surface, deep, and periventricular regions and error types from the NAT (e.g., omissions, commissions, and additions). NAT commissions showed a significant association with white matter integrity, specifically in the deep region. In contrast, addition errors (e.g., off-task actions) appeared to be multidetermined, showing a relation to both intact deep white matter and gray matter structures (cortex and hippocampus). Omissions were most related to hippocampal volumes. Bailey and colleagues (2013) examined volumes of the dorsolateral prefrontal cortex (DLPFC), medial temporal lobes (MTL), posterior cortex, and anterior cingulate cortex (ACC) in a group of healthy, MCI, and AD participants who had completed the NAT. Results showed omission errors correlated significantly with MTL volume and ACC volume, but MTL volume was the only significant predictor of omission errors when entered into a regression. Commission errors were related to DLPFC volume, in the unexpected direction, such that larger DLPFC volumes were associated with more commission errors. Action addition errors were correlated with both posterior volume and ACC volume, but in a regression only ACC volume significantly predicted action additions.

The omission–commission model is also relevant for identifying effective behavioral interventions. The notion of matching specific deficits to treatment approach makes theoretical sense and has been proven to be the most prudent approach to intervention for other complex neuropsychological disorders, including amnesia and aphasia (Riddoch & Humphreys, 1994; Sohlberg & Mateer, 2001; Wilson, Gracey, & Evans, 2009). We argue that a similar, theoretically motivated approach should inform interventions for everyday functioning. Work from our group has shown that Parkinson's dementia and AD participants with comparable overall impairment but significantly different functional impairment profiles on performance-based measures (Giovannetti et al., 2012) responded differently to goal cues (i.e., reminders of the task goal). The goals cues had a significant effect in reducing only omission errors, which have been associated with episodic memory impairment and were more frequent among participants with AD. By contrast, significant numbers of commission errors, which have been associated with executive function impairment (Giovannetti et al., 2008b, 2012; Kessler et al., 2007), were not corrected after presentation of the goal cues, and additional commission errors were sometimes made after the cues. These findings further support the omission–commission model and imply that interventions should be tailored to match patient's unique neuropsychological and functional deficits to optimize everyday functioning and independence. A "one-size fits all" approach to functional interventions will likely fail for some patients.

As stated earlier, overt errors are infrequent in people with MCI who demonstrate more mild functional difficulties. Therefore, there is no current evidence to support the omission–commission model in MCI. Our group is currently working on identifying meaningful subtypes of microerrors to determine whether there are differential profiles of functional difficulty in MCI. However, there is some evidence for differential functional profiles depending on which cognitive domain(s) are affected across MCI subtypes. MCI is commonly divided into amnestic single-domain (impaired only in memory domain), amnestic multiple-domain (impaired in memory and at least one other domain), nonamnestic single-domain (impaired in one domain other than memory), and nonamnestic multiple-domain (impaired in two or more domains, but not memory) subtypes (Petersen et al., 2001, 2009). In the Farias et al. (2006) study described earlier, the MCI group's greater difficulties in the domain of everyday memory could be related to the composition of the MCI sample. Approximately 45% of the sample was classified as amnestic single-domain MCI, which could account for the group's greater informant-reported difficulties with activities related to episodic memory. Another 39% of the MCI sample was classified as multiple domain MCI, although these participants were not further subdivided into amnestic or nonamnestic groups.

Other studies suggest there is some evidence for differential functional profiles based on task across MCI subtypes. Bangen and colleagues (2010) found that amnestic MCI participants were impaired on a performance-based measure of financial ability, while nonamnestic MCI participants were impaired on measures relating to health and safety. Similarly, Kim and colleagues (2009) found that, in a sample of older South Korean adults, the items on which MCI participants were impaired when compared to a control group varied based on MCI subtype. Nonamnestic single domain participants were impaired on items relating to using the telephone and using household appliances, while amnestic multiple-domain participants were impaired on items relating to using the telephone, using transportation, and managing finances. Whether the functional difficulties in the amnestic MCI groups in Bangen et al. (2010) and Kim et al. (2009) were due to episodic memory deficits per se or to other impaired cognitive abilities remains to be determined. Although amnestic MCI groups in both studies demonstrated impairments in financial abilities, other studies examining the cognitive correlates of financial abilities have noted relationships with a variety of cognitive abilities, including executive functioning (Griffith et al., 2003; Marson, 2001; Han et al., 2015).

3.4. Conceptual Knowledge

Relative to executive function and episodic memory, the role of semantic knowledge has not been extensively studied in relation to everyday function. It is well documented that semantic difficulties are the core deficit in semantic dementia (Neary et al., 1998) and are commonly reported in dementia due to AD (Adlam, Bozeat, Arnold, Watson, & Hodges, 2006; Verma & Howard, 2012). Semantic impairment that could not be explained solely by retrieval deficits also has been reported in people with other forms of neurodegenerative disease (e.g., Parkinson's disease without dementia (Portin, Laatu, Revonsuo, & Rinne, 2000).

Knowledge of tools and their actions and associate objects is degraded in patients with AD (Ochipa et al., 1992; Roll, Giovannetti, Libon, & Eppig, 2019) and those with semantic dementia (Chrysikou et al., 2011). The necessity of intact object knowledge for successful completion of everyday activities has been investigated in case reports of semantic dementia (Buxbaum, Schwartz, & Carew, 1997; Funnell, 2001; Hodges, Bozeat, Ralph, Patterson, & Spatt, 2000; Lauro-Grotto, Piccini, & Shallice, 1997; Snowden et al., 2001), but results have been inconclusive. Some investigators have argued that deficient object knowledge may be compensated for by intact mechanical knowledge or script knowledge (Hodges et al., 2000; Lauro-Grotto et al., 1997). Few studies have examined the relation between semantic knowledge for everyday objects and everyday function in people with other types of dementia. Recently Kirchberg and colleagues (2012) reported a significant association between measures of semantic knowledge and the percent of steps correctly executed on a performance-based test of everyday functioning in people with AD and amnestic MCI, although the relation between everyday function and semantic knowledge was not as strong as the relation between episodic memory and everyday function. One drawback of this Kirchberg study is that the measure of semantic knowledge (i.e., a novel semantic distance task) included animals and other objects that are not directly related to everyday function. Semantic deficits may be circumscribed to specific categories; consequently, it is reasonable to assume that deficits in animal knowledge may not affect everyday function.

Our laboratory has developed a series of tasks to evaluate knowledge of everyday tasks, including the knowledge of tasks steps and their order. These novel tasks were informed by the literature on semantic knowledge and borrowed test formats developed to minimize retrieval deficits (e.g., probe tasks, serial ordering of cards, etc.). Results obtained with these tests of everyday task knowledge showed significant associations with performance-based tests of everyday function. Specifically, scores on semantic tasks, along with measures of episodic memory, significantly predicted omission errors on the NAT. Performance on a picture sequencing task was associated with omissions as well as commission errors, suggesting knowledge of serial ordering is also associated with commission errors, of which the majority involve mis-sequencing of task steps (Roll et al., 2019).

4. Conclusions and Future Directions

4.1. Conclusions

Terminology and methodology differ widely across studies of everyday functioning. Various methods have unique strengths and weaknesses, and lack of consistency across studies will stall our progress in fully understanding the nature of functional changes, difficulties, and impairment. There is a strong influence of level of cognitive impairment on everyday functioning, with greater cognitive deficits associated with greater functional impairments. MCI is associated with minor errors that reduce efficiency of performance, while more severe cognitive impairment is associated with the omission of large task segments that may ultimately preclude successful completion of the task. Even among healthy older adults, everyday functioning is not as efficient and is more error-prone when compared to younger adults.

Among individuals with the same overall level of cognitive impairment, however, specific cognitive processes have been associated with varying patterns of functional errors. On performance-based tests, impairments in episodic memory are associated with errors of omission, while executive functioning deficits are associated with commission errors (i.e., omission–commission model). Evidence from questionnaire-based methodologies also suggests that impairments in particular everyday activities are differentially associated with episodic memory abilities versus executive functioning abilities. Other forms of cognition, which are not as frequently studied, also are associated with everyday action functioning; for example, degradation in semantic knowledge are also related to impaired performance of everyday activities and particularly with omission errors.

In conclusion, individuals with different dementia syndromes (e.g., AD, VaD) will likely exhibit different error profiles to the extent to which they also show different cognitive impairment patterns. However, due to heterogeneity across individuals diagnosed with the same dementia syndrome, a more prudent approach to characterizing functional deficit profiles is to consider both level of cognitive impairment along with type of cognitive impairment, regardless of diagnosis. Thus, individuals with greater episodic and semantic memory impairment may be expected to have difficulty completing meaningful task segments, due to premature decay or degraded task goals. These individuals also may benefit from reminders of task goals. On the other hand, individuals with greater executive function impairment may experience greater disorganization and interference from distractors and may benefit less from reminder cues and more from environmental adaptations that reduce clutter and provide more structure to prevent derailment.

4.2. Future Directions

Studies currently use a variety of methods to assess everyday functioning with little consistency between research groups. Going forward, it is essential to identify which methods are most accurate at detecting and quantifying functional changes in older adults. Identification of the most valid and reliable measures should inspire researchers to adopt the same measures in longitudinal studies of diverse populations, thus allowing for more interpretable comparisons between studies and greater generalizability of findings. Publication of longitudinal studies using such measures would also be valuable to our understanding of functional change in both healthy and dysfunctional aging.

MCI remains an exciting area for further study of everyday functioning. Given the potential predictive power of functional difficulties in predicting risk for dementia, it will be important to develop sensitive measures to detect early functional difficulties occurring in individuals with MCI (Seligman et al., 2014; Seligman & Giovannetti, 2015; Rycroft, Giovannetti, Divers, & Hulswit, 2018; Rycroft et al., 2018; Giovannetti et al., 2019). Using such measures, norms and cut points for defining functional changes, functional difficulties, and functional impairment could be more clearly identified. Given the heterogeneity in patterns of cognitive impairments in MCI, this remains a promising area in which to look for specific patterns of functional difficulties and their relation to particular cognitive profiles and risk for future decline.

Our review of the literature indicates that in addition to the role of level of cognitive functioning, it is also important to consider cognitive profiles in understanding functioning. Indeed, we suggest that everyday functioning should not be investigated in specific dementia syndromes (e.g., AD and VaD), but rather in heterogeneous dementia populations. Such diverse samples will uncover the particular cognitive processes associated with specific everyday activities and specific everyday action errors. Although studies so far have largely focused on executive functioning and episodic memory, it is important to keep in mind that everyday functioning is highly complex and thus likely requires a combination of many diverse cognitive operations. Precisely which cognitive processes are involved and the specific role they play remains to be fully mapped across the span of cognitive impairment, from healthy aging to dementia. Additionally, existing literature on everyday function has largely neglected the consideration that executive functioning is not a unitary construct. Utilization of measures, such as the NIH EXAMINER (Kramer, 2014; Kramer et al., 2014), that assess specific components of executive functioning like working memory, inhibition, etc. will allow researchers to identify which components of executive functioning are most strongly associated with everyday functioning. We posit that a detailed understanding of the cognitive processes required for successful everyday action performance, as well as the consequences for functioning of cognitive impairment, will contribute to the development of effective interventions for functional decline.

It is important not to forget that the ultimate goal of understanding the cognitive processes that explain the breakdown of everyday action is to improve functioning in people with dementia and prevent decline in those with MCI and healthy older adults. As technology offers a plethora of new assistive devices, it will be critical to assist older adults in identifying the assistive devices and strategies that most effectively match their cognitive profile and serve to promote accurate and efficient functioning. A precision approach to selecting interventions that address an individual's specific underlying cognitive impairment(s) will assist older adults in navigating the sea of new promising devices an apps and reduce the risk of wasting effort and imposing additional cognitive burden on ineffective adaptations, interventions, and strategies.

References

Adam, S., De Linden, M. V., Juillerat, A. C., & Salmon, E. (2000). The cognitive management of daily life activities in patients with mild to moderate Alzheimer's disease in a day care centre: A case report. *Neuropsychological rehabilitation*, *10*(5), 485–509.

Adlam, A. L. R., Bozeat, S., Arnold, R., Watson, P., & Hodges, J. R. (2006). Semantic knowledge in mild cognitive impairment and mild Alzheimer's disease. *Cortex*, *42*(5), 675–684.

Albert, M. S., DeKosky, S. T., Dickson, D., Dubois, B., Feldman, H. H., Fox, N. C., . . . Phelps, C. H. (2011). The diagnosis of mild cognitive impairment due to Alzheimer's disease: Recommendations from the National Institute on Aging-Alzheimer's Association workgroups on diagnostic guidelines for Alzheimer's disease. *Alzheimers Dement, 7*(3), 270–279. doi:10.1016/j.jalz.2011.03.008

Albert, S. M., Michaels, K., Padilla, M., Pelton, G., Bell, K., Marder, K., . . . Devanand, D. P. (1999). Functional significance of mild cognitive impairment in elderly patients without a dementia diagnosis. *American Journal of Geriatric Psychiatry, 7*, 213–220.

Alexopoulos, P., Grimmer, T., Perneczky, R., Domes, G., & Kurz, A. (2006). Progression to dementia in clinical subtypes of mild cognitive impairment. *Dementia and Geriatric Cognitive Disorders, 22*(1), 27–34.

Allain, P., Foloppe, D. A., Besnard, J., Yamaguchi, T., Etcharry-Bouyx, F., Le Gall, D., Nolin, P., & Richard, P. (2014). Detecting everyday action deficits in Alzheimer's disease using a nonimmersive virtual reality kitchen. *Journal of the International Neuropsychological Society, 20*(5), 468–477.

Arguelles, S., Loewenstein, D. A., Eisdorfer, C., & Arguelles, T. (2001). Caregivers' judgments of the functional abilities of the Alzheimer's disease patient: Impact of caregivers' depression and perceived burden. *Journal of Geriatric Psychiatry and Neurology, 14*(2), 91–98.

Bailey, H. R., Kurby, C. A., Giovannetti, T., & Zacks, J. M. (2013). Action perception predicts action performance. *Neuropsychologia*, 51(11), 2294–2304.

Bangen, K. J., Jak, A. J., Schiehser, D. M., Delano-Wood, L., Tuminello, E., Han, S. D., . . . Bondi, M. W. (2010). Complex activities of daily living vary by mild cognitive impairment subtype. *Journal of the International Neuropsychological Society, 16*(4), 630–639. doi:10.1017/S1355617710000330

Bettcher, B. M., Giovannetti, T., Macmullen, L., & Libon, D. J. (2008). Error detection and correction patterns in dementia: A breakdown of error monitoring processes and their neuropsychological correlates. *Journal of the International Neuropsychological Society*, 14(2), 199–208. doi:10.1017/S1355617708080193

Bickerton, W. L., Humphreys, G. W., & Riddoch, M. J. (2007). The case of the unfamiliar implement: Schema-based over-riding of semantic knowledge from objects in everyday action. *Journal of the International Neuropsychological Society*, 13(6), 1035–1046. doi:10.1017/ S1355617707071585

Boyle, P. A., Malloy, P. F., Salloway, S., Cahn-Weiner, D. A., Cohen, R., & Cummings, J. L. (2003a). Executive dysfunction and apathy predict functional impairment in Alzheimer disease. *American Journal of Geriatric Psychiatry*, 11(2), 214–221.

Boyle, P. A., Paul, R. H., Moser, D. J., & Cohen, R. A. (2004). Executive impairments predict functional declines in vascular dementia. *Clinical Neuropsychologist, 18*(1), 75–82. doi:10.1080/13854040490507172

Boyle, P. A., Paul, R., Moser, D., Zawacki, T., Gordon, N., & Cohen, R. (2003b). Cognitive and neurologic predictors of functional impairment in vascular dementia. *American Journal of Geriatric Psychiatry*, 11(1), 103–106.

Boyle, P. A., Yu, L., Wilson, R. S., Segawa, E., Buchman, A. S., & Bennett, D. A. (2013). Cognitive decline impairs financial and health literacy among community-based older persons without dementia. *Psychology and Aging*, 28(3), 614–625.

Brown, P. J., Devanand, D. P., Liu, X., & Caccappolo, E., for the Alzheimer's Disease Neuroimaging Initiative. (2011). Functional impairment in elderly patients with mild cognitive impairment and mild Alzheimer disease. *Archives of General Psychiatry, 68*(6), 617–626. doi:10.1001/archgenpsychiatry.2011.57

Buxbaum, L. J. (1998). Ideational apraxia and naturalistic action. *Cognitive Neuropsychology*, 15(6-8), 617–643.

Buxbaum, L. J., Schwartz, M. F., & Carew, T. G. (1997). The role of semantic memory in object use. *Cognitive Neuropsychology*, 14(2), 219–254.

Buxbaum, L., Schwartz, M., & Montgomery, M. (1998). Ideational apraxia and naturalistic action. *Cognitive Neuropsychology*, 15, 617–643.

Cahn-Weiner, D. A., Farias, S. T., Julian, L., Harvey, D. J., Kramer, J. H., Reed, B. R., . . . Chui, H. (2007). Cognitive and neuroimaging predictors of instrumental activities of daily living. *Journal of the International Neuropsychological Society, 13*(5), 747–757. doi:10.1017/S1355617707070853

Chrysikou, E. G., Giovannetti, T., Wambach, D. M., Lyon, A. C., Grossman, M., & Libon, D. J. (2011). The importance of multiple assessments of object knowledge in semantic dementia: The case of the familiar objects task. *Neurocase, 17*(1), 57–75.

Cook, D. J., & Schmitter-Edgecombe, M. (2009). Assessing the quality of activities in a smart environment. *Methods of Information in Medicine, 48*(5), 480–485. doi:10.3414/ME0592

DeBettignies, B. H., Mahurin, R. K., & Pirozzolo, F. J. (1990). Insight for impairment in independent living skills in Alzheimer's disease and multi-infarct dementia. *Journal of Clinical and Experimental Neuropsychology, 12*, 355–363.

Dodge, H. H., Mattek, N. C., Austin, D., Hayes, T. L., & Kaye, J. A. (2012). In-home walking speeds and variability trajectories associated with mild cognitive impairment. *Neurology, 78*(24), 1946–1952. doi:10.1212/WNL.0b013e318259e1de

Edmonds, E. C., Delano-Wood, L., Galasko, D. R., Salmon, D. P., Bondi, M. W., for the Alzheimer's Disease Neuroimaging Initiative. (2014). Subjective cognitive complaints contribute to misdiagnosis of mild cognitive impairment. *Journal of the International Neuropsychological Society, 20*(8), 836–847. doi:10.1017/S135561771400068X

Espiritu, D. A. V., Rashid, H., Mast, B. T., Fitzgerald, J., Steinberg, J., & Lichtenberg, P. A. (2001). Depression, cognitive impairment and function in Alzheimer's disease. *International Journal of Geriatric Psychiatry*, 16(11), 1098–1103.

Farias, S. T., Mungas, D., Harvey, D. J., Simmons, A., Reed, B. R., & DeCarli, C. (2011). The measurement of everyday cognition: Development and validation of a short form of the Everyday Cognition scales. *Alzheimer's & Dementia*, 7(6), 593–601.

Farias, S. T., Mungas, D., Reed, B. R., Cahn-Weiner, D., Jagust, W., Baynes, K., & DeCarli, C. (2008). The measurement of everyday cognition (ECog): scale development and psychometric properties. *Neuropsychology*, 22(4), 531–544.

Farias, S. T., Mungas, D., Reed, B. R., Harvey, D., Cahn-Weiner, D., & Decarli, C. (2006). MCI is associated with deficits in everyday functioning. *Alzheimer Disease and Associated Disorders, 20*(4), 217–223. doi:10.1097/01.wad.0000213849.51495.d9

Farias, S. T., Park, L. Q., Harvey, D. J., Simon, C., Reed, B. R., Carmichael, O., & Mungas, D. (2013). Everyday cognition in older adults: associations with neuropsychological performance and structural brain imaging. *Journal of the International Neuropsychological Society, 19*(4), 430–441. doi:10.1017/S1355617712001609

Forde, E. M. E., & Humphreys, G. W. (2002). Dissociations in routine behaviour across patients and everyday tasks. *Neurocase, 8*, 151–167.

Foundas, A. L., Macauley, B. L., Raymer, A. M., Maher, L. M., Heilman, K. M., & Roth, L. J. G. (1995). Ecological implications of limb apraxia: Evidence from mealtime behavior. *Journal of the International Neuropsychological Society, 1*, 62–66.

Funnell, E. (2001). Evidence for scripts in semantic dementia: Implications for theories of semantic memory. *Cognitive Neuropsychology*, *18*(4), 323–341.

Giovannetti, T., Bettcher, B. M., Brennan, L., Libon, D. J., Burke, M., Duey, K., . . . Wambach, D. (2008a). Characterization of everyday functioning in mild cognitive impairment: a direct assessment approach. *Dementia and Geriatric Cognitive Disorders*, *25*(4), 359–365. doi:10.1159/000121005

Giovannetti, T., Bettcher, B. M., Brennan, L., Libon, D. J., Kessler, R. K., & Duey, K. (2008b). Coffee with jelly or unbuttered toast: Commissions and omissions are dissociable aspects of everyday action impairment in Alzheimer's disease. *Neuropsychology*, 22(2), 235.

Giovannetti, T., Bettcher, B. M., Brennan, L., Libon, D. J., Wambach, D., & Seter, C. (2010). Target-related distractors disrupt object selection in everyday action: Evidence from participants with dementia. *Journal of the International Neuropsychological Society*, 16(3), 484–494. doi:S1355617710000081 [pii]10.1017/S1355617710000081

Giovannetti, T., Bettcher, B. M., Libon, D. J., Brennan, L., Sestito, N., & Kessler, R. K. (2007). Environmental adaptations improve everyday action performance in Alzheimer's disease: Empirical support from performance-based assessment. *Neuropsychology*, 21(4), 448.

Giovannetti, T., Britnell, P., Brennan, L., Siderowf, A., Grossman, M., Libon, D. J., . . . Seidel, G. A. (2012). Everyday action impairment in Parkinson's disease dementia. Journal of the *International Neuropsychological Society*, *18*(05), 787–798.

Giovannetti, T., Libon, D. J., Buxbaum, L. J., & Schwartz, M. F. (2002). Naturalistic action impairments in dementia. *Neuropsychologia*, *40*(8), 1220–1232.

Giovannetti, T., Libon, D. J., & Hart, T. (2002). Awareness of naturalistic action errors in dementia. *Journal of the International Neuropsychological Society*, *8*(5), 633–644.

Giovannetti, T., Schmidt, K. S., Gallo, J. L., Sestito, N., & Libon, D. J. (2006). Everyday action in dementia: Evidence for differential deficits in Alzheimer's disease versus subcortical vascular dementia. *Journal of the International Neuropsychological Society*, *12*(01), 45–53.

Giovannetti, T., Schwartz, M. F., & Buxbaum, L. J. (2007). The Coffee Challenge: A new method for the study of everyday action errors. *Journal of Clinical and Experimental Neuropsychology*, *29*, 690–705.

Giovannetti, T., Sestito, N., Libon, D. J., Schmidt, K., Gallo, J., Gambino, M., & Chrysikou, E. G. (2006). The influence of personal experience on object knowledge in dementia. *Archives of Clinical Neuropsychology*, *21*, 607–614.

Giovannetti, T., Yamaguchi, T., Roll, E., Harada, T., Rycroft, S.S., Divers, R. . . . Mis, R. (2019). The Virtual Kitchen Challenge: Preliminary data from a novel virtual reality test of mild difficulties in everyday functioning, *Aging Neuropsychology, and Cognition*, 26(6), 823–841. doi:10.1080/13825585.2018.1536774

Gitlin, L. N., Corcoran, M., Winter, L., Boyce, A., & Hauck, W. W. (2001). A randomized, controlled trial of a home environmental intervention effect on efficacy and upset in caregivers and on daily function of persons with dementia. *Gerontologist*, *41*(1), 4–14.

Green, C. R., Mohs, R. C., Schmeidler, J., Aryan, M., & Davis, K. L. (1993). Functional decline in Alzheimer's disease: a longitudinal study. *Journal of the American Geriatrics Society*, *41*(6), 654–661.

Griffith, H. R., Belue, K., Sicola, A., Krzywanski, S., Zamrini, E., Harrell, L., & Marson, D. C. (2003). Impaired financial abilities in mild cognitive impairment A direct assessment approach. *Neurology*, *60*(3), 449–457.

Han, S. D., Boyle, P. A., James, B. D., Yu, L., & Bennett, D. A. (2015). Poorer financial and health literacy among community-dwelling older adults with mild cognitive impairment. *Journal of Aging and Health, 27*(6), 1105–1117.

Hargrave, R., Reed, B., & Mungus, D. (2000). Depressive symptoms and functional ability in dementia. *Journal of Geriatric Psychiatry and Neurology, 13*, 72–77.

Hodges, J. R., Bozeat, S., Ralph, M. A. L., Patterson, K., & Spatt, J. (2000). The role of conceptual knowledge in object use evidence from semantic dementia. *Brain, 123*(9), 1913–1925.

Hoeymans, N., Feskens, E. J., van den Bos, G. A., & Kromhout, D. (1996). Measuring functional status: cross-sectional and longitudinal associations between performance and self-report (Zutphen Elderly Study 1990–1993). *Journal of Clinical Epidemiology*, 49(10), 1103–1110.

Humphreys, G. W., & Forde, E. M. E. (1998). Disordered action schema and action disorganisation syndrome. *Cognitive Neuropsychology, 15*, 771–811.

Hurley, R. S., Paller, K. A., Rogalski, E. J., & Mesulam, M. M. (2012). Neural mechanisms of object naming and word comprehension in primary progressive aphasia. *Journal of Neuroscience, 32*(14), 4848–4855.

Jefferson, A. L., Cahn-Weiner, D., Boyle, P., Paul, R. H., Moser, D. J., Gordon, N., & Cohen, R. A. (2006). Cognitive predictors of functional decline in vascular dementia. *International Journal of Geriatric Psychiatry, 21*(8), 752–754.

Kaye, J., Mattek, N., Dodge, H. H., Campbell, I., Hayes, T., Austin, D., . . . Pavel, M. (2014). Unobtrusive measurement of daily computer use to detect mild cognitive impairment. *Alzheimer's & Dementia, 10*(1), 10–17. doi:10.1016/j.jalz.2013.01.011

Kazui, H., Matsuda, A., Hirono, N., Mori, E., Miyoshi, N., Ogino, A., Tokunaga, H., Ikejiri, Y., & Takeda, M. (2005). Everyday Memory Impairment of Patients with Mild Cognitive Impairment. *Dementia and Geriatric Cognitive Disorders, 19*(5-6), 331–337.

Kempen, G. I., Steverink, N., Ormel, J., & Deeg, D. J. (1996). The assessment of ADL among frail elderly in an interview survey: self-report versus performance-based tests and determinants of discrepancies. *Journals of Gerontology Series B: Psychological Sciences and Social Sciences, 51*(5), P254–P260.

Kessler, R. K., Giovannetti, T., & MacMullen, L. R. (2007). Everyday action in schizophrenia: Performance patterns and underlying cognitive mechanisms. *Neuropsychology, 21*(4), 439.

Kim, K. R., Lee, K. S., Cheong, H. K., Eom, J. S., Oh, B. H., & Hong, C. H. (2009). Characteristic profiles of instrumental activities of daily living in different subtypes of mild cognitive impairment. *Dementia and Geriatric Cognitive Disorders, 27*(3): 278–285.

Kirchberg, B. C., Cohen, J. R., Adelsky, M. B., Buthorn, J. J., Gomar, J. J., Gordon, M., . . . Goldberg, T. E. (2012). Semantic distance abnormalities in mild cognitive impairment: their nature and relationship to function. *American Journal of Psychiatry, 169*(12), 1275–1283.

Kiyak, H. A., Teri, L., & Borson, S. (1994). Physical and functional health assessment in normal aging and in Alzheimer's disease: Self-reports vs family reports. *Gerontologist, 34*(3), 324–331.

Knopman, D. S., Berg, J. D., & Thomas, R. (1999). Nursing home placement is related to dementia progression: Evidence from a clinical trial. *Neurology, 52*, 714–718.

Knopman, D. S., Kitto, J., Deinard, S., & Heiring, J. (1988). Longitudinal study of death and institutionalization in patients with primary degenerative dementia. *Journal of the American Geriatrics Society, 36*(2), 108–112.

Kramer, J. H. (2014). Special series introduction: NIH EXAMINER and the assessment of executive functioning. *Journal of the International Neuropsychological Society, 20*(1), 8–10.

Kramer, J. H., Mungas, D., Possin, K. L., Rankin, K. P., Boxer, A. L., Rosen, H. J., . . . Widmeyer, M. (2014). NIH EXAMINER: Conceptualization and development of an executive function battery. *Journal of the International Psychological Society, 20*(1), 11–9.

Lauro-Grotto, R., Piccini, C., & Shallice, T. (1997). Modality-specific operations in semantic dementia. *Cortex, 33*(4), 593–622.

Lawton, M. P., & Brody, E. M. (1969). Assessment of old people: Self-maintaining and instrumental activities of daily living. *Gerontologist, 9*, 179–186.

Lechowski, L., Dieudonne, B., Tortrat, D., Teillet, L., Robert, P. H., Benoit, M., Forette, B., & Vellas, B. (2003). Role of behavioural disturbance in the loss of autonomy for activities of daily living in Alzheimer patients. *International Journal of Geriatric Psychiatry, 18*(11), 977–982.

Li, Y., Gao, J., Enkavi, A. Z., Zaval, L., Weber, E. U., & Johnson, E. J. (2015). Sound credit scores and financial decisions despite cognitive aging. *Proceedings of the National Academy of Sciences, 112*(1), 65–69.

Loewenstein, D. A., Amigo, E., Duara, R., Gutteman, A., Hurwitz, D., Berkowitz, D., . . . Eisdorfer, C. (1989). A new scale for the assessment of functional status in Alzheimer's disease and related disorders. *Journal of Gerontology, 4*, 114–121.

Loewenstein, D. A., Ardila, A., Rosselli, M., Hayden, S., Duara, R., Berkowitz, N., . . . Eisdorfer, C. (1992). A comparative analysis of functional status among Spanish- and English-speaking patients with dementia. *Journal of Gerontology, 47*(6), 389–394.

Loewenstein, D. A., Argüelles, S., Bravo, M., Freeman, R. Q., Argüelles, T., Acevedo, A., & Eisdorfer, C. (2001). Caregivers' judgments of the functional abilities of the Alzheimer's disease patient: A comparison of proxy reports and objective measures. *Journals of Gerontology Series B: Psychological Sciences and Social Sciences, 56*(2), P78–P84.

Lukovits, T. G., & McDaniel, K. D. (1992). Behavioral disturbance in severe Alzheimer's disease: A comparison of family member and nursing staff reporting. *Journal of the American Geriatrics Society*, 40(9), 891–895.

Mangone, C. A., Sanguinetti, R. M., Baumann, P. D., Gonzalez, R. C., Pereyra, S., Bozzola, F. G., . . . Sica, R. E. P. (1993). Influence of feelings of burden on the caregiver's perception of the patient's functional status. *Dementia and Geriatric Cognitive Disorders, 4*(5), 287–293.

Marcotte, T. D., & Grant, I. (Eds.). (2009). *Neuropsychology of everyday functioning*. New York, NY: Guilford Press.

Marson, D. C. (2001). Loss of financial competency in dementia: Conceptual and empirical approaches. *Aging, Neuropsychology, and Cognition, 8*(3), 164–181.

Martyr, A., & Clare, L. (2018). Awareness of functional ability in people with early-stage dementia. *International Journal of Geriatric Psychiatry, 33*(1), 31–38.

McAlister, C., & Schmitter-Edgecombe, M. (2013). Naturalistic assessment of executive function and everyday multitasking in healthy older adults. *Aging, Neuropsychology, and Cognition, 20*(6), 735–756.

McKhann, G. M., Knopman, D. S., Chertkow, H., Hyman, B. T., Jack, C. R., Kawas, C. H., . . . Phelps, C. H. (2011). The diagnosis of dementia due to Alzheimer's disease: Recommendations from the National Institute on Aging-Alzheimer's Association workgroups on diagnostic guidelines for Alzheimer's disease. *Alzheimer's & Dementia, 7*(3), 263–269.

Meyer, J. S., Xu, G., Thornby, J., Chowdhury, M., & Quach, M. (2002). Longitudinal analysis of abnormal domains comprising mild cognitive impairment (MCI) during aging. *Journal of the Neurological Sciences, 201*(1), 19–25.

Neary, D., Snowden, J. S., Gustafson, L., Passant, U., Stuss, D., Black, S. A., . . . Boone, K. (1998). Frontotemporal lobar degeneration A consensus on clinical diagnostic criteria. *Neurology, 51*(6), 1546–1554.

Newens, A. J., Forster, D. P., & Kay, D. W. (1995). Dependency and community care in presenile Alzheimer's disease. *British Journal of Psychiatry, 166*(6), 777–782.

Nowrangi, M. A., Rosenberg, P. B., & Leoutsakos, J. S. (2016). Subtle changes in daily functioning predict conversion from normal to mild cognitive impairment or dementia: An analysis of the NACC database. *International Psychogeriatrics, 28*(12), 2009–2018. doi:10.1017/S1041610216000995

Ochipa, C., Rothi, L. J. G., & Heilman, K. M. (1992). Conceptual apraxia in Alzheimer's disease. *Brain, 115*, 1061–1072.

Okonkwo, O., Wadley, V. G., Griffith, H. R., Belue, K., Lanza, S., Zamrini, E. Y., . . . Marson, D.C. (2008). Awareness of deficits in financial abilities in patients with mild cognitive impairment: Going beyond self-informant discrepancy. *American Journal of Geriatric Psychiatry,16*(8), 650–659.

Østbye, T., Tyas, S., McDowell, I., & Koval, J. (1997). Reported activities of daily living: agreement between elderly subjects with and without dementia and their caregivers. *Age and Ageing, 26*(2), 99–106.

Park, N. W., Lombardi, S., Gold, D. A., Tarita-Nistor, L., Gravely, M., Roy, E. A., & Black, S. E. (2012). Effects of familiarity and cognitive function on naturalistic action performance. *Neuropsychology, 26*(2), 224–237. doi:2011-29861-001

Paul, R. H., Cohen, R. A., Ott, B. R., Zawacki, T., Moser, D. J., Davis, J., Gordon, N., & Stone, W. (2000). Cognitive and functional status in two subtypes of vascular dementia. *NeuroRehabilitation, 15*(3), 199–205.

Petersen, R. C., Doody, R., Kurz, A., Mohs, R. C., Morris, J. C., Rabins, P. V., . . . Winblad, B. (2001). Current concepts in mild cognitive impairment. *Archives of* Neurology, 58(12), 1985–1992.

Petersen, R. C., Roberts, R. O., Knopman, D. S., Boeve, B. F., Geda, Y. E., Ivnik, R. J., . . . Jack, C. R. (2009). Mild cognitive impairment: Ten years later. *Archives of Neurology, 66*(12), 1447–1455.

Pfeffer, R. I., Kurosaki, T. T., Harrah, C. H., Chance, J. M., & Filos, S. (1982). Measurement of functional activities in older adults in the community. *Journal of Gerontology, 37*(3), 323–329.

Portin, R., Laatu, S., Revonsuo, A., & Rinne, U. K. (2000). Impairment of semantic knowledge in Parkinson disease. *Archives of Neurology, 57*(9), 1338–1343.

Ramsden, C. M., Kinsella, G. J., Ong, B., & Storey, E. (2008). Performance of everyday actions in mild Alzheimer's disease. *Neuropsychology, 22*(1), 17–26. doi:2008-00382-004

Riddoch, M. J., & Humphreys, G. W. (1994). Toward an understanding of neglect. In M. J. Riddoch & G. W. Humphreys (Eds.), *Cognitive neuropsychology and cognitive rehabilitation* (pp. 125–149). Hillsdale, NJ: Erlbaum.

Roll, E. E., Giovannetti, T., Libon, D. J., & Eppig, J. (2019). Everyday task knowledge and everyday function in dementia. *Journal of Neuropsychology, 13*(1), 96–120. doi:10.1111/jnp.12135.

Rothi, L. J. G., Ochipa, C., & Heilman, K. M. (1991). A cognitive neuropsychological model of praxis. *Cognitive Neuropsychology, 8*, 443–458.

Royall, D. R. (2006). Mild cognitive impairment and functional status. *Journal of the American Geriatrics Society, 54*(1), 163–165.

Royall, D. R., Palmer, R., Chiodo, L. K., & Polk, M. J. (2004). Declining executive control in normal aging predicts change in functional status: The Freedom House Study. *Journal of the American Geriatrics Society, 52*(3), 346–352.

Royall, D. R., Palmer, R., Chiodo, L. K., & Polk, M. J. (2005). Executive control mediates memory's association with change in instrumental activities of daily living: The Freedom House Study. *Journal of the American Geriatrics Society, 53*(1), 11–17.

Rubenstein, L. Z., Schairer, C., Wieland, G. D., & Kane, R. (1984). Systematic biases in functional status assessment of elderly adults: Effects of different data sources. *Journal of Gerontology, 39*(6), 686–691.

Rycroft, S. S., Giovannetti, T., Divers, R., & Hulswit, J. (2018). Sensitive performance-based assessment of everyday action in older and younger adults. *Aging, Neuropsychology, and Cognition, 25*(2), 259–276.

Rycroft, S. S., Giovannetti, T., Shipley, T. F., Hulswit, J., Divers, R., & Reilly, J. (2018). Windows to functional decline: Naturalistic eye movements in older and younger adults. *Psychology and Aging*, 33(8):1215–1222.

Sanders, C., & Schmitter-Edgecombe, M. (2012). Identifying the nature of impairment in planning ability with normal aging. *Journal of Clinical and Experimental Neuropsychology, 34*(7), 724–737.

Sands, L. P., Ferreira, P., Stewart, A. L., Brod, M., & Yaffe, K. (2004). What explains differences between dementia patients' and their caregivers' ratings of patients' quality of life? *American Journal of Geriatric Psychiatry, 12*(3), 272–280.

Schmitter-Edgecombe, M., McAlister, C., & Weakley, A. (2012). Naturalistic assessment of everyday functioning in individuals with mild cognitive impairment: The day-out task. *Neuropsychology, 26*(5), 631.

Schwartz, M. F. (2006). The cognitive neuropsychology of everyday action and planning. *Cognitive Neuropsychology, 23*(1), 202–221. doi:10.1080/02643290500202623

Schwartz, M. F., & Buxbaum, L. J. (1997). Naturalistic action. In L. J. G. Rothi & K. M. Heilman (Eds.), *Apraxia: The neuropsychology of action* (pp. 269–290). East Sussex, England: Psychology Press.

Schwartz, M. F., Buxbaum, L. J., Ferraro, M., Veramonti, R., & Segal, M. (2003). *The Naturalistic Action Test*. Bury St. Edmunds, England: Thames Valley Test Company.

Schwartz, M. F., Buxbaum, L. J., Montgomery, M. W., Fitzpatrick-DeSalme, E., Hart, T., Ferraro, M., . . . Coslett, H. B. (1998). Naturalistic action production following right hemisphere stroke. *Neuropsychologia, 37*, 51–66.

Schwartz, M. F., Fitzpatrick-DeSalme, E. J., & Carew, T. G. (1995). The multiple objects test for ideational apraxia: Etiology and task effects on error profiles [Abstract]. *Journal of the International Neuropsychological Society, 1*, 149.

Schwartz, M. F., Montgomery, M. W., Buxbaum, L. J., Lee, S. S., Carew, T. G., Coslett, H., . . . Mayer, N. (1998). Naturalistic action impairment in closed head injury. Neuropsychology, 12(1), 13.

Schwartz, M. F., Montgomery, M. W., Fitzpatrick-DeSalme, E. J., Ochipa, O., Coslett, H. B., & Mayer, N. H. (1995). Analysis of a disorder of everyday action. *Cognitive Neuropsychology, 12*, 863–892.

Schwartz, M. F., Reed, E. S., Montgomery, M. W., Palmer, C., & Mayer, M. H. (1991). The quantitative description of action disorganization after brain damage: A case study. *Cognitive Neuropsychology, 8*, 381–414.

Schwartz, M. F., Segal, M., Veramonti, T., Ferraro, M., & Buxbaum, L. J. (2002). The Naturalistic Action Test: A standardised assessment for everyday action impairment. *Neuropsychological Rehabilitation, 12*(4), 311–339.

Seidel, G. A., Giovannetti, T., Price, C. C., Tanner, J., Mitchell, S., Eppig, J., & Libon, D. J. (2013). Neuroimaging correlates of everyday action in dementia. *Journal of Clinical and Experimental Neuropsychology, 35*(9), 993–1005.

Seligman, S. C., & Giovannetti, T. (2015). The potential utility of eye movements in the detection and characterization of everyday functional difficulties in mild cognitive impairment. *Neuropsychology Review, 25*(2), 199–215.

Seligman, S. C., Giovannetti, T., Hulswit, J., & Divers, R. (2017). Sensitive performance-based assessment of everyday action in older and younger adults, *Aging Neuropsychology, and Cognition, 25*(2), 259–276.

Seligman, S. C., Giovannetti, T., Sestito, J., & Libon, D. J. (2014). A new approach to the characterization of subtle errors in everyday action: implications for mild cognitive impairment. *Clinical Neuropsychologist*, 28(1), 97–115. doi:10.1080/13854046.2013.852624

Sestito, N., Schmidt, K. S., Gallo, J., Giovannetti, T., & Libon, D. J. (2005). Using the Naturalistic Action Test (NAT) to assess everyday action in healthy older adults and patients with dementia. Journal of the International Neuropsychological Society, *11*(Suppl. 1), 90–91.

Smith, G. E., Kokmen, E., & O'Brien, P. C. (2000). Risk factors for nursing home placement in a population-based dementia cohort. *Journal of the American Geriatric Society, 48*, 519–525.

Snowden, J. S., Bathgate, D., Varma, A., Blackshaw, A., Gibbons, Z. C., & Neary, D. (2001). Distinct behavioural profiles in frontotemporal dementia and semantic dementia. *Journal of Neurology, Neurosurgery & Psychiatry, 70*(3), 323–332.

Sohlberg, M. M., & Mateer, C. A. (Eds.). (2001). *Cognitive rehabilitation: An integrative neuropsychological approach*. New York, NY: Guilford Press.

Tekin, S., Fairbanks, L. A., O'connor, S., Rosenberg, S., & Cummings, J. L. (2001). Activities of daily living in Alzheimer's disease: Neuropsychiatric, cognitive, and medical illness influences. *American Journal of Geriatric Psychiatry*, 9(1), 81–86.

Tucker-Drob, E. M. (2011). Neurocognitive functions and everyday functions change together in old age. *Neuropsychology, 25*(3), 368–377. doi:10.1037/a0022348

Tuokko, H., Morris, C., & Ebert, P. (2005). Mild cognitive impairment and everyday functioning in older adults. *Neurocase, 11*(1), 40–47.

U.S. Department of Health and Human Services. (2014). *A profile of older Americans: 2014*. Washington, DC: Author.

Vitaliano, P. P., Echeverria, D., Yi, J., Phillips, P. E., Young, H., & Siegler, I. C. (2005). Psychophysiological mediators of caregiver stress and differential cognitive decline. *Psychology and Aging, 20*(3), 402–411.

Verma, M., & Howard, R. J. (2012). Semantic memory and language dysfunction in early Alzheimer's disease: a review. *International Journal of Geriatric Psychiatry, 27*(12), 1209–1217.

Wilson, B. A., Gracey, F., & Evans, J. J. (2009). *Neuropsychological rehabilitation: Theory, models, therapy and outcome*. Cambridge, England: Cambridge University Press.

Wolinsky, F. D., Callahan, C. M., Fitzgerald, J. F., & Johnson, R. J. (1993). Changes in functional status and the risks of subsequent nursing home placement and death. *Journal of Gerontology, 48*(3), S94–101.

Xiao, J. J., Chen, C., & Sun, L. (2015). Age differences in consumer financial capability. *International Journal of Consumer Studies*, *39*(4), 387–395.

Yu, L., Wilson, R. S., Schneider, J. A., Bennett, D. A., & Boyle, P. A. (2017). Financial and health literacy predict incident Alzheimer's disease dementia and pathology. *Journal of Alzheimer's Disease*, *56*(4), 1485–1493.

Zanetti, O., Frisoni, G. B., Deleo, D., Dellobuono, M., Bianchetti, A., & Trabucchi, M. (1995). Reality orientation therapy in Alzheimer-disease—useful or not: A controlled-study. *Alzheimer Disease & Associated Disorders*, 9(3), 132–138.

Zanetti, O., Geroldi, C., Frisoni, G. B., Bianchetti, A., & Trabucchi, M. (1999). Contrasting results between caregiver's report and direct assessment of activities of daily living in patients affected by mild and very mild dementia: The contribution of the caregiver's personal characteristics. *Journal of the American Geriatrics Society*, *47*(2), 196–202.

6

Heterogeneity in Dementia and Mild Cognitive Impairment

Using Statistical Modeling Techniques

Deborah A. G. Drabick and Jill Rabinowitz

1. Introduction

Mild cognitive impairment (MCI) and dementing diseases such as Alzheimer's disease (AD) and vascular dementia (VaD) are associated with significant impairments in cognition that adversely influence their ability to perform their occupation, their instrumental activities, and their activities of daily living. The alterations also have a strong negative impact on psychosocial activities (Apostolova & Cummings, 2007; Beeber, Thorpe, & Clipp, 2008; Eppig et al., 2017; Fiest et al., 2016; Forrester et al., 2015; Hanfelt et al., 2011; Libon et al., 2014; Mirza et al., 2017; Moran et al., 2004; Peter et al., 2014; Youn et al., 2011). There is, however, tremendous heterogeneity in terms of pathophysiology, presentation, correlates, clinical course, and outcomes among individuals with MCI or dementia (Eppig et al., 2017; Forrester et al., 2015; Jellinger, 2008; Libon et al., 2014; Moran et al., 2004; Peter et al., 2014). This heterogeneity suggests that efforts at identifying more homogeneous subgroups may be useful for many purposes, including informing intervention efforts and research.

MCI refers to a noticeable decrease in cognitive functioning that often exceeds those changes associated with normal aging but is not severe enough to meet diagnostic criteria for dementia or major neurocognitive disorder (Gallagher, Fischer, & Iaboni, 2017; Sachs-Ericsson & Blazer, 2015). MCI may be characterized by impairments in a single domain (e.g., memory deficits; amnesic MCI), impairments in cognitive functioning other than memory (nonamnestic MCI), or multiple domains (e.g., impairments in memory, executive function, visuospatial/language abilities; Brambati et al., 2009; Ward, Arrighi, Michels, & Cedarbaum, 2012). The prevalence rates for these different types of MCI range from 2.15% to 7.13% among adults 65 or older (Juncos-Rabadán et al., 2014; Ward et al., 2012) and 4.02% among adults aged 60 and older (Fiest et al., 2016).

Deborah A. G. Drabick and Jill Rabinowitz, *Heterogeneity in Dementia and Mild Cognitive Impairment* In: *Vascular Disease, Alzheimer's Disease, and Mild Cognitive Impairment.* Edited by: David J. Libon, Melissa Lamar, Rodney A. Swenson, Kenneth M. Heilman, Oxford University Press (2020).
DOI: 10.1093/oso/9780190634230.003.0007

MCI may precede dementia, which can be characterized by deficits in episodic memory, executive functioning, language, and visuospatial abilities (Peter et al., 2014; Sachs-Ericsson & Blazer, 2015). In addition, many adults with dementia display depressive symptoms, irritability, and behavior dysregulation, issues that are likely to persist over time (Wetzels et al., 2010; Youn et al., 2011). Dementia is primarily caused by AD and/or VaD (Jellinger, 2007, 2008). Annual incidence of VaD is 0.38%, and the risk for this dementia increases with age (Jellinger, 2008). VaD has variable pathophysiology and numerous potential causes, including multifocal small cerebral lesions (lacuna state), ischemic demyelination (leukoaraiosis), large focal strokes, and hippocampal sclerosis (Jellinger, 2008). These cerebrovascular disorders can be caused by large or small vessel disease, cardiac arrhythmias, heart failure with embolization, and clotting disorders. In contrast to VaD, AD is primarily caused by neurofibrillary tangles, plaques, and synaptic and neuronal deterioration and has been associated with the apolipoprotein ε4 (APOE4) polymorphism (van der Flier, Shoonenboom, Pijnenburg, Fox, & Scheltens, 2006; von Gunten, Bouras, Kövari, Giannakopoulos, & Hof, 2006). In 2003, worldwide about 27.7 million people were affected by AD, and this number is expected to increase fourfold by 2050 (Brookmeyer, Johnson, Ziegler-Graham, & Arrighi, 2007; Wimo, Jonsson, & Winblad, 2006). Unfortunately, available interventions for MCI and dementia have limited success in attenuating symptoms or further cognitive impairments and their sequelae (Gallagher, 2017). Given these prevalence rates, heterogeneity in presentation and deficits, poor prognosis, and deleterious correlates, characterizing MCI and dementia more precisely is an important goal. Such knowledge can inform prevention and intervention efforts, as well as predictions regarding course, correlates, and outcomes.

2. Variable- and Person-Centered Techniques

Heterogeneity in pathophysiology, phenotypic presentation, and deficits is expected among individuals with MCI or dementia. Nevertheless, much of the earlier research involving MCI and dementia has used variable-centered statistical approaches (e.g., Devanand et al., 2008; Petersen et al., 1999; Rowe et al., 2007). Variable-centered techniques (e.g., structural equation modeling, factor analysis, regression) assume that the influence of predictors on outcomes is homogeneous across the sample (Laursen & Hoff, 2006; Masyn et al., 2013). In contrast to variable-centered approaches, person-centered techniques (e.g., latent profile analysis [LPA], growth mixture modeling) assume that the population of interest is heterogeneous and thus focus on differences among individuals; these analytic approaches evaluate whether the relations between predictors and outcomes vary across individuals (Laursen & Hoff, 2006; Masyn et al., 2013).

Person-centered approaches may be especially useful for classifying individuals that exhibit a particular set of cognitive, behavioral, and/or neurological symptoms. Although MCI may precede the development of dementia, not all individuals with MCI go on to develop this disease. Individuals with MCI that also exhibit neuropsychiatric symptoms (e.g., depressive symptoms, irritability) are more likely to develop AD relative to individuals without neuropsychiatric symptoms (Apostolova & Cummings, 2007; Forrester, Gallo, Smith, & Leoutsakos, 2015; Modrego & Ferrández, 2012). Other research indicates that differences in cortical atrophy and regional gray matter volumes may partially underlie progression to dementia. For example, adults with MCI that exhibited higher levels of baseline atrophy in the left entorhinal cortex, bilateral superior temporal gyri, and right inferior frontal gyrus were more likely to develop AD relative to individuals who displayed lower levels of atrophy in these regions (Bell-McGinty et al., 2005). Similarly, altered levels of pathological cerebrospinal fluid markers (e.g., tau proteins, beta-amyloid 42 concentrations) are associated with greater risk for developing AD (Hansson et al., 2006). Taken together, these examples illustrate the heterogeneity in pathophysiology, neurocognitive and psychological impairments, and clinical course among these conditions and suggest that different risk profiles can potentially be characterized (Davidson et al., 2010; Eppig et al., 2017).

3. Applying Latent Class and Latent Profile Analyses

Given this recognition of the heterogeneity across numerous domains among these conditions, more recent research with MCI and dementia has used person-centered analytic strategies. Two approaches that permit categorizing individuals exhibiting different cognitive, behavioral, or neurological symptoms are LPA and latent class analysis (LCA). LPA is used when indicators are continuous, whereas LCA can include both continuous and categorical indicators (Masyn, 2013). As opposed to variable-centered approaches, LPA and LCA group individuals into homogeneous "profiles" or "classes," respectively (Muthén & Muthén, 2000). These approaches confer several advantages. First, LPA and LCA employ a variety of model fit indices, which may help researchers determine the appropriate number of classes or profiles that best fit the data (Libon et al., 2014). The LCA and LPA procedures permit identification of quantitative and/or qualitative differences among subgroups of individuals as well. In addition, these analytic approaches allow evaluation as to whether and to what extent external validators (e.g., demographic characteristics, response to intervention, indicators of course) are associated with class or profile membership (Libon et al., 2014). Lastly, LCA and LPA models are probabilistic, permitting the replication of subgroup findings in other samples (Muthén & Muthén, 2000).

Both LCA and LPA procedures begin with a one profile or class (unconditional) model. The number of profiles or classes is increased until there is no additional improvement in model fit (Nylund, Asparouhov, & Muthén, 2007; Nylund, Bellmore, Nishina, & Graham, 2007). Several model fit indices are often examined, including the Akaike information criterion (Akaike, 1987), Bayesian information criterion (BIC; Schwartz, 1978), and sample-size adjusted BIC (Sclove, 1987). The model that generates the smallest values on these fit indices is considered to have the best fit to the data. The bootstrap likelihood ratio test (BLRT) and Vuong–Lo–Mendell–Rubin likelihood ratio test also can be used to evaluate model fit, the latter of which is more stringent (Masyn, 2013; Nylund, Asparouhov et al., 2007; Nylund, Bellmore et al., 2007), although the BLRT is not available if all predictors are categorical. Both tests compare the fit of the model with k profiles to the model with $k-1$ profiles. The size of the smallest profile or class is considered as well, as small sizes (e.g., less than 5% of the sample) may indicate overfitting of the data and potential problems with replication and generalizability of the LPA/LCA solution. Another model fit index that is often considered is entropy, a measure of classification uncertainty. Entropy ranges from zero to 1 and higher values (e.g., > 0.7) indicate better classification of individuals. Although all of the model fit indices referenced above are evaluated, Monte Carlo simulation studies indicate that the BIC and BLRT are the most robust predictors of model fit (Nylund, Asparouhov et al., 2007). Last, models should also be examined to determine whether profiles or classes are distinct, as well as conceptually meaningful and consistent with the theoretical rationale that underpins the research questions. Examination of means among the classes or profiles permits consideration of whether identified subgroups are consistent with previous research and conceptual models. In addition, after determining the appropriate number of subgroups, tests of equality of means can be conducted to determine the external validity of the identified profiles or classes. These tests hold subgroup membership constant and generate chi-square statistics for omnibus and pairwise comparisons across latent classes or profiles. Pairwise comparisons are explored only if the omnibus tests are significant.

4. Examples of Research Using Person-Centered Approaches

Recently, more studies have begun to use LPA and LCA to characterize individuals with MCI or dementia who may quantitatively and qualitatively differ in term of biological, cognitive, and behavioral features. Most of this work has attempted to externally validate observed profiles/classes by examining whether these subgroups are associated with different risk factors, correlates, courses, and/or outcomes. Studies that have used LPA/LCA generally have found three to four profiles/classes that are often at differential risk for exacerbation of neurocognitive difficulties over time. The following discussion provides some examples of recent research that has used LCA or LPA to characterize adults with MCI or dementia. Given the dearth of clear diagnostic criteria for these disorders, the findings reviewed herein provide a foundation for using actuarial data drawn from multiple sources and using multiple levels of analysis to characterize more homogeneous subgroups of individuals with MCI or dementia (Eppig et al., 2017).

As a first example, Forrester et al. (2015) identified three symptom profiles among adults with MCI. These included a "severe" profile that reported high rates of symptoms (e.g., delusions, anxiety, apathy, disinhibition, irritability); an "affective" profile characterized primarily by high rates of depression, anxiety, and irritability; and an "asymptomatic" group, who exhibited low symptom levels (Forrester et al., 2015). When using the asymptomatic profile as the reference group, auxiliary analyses indicated that individuals in the severe group were almost twice as likely, and individuals in the affective profile were about 1.5 times more likely, to develop dementia 2 years after the initial assessment (Forrester et al., 2015). A second study similarly identified three profiles of individuals with MCI: a "memory deficit" profile, a "least cognitively impaired" profile, and a "multiple deficits" profile (e.g., reduced category and letter fluency, visuospatial function, and executive function ability; McGuinness, Barrett, McIlvenna, Passmore, & Shorter, 2015). Auxiliary analyses indicated that in comparison to the multiple deficits profile, the least cognitively impaired profile was younger and had a higher IQ. The memory deficit profile was less likely to convert to dementia than the multiple deficits profile; the least cognitively impaired profile was less likely to develop dementia than the other two profiles (McGuiness et al., 2015).

In a third example examining individuals with MCI, Eppig et al. (2017) identified three profiles based on variables derived from a comprehensive neuropsychological protocol (i.e., visuoconstructional ability, language, attention/executive function, episodic memory): a "mixed impairment MCI" profile, an "amnestic MCI" profile, and a "normal" profile. In terms of external validation of these profiles, the amnestic and mixed classes were more likely to be apolipoprotein e4+, as well as having cerebrospinal fluid biomarkers consistent with AD, than individuals with the normal profile. Thus, research involving individuals with MCI identifies more homogeneous subgroups that exhibit different profiles with regard to neuropsychological functioning that also can be distinguished based on course and illness markers.

Other work using person-centered analyses has identified three subgroups of individuals with AD. These profiles included (a) a low behavioral and psychological symptoms of dementia profile; (b) an affective profile characterized by a greater probability of depression and irritability; and (c) a high behavioral and psychological symptoms of dementia (e.g., irritability, delusions, aggression, unusual motor behaviors) profile (Lam, Leung, Lui, Leung, & Chiu, 2006; Lyketsos et al., 2001). Similar profiles were observed in another study that found a "low symptomatic" class that reported very few symptoms and an "anxiety/depressive" symptoms class characterized by higher endorsement of affective disturbance, anxiety, and agitation (Moran, Lynch, Coen, Coakley, & Lawlor, 2004). However, unlike the Lam et al. (2006) and Lyketsos et al. (2001) studies, Moran et al. (2004) found a distinct subgroup of Alzheimer's patients who endorsed engaging in higher levels of aggressive behavior relative to the other classes (i.e., an "aggressive" class).

Another study that examined sleep patterns (e.g., daytime sleepiness, frequent awakenings during sleep) among adults with AD also found three profiles (Ownby, Peruyera, Acevedo, Loewenstein, & Sevush, 2012), who were labeled as experiencing no, moderate, or severe sleep problems. Auxiliary analyses indicated that compared to the class with no sleep problems, adults with moderate sleep problems were older, attained fewer years of education, and exhibited reduced cognitive functioning and higher levels of depressive symptoms. Adults in the severe sleeping problems class also had less education and had more cognitive deficits compared to adults in the moderate sleeping group (Ownby et al., 2012).

Some analyses have considered service utilization among individuals with dementia as opposed to processes associated with this condition. For example, Beeper et al. (2008) identified three profiles of engagement in community-based services among individuals with dementia: individuals with a low, average, or high probability of using these services. Subsequent analyses indicated that adults who were more likely to use community-based support services were more likely to report financial stability, private insurance, difficulties with daily activities, and higher concurrent symptoms (e.g., depression, psychosis); live in counties with a greater number of skilled nursing centers and physicians; and have AD rather than VaD (Beeber et el., 2008). Thus, meaningful, more homogeneous profiles have been identified among individuals with dementia that are characterized by cognitive, psychological, and service utilization variables. External validation supports the predictive utility and concurrent validity of the identified profiles and provides potentially important implications for course and intervention recommendations.

Other studies among individuals with MCI or dementia have identified four profiles. For example, Davidson et al. (2010) identified four subgroups of Alzheimer's patients: a "mild" group characterized by a low probability of memory problems, perseverations, language difficulties, and praxis; an "attention/construction" class that had a moderate to high probability of attention, conceptualization, and construction difficulties; a "memory" class that exhibited a high probability of memory, construction, and orientation problems; and a "severe" class categorized by a very high probability of memory, orientation, and perseveration impairments. In terms of external validation, individuals in the mild class were categorized as (a) having a high probability of possessing the APOE4 genotype relative to the other classes; (b) being younger than the severe and memory classes, but older than the attention/construction classes; and (c) being more educated than the severe class. The severe class also had a greater likelihood of experiencing visuospatial deficits and showing grasp reflexes, an indicator of disease progression, than the other classes. The attention/concentration class was the least likely to have the APOE4 genotype and was more likely to have significant visuospatial impairments relative to individuals in the other classes. In addition, the memory class had a low likelihood of experiencing visuospatial problems and white matter changes compared to the other groups (Davidson et al., 2010).

Ferriera et al. (2017) similarly identified four distinct subgroups of Alzheimer's patients: a "typical" AD group, a "hippocampal-sparing" group, a "limbic-predominant" group, and a "no atrophy" group. In terms of external validation of these profiles, individuals in the typical AD group exhibited more difficulties in learning and had greater increases in disease progression than the hippocampal-sparing and no atrophy groups. The limbic-predominant group also exhibited greater increases in cognitive deficits compared to the hippocampal-sparing and no atrophy groups (Ferriera et al., 2017).

In another recent example, Hayden et al. (2014) identified four subgroups of individuals varying in AD symptoms, including groups that exhibited (a) very low memory, attention, executive function, and language abilities; (b) low to moderate memory, attention, executive function, and language abilities; (c) moderate memory, attention, executive function, and language abilities; and (d) high memory, attention, executive function, and language abilities. The low memory, attention, executive function, and language profile was the least likely to remain cognitively typical 3 years later, whereas the low to moderate memory, attention, executive function, and language profile had increased odds of impairment, except in the nonamnestic areas. The moderate and high memory, attention, executive function, and language profile had very low odds of developing cognitive impairments 3 years later relative to the other classes (Hayden et al., 2014).

Four classes of individuals with dementia were also identified by Libon et al. (2014). These included (a) a "moderate/mixed" group characterized by delayed recognition and lower levels of lexical retrieval and naming; (b) a "mild/mixed" group that exhibited relatively high performance on neuropsychological measures; (c) an "amnestic" profile that exhibited poor performance on delayed free recall and recognition and higher levels of lexical retrieval and naming; and (d) a "dysexecutive" class that manifested poor performance on executive functioning measures, but higher performance on memory-related tests. In terms of external validation of these classes, the dysexecutive and moderate/mixed classes exhibited lower executive functioning performance than the mild/mixed and amnestic groups, and the mild/mixed group also performed less well than the amnestic group. The moderate/mixed group performed less well on lexical retrieval/naming tasks than the other profiles, whereas the mild/mixed group exhibited lower performance than the amnestic group. In terms of memory functioning, two main findings emerged: (a) the amnestic and moderate/mixed profiles exhibited greater memory deficits than the mild/mixed and dysexecutive profiles, and (b) the mild/mixed group exhibited reduced performance on memory tasks relative to the dysexecutive profile (Libon et al., 2014).

In another study conducted by Libon et al. (2016), the authors examined performance on neuropsychological tests as an indicator of MCI among individuals with chronic regional pain syndrome. Four profiles were identified: (a) moderate neuropsychological test performance, (b) amnestic, (c) low/average neuropsychological test performance, and (d) average/high neuropsychological test performance (Libon et al., 2016). Auxiliary analyses revealed that the low/average and moderate neuropsychological test performance profiles had fewer years of education than the average/high neuropsychological test performance group; the moderate neuropsychological test performance profile also had less education than the amnestic profile. Profiles also differed in depressive symptoms such that individuals with average/high neuropsychological test performance exhibited higher depressive symptoms than individuals with low/average neuropsychological test performance. Further, the amnestic profile exhibited higher pain levels than the average/high and low/average neuropsychological test performance profiles (Libon et al., 2016).

In a study that sought to examine risk for MCI and dementia based on neuropsychiatric variables, Leoutsakos, Forrester, Lyketsos, and Smith (2015) identified four profiles of individuals, including profiles with (a) a high probability of agitation and irritability, (b) a high probability of several neuropsychiatric symptoms (e.g., hallucinations, anxiety), (c) a high likelihood of depression, and (d) a low probability of symptoms. Using the group with a low probability of symptoms as the reference class, the group with the highest probability of neuropsychiatric symptoms was three times more likely to develop dementia, followed by the other profiles, which were about twice as likely to develop dementia (Leoutsakos et al., 2015).

Norton et al. (2012) used LCA to identify subgroups of adults with AD who differed based on lifestyle patterns (i.e., social activities, smoking, diet, alcohol use, church attendance, and physical activity). Four classes were found, including (a) an unhealthy–religious class, (b) an unhealthy–nonreligious group, (c) a moderately healthy–religious class, and (4) a healthy–very religious class. Compared to the unhealthy–religious class, the moderately healthy–religious and healthy–very religious classes had a lower probability of developing dementia (Norton et al., 2012). Thus, in terms of phenotypic presentation, neuropsychological performance, co-occurring symptoms, and community activities, previous research has identified three to four profiles or classes among individuals experiencing or at risk for MCI or dementia.

Nevertheless, some studies have identified more than four profiles or classes among individuals with MCI or dementia. For example, Köhler et al. (2013) created profiles using scores for immediate and delayed recall, delayed recognition, speed of information processing, attention, verbal fluency, and executive function abilities among individuals with MCI. Five profiles were identified: (a) high normal cognition, (b) low normal cognition, (c) primary memory impairment in recall, (d) memory impairment in recall and deficits in delayed recognition, and (e) primary nonmemory impairments. Auxiliary analyses indicated that individuals in the memory impairment classes prospectively exhibited elevated rates of AD, whereas most participants with nonmemory impairments developed non-Alzheimer's dementia.

In a study examining individuals with AD, Iqbal et al. (2005) identified six profiles that involved different patterns of cerebrospinal fluid molecular markers (tau, ubiquitin, and amyloid β peptide 1-42 [AB_{1-42}]) and APOE alleles. Specifically, these profiles included (a) a group with low AB_{1-42}, low tau, average ubiquitin, and high APOE4; (b) a "normal" group characterized by high AB_{1-42}, low tau, average ubiquitin, and levels of APOE allele distribution similar to the typically developing population; (c) a profile that displayed low AB_{1-42}, high tau and average ubiquitin and was not more likely to possess APOE4 alleles; (d) a group characterized by low AB_{1-42}, tau, and ubiquitin; (e) a profile characterized by high AB_{1-42}, average tau, and average ubiquitin; and (f) a group with low AB_{1-42}, high tau, and high ubiquitin.

Hanfelt et al. (2011) identified seven profiles among adults with MCI that differed in their risk for developing VaD. These profiles were (a) a "minimally impaired" group that exhibited similar patterns of memory functioning as typically developing individuals; (b) an "amnestic only" group characterized by subtle impairments in delayed memory; (c) an "amnestic with functional and neuropsychiatric features" group that exhibited difficulties in immediate and delayed memory, challenges with performing daily living activities, and neuropsychiatric disturbances; (d) an "amnestic multidomain" profile that exhibited multiple deficits in episodic/semantic memory, executive function, and language; (e) an "amnestic multidomain with functional and neuropsychiatric features" group that displayed challenges in performing daily living activities, neuropsychiatric deficits, and difficulties with attention and visual motor skills; (f) a "functional and neuropsychiatric features" group that exhibited functional and behavioral deficits without cognitive impairments; and (g) an "executive function and language impairments" group that displayed impairments in nonmemory related areas. In terms of external validation, individuals in the amnestic multidomain with functional and neuropsychiatric features profile, as well as the functional and neuropsychiatric features profiles, were about four times more likely to exhibit signs of cerebrovascular disease (e.g., deterioration of cognitive abilities, hypertension, stroke) than the minimally impaired group (Hanfelt et al., 2011).

In another illustration of the significant neurocognitive heterogeneity among individuals with AD, Scheltens et al. (2016) identified eight profiles: mild memory impaired, moderate memory impaired, mild visuospatial/language impaired, moderate visuospatial language impaired, mild executive functioning impaired, moderate language impaired, mild diffuse impaired, and severe diffuse impaired profiles. Using the mild memory impaired group as the reference class, younger adults were twice as likely to be in the severe diffuse group, three times as likely to be in the moderate visuospatial class, and six times more likely to be in the mild executive functioning class. In addition, patients with AD with higher tau concentrations were more likely to be a member of the moderate language class, whereas individuals with higher tau phosphorylated at threonine-181 (pT) concentrations were half as likely to be members of the mild executive and mild diffuse classes. The moderate visuospatial group was associated with younger age, APOE e4 negative genotype, and posterior cortical atrophy. Individuals with prominent medial temporal lobe atrophy were half as likely to be in the mild executive profile. Like the moderate visuospatial profile, the severe diffuse profile was associated with atrophy in the posterior cortex. Lastly, patients with more white matter hyperintensities were about three times more likely to be in the moderate language group relative to the other profiles (Sheltens et al., 2016).

Across studies that have found multiple profiles of individuals with MCI and dementia, important similarities can be observed. For example, the severe class identified by Forrester et al. (2015) and Davidson et al. (2010), the multiple deficits group identified by McGuiness et al. (2015), the high memory and executive functioning impaired class identified by Hayden et al. (2014), the severe diffuse group identified by Sheltens et al. (2016), and the high behavioral and psychological symptoms profile identified by Lam et al. (2006), Lyketsos et al. (2001), and Leoutsakos et al. (2015) exhibited significant impairments in several domains (e.g., irritability, delusions). Adults included in these profiles also possessed features (e.g., higher levels of cortical atrophy, APOE4 polymorphism) that were associated with cognitive impairments and prospective decline, more so than individuals without these features (Davidson et al., 2010; Forrester et al., 2015; Hayden et al., 2014; McGuiness et al., 2015; Sheltens et al., 2016). Thus, despite significant heterogeneity in presentation, person-centered approaches permitted identification of subgroups of individuals who were at elevated risk for negative cognitive outcomes and a more challenging course.

Many studies also identified a profile characterized by memory problems specifically, which is unsurprising given the high rates of memory problems among individuals with MCI or AD. These profiles have been referred to in different ways, including the memory deficit group (McGuinness et al., 2015), low to moderate memory and executive functioning impaired group (Hayden et al., 2014), and an amnestic profile (Hanfelt et al., 2011; Libon et al., 2014, 2016). In addition, among individuals with MCI or AD in the studies reviewed, adults that were least cognitively impaired were reflected in the asymptomatic group identified by Forrester et al. (2015), the low behavioral and psychological symptoms of dementia identified by Lam et al. (2006) and Lyketsos et al. (2001), the least cognitively impaired by McGuinness et al. (2015), the mild class identified by Davidson et al. (2010), the high memory and executive functioning profiles identified by Hayden et al. (2014) and Kohler et al. (2013), the mild diffuse impaired profile identified by Sheltens et al. (2016), the minimally impaired group identified by Hanfelt et al. (2011), and the low symptomatic profiles coined by Moran et al. (2004) and Leoutsakos et al. (2015). Individuals with these profiles were often at reduced risk for further impairments in cognitive functioning over time (Eppig et al., 2017; Forrester et al., 2015; Hanfelt et al., 2011; McGuinness et al., 2015).

It is clear that there is significant heterogeneity not only in presentation of MCI and AD, but also in the profiles and classes identified across studies examining individuals with MCI or AD. There are several potential reasons that may underpin these differences across studies. First, variability among samples may have influenced the number of observed classes and profiles; for example, heterogeneity among individuals with MCI, AD, or VaD may have influenced observed subgroups. Second, the variables considered in the LCA/LPA, as well as the auxiliary variables explored, may influence the quantitative and qualitative differences among studies in terms of the subgroups identified. Many of the studies that found three profiles focused on memory and neuropsychiatric symptom domains (e.g., depression, psychosis; Lam et al., 2006; Lyketsos et al., 2001). However, authors that examined additional characteristics (e.g., executive functioning, language, visuospatial abilities) have reported between four (Hayden et al., 2014; Libon et al., 2014, 2016) and eight (Scheltens et al., 2016) profiles, suggesting that the inclusion of other features relevant to MCI and dementia may influence the observed heterogeneity in terms of model selection across studies. Similarly, a wide variety of auxiliary variables were considered (e.g., demographic characteristics, presence of APOE e4 cortical atrophy), which, if the authors were concerned with external validation of the statistical solution, potentially could influence the final model selected. Third, the informant and method of assessment (e.g., questionnaires, immunoassay) may have led to some discrepancies between identified classes or profiles. Nevertheless, the use of multiple levels of analysis for characterizing strengths and challenges among individuals with MCI or dementia can shed critical light on these profiles and provide information that can bolster etiological and intervention models.

5. Conclusions and Implications

MCI, AD, and VaD are deleterious conditions that may result in significant, chronic impairment across a multitude of domains and are often associated with a deteriorating course. Until relatively recently, much research has relied on variable-centered techniques to study these conditions. Although studies that have employed variable-centered statistical approaches have enhanced our understanding of etiological factors and correlates that contribute to or exacerbate MCI and dementia, variable-centered techniques assume that the influence of predictors on outcomes is homogenous across the population (Laursen & Hoff, 2006; Masyn et al., 2013). Given evidence that MCI and dementia are heterogeneous conditions (e.g., Forrester et al., 2015; Garre-Olmo et al., 2010; Libon et al., 2014), person-centered procedures, such as LCA and LPA, are useful analytic approaches for identifying more homogeneous subgroups or profiles that may have distinct correlates, courses, and potentially different responses to treatments. Indeed, the research reviewed in this chapter indicates that these strategies permit one to (a) identify subgroups of individuals who differ in the frequency and/or quality of neurocognitive symptoms, correlates, course, or outcomes and (b) identify differences among subgroups that can externally validate and provide support for the predictive validity and utility of these profiles or classes.

Available person-centered research among individuals with MCI or dementia has identified three to eight subgroups varying in neurocognitive (e.g., executive functioning, memory, language), lifestyle, neuropsychiatric, neurobiological (e.g., cerebrospinal fluid markers), and/or genetic (e.g., APOE e4 genotype) features. In terms of external validation, studies have considered an extensive range of variables, including the course and development of further cognitive impairments (e.g., conversion to AD), demographic characteristics (e.g., age, socioeconomic status, area of residency), genetic features (e.g., presence of APOE e4 polymorphism), neurocognitive correlates (e.g., visuospatial, memory, or executive functioning abilities), depressive symptoms, pain, and neurobiological markers (e.g., indicators of cerebrovascular disease, cortical atrophy). There are some similarities across studies in terms of groups identified and patterns of external validation, and these results can inform identification of individuals at greatest risk for negative outcomes and intervention efforts among individuals with MCI or dementia.

The use of person-centered approaches to identify more homogeneous subgroups of individuals with MCI or dementia is relatively new, but this approach holds great promise for increasing our understanding about these disorders. Future research should continue to use LCA and LPA to decrease heterogeneity and identify meaningful subgroups, although it will be important to seek to replicate previous work using similar variables to test the generalizability of the subgroups identified. The breadth of person-centered research reviewed in this chapter illustrates this exciting method for the better understanding of the heterogeneity associated with MCI or dementia. Nevertheless, it also points to the fact that using similar variables across studies and in clinical assessments would be helpful for building actuarial approaches that can improve diagnostic accuracy and predictive utility (Eppig et al., 2017). Future research that uses other person-centered approaches would be helpful for extending knowledge regarding more homogeneous subgroups of individuals with MCI or dementia; for example, growth mixture modeling would be particularly useful for longitudinal, repeated-measures data, as it allows for the identification of subgroups that follow similar trajectories (Garre-Olmo, et al., 2010). Future work also could extend to intervention variables as external validators, given that there is also variability in terms of responses to prevention and treatment efforts. For example, identifying profiles with particular neurobiological, neurocognitive, or neuropsychological features can speak not only to course but also to prevention and intervention strategies, such as targeted pharmacological treatments or psychosocial interventions based on an individual's profile.

References

Akaike, H. (1987). Factor analysis and AIC. *Psychometrika*, *52*, 317–332.

Apostolova, L. G., & Cummings, G. L. (2007). Neuropsychiatric manifestations in mild cognitive impairment: A systematic review of the literature. *Dementia and Geriatric Cognitive Disorders*, *25*, 115–126.

Beeber, A. S., Thorpe, J. M., & Clipp, E. C. (2008). Community-based service use by elders with dementia and their caregivers. *Nursing Research*, *57*, 312–321.

Bell-McGinty, S. Lopez, O. L., Meltzer, C. C., Scanlon, J. M., Whyte, E. M., DeKosky, S. T., & Becker, J. T. (2005). Differential cortical atrophy in subgroups of mild cognitive impairment. *Archives of Neurology*, *62*, 1393–1397.

Brambati, S. M., Belleville, S., Kergoat, M-J., Chayer, C., Gauthier, S., & Joubert, S. (2009). Single- and multiple-domain amnestic mild cognitive impairment: Two sides of the same coin? *Dementia and Geriatric Cognitive Disorders, 28*, 541–549.

Brookmeyer, R., Johnson, E., Ziegler-Graham, K., & Arrighi, H. M. (2007). Forecasting the global burden of Alzheimer's disease. *Alzheimer's and Dementia, 3*, 186–191.

Davidson, J. E., Irizarry, M. C., Bray, B. C., Wetten, S., Galwey, N., Gibson, R., . . . Monsch, A. U. (2010). An exploration of cognitive subtypes in Alzheimer's disease. *Journal of the International Neuropsychological Society, 16*, 233–243.

Devanand, D. P., Liu, X., Tabert, M. H., Pradhaban, G., Cuasay, K., de Leon, M. J., . . . Pelton, G. H. (2008). Combining early markers strongly predicts conversion from mild cognitive impairment to Alzheimer's disease. *Biological Psychiatry, 15*, 871–879.

Eppig, J.S., Edmonds, E.C., Campbell, L., Sanderson-Cimino, M., Delano-Wood, L., & Bondi, M.W.; Alzheimer's Disease Neuroimaging Initiative. (2017). Statistically derived subtypes and associations with cerebrospinal fluid and genetic biomarkers in mind cognitive impairment: A latent profile analysis. *Journal of the International Neuropsychological Society, 23*, 1–13.

Ferriera, D., Verhagen, C., Hernández-Cabrera, J. A., Cavallin, L., Guo, C-J., Ekman, U., . . . Westman, E. (2017). Distinct subtypes of Alzheimer's disease based on patterns of brain atrophy: Longitudinal trajectories and clinical applications. *Scientific Reports, 7*, 1–13.

Fiest, K. M., Roberts, J. I., Maxwell, C. K., Hogan, D. B., Smith, E. E., Frolkis, A., . . . Jetté, N. (2016). The prevalence and incidence of dementia due to Alzheimer's disease: A systematic review and meta-analysis. *Canadian Journal of Neurological Sciences, 43*, S51–S82.

Forrester, S. N., Gallo, J. J., Smith, G. S., & Leoutsakos, J-M. S. (2015). Patterns of neuropsychiatric symptoms in mild cognitive impairment and risk of dementia. *American Journal of Geriatric Psychology, 24*, 117–125.

Gallagher, D., Fischer, C. E., & Iaboni, A. (2017). Neuropsychiatric symptoms in mild cognitive impairment: An update on prevalence, mechanisms, and clinical significance. *Canadian Journal of Psychiatry, 62*, 161–169.

Garre-Olmo, J., López-Pousa, S., Vilalta-Franch, J., de Garcia-Blanco, M., & Vilarrasa, A. B. (2010). Grouping and trajectories of neuropsychiatric symptoms in patients with Alzheimer's disease. Part II: Two-year patient trajectories. *Journal of Alzheimer's Disease, 22*, 1169–1180.

Hanfelt, J. J., Wuu, J., Sollinger, A. B., Greenaway, M. C., Lah, J. J., Levey, A. I., & Goldstein, F. C. (2011). An exploration of subgroups of mild cognitive impairment based on cognitive, neuropsychiatric, and functional features: Analysis of data from the National Alzheimer's Coordinating Center. *American Journal of Geriatric Psychiatry, 19*, 940–950.

Hansson, O., Zetterberg, H., Buchhave, P., Londos, E., Blennow, K., & Minthon, L. (2006). Association between CSF biomarkers and incipient Alzheimer's disease in patients with mild cognitive impairment: A follow-up study. *Lancet Neurology, 5*, 228–234.

Hayden, K. M., Kuchibhatla, M., Romero, H. R., Plassman, B. L., Burke, J. R., Browndyke, J. N., & Welsh-Bohmer, K. A. (2014). Pre-clinical cognitive phenotypes for Alzheimer's disease: A latent profile approach. *American Journal of Geriatric Psychiatry, 22*, 1364–1374.

Iqbal, K., Flory, M., Khatoon, S., Soininen, H., Pirttila, T., Lehtovirta, M., . . . Vanmechelen, E. (2005). Subgroups of Alzheimer's disease based on cerebrospinal fluid molecular markers. *Annals of Neurology, 58*, 748–757.

Jellinger, K. A. (2007). The enigma of vascular cognitive disorder and vascular dementia. *Acta Neuropathology, 113*, 349–388.

Jellinger, K. A. (2008). Morphological diagnosis of vascular dementia: A critical update. *Journal of the Neurological Sciences, 270*, 1–12.

Juncos-Rabadán, O., Periero, A. X., Facal, D., Lojo, C., Camaño, J. A., Sueiro, J., . . . Eiroa, P. (2014). Prevalence and correlates of mild cognitive impairment in adults aged over 50 years with subjective cognitive complaints in primary care centers. *Geriatrics and Gerontology International, 14*, 667–673.

Köhler, S., Hamel, R., Sistermans, N., Koene, T., Pijnenburg, Y. A. L., van der Flier, W. M., . . . Ramakers, I. (2013). Progression to dementia in memory clinic patients without dementia: A latent profile analysis. *Neurology, 81*, 1342–1349.

Lam, L. C. W., Leung, T., Lui, V. W. C., Leung, V. P. Y., & Chiu, H. F. K. (2006). Association between cognitive function, behavioral syndromes, and two-year clinical outcomes in Chinese subjects with late-onset Alzheimer's disease. *International Psychogeriatrics, 18*, 517–526,

Laursen, B., & Hoff, E. (2006). Person-centered and variable-centered approaches to longitudinal data. *Merrill-Palmer Quarterly, 52*, 377–389.

Leoutsakos, J-M. S., Forrester, S. N., Constantine, G. L., & Smith, G. W. (2015). Latent classes of neuropsychiatric symptoms in NACC controls and conversion to MCI or dementia. *Journal of Alzheimer's Disease, 48*, 483–493.

Libon, D., Drabick, D. A., Giovanetti, T., Price, C. C., Bondi, M. W., Eppig, J., . . . Swenson, R. (2014). Neuropsychological syndromes associated with Alzheimer's/vascular dementia: A latent class analysis approach. *Journal of Alzheimer's Disease, 42*, 999–1014.

Libon, D. J., Eppig, J., Drabick, D. A. G., Erwin, K., Annibali, C., Durmala, L., . . . Schwartzmann, R. J. (2016). Neuropsychological and related clinical features associated with complex regional pain syndrome: A latent class analysis. *British Journal of Medicine and Medical Research, 18*, 1–12.

Lyketsos, C. G., Sheppard, J-M. E., Steinberg, M., Tschanz, J. A. T., Norton, M. C., Steffens, D. C., & Breitner, J. C. S. (2001). Neuropsychiatric disturbance in Alzheimer's disease clusters into three groups: The Cache County study. *International Journal of Geriatric Psychiatry, 16*, 1043–1053.

Masyn, K. (2013). Latent class analysis and finite mixture model. In T. D. Little (Ed.), *The Oxford handbook of quantitative methods: Vol. 2, Statistical analysis.* New York, NY: Oxford University Press. doi:10.1903/oxfordhb/9780199934898.013.0025

McGuinness, B., Barrett, S. L., McIlvenna, J., Passmore, A. P., & Shorter, G. W. (2015). Predicting conversion to dementia in a memory clinic: A standard clinical approach compared with an empirically defined clustering method (latent profile analysis) for mild cognitive impairment subtyping. *Alzheimer's and Dementia: Diagnosis, Assessment, and Disease Monitoring, 1*, 447–454.

Mirza, S.S., Ikram, M. A., Bos, D., Mihawscu, R., Hofman, A., & Tiemeier, H. (2017). Mild cognitive impairment and risk of depression and anxiety: A population-based study. *Alzheimer's and Dementia, 13*, 130–139.

Modrego, P. J., & Ferrández, J. (2012). Depression in patients with mild cognitive impairment increases the risk of developing dementia or Alzheimer type. *Archives of Neurology, 61*, 1290–1293.

Moran, M., Walsh, C., Lynch, A., Coen, R. F., Coakley, D., & Lawlor, B. A. (2004). Syndromes of behavioural and psychological symptoms in mild Alzheimer's disease. *International Journal of Geriatric Psychiatry, 19*, 359–364.

Muthén, B., & Muthén, L. K. (2000). Integrating person-centered and variable-centered analyses: Growth mixture modeling with latent trajectory classes. *Alcoholism: Clinical and Experimental Research, 24*, 882–891.

Norton, M. C., Dew, J., Smith, H., Fauth, E., Piercy, K. W., Breitner, J. C. S., . . .Welsh-Bohmer, K. (2012). Lifestyle behavior pattern is associated with different levels of risk for incident dementia and Alzheimer's disease: The Cache County study. *Journal of American Geriatric Society, 60*, 405–412.

Nylund, K. L., Asparouhov, T., & Muthén, B. O. (2007). Deciding on the number of latent classes in latent class analysis and growth mixture modeling: A Monte Carlo simulation study. *Structural Equation Modeling, 14*, 535–569.

Nylund, K. L., Bellmore, T., Nishina, A., & Graham, S. (2007). Subtypes, severity, and structural stability of peer victimization: What does latent class analysis say? *Child Development, 78*, 1706–1722.

Ownby, R. L., Peruyera, G., Acevedo, A., Loewenstein, D., & Sevush, S. (2012). Subtypes of sleep problems in patients with Alzheimer disease. *American Journal of Geriatric Psychiatry, 22*, 148–156.

Peter, J., Abdulkadir, A., Kaller, C., Kümmer, D., Hüll, M., Vach, W., & Klöppel, S. (2014). Subgroups of Alzheimer's disease: Stability of empirical clusters over time. *Journal of Alzheimer's Disease, 42*, 651–661.

Petersen, R. C., Smith, G. E., Waring, S. C., Ivnik, R. J., Tangalos, E. G., & Kokmen, E. (1999). Mild cognitive impairment: Clinical characterization and outcome. *Archives of Neurology, 56*, 303–308.

Rowe, C. C., Ng, S., Ackermann, U., Gong, S. J., Pike, K., Savage, G., . . . Villemagne, V. L. (2007). Imaging β-amyloid burden in aging and dementia. *Neurology, 68*, 1718–1825.

Sachs-Ericcson, N., & Blazer, D. G. (2015). The new DSM-5 diagnosis of mild neurocognitive disorder and its relation to research in mild cognitive impairment. *Aging and Mental Health, 19*, 2–12.

Schwartz, G. (1978). Estimating the dimension of a model. *Annals of Statistics, 6*, 461–464.

Scheltens, N. M., Galindo, Garre, F., Pijnenburg, Y. A. L., van der Vlies, A. E., Smits, L. L., & . . . van der Flier, W. M. (2016). The identification of cognitive subtypes in Alzheimer's disease dementia using latent class analysis. *Journal of Neurology, Neurosurgery, and Psychiatry, 87*, 235–243.

Sclove, S. L. (1987). Application of model-selection criteria to some problems in multivariate analysis. *Psychometrika, 52*, 333–343.

van der Flier, W. M., Schoonenboom, S. N. M., Pijnenburg, Y. A. L., Fox, N. C., & Scheltens, P. (2006). The effect of APOE genotype on clinical phenotype in Alzheimer disease. *Neurology, 67*, 526–527.

von Gunten, A., Bouras, C., Kövari, E., Giannakopoulos, P., & Hof, P. R. (2006). Neural substrates of cognitive and behavioral deficits in Alzheimer's disease. *Brain Research Reviews, 51*, 176–211.

Ward, A., Arrighi, M. H., Michels, S., & Cedarbaum, J. M. (2012). Mild cognitive impairment: Disparity of incidence and prevalence estimates. *Alzheimer's and Dementia, 8*, 14–21.

Wetzels, R. B., Zuidema, S. U., de Jonghe, J. F. M., Verhey, F. R. J., & Koopmans, R. T. C. M. (2010). Course of neuropsychiatric symptoms in residents with dementia in nursing homes over 2-year period. *American Journal of Geriatric Psychiatry, 18*, 1054–1065.

Wimo, A., Jonsson, L., & Winblad, B. (2006). An estimate of the worldwide prevalence and direct costs of dementia in 2003. *Dementia and Geriatric Cognitive Disorders*, *21*, 175–181.

Youn, J. C., Lee., D. Y., Jhoo, J. H., Kim, K. W., Choo, I. H., & Woo, J. I. (2011). Prevalence and neuropsychiatric syndromes of Alzheimer's disease (AD). *Archives of Gerontology and Geriatrics*, *52*, 258–263.

7

Apraxic and Action-Intentional Disorders Associated With Vascular and Degenerative Dementing Diseases

Kenneth M. Heilman

1. Introduction

All animals move, and these movements allow them to successfully interact with their environment, other animals, themselves and their families. Humans have a great repertoire of movements and the human motor system can mediate an almost infinite number of movements. Therefore, to have successful interactions, the human motor system needs to be guided by programs, and there are two major forms of programs that that are important in human performance, praxic and intentional. The praxic-movement programs provide the human motor system, including the corticospinal system, with the knowledge of "how" to perform purposeful skilled movements, including the spatial component of both the egocentric (body centered) and allocentric (object or environmentally centered) movements as well as the temporal aspects of movements, and the force exerted. It is not only is important to know "how" to move, but it is also important to know "when" to move and the action-intentional programs provide the motor system with information about "when" to move. In this chapter we will discuss both disorders of the praxic, "how" and intentional "when" systems.

Many patients with dementia from vascular disease or degenerative disease have disorders of these "how" praxic and "when" intentional networks. Unfortunately, few clinicians test patients for the different forms of apraxia or action intentional disorders. The diagnosis of apraxia, as well as the type of apraxia may be important for several reasons. Determining the presence of apraxia and the type of apraxia, as well as the presence of an intentional disorder, may help the clinician determine the form of dementia with which a patient's is suffering. In addition, the limb apraxic and action intentional disorders can often cause a disability. The detection of these disorders may help reduce disability by informing patients and caregivers about the types of activities that may be dangerous and

Kenneth M. Heilman, *Apraxic and Action-Intentional Disorders Associated With Vascular and Degenerative Dementing Diseases* In: *Vascular Disease, Alzheimer's Disease, and Mild Cognitive Impairment.* Edited by: David J. Libon, Melissa Lamar, Rodney A. Swenson, Kenneth M. Heilman, Oxford University Press (2020). © Oxford University Press.
DOI: 10.1093/oso/9780190634230.003.0008

aid them in the development of strategies that may help them to overcome these disabilities. In the following sections, the signs of these programming disorders, the tests used to assess patients for these disorders, as well as their pathophysiology will be reviewed. Although we would like to discuss treatment, unfortunately, little is known about the treatment/rehabilitation of these disorders.

2. Apraxia

Humans primarily use their upper limbs to interact with their environment, other people, and themselves. To successfully perform these interactions a person needs to know "how" to correctly perform meaningful and purposeful actions. There are several major components of performing purposeful actions. First, a person needs to know the final goal of an action or series of actions, how to organize and sequence these actions, and the tools that are required to provide the mechanical advantage required to successfully complete these action. In addition, a person needs to know how to correctly posture their forelimb to perform a direct action with their hands or hold a tool/implement that will allow a person to perform this action. They also need to know how to contract their muscles to properly move their joints to accomplish the required actions. In addition, to correctly interact with an object, a person also needs to how to spatially direct their hand and fingers, or the tool they are using, to the object with which they want to act upon, as well as how fast to move portions of the their forelimb, and how much force to use. A loss of the ability to correctly use the limbs to perform a desired goal is called apraxia. In this chapter, we will review the several forms of apraxia that vascular and degenerative diseases may cause, including the means of testing for these different forms of apraxia, the signs and symptoms of the different forms of apraxia, the diseases that may cause these disorders, and the possible brain mechanisms that may account for these disorders.

Whereas apraxia is a major cause of disability, there are many other disorders associated with dementing diseases that can cause an impaired ability to perform purposeful skilled movements, including abnormal movements such as tremor, chorea, ballismus, and myoclonus. In addition, severe sensory-perceptual deficits, attentional deficits, and cognitive impairments, such as an impaired speech comprehension, may also impair a person's ability to perform purposeful goal oriented actions. Whereas the presence of these nonapraxic disorders may cause an impairment in the ability to perform purposeful skilled movements, these disorders may also interfere with the clinician's ability to test for apraxia; however, the presence of these disorders does not preclude the possibility that these patients also have an apraxia.

3. Task-Specific Forms of Limb Apraxia: Dressing and Construction

Often when a clinician views a patient who is performing abnormal movements and does not know the cause of this disorder, they will also call this disorder apraxia. For example, when seeing a patient with impaired walking, they will call this disorder apraxia of gait. However, in regard to the forelimbs, there are two major task specific impairments of purposeful movement that are called apraxia. These are impairments of "how" to dress, called dressing apraxia, and "how" to draw, called construction apraxia. Although these disorder appear to be "how" deficits, they can be caused by disorders other than motor programming. For example, dressing apraxia or constructional apraxia can be caused by unilateral inattention or neglect, such that the person with this disorder does not dress their left side (neglected) side of their body or draw on one side of the page. Therefore, while disorders such as constructional apraxia are commonly associated with dementia and are often assessed in neuropsychological batteries such as the Mini-Mental Status Examination and the Montreal Cognitive Assessment, these task-specific apraxic disorders will not be discussed in this chapter.

4. Forms of Upper Limb Apraxia

Whereas the term "apraxia" was a term was originally used by Steinthal (1871) to describe impairments in the ability of patients to correctly carry out "how" motor programs, it was primarily Hugo Liepmann (1920) who made the first important contributions to the understanding of these "how" disorders including describing three major forms of upper limb apraxia including: (a) limb-kinetic apraxia, (b) ideomotor apraxia, and (c) ideational apraxia. Although most of the patients described by Liepmann had their apraxia caused by a cerebral infarction, these three forms of apraxia can also be seen with patients who have degenerative diseases.

We described a fourth type of upper limb apraxia that we call conceptual apraxia (Heilman et al., 1997; Ochipa et al., 1992). This disorder can also be caused by vascular as well as degenerative diseases that are associated with dementia. There is another form of apraxia that we initially misnamed "ideational apraxia" (Heilman, 1973) and we now call "dissociation apraxia" (Heilman et al., 2012). These different forms of apraxia are clinically distinguished by the types of motor programming errors made by the patients who exhibit these different form of apraxia described by Liepmann. The following sections will contain descriptions of how patients may be tested as well as the type of errors made by the patients who exhibit each of these forms of apraxia. The brain mechanisms that may account for these forms of apraxia will also be discussed as well as the different diseases that can cause each of these apraxic disorders.

5. Conceptual Apraxia

5.1. Clinical Signs

Whereas there are many changes in the environment that humans can make by using their hands, there are also changes that cannot be made by only using their hands. Even without taking a course in physics, humans have forms of mechanical knowledge that are based on laws of physics. For example to crack ice into small pieces, much pressure is needed and often the ice cannot be cracked by pressing the hand or finger against this ice. However, we do know that we can increase pressure by reducing the area to which this pressure is applied. If we use a tool that has a very small area, such as the tip of an ice pick, with the same force we used with our finger, we can crack ice. Therefore, when a person needs to alter something, they need to know the correct tool that would allow them to accomplish their goal, and patients with conceptual apraxia may not know the correct tool. Since humans have mechanical knowledge if the proper tool is not available, we are able to use alternative tools, such as using a screwdriver to crack the ice, and patients with conceptual apraxia may also have an impairment of selecting alternative tools. If there is no tool to use for making the desired alteration, humans often develop new tools, and patients with conceptual apraxia may be impaired at developing tools.

When assessing patients for conceptual apraxia, they may be tested by learning if they can select the specific tool (e.g., hammer) that is designed to work with a specific object (e.g., nail; tool–object associative knowledge). To further test for a loss of mechanical knowledge, a more sensitive test is the "alternative tool use task." For example, when attempting to drive a nail into a piece of wood and there is no hammer available, which of the three tools would be best to accomplish this goal: a wrench, a screwdriver or hacksaw? The patient with conceptual apraxia might select a screwdriver rather than a wrench to pound in this nail (Ochipa, Rothi, & Heilman, 1992). The most sensitive test for mechanical knowledge is to learn if a patient can successfully develop a tool. For example, bending a wire to make a hook to retrieve an item in the bottom of a tube (Ochipa et. al., 1992, Heilman et al., 1997).

In addition to knowing and selecting the tool can provide the needed mechanical advantage to make the desired changes, a person needs to know the type of movements that are associated with specific tools, utensils, or objects (tool–object movement associative knowledge). For example, after selecting the ice pick, the person who wants to crack ice also needs to know that they have to make pounding movements. When shown a picture of an ice pick and asked to demonstrate by pantomiming the use of this tool, patients with conceptual apraxia may make twisting movements of their hand, like that used to use a screwdriver.

5.2. Pathophysiology

Right-handed patients with a callosal disconnection can demonstrate conceptual apraxia of their nonpreferred, nondominant left hand (Watson & Heilman, 1983). This observation suggests that in people who are right-handed, it is their left hemisphere that stores this tool–object, tool–movement, and mechanical knowledge. In prior research (Heilman et al., 1997), we wanted to learn the localization of injury that induces conceptual apraxia and to confirm that the left hemisphere is dominant for storing mechanical knowledge. We studied right-handed subjects with unilateral hemispheric strokes. Although we found that conceptual apraxia was most commonly associated with left hemisphere lesions, our analysis of lesion sites did not reveal where in the left hemisphere this information might be stored. The failure to find a specific locus could have been caused by an insufficient number of subjects; however, it is possible that tool–object, tool–movements, and mechanical knowledge are each stored in widely distributed left hemisphere networks. A subsequent functional imaging study appears to support this hypothesis. This study revealed that when the conceptual tasks were compared with the control tasks, there was overlapping activation in left parietal temporal occipital junction and prefrontal, dorsal premotor, cuneus, and inferior temporal areas (Ebisch et al., 2007).

5.3. Diseases That Can Cause Conceptual Apraxia

Although patients with Alzheimer's disease (AD) are rarely tested for conceptual apraxia, this disorder is often present (Ochipa et al., 1992). When taking a history, the family of these patients will often explain that the patient has difficulty performing instrumental activities, and this disability is often related to the presence of conceptual apraxia. In some patients, the signs of conceptual apraxia might be one of the earliest cognitive signs in this disease. There is also some evidence that patients with semantic dementia, a form of frontotemporal lobar degeneration may also have conceptual apraxia (Silveri & Ciccarelli, 2009). As previously mentioned, this disorder may also be seen with vascular disease that damages the left hemisphere.

6. Ideomotor Apraxia

6.1. Clinical Signs

When obtaining a history from either the patient or the patient's caregiver, clinicians rarely ask about a patients ability to perform goal-directed purposeful instrumental activities; however, the caregiver or patient may provide this information when asked. Some patients can have apraxia primarily in one upper limb or one upper limb may have a more severe apraxic deficit, and thus both limbs, when possible, should be test. Most often when testing patients, clinicians request that patients perform a series of pantomimes to verbal commands as well as to imitate the examiner making pantomimes. There are two forms of pantomimes, transitive and intransitive. When examining transitive pantomimes the patient is asked to make believe they are performing a task with a specific tool. "Make believe you are holding scissor and you are going cut a piece of paper." They are also told not to use their hand as if it were the tool. When performing intransitive gesture, they are asked to show how they communicate using their arm and hand. For example, "When hitch-hiking, show me how you would let drivers that you would like to ride with them." Patients with ideomotor apraxia often perform more poorly with transitive ("Show me how would you scramble eggs with a fork") than intransitive acts ("Wave bye-bye") (Haaland et al., 2000; Rothi et al., 1988), and thus patients should be assess by having them pantomime transitive actions. When testing patients with imitation, the examiner can either use pantomimes of actual actions (such as using scissors) or novel actions. Patients can also be tested by having them use actual tools; however, seeing and holding tools may provide the patient with cues that may help them perform the correct actions, and therefore this method is the least sensitive for determining the presence of ideomotor apraxia. When performing learned purposeful actions such as pantomiming how to use a screwdriver to insert a screw into the wall, patients with ideomotor apraxia can make several types of spatial errors. They can make (a) postural errors, (b) egocentric spatial movement errors, and (c) allocentric spatial movement errors.

Postural errors, which are also called internal configuration errors, are most likely seen when a patient is asked to pantomime a transitive act. Goodglass and Kaplan (1963) reported that when patients are asked to pantomime the use of a tool or implement, such as scissors or a screwdriver, patients often use their hand and fingers as the tool. For example, when the patients with ideomotor apraxia are asked to demonstrate how they would use a screwdriver to put a screw in the wall they often will use their index finger as if it was the screwdriver, and when asked to use pair of scissors to cut a piece of paper in half, they will often extend their forefinger and middle finger and then repeatedly move these two fingers together and apart like they are the blades of the scissors. Goodglass and Kaplan called these types of errors "body-part as object errors," but in our papers we have called these errors "body part as the tool errors." Making body part as tool errors is not always a sign of the presence of ideomotor apraxia, because even normal people, when asked to pantomime a transitive action, will often make these types of errors. It is rare that healthy people perform transitive pantomimes but commonly do use emblems. Using the finger as blades is an emblem of scissors rather than a pantomime. However, Raymer et al. (1997) demonstrated that although normal people when asked to pantomime transitive acts do frequently produce emblems (body part as tool errors), when they are asked to not use their hands or other body parts as the actual tools, they then perform correct pantomimes.

Some patients with ideomotor apraxia when asked not to use their body parts as the tool will stop making body part as tool errors and will attempt to pantomime, but they will often incorrectly posture their fingers, hand, forearm, and arm. When performing transitive pantomime to verbal command or imitating the examiner performing a transitive or meaningless action, as well as even when using actual objects, a person needs to correctly move the joints in their upper limb. There are two major aspects of these movements, one being egocentric and the other allocentric. The egocentric movements such as rotation at the elbow when using a screwdriver or flexion and extension at the wrist when using a hammer are the egocentric components, and moving the arm so that the hammer will hit the nail is the allocentric component. The patient with ideomotor apraxia often will move the incorrect joints. For example, if asked to pantomime using a screw-driver to insert a screw into a wall, patients with ideomotor apraxia may rotate their wrist rather that rotating their arm at their elbow.

Whereas hitting a nail with a hammer and turning a screw with a screwdriver can be performed with movements at just one joint (i.e., wrist movements for hammering and elbow rotation for screwing), many purposeful skill acts require coordinated movements of two or more joints. For example, if a person is asked to use a bread knife to slice a piece of bread from a loaf of bread, a person will usually bring their arm at their shoulder forward and at the same time extend their arm at their elbow, but not move their wrist. Then, after they have made this forward movement with the bread knife, they would have to reverse these movements to move the knife backward, and as they move their arm backwards at their shoulder, they have to flex their arm at the elbow; however, with each stroke with the knife, they should also reduce their flexion at the elbow to permit the knife to move downward. Patients with ideomotor apraxia when pantomiming, imitating, or actually using a knife will often just move one joint such as the elbow and instead of making slicing movement they may make chopping movements (Rothi et al., 1988; Poizner et al., 1990).

Patients with ideomotor apraxia can also make errors in their allocentric or target-oriented movements (Rothi et al., 1988; Poizner et al., 1990). Therefore, when demonstrating how to slice bread they may not keep their knife on the same sagittal plane. Although it is usually easiest for the clinician to detect postural and spatial movement errors, patients with ideomotor apraxia may also make errors in the speed with which they move their limb. For example, Poizner et al. (1990) reported that when patients with ideomotor apraxia demonstrate how they would use a knife to slice turkey, unlike healthy participants who move their arm more slowly as the knife approaches it turning point, patients with apraxia will often not reveal this speed pattern.

Finally, patients with ideomotor apraxia may also have praxis recognition disorders, including having an impairment of comprehending other people's meaningful pantomimes, and they may also be impaired at discriminating correct form incorrect postures (Mozaz et al., 2002), as well as pantomimed actions (Heilman et al., 1982). Patients with deficits of error detection and a failure to understand other peoples' gestures may have their brain dysfunction in different areas of the brain than those apraxic patients who are able to correctly perform these recognition tasks. Therefore, tests of comprehension of well-performed pantomimes and discrimination between correctly and incorrectly performed pantomimes should also be tested.

6.2. Pathophysiology

The first person to systematically study ideomotor apraxia was Hugo Liepmann. In one of his earliest papers Liepmann (1907) studied a population of right-handed patients who had damage confined to either their left or right hemisphere and reported that whereas ideomotor apraxia was rare in those patients with a right hemisphere injury, ideomotor apraxia was present in about 50% of those patients with left hemispheric strokes. Based on the frequent co-existence of aphasia and ideomotor apraxia in patients with left hemisphere lesions, it was posited that that both aphasia and apraxia are signs of an impairment in using symbols, a deficit that has been termed asymbolia (Finkelburg, 1873). Liepmann (1907), however, reported that these two disorders are dissociable. He had observed some patients who were aphasic who did not have ideomotor apraxia and others with ideomotor apraxia who were not aphasic. Thus, at least in part, the networks that mediate these two functions are independent, but the frequent co-occurrence of these two disorders is probably related to two factors. Both networks can be served by the same artery, such as the middle cerebral artery, and certain portions of the cerebral cortex may have neuronal networks that perform more than one function.

Liepmann (1920) reported that when a person with a left hemisphere injury developed ideomotor apraxia, they often had an injury to the inferior parietal lobe. Geschwind (1965) posited that a lesion of the left supramarginal gyrus was likely to injure the arcuate fasciculus that connects Wernicke's area, located in the posterior-superior temporal lobe, with the left hemisphere's convexity premotor cortex. This lesion would produce an ideomotor apraxia because the area of the brain important in verbal comprehension (Wernicke's area) is disconnected from the premotor cortex important in providing the motor cortex with the movement program; however, patients with ideomotor apraxia from an inferior parietal lobe lesion are also impaired at imitating pantomimes and gestures as well as performing with actual tools (Poizner et al., 1990), and Geschwind's (1965) verbal–motor disconnection hypotheses cannot explain these observations. As an alternative hypothesis, we suggested that the inferior parietal lobe may contain the three-dimensional visual and kinesthetic spatial-temporal movement representations (Heilman et al., 1982; Rothi et al., 1985) that are critical for programming purposeful skilled movements. Rather than cause a verbal comprehension-premotor disconnection as suggested by Geschwind, we proposed that left inferior parietal lesions degraded these movement representations that we have also called "praxicons," and without these spatial and temporal representation, patients cannot correctly perform pantomimes to command, imitate, or even correctly use tools and implements.

Ungerleider and Mishkin (1982) proposed that there are two visual processing networks. One network is ventral and is important for object recognition and has been called the "what" system. The other system is more dorsal and is important for determination of object's spatial position in relation to the viewer. This dorsal system, is often called the "where" system. The left hemisphere's inferior parietal lobe receives visual information from both of these systems. Whereas the ventral "what" system allows a person to recognize the object that will be altered and the tool that will aid the participant in performing this alteration, the dorsal "where" visual network provides information about the location of the object in relationship to the participant's body. The left inferior parietal lobe also receives input from the superior parietal association areas that processes proprioceptive-kinesthetic information from the somatosensory cortex, stores proprioceptive-kinesthetic representations of upper limb movements and sends this information to the inferior parietal lobe.

Based on this visual "what" and "where" information together with the proprioceptive-kinesthetic information, the left inferior parietal lobe develops three-dimensional visual and kinesthetic spatial-temporal movement representations of skilled movements. Therefore, if a patient has an injury to the left inferior parietal lobe and a degradation of these movement representations, the patient will demonstrate deficits when pantomiming to command, imitating both meaningful and meaningless gestures, and even when using their hands or tool to alter object or to communicate. Furthermore, in addition to these spatial and temporal performance deficits when these representations are degraded, patients with this injury may unable to comprehend other people's gestures or pantomimes.

These praxis representations (praxicons) may be analogous to sheet music, which for musician, such a pianist, contains spatial information about the piano keys that must be pressed, as well as the timing information about how long and how hard to press each of the piano keys. In the human brain, whereas the praxicons or movement representations are stored in the left inferior parietal lobe, it is the premotor cortex that translates these visual and kinesthetic spatial-temporal movement representations into the programs that will excite the specific cortical motor neurons required to make the correct arm and hand movements.

Based on this model, if the movement representations, or praxicons, are intact and a person has an injury to their premotor cortex, they should also demonstrate the errors associated with ideomotor apraxia; however, in contrast to patients with left hemispheric inferior parietal lesions, patients with a premotor injury who have intact praxicons should be able to discriminate between incorrect and correct pantomimes performed by the examiner. Heilman et al. (1982) and Rothi et al. (1985) reported the results of the patients they tested who had either anterior or posterior left hemisphere cerebral cortical lesions for the presence of ideomotor apraxia. In addition to having these patients produce transitive pantomimes, they were also tested for their ability to detect correct from incorrect pantomimes. We found that some of the patients with a left hemispheric lesion that was either anterior or posterior had evidence for the presence of ideomotor apraxia; however, we also found that unlike the patients with anterior lesions who just had production deficits, the patients with just posterior damage had both production and discrimination impairments. Subsequently, Halsband and co-workers (2001) also reported similar results. These results provided support the hypothesis that injury of the left inferior parietal lobe induces ideomotor apraxia because injury to this area degrades the movement representations that are stored in the inferior parietal lobe. Converging evidence for the role of the left inferior parietal lobe in the storage of movement representations also comes from functional imaging studies (Mool et al., 2000).

6.3. Superior Longitudinal Fasciculus

According to the model presented here, the praxis movement information stored in inferior parietal lobe has to be transmitted to the premotor cortex. Pramstaller and Marsden (1996) reported that subcortical lesions that injure the superior longitudinal fasciculus are associated with ideomotor apraxia. Therefore, ideomotor apraxia can be induced by an intrahemispheric disconnection syndrome.

6.4. The Supplementary Motor Area

The spatial temporal information being transmitted from the inferior parietal lobe is carried to the premotor cortex (Brodmann's area 6). The premotor cortex has two portions one in the lateral portion of the frontal lobes and the other medial. This medial division, called the supplementary motor area (SMA) receives projections from parietal neurons and projects to the convexity (lateral) premotor cortex as well as to the primary motor cortex. When the primary motor cortex in the hand area is stimulated, one or more fingers may twitch. In contrast, when the SMA is stimulated, the person will perform complex arm, forearm, hand, and finger movements. In addition, during functional imaging studies when normal people move just one finger in a repetitive motion, the hand area in the contralateral, the primary motor cortex, will demonstrate activation; however, when performing transitive pantomimes there is activation of the SMA, as well as primary motor cortex (Lauritzen et al., 1981; Rao et al., 1993). In addition, electrophysiological studies have demonstrated that when performing movements the SMA activates before the primary motor cortex. Based on these reports, it would appear that the SMA is the area of the brain that converts the visual-kinesthetic temporo-spatial movement representations into a motor programs that direct the activation of the motor neurons in primary motor cortex. Support for the hypothesis come from a report by Watson et al. (1986) who reported several patients with ideomotor apraxia from left-sided medial frontal lesions that included the SMA. These patients, unlike the patients with left parietal lesions, were able to discriminate between correctly and incorrectly performed pantomimes suggesting that these patients preserved their visuo-kinesthetic spatial temporal movement representations.

6.5. Convexity Premotor Cortex

The role of injury/degeneration of the convexity premotor cortex in the development of ideomotor apraxia has not been entirely elucidated. Faglioni and Basso (1985) wrote that they had difficulty finding any well-documented cases where patients had IMA as a result of injury to convexity premotor region. In addition, Freund and Hummelsheim (1985) studied a population of patients with convexity premotor lesions. Whereas they found that these patients were apraxic, they had limb-kinetic apraxia rather than ideomotor apraxia. Subsequently, Barrett et al. (1998) and Haaland et al. (2000) described patients with frontal convexity premotor injury who appeared to have an ideomotor apraxia. Barrett et al.'s report described one patient who could properly make a movement if it only required the movement of one joint of the upper limb; however, when this patient was required to make coordinated movements of multiple joints, she was impaired.

The medial (SMA) and lateral (convexity) premotor areas are strongly interconnected with each other and with the primary motor cortex, and while both appear to be important in converting the visual-kinesthetic spatial-temporal representations stored in the left inferior parietal lobe into the movement programs that active the motor neurons in the primary motor cortex, the role of each of these is unclear. In general, whereas the more medial portions of the frontal cortex appear to be important for mediating egocentric activities, the lateral convexity portions of the frontal lobes appear important for mediating allocentric activities. Perhaps, the medial premotor cortex primarily programs the egocentric component of purposeful movements and the convexity premotor cortex primarily programs the allocentric component; however, further research will have to be performed to test this hypothesis.

6.6. Basal Ganglia and Thalamus

There have been many paper that have reported subcortical lesions can also induce ideomotor apraxia (Agostoni et al., 1983; Kertesz & Ferro, 1984; Kleist, 1907; von Monakov, 1914; Basso & Della Sala, 1986; De Renzi et al., 1986; Della Sala et al., 1992). To learn if subcortical lesions produced different signs than cortical lesions, Hanna-Pladdy et al. (2001) compared patients with cortical and subcortical strokes. We found that both the group of patients with cortical and the group with subcortical lesions made the spatial and temporal errors associated with ideomotor apraxia; however, we also found some differences. The patients with cortical lesions were impaired in both the production of transitive and intransitive gestures-to-verbal command and imitation. In addition, they were also impaired in discriminating correct from incorrect gestures. In contrast, the participants who had subcortical lesions only demonstrated mild production errors performing transitive pantomimes to verbal command. These findings are consistent with the report of Pramstaller and Marsden (1996) who also reported that the patients with subcortical lesions had normal imitation. In addition, unlike the patients with cortical lesions, the group of patients with the subcortical lesions were unimpaired on a gesture discrimination, and the patients with subcortical lesions made more postural errors than those with cortical lesions. Unfortunately, we have not entirely learned the role of the specific subcortical structures in controlling the performance of purposeful skilled upper limb movements.

Pramstaller and Marsden (1996) performed a meta-analysis and concluded that lesions confined to the basal ganglia rarely, if ever, cause an ideomotor apraxia. However, subcortical injury can also injure portions of the thalamus and there have been reports of patients who developed an ideomotor apraxia from lesions of the left thalamus that appeared to have damaged the left pulvinar nucleus (Shuren et al., 1994; Nadeau et al., 1994). As previously mentioned, the left inferior parietal lobe appear to be critical for the programming of skilled purposeful movements and the pulvinar nucleus has strong connections with the inferior parietal lobes. Therefore, damage to the pulvinar may have impaired the patients' ability to activate the visual-kinesthetic spatial-temporal movement representations.

7. Degenerative and Vascular Diseases Associated With Ideomotor Apraxia

7.1. Vascular Diseases

In most of the published studies of ideomotor apraxia, the patients had vascular disease with cerebral infarctions. The most common vascular lesion to cause this disorder is a thrombosis in the distribution of the left-middle cerebral artery that damages the parietal cortex. Infarction of the left hemisphere's premotor cortex either medially caused by a left anterior cerebral artery distribution infarction or laterally caused by an infarction in the anterior branches of the middle cerebral artery can also cause ideomotor apraxia. In addition, Oskar et al. (2013) studied patients with subcortical vascular dementia and found that about 17% of these patient had ideomotor apraxia. Studies of disability from vascular disease have revealed that the presence of ideomotor apraxia is one of the major reasons patients with strokes cannot live independently (Hanna-Pladdy et al., 2003) and often cannot return to work (Saeki & Hachisuka, 2004).

7.2. Alzheimer's Disease

Along with impairments of episodic memory and language (e.g., anomia), ideomotor apraxia is one of the most common deficits observed in patients with AD. In addition to making postural, spatial, and temporal errors that are typical of ideomotor apraxia, patients with AD are also frequently impaired at pantomime recognition and discrimination (Mozaz et al. 2006; Rousseaux et al., 2012). These impairments in comprehension and discrimination suggest that patients with AD have a decrement in their movement representations, and this decrement may be related to the atrophy of the inferior parietal lobe that is often associated with AD. Prior studies have revealed that patients with AD have degeneration of their corpus callosum and Cimino-Knight, Gonzalez-Rothi, and Heilman (2017) reported that right-handed patients with AD often have a more severe ideomotor apraxia of their left than right hand. This asymmetry suggests that in addition to degeneration of their left inferior parietal lobe, these patients asymmetrical apraxia have a degeneration of their corpus callosum. Posterior cortical atrophy, or Benson's disease, is a form of AD that often starts with visuospatial disabilities and forms of visual agnosia. Patients with this disorder can also have an ideomotor apraxia (Goethals & Santens, 2001).

7.3. Parkinson's Disease

Patients with Parkinson's disease (PD) can have an ideomotor apraxia (Goldenberg et al., 1986; Leiguarda et al., 1997). Leiguarda et al. (1997) found that these patients' ideomotor apraxia did not improve with dopaminergic treatment. Goldenberg et al. (1986) reported that the severity of these patients' apraxia did not appear to be directly related to the severity of these patients' motor signs. The patients with PD who had ideomotor apraxia had normal pantomime recognition and were able discriminate well-performed from improperly performed pantomimes. These observations suggest that their impairment was not related to degradation of their movement representation stored in their inferior parietal lobe but rather to an inability to translate these representation into motor programs. Thus, their deficit appear to be related to premotor dysfunction. In addition, these patients' apraxia appeared to be frequently associated with other deficits of frontal-executive functions.

7.4. Parkinson Plus Syndromes

One of the earliest and most prominent signs associated with corticobasal degeneration is an asymmetrical or even a unilateral ideomotor apraxia. We have noted that many patients with corticobasal degeneration who demonstrate severe ideomotor apraxia on tests of pantomime, imitation, and object use can still discriminate incorrect from properly formed gestures performed by the examiner, and this preserved ability suggests that that these patients movement representation are still intact. Therefore, their ideomotor apraxia may be related to degeneration of premotor cortex. Leiguarda et al. (1997) also reported that the majority of patients with progressive supranuclear palsy demonstrate an ideomotor apraxia. These patient's apraxia was characterized by spatial errors including postural errors as well as ego and allocentric movement errors. Whereas corticobasal degeneration and supranuclear palsy are often difficult to clinically differentiate, Pharr et al. (2001) reported that patients with supranuclear palsy had less severe apraxia than those with corticobasal degeneration. Although Leiguarda et al. reported that patients with multisystem atrophy did not exhibit ideomotor apraxia, Monza et al. (1998) as well as Uluduz et al. (2010) reported that patients with multisystem atrophy do exhibit ideomotor apraxia. These investigators also found that the patients with multisystem atrophy who have an ideomotor apraxia often also have executive dysfunction. Finally, patients with Huntington's disease also commonly demonstrate ideomotor apraxia (Hödl et al., 2008).

8. Limb-Kinetic Apraxia (Melokinetic Apraxia, Innervatory Apraxia)

8.1. Clinical Signs

Patients with what Liepmann (1929) called limb-kinetic apraxia, also called innervatory apraxia, have a loss of hand/finger deftness and are impaired in making precise movements of the upper limb, especially their fingers, as well as being impaired in making independent but coordinated finger movements. There are many activities that require such movements such as buttoning a shirt or tying shoe laces.

Although there are several tests that measure deftness or dexterity such as having patients button a shirt, we assess patients using the coin rotation task. When performing this test, the patient is asked to rotate a nickel between their thumb, index, and middle fingers, as rapidly as possible for 20 revolutions and the time taken to perform this test is measured (Hanna-Pladdy, Mendoza, Apostolos, & Heilman, 2002). Although this test is easy to perform, gives quantitative results, and appears to be sensitive, a possible confound is the presence of bradykinesia. Therefore, when performing the coin rotation, it is valuable to view the patient's performance to learn if the only problem is slow movements or if the finger movements are not precise and well-coordinated. A test that is more qualitative is having patients pick up dimes from a table. Normal adults pick up these dimes using their thumb and forefinger using a pincher grasp. In contrast, patients with limb-kinetic apraxia will often either attempt to pick up the dime using a palmer grasp or slide the dime off the table into their palm. Another test that can be used to assess for limb-kinetic apraxia is the pegboard. Lifting the peg from a well cannot be performed with a palmar grasp and requires a pincer grasp. In addition, these pegs have to be placed into small holes that also requires precise movements; however, this test is also timed and patients may perform poorly for many other reasons other than having a limb-kinetic apraxia.

8.2. Pathophysiology

Liepmann (1920) posited that it was injury of the primary sensorimotor cortex that caused limb-kinetic apraxia. Lawrence and Kuypers (1968) trained monkeys to retrieve food from different-sized holes. After performing lesions of the brain stem (medulla) pyramid that injured the corticospinal tract, these animals were not hemiparetic and by using a palmer grasp could get food from large holes. In contrast, they could not retrieve food from the narrow holes because of a loss of a precision pincher grasp. Freund and Hummelsheim (1985), and then Fogassi and colleagues (2001) reported that damage to the premotor cortex (Brodmann's area 6) also produce a loss of finger deftness. Functional imaging provided convergent evidence for the role of premotor cortex in programming deft finger movements. Nirkko and co-workers (2001) performed functional magnetic resonance imaging while participants were performing unilateral deft finger movements and found that performance of these movements were associated with activation of the convexity premotor cortex.

Heilman, Meador, and Loring (2000) and Hanna-Pladdy and colleagues (2002) reported that right-handed people with left hemispheric dysfunction are more likely to have an ipsilateral loss of deftness (limb-kinetic apraxia of their left hand) than patients with right hemispheric dysfunction have with their ipsilateral right hand. These observations suggest that the left hemisphere of right-handed people plays a critical role in programing deft movements of the left hand. Ghacibeh et al. (2007) studied healthy right-handed participants using motor-evoked potentials of one hand while the other hand (task hand) performed motor tasks such as the Perdue peg board and found that in right-handers the left motor cortex appears to be more active with ipsilateral left-hand movements. There are at least two possible means by which the left hemisphere may influence the deftness/dexterity of the left hand, either by callosal connections or by ipsilesional corticospinal projections. Acosta, Bennett, and Heilman (2014) described a 57-year-old right-handed man who had a memory impairment, and upon brain imaging he was found to have a septum pellucidum cyst that was causing mild ventricular obstruction. He underwent an endoscopic-assisted fenestration of the septum pellucidum. Postoperative imaging revealed a lesion of the mesial portion of his corpus callosum and an assessment of praxis revealed that he had both a limb-kinetic and ideomotor apraxia of his left but not his right hand. The observation that this man had a callosal disconnection limb-kinetic apraxia of his left hand suggests that in some people it is the left hemisphere's premotor or motor cortex that enables the right hemisphere's motor system to program deft movements of the left hand. However, we also described a patient who had a callosal infarction secondary to an interhemispheric hemorrhage that caused spasm of her anterior cerebral artery (Watson & Heilman, 1983). Although this woman had a ideomotor apraxia of her left hand, she did not have a limb-kinetic apraxia of her left hand. There are at least two means by which this woman was able to perform deft/dexterous movement of her left hand. Either she had ipsilateral pathways from the left hemisphere that traveled to the motor neurons that control the left hand, or both the left and right hemispheres were able to program deft/dexterous movements of the contralateral hand. Further research will have to investigate these two alternative hypotheses.

8.3. Diseases That Can Cause Limb-Kinetic Apraxia

As previously mentioned, limb-kinetic apraxia can often be associated with cerebrovascular disease when there is ischemia to the premotor cortex as well as the motor cortex and corticospinal pathways. We have also found that many patients with PD have limb-kinetic apraxia and this limb-kinetic apraxia does not appear to be related to their bradykinesia (Quencer et al., 2007). In addition, unlike bradykinesia, limb-kinetic apraxia does not appear to be responsive to dopaminergic treatment (Gebhardt et al., 2008). The limb-kinetic apraxia that is associated with diseases such as PD has been shown to interfere with activities of daily living (Foki et al., 2016). Limb-kinetic apraxia can also be seen with the Parkinson's plus syndromes such corticobasal degeneration and progressive supranuclear palsy (Leiguardia et al., 1997), and in these conditions the limb-kinetic apraxia may be asymmetrical.

9. Ideational and Dissociation Apraxia

9.1. Clinical Signs

Unfortunately, the term "ideational apraxia" has been used to label several different disorders. We used this term for patients who have a loss of mechanical and tool knowledge, and we now call this disorder "conceptual apraxia" (Ochipa, Rothi, & Heilman, 1989). In contrast, DeRenzi et al. (1968) used this same term for patients whose ideomotor apraxia was so severe that they were impaired even when they attempted to use actual tools. To make matter even worse, I also used this term for patients who could not produce the correct transitive pantomime to verbal command but could perform normally when seeing the tool or the object upon which the tool normally works (Heilman, 1973). Since it appears that these patients have a dissociation between the systems important in comprehending speech and those important in programming movements, we now call this disorder "verbal dissociation apraxia" (Heilman et al., 2008). Leipmann (1920) initially used the term "ideational apraxia" for a disorder that was first described by Marcuse, (1904) and Pick, (1905) who described patients that had an inability to correctly sequence a series of acts, an ideational plan, that would be required to successfully complete a task. Many patients with frontal-subcortical executive dysfunction often have an impaired ability to disengage and thus perseverate. Poeck (1983) noted that whereas some patients may fail to complete a task because they perseverate one or more of the actions needed to complete the task, ideational apraxia is not solely caused by perseveration, but rather is a disturbance in the conceptual organization of actions. Some investigators now call ideational apraxia the "action disorganization syndrome" (Forde & Humphreys, 2002). Thus, the most important test for making the diagnosis of ideational apraxia is having the patient perform and complete a task that requires several orderly sequential motor actions. For example, some clinicians test patients for ideational apraxia by having them verbally describe the means by which they would make something such as a sandwich. To assess for ideational apraxia, Qureshi et al. (2011) presented participants with sets of pictures that showed the steps required to completing a variety tasks, but these critical steps were not shown in the correct order. The participants were asked to point to the pictures in the correct sequence to complete each task. There are other tests that also assess for ideational apraxia. For example, another test used to assess for this disorder is the "natural action test." In this test, the patients are presented with real objects and are required to perform multistep tasks that lead to a completed goal (Schwartz et al., 2002).

9.2. Pathophysiology

Hugo Liepmann (1920) thought that the lesion that induced ideational apraxia was located in the left occipital-parietal region. A functional imaging study performed when healthy participants were performing a sequential action task revealed activation of the parietal lobe as suggested by Liepmann; however, the critical anatomic focus of the lesions that can induce an ideational apraxia still needs be further investigated (Humphreys & Forde, 1998). The frontal lobes are thought to be important in sequencing, and Niki et al (2009) reported several patients with frontal lobe tumors who had evidence of the "action disorganization syndrome" or ideational apraxia.

9.3. Diseases Associated With Ideational Apraxia

Most often the patients with ideational apraxia have some form of dementia such as AD (Chainay et al., 2006). Crutch, Rossor, and Warrington (2007) assessed 35 patients with AD and 75 healthy controls for the presence of ideational apraxia using two tests that required three-item sequential movements and found that patients with AD were impaired. Giovannetti et al. (2006) demonstrated that patients with vascular dementia were even more likely to have ideational apraxia (deficits on the natural action test) than patients with AD. We tested patients with PD for the presence of ideational apraxia by having them arrange pictures of the actions needed to complete a task and found that patients with PD often had an ideational apraxia. The predominant errors produced by patients with PD were in sequencing rather than repetition or omission of actions, indicating that the poor performance was not caused by perseveration (Qureshi et al., 2011). In addition, Leiguarda et al. (1997) reported that some patients with Parkinson's plus syndromes such as progressive supranuclear palsy also had problems with tasks requiring the sequential ordering of multiple steps.

10. Action-Intentional Disorders

As mentioned in the introduction, to successfully interact with stimuli in the environment, with other people, or with oneself, in addition to knowing "how" to move, it is also important to know "when" to move. The action-intentional programs provide the motor system with information about "when" to move. When interacting with people and objects in the environment as well as oneself, there are four major "when" decisions that a person will have to make to guide their behavior including (a) when to initiate an action or a series of actions, (b) when to persist at an action or series of actions, (c) when to end a movement or an action as well when to end a series of actions, and (d) when not to move or act. Disease that damages the cortical motor neurons, the corticospinal track, the spinal motor neurons, the motor nerves, the myo-neural junction, and the muscles may all cause a failure to move, but the failure to move in these patients is caused by weakness rather than not knowing "when" to move. Patients who have severe rigidity and cannot relax their antagonist muscles may also have a failure to move. A failure to move may also be caused by impaired levels of consciousness and comprehension and inattention/unawareness. In the absence of these disorders, the inability or failure to initiate a movement or action when the need for this action is recognized, is called "akinesia." Some patients are unable to initially initiate a movement, but are able to move after a delay. This delay of action initiation is called "hypokinesia."

There are some patients who can initiate a movement but cannot sustain a movement or a series of movements that are needed to complete a task, and this disorder is called "motor impersistence." When an action or series of actions have been completed such that the goal of this action or series of actions has been completed or when this action or series of actions are not producing the desired effect, a person normally should stop performing this action or series of actions. The inability to stop a movement or series of movements when the task is completed or when these movements are not accomplishing their goal is called "motor perseveration."

Finally, the inability to withhold a specific response to a sensory stimulus when either no response is required or when a response is detrimental to a person's goals, is called "defective response inhibition." In many respects, these four major forms of action-intentional disorders have similarities or parallels to disorders of sensory attention. Whereas attention relates to the processing of input (sensory or afferent processing), intention relates to the processing of output (motor or efferent processing). The human brain is the most complex and highly developed processing apparatus that is known; however, the brain still has a limited ability to perform parallel processing. For example, the brain receives complex information from all our sensory systems, and we are incapable of simultaneously processing all this information. Therefore, based on long- and short-term goals, our brain must select/triage from all this incoming information those stimuli that will be further processed. Thus, while reading this material, you are attending to the letters and words on this page, but not attending to feeling the tactile pressure on the soles of your feet, but after reading this you will feel this pressure. In few minutes, however, you will again focus on the words and no longer be aware of the feelings in your feet.

In a similar manner, humans can perform an almost unlimited variety of different actions but can only perform a limited number of simultaneous actions.

In addition, as we have learned in physics, pressure equals force divided by the area to which this force is applied. Thus, with the same force, if increased pressure is needed, the area to which this force is applied must be reduced. Similarly, a person can perform only a limited number of actions simultaneously (e.g., parallel to limited force), and the more novel and difficult an action (e.g., parallel to a need for more pressure), the fewer the number of simultaneous actions that can be successfully performed (e.g., parallel to a reduced area). Therefore, based on long- and short-term goals humans also have to triage the actions we select to perform. Based on the concept of triage, in the action-intentional domain akinesia may be parallel to the attentional state of unawareness, impersistence being the intentional parallel of decreased vigilance, motor perseveration being parallel to failures of sensory habituation (or extinction), and defective response inhibition being parallel to attentional distractibility.

11. Subtypes of Motor Intentional Disorders

11.1. Akinesia and Hypokinesia

11.1.1. Clinical Signs

Whereas akinesia is a failure to initiate movements, hypokinesia is a delay in initiation. There are several reasons why a person may fail to act or be delayed in the initiation of an action. A failure to rapidly initiate a movement can be caused by cognitive disorders, such as not knowing that an action is necessary or would be beneficial, not understanding a command, or being unaware of the circumstances that would require an action. In addition to cognitive disorders, a failure to initiate a movement can also be caused by sensory or attentional disorders. As mentioned, disorders of portions of the motor systems such as the corticospinal system can also produce a failure to or delay in the initiate an action. In contrast to these cognitive and sensorimotor disorders, akinesia and hypokinesia are caused by a failure of the networks that are responsible for activating the motor system.

11.1.2. Subtypes of Akinesia

There are several forms of akinesia. Akinesia may involve a variety of body parts including a limb on one side of the body or both sides of the body, the eyes, the head, or the whole body. Akinesia may be present when a limb is used on one side of the body, but not the other side and this is called *body-centered hemispatial akinesia.* For example, in the patient described by Meador et al. (1986), the arm contralateral to a brain lesion was less akinetic in ipsilesional than in contralesional hemispace, independent of the direction of movement. Akinesia may vary depending upon the right versus left movement direction of the arm, head, or eyes, and this disorder is called *directional akinesia* (Heilman, 2004). Directional akinesia of the eyes, head, and neck as well as the upper limb may cause deviation of one more of these body parts in one direction (Heilman, Bowers and Watson. 1983).

There are patients who may be able to initiate an action to an external stimulus but cannot initiate goal-oriented actions in the absence of a stimulus. This disorder is called *endogenously (endo-evoked) akinesia* and this is also called *abulia* or a *loss of volition.* In contrast, there are patients who can initiate self-willed movements, but not initiate movements in response to certain stimuli. We call this unusual disorder *exogenously evoked (exo-evoked) akinesia.* A patient may have both exo-evoked and endo-evoked akinesia called *global akinesia.*

Whereas patients with akinesia have a failure to move certain parts of their body or their entire body or cannot move in a specific direction or in a portion of space, there are also patients have a disorder of movement initiation where they are able to move, but they have a delay of initiation. This disorder is called *hypokinesia.* Like akinesia, hypokinesia can also be subtyped into body part (e.g., limb, eyes, entire body) and action space (e.g., directional and hemispatial).

11.1.3. Testing

As previously mentioned. akinesia may affect different body parts; therefore, the clinician should assess movements of the eyes, neck/head, trunk, and limbs as well as whole body actions. If a patient has akinesia of a limb, such as their arm, it may be difficult to distinguish this akinesia from weakness, and the clinician may have to rely on imaging or motor-evoked potentials. To detect endo-evoked akinesia, it is important to observe spontaneously initiated behaviors. Patients with endo-evoked akinesia often have symptoms of abulia (decreased drive, with psychomotor retardation). Exo-evoked akinesia, also called "motor neglect" results in failure to move in response to a stimulus, when this failure to respond is not the result of an elemental sensory defect or sensory inattention. Watson, Miller, and Heilman (1978) devised the crossed-response task to distinguish between these deficits. Although originally used in monkeys, it can also be used with humans. Participants who have their eyes closed and their hands on a table or on their lap are trained to respond by raising their right hand when the left hand is touched and raising their left hand when the right hand is touched. A patient is considered to have a unilateral exo-evoked akinesia if this patient fails to move the contralesional extremity in response to stimuli presented to the "normal" (ipsilesional) side, despite intact spontaneous movements and normal strength of the contralesional arm. The crossed-response task can also be used to test for exo-evoked akinesia of the eyes or the head, as well as defective response inhibition.

To assess whether the spatial coordinates of actions influence akinesia, the examiner needs to observe directional and hemispatial movements that are both endo-evoked (spontaneous) and exo-evoked (in response to stimuli). When attempting to determine if there is a directional akinesia of the eyes, the clinician should observe spontaneous eye movements to detect eye deviation or bias toward one side, as well as determine how well the patient performs eye movement in response to the examiner's verbal commands. A failure to move the eyes to one side to command cannot be explained by a hemianopia or sensory inattention (sensory neglect). An exo-evoked directional akinesia of the eyes can be assessed by a modification of the Watson, et al. (1978) paradigm where the examiner stands directly in front of a patient and places their left hand in the patient's right visual field and the right hand in the left visual field, at eye level. The patient is instructed to fixate on the examiner's nose, and when the examiner moves their hand they are to look to the hand on the side opposite the moving hand, as quickly as possible. An impairment in looking to one side may be related to a hemianopia, hemispatial sensory inattention, or a directional akinesia and these disorders can be dissociated by then asking the patient to look at the moving hand. If on one side they can move their eyes and look at the moving hand but cannot look away (to the opposite side), they have a directional akinesia (Butter et al., 1988).

Similar tests can be used to detect directional and hemispatial akinesia of the head or arm. One means to test for a directional bias of an arm is place a patients forefinger on the middle of their chest and then to ask the patient to close their eyes and to point with their index finger to the position in space that is directly in front of them (perpendicular to their sternum or their the midsagittal plane). If a patient has a directional motor (intentional) bias, they will deviate their arm in the direction of their bias (Heilman et al., 1983). De Renzi et al. (1970) developed a test for assessing patients for hemispatial neglect that we have modified and can be used to test for endo-evoked directional and hemispatial limb akinesia. In our modification, the patient is blindfolded and a small object such as a coin is placed or not placed on a table in front of the patient within arm's reach. The coin is randomly placed to the left of right of the patient's midline. The patient's hand (right or left) is placed on the table to the right or to the left of the coin, and the patient is told that there might be or not be a coin on the table, and they asked to find and pick up the coin on the table, if there is one present. This task is more endo-evoked because the patient cannot see the coin and must initiate exploratory behavior in the absence of an external stimulus. Patients with an endo-evoked hemispatial akinesia of the arm may fail to move their arm fully into one side of space to explore for the coin. Patients with directional akinesia may explore primarily in one direction.

In some conditions, a patient's failure to move a limb may not be limited to a portion of space or in a direction and the patient may appear to have a hemiparesis; however, this failure to move may be related to a limb akinesia or motor neglect rather than weakness caused by damage to the corticospinal system or motor nerves. Usually, when patients are hemiparetic and attempt to move, they may show expressions of effort and move more proximal parts of their body (Gold et al. 1994). Therefore, a failure to show these signs of effort may suggest the diagnosis of akinesia. The diagnosis of akinesia or motor neglect versus a paresis may have to depend on brain imaging or physiological techniques such as transcranial magnetic stimulation of the motor cortex that will allow the clinician to learn if the brain lesion did or did not involve the motor system (Triggs et al.,1994).

To assess for hypokinesia (a delay in movement initiation), a form of a reaction time task is most frequently used. Unfortunately, although measuring reaction times is the best mean of testing for hypokinesia, when patients have a delay of their reaction times, this delay can also be caused by several other disorders. To respond to a stimulus, a person has to be aware of this stimulus and thus sensory and attention deficits can also cause a delay reaction times.

11.2. Motor Impersistence

11.2.1. Clinical Signs

The completion of many goal-oriented activities requires either sustaining action or sustaining a series of actions. The inability to sustain an action or a series action that are required to complete a task is called motor impersistence (Fisher, 1956, Kertesz et al., 1985). Motor impersistence can be associated with various body parts (e.g., the limbs, eyes, neck, eyelids, jaw, and tongue) and also may be directional (e.g., unable to maintain a leftward gaze), hemispatial, or global.

11.2.2. Testing

There are many means of testing for motor impersistence. Most often patients are asked to keep their eyes closed for 20 seconds; however, having patients perform two simultaneous actions appears to be more sensitive, and thus often patients are asked to protrude their tongue and keep their eyes closed for 20 seconds. To test for directional impersistence patients may be asked to look to one side for 20 seconds and for limb impersistence to elevate one arm at the shoulder and to dorsiflex their arm at the wrist.

11.3. Defective Response Inhibition

11.3.1. Clinical Signs

Defective response inhibition is the performance of an inappropriate action in response to a stimulus. Like the other disorders of action intention discussed in this chapter, defective response inhibition can be seen in a variety of body parts such as the upper limbs and eyes and might also be directional.

11.3.2. Testing

One of the oldest means of testing for a form of defective response inhibition is the Myerson's sign also called the glabella reflex. The examiner tells the patient that they are going to tap their forehead between their eyebrows and that they (the patient) is to try keep their eyes open and try not to blink. The examiner repeatedly taps this region with their forefinger or middle finger at a rate of about one tap each second. Normally, people will blink with the first two or three taps and then stop blinking, but patients with frontal-subcortical and basal ganglia dysfunction, appear to continue to blink with repeated taps.

One of the best means for testing defective response inhibition of the upper limbs is to use the previously mentioned crossed-response inhibition task that was initially devised to test monkeys with frontal lesions for defective response inhibition (Heilman et al., 1995). When stimulated on one side the monkey was trained to respond on the opposite side, but several weeks to months after a unilateral frontal lobe ablation we found that the monkeys incorrectly responded on the contralesional side they were stimulated. When we use this test for assessing patients, the patient, who is sitting with their eyes closed or blindfolded, is told to place their hands on their lap with their palms down and that when they are touched on the back of their left or right hand they are to lift the hand opposite to that touched as rapidly as possible after detecting the touch (Crucian et al., 2007). On this test even healthy people may make errors, but with 10 trials they usually make two or less errors.

A similar test that is directional can be performed with the eyes. There are two means of performing this test. In one form the examiner tells the patient that they are to fixate on the examiner's eyes and to tell the examiner when s/he moves their finger, but to continue to look at the examiner. Patients with defective response inhibition will often look at the examiner's moving finger. The visual eye movement crossed-response task may be a little more sensitive. The examiner asks the patient to look at the examiner's eyes, but when the examiner waves the hand on the left side of their head they are to look toward the examiner's right hand, and vice versa; however, in patients with PD, the eye movement test was found not to be as sensitive as the limb test (Crucian et al., 2007).

As described by Luria (1980), another test for defective response inhibition is the "go/no-go" test. In this test, the patient is asked to put up (extend) two fingers when the examiner puts up one finger and to put up no fingers if the examiner puts up two fingers. Patients with defective response inhibition will often put up one or two fingers when the examiner put up two fingers. Luria (1980) also described a test for another form of defective response inhibition called echopraxia. The patient is told if the examiner puts up one finger the patient is to put up two fingers, and if the examiner puts up two fingers the patients is to put up one finger. An error on this task is when the patient mimics the examiner, such that when the examiner puts up two fingers, the patient puts up two fingers rather than one.

Cohen et al. (2015) demonstrated another form of defective response inhibition. Many individuals with PD have kinesia paradoxica, with more difficulty self-initiating movements (i.e., endo-evoked movement) than moving in response to environmental stimuli (i.e., exo-evoked movement). In many situations, planned and prepared actions are recognized as being incorrect and must be terminated so that the proper action can be initiated. Cohen et al. wanted to learn if patients with PD had more difficulty terminating, disengaging, and reprogramming self-selected but invalid preparations for an action versus those preparations made in response to an external warning stimulus that during preparation is found to be invalid (e.g., termination of incorrect movement in response to stimuli versus termination of a self-initiated movement). When performing this reaction time test, the patients with PD were on their dopaminergic medications. We found that, when compared to healthy participants, the patients with PD produced similar reaction times as did the controls following endogenous and exogenous valid cues. There was also no group differences following invalid exogenous cues. However, following invalid endogenous action preparation, the participants with PD were slower than the heathy participants to terminate their endogenous preparation and execute the correct alternative action. These results suggest that patients with PD have a form of defective response inhibition of self-initiated (endo-evoked) action plans.

11.4. Motor Perseveration

11.4.1. Clinical Signs

There are several forms of motor perseveration. One form of perseveration is when a task is completed, a patient continues to perform the same action. Luria (1980) called this efferent perseveration; however, Sandson and Albert's (1987) called this same "disorder continuous perseveration." Many tasks require as series of different movements, and another form of perseveration is when a patient incorrectly and inappropriately repeats a prior response when a different action is required. Whereas Luria (1965) called this disorder "inertia of program action," Sandson and Albert (1987) call this "recurrent perseveration."

11.4.2. Testing

There are several means of testing for perseveration. One of the most popular tests is Dubois et al.'s (2005) "applause test." In this test, the patient is asked to imitate the examiner's actions, and the examiner rapidly claps three times. The performance of the patient is normal when she or he claps only three times or is abnormal when he or she clap more than three times. Another method of testing for motor perseveration is the "n–m" test where the patient is asked to alternate writing the letters "n" and "m" or the ramparts test where the person is asked to draw a series of squares with each square followed by the drawing of a triangle. During these tests, the patient should be instructed not to take the pen off the paper. If a patient writes two or more of the same letters together or draws two or more triangles or squares together, it is a sign of perseveration.

One means of determining if a patient has recurrent (also called return perseveration) or continuous (also called consecutive) perseveration is by using the cancellation test. In this task, patients are presented with short lines (approximately 1 inch long) that are oriented in a variety of directions and randomly distributed over a page. The patient is asked to cross out all the lines. Although this test is most often used to assess patients for spatial neglect, many patients will often reveal both continuous perseveration where they repeatedly cross out the same line or recurrent perseveration where, after crossing out another line, they return to a line that had been earlier crossed out, and they cross it out again (Kim et al., 2009).

11.5. Diseases Associated With Action Intentional Deficits

Strokes and other forms of injury to critical areas of the brain can cause action intentional deficits. For example, strokes in an anterior cerebral artery distribution that injure structures such as the anterior cingulate gyrus and the SMA can produce akinesia as well as mutism. In addition, strokes that injury the dorsomedial nucleus of the thalamus can also cause a kinetic mutism. Cairns (1941) reported a patient with akinetic mutism from an epidermoid cyst of the third ventricular, and this cyst may have been putting pressure on the medial thalamus.

In addition, infarctions of the caudate have also been reported to cause akinesia (Bhatia & Marsden, 1994; Caplan et al., 1990). However, microvascular disease with lacunes and widely distributed leukoaraiosis is a frequent cause of akinesia and other intentional deficits. There are many other diseases that cause injury to the white matter connections between the basal ganglia, thalamus, and frontal cortex, such as multiple sclerosis, and these diseases can also cause action intentional deficits.

Akinesia, and other intention deficits are not frequently observed in the earlier or even middle stages of AD. Whereas tremor and rigidity are often associated with PD, often the most disabling disorder are the action-intentional deficits. These action-intentional deficits are also often seen in other movement disorders (e.g., Parkinson plus syndromes, such as striatonigral degeneration, olivopontocerebellar atrophy, progressive nuclear palsy, corticobasal degeneration, and Huntington's disease). Often these signs can be subtle, such as a reduction of facial movements (masked-like face) to complete immobility.

Moderate to severe head trauma and central nervous system infections are other common causes of intentional disorders. Some infections and inflammatory diseases that can cause akinesia and other intentional disorders include acquired immunodeficiency syndrome (AIDs), syphilis, Lyme, prion diseases such as Creutzfeldt–Jakob disease, chronic meningitis (e.g., fungal infections such as cryptococcosis and sarcoidosis), Whipple's disease, and progressive multifocal leukoencephalopathy.

Autoimmune diseases including demyelinating diseases such as multiple sclerosis, Behçet's disease, lupus, and the leukodystrophies may also have intentional components. Endocrine disorders such as hypothyroidism and hypoparathyroidism have be associated with intentional disorders. Several toxic/metabolic/deficiency disorders may have signs of intentional disorders (e.g., Marchiafava–Bignami disease, vitamin B12 deficiency, anoxia, Wilson's disease, and status dysmyelinatus with iron deposition in the basal ganglia).

11.6. Pathophysiology of Action Intentional Disorders

Intentional motor disorders, are often caused by bilateral hemispheric lesions, but when these disorders are caused by a unilateral hemispheric lesion, they appear to be more commonly associated with right rather than left hemisphere lesions. The intentional disorders that have been reported to be induced by primarily right hemisphere lesions including left-sided limb akinesia (Coslett & Heilman, 1989), directional akinesia with leftward arm movements (Heilman et al., 1985) and even left horizontal gaze "paralysis" (De Renzi et al., 1982).

Many of the intentional defects associated with right hemisphere dysfunction, however, are not just limited to the left side of the body or to leftward movements. Patients with right hemisphere lesion are more often abulic and have hypokinesia (slowed reaction times; Howes & Boller, 1975), even with their ipsilesional right hand. Kertesz et al. (1985) reported that impersistence was also most frequently caused by right hemispheric lesions, and these lesions are most commonly have injured the frontal lobe. More recently, Kim et al. (2013) examined patients with stroke for the presence of hypokinesia and impersistence and found that these deficits were more common in those patients with right than left hemisphere strokes and that it was primarily the patients with frontal and subcortical lesions that were most likely to demonstrate these deficits. Sandson and Albert (1987) found that whereas patients with aphasia produced significantly more recurrent perseveration than did patients with right hemisphere damage or healthy controls, patients with right hemisphere lesions were more likely to demonstrate continuous perseveration.

Overall, based on the clinical studies as just reviewed, it appears as though the right hemisphere may be dominant for intentional control of the motor systems. To help learn if the right hemisphere played a dominant role in mediating motor intention, we studied healthy participants using a reaction time task where the participants were randomly provided with a warning stimulus before the imperative reaction time stimulus. These warning stimuli were either presented to the left or right hemisphere (in the right or left visual fields and hemispaces). We found that warning stimuli presented to the right hemisphere reduced the reactions times more than warning stimuli presented to the left hemisphere (Heilman & Van Den Abell, 1979). Therefore, it appears that this study with normal participants provides further evidence for right hemispheric dominance in mediating action intention.

Marcel Kinsbourne once told me that since humans like dichotomies, it is ideal that we have two hemispheres (personal communication). There appears to be many domains where there are functional left versus right hemispheric dichotomies, such as proposition language versus emotional prosodic communication, verbal versus visuospatial memory, recognition of faces versus objects, focal attention versus global attention, and melody versus rhythm. These forms of hemispheric specialization allow people to perform parallel processing. For example, when listening to someone speak while the left hemisphere is analyzing the meaning of the propositional message transmitted by words, the right hemisphere is analyzing the emotions that the speaker is communicating by listening to the emotional prosody. Thus, in regard to actions, whereas the left hemisphere programs "how" to perform the action or actions, the right programs "when" to perform the action or actions.

Whereas the anatomic and physiological basis for this "when" action-intentional dominance is not entirely understood, overall, it appears that to successfully interact with stimuli in the environment, with other people, and with oneself, a person needs to know both "how" to move as well as "when" to move, and it appears that whereas the left hemisphere is dominant for the processing and programming of "how" to move, the right hemisphere appears to be dominant get for determining "when" to move.

Franz Josef Gall, best known as the founder of phrenology, developed two important hypotheses about the brain organization and function: modularity and magnitude. He posited that different areas of the brain are important for mediating different cognitive activities, and the larger this area is, the better the performance of this module is (i.e., bigger is better). The modularity hypotheses was first supported by work of Paul Broca (1865) who demonstrated that the left hemisphere is most often dominant for the mediation of speech. The magnitude hypothesis was supported by Geschwind and Levinski (1968) who demonstrated that Wernicke's area (planum temporale), important for storing the sequence of phonemes that compose previously learned words, is often larger in the left, language-dominant, hemisphere than in the right hemisphere.

About two decades ago in an important theoretical article, Mountcastle (1997) wrote that a critical factor in determining the functions of a module is its connectivity. In regard to the network mediating "when" to move (intention), studies of patients with a stroke have revealed that often there is disruption of the frontal-subcortical neural networks. In the human posterior cerebral cortex, each of the primary sensory cortical areas such as vision, audition, and touch project only to their modality specific association areas, and then these sensory association areas converge in the inferior parietal lobe as well as in portions of the posterior temporal lobe in multimodal and polymodal cortical areas (Chavis & Pandya, 1976). The frontal lobes by means of the longitudinal fasciculi connect with these neocortical sensory association and sensory convergence areas. These connections with the frontal lobe provide the frontal lobes with information about the external stimuli that may call the individual to action. In addition, the posterior temporal and parietal polymodal areas that are connected to the frontal lobes store the cognitive information often important in making decisions about the need for action. Furthermore, limbic connections with the amygdala and cingulate gyrus can provide the frontal lobes with emotional and motivational information. Therefore, because portions of the frontal lobes have strong connections with sensory association areas, polymodal association areas, and portions of the limbic system, these frontal networks would appear to be an ideal candidate for initiating as well as completing actions that may help fulfill long-term goals (endo-evoked). These frontal networks also appear to be critical for initiating those actions that are in response to those significant external stimuli that require alteration (exo-evoked; Heilman et al., 1987).

The lateral frontal lobes also have strong connections with portions of the thalamus such as the nonspecific intralaminar thalamic nuclei, including the central median-parafascicular (CM-Pf) nucleus. When we unilaterally ablated this area in monkeys, these animals developed contralesional motor-intentional neglect (Watson et al., 1978). This action-intentional disorder has subsequently also been reported in patients with thalami lesions (Bogousslavsky et al., 1986; Mills & Swanson, 1978). Therefore, it appears that the lateral prefrontal lobes together with intralaminar and dorsolateral thalamic nuclei (CM Pf) play a critical role in mediating responses to meaningful stimuli and that damage to this network, including the subcortical white matter connections, can induce exo-evoked akinesia and hypokinesia. Injury to the dorsomedial thalamic nuclei, such as stroke, can also induce akinesia and hypokinesia; however, whereas with the akinetic mutism-associated medial frontal lesions where the patients appear vigilant, those patients with the akinetic mutism from thalamic lesions often appear to be somewhat lethargic (Segarra, 1970).

In regard to the medial frontal lobes, a portion of the limbic system, the anterior cingulate gyrus along and the supplementary premotor area when injured also produce akinesia and bilateral lesions of this area cause a kinetic mutism (Nagaratnam et al., 2004; Nielsen 1951). The SMA has connections with the motor cortex, the lateral premotor cortex, and direct connections with the motor neurons in the spinal cord. Several studies have revealed that the supplementary premotor area reveals activity before an action is initiated, and therefore this area may be important in the self-mediated initiation of actions.

The anterior cingulate gyrus has connections with the ventral striatum, including the nucleus accumbens, and this ventral striatal network plays a critical role in reward. The desire for reward often leads to the initiation of actions and the persistence of action until the task is completed. The anterior cingulate gyrus also has reciprocal connections with other limbic structures and the frontal cortex. Therefore, the anterior cingulate gyrus, with its connections to the limbic-emotional networks and to the frontal lobes, appears to play a critical role in uniting the action decision-making processes with the limbic-emotional networks.

The supplementary motor and cingulate gyrus of the medial frontal lobe are the cortical elements of the motor and anterior consulate basal ganglia networks described by Alexander, DeLong, and Strict (1986). These basal ganglia networks receive dopaminergic input from the substantial nigra. There is much evidence that interruption of the dopaminergic system induced by diseases such as PD, or certain toxins and medications (e.g., haloperidol), can produce motor intentional disorders. There appears to be three major dopaminergic pathways (Williams and Goldman-Rakic, 1998). The nigrostriatal dopaminergic system originates in the dopaminergic neurons of the pars compacta of the substantia nigra. This system primarily projects to the basal ganglia (e.g., the caudate and putamen). The mesolimbic system originates principally in the dopaminergic neuron located in ventral tegmental area in the midbrain and terminates in portions of the ventral striatum such as nucleus accumbens. This network appears to be critical for reward. The mesocortical pathway originates principally in dopaminergic neurons located more laterally in the midbrain and projects to the frontal and cingulate cortex. Although the dopaminergic deficit associated with PD can account for the action-intentional deficits that are a major cause of the disability associated with PD, the reason that many patients with PD reveal kinesia paradoxica is not entirely known.

The influence of dopaminergic treatment on the akinesia and hypokinesia associated with PD is well known and will not be discussed in this chapter. The severe perseveration disorders that can be associated with PD do not seem to be helped by dopaminergic treatment, but subthalamic deep brain stimulation appears to help reduce perseveration in these patients (Herzog et al., 2009).

Whereas patients with PD do reveal defective response inhibition (Crucian et al., 2007), there were no studies about the influence of treatment on this disorder or about treatment of impersistence. In regard to vascular disease, there have been several reports of patients with akinesia who appeared to also benefit from dopaminergic medications. For example, Alexander (2001) reported a patient with a mesencephalic-diencephalic infarction who improved with dopaminergic medications, and Comnarros et al. (2000) also reported that patients with akinetic mutism responded to treatment with levodopa. Jorge et al. (2010) reported that after stroke treatment with cholinesterase, inhibitors reduced apathy. Although the deficits in the praxis "how" as well as the action-intentional "when" networks are a major cause of disability, there has been a paucity of studies that have investigated the best means of treating and rehabilitating these disorders. Hopefully, future studies will begin to learn how and when we can help these unfortunate patients.

References

Acosta, L. M., Bennett, J. A., & Heilman, K. M. (2014). Callosal disconnection and limb-kinetic apraxia. *Neurocase, 20*(6), 599–605.

Agostoni, E., Coletti, A., Orlando, G., & Tredici, G. (1983). Apraxia in deep cerebral lesions. *Journal of Neurology, Neurosurgery, and Psychiatry, 46*, 804–808.

Alexander, M. P. (2001). Chronic akinetic mutism after mesencephalic-diencephalic infarction: Remediated with dopaminergic medications. *Neurorehabilitation and Neural Repair,15*(2), 151–156.

Alexander, G. E., DeLong, M. R., & Strick, P. L. (1986). Parallel organization of functionally segregated circuits linking basal ganglia and cortex. *Progress in Brain Research, 9*, 357–81.

Barrett, A. M., Schwartz, R. L., Raymer, A. L., Crucian, G. P., Rothi, L. J. G., & Heilman, K. M. (1998). Dyssynchronous apraxia: Failure to combine simultaneous preprogrammed movements. *Cognitive Neuropsychology, 15*, 685–703.

Basso, A., & Della Sala, S. (1986). Ideomotor apraxia arising from a purely deep lesion [letter]. *Journal of Neurology, Neurosurgery, and Psychiatry, 49*(4), 437–454.

Bhatia, K. P., & Marsden, C. D. (1994). The behavioural and motor consequences of focal lesions of the basal ganglia in man. *Brain, 117*(Pt 4), 859–876.

Bogousslavsky, J., Miklossy, J., Deruaz, J. P., Regli, F., & Assal, G. (1986). Unilateral left paramedian infarction of thalamus and midbrain: a clinico-pathological study. *Journal of Neurology, Neurosurgery, and Psychiatry, 49*(6), 686–694. http://doi.org/10.1136/jnnp.49.6.686

Broca, P. (1865). Sur le siege de la faculte du langage articule. *Bulletin de la Societe d'anthropologie, 6*, 37–93.

Butter, C. M., Rapcsak, S., Watson, R. T., & Heilman, K. M. (1988). Changes in sensory inattention, directional motor neglect and "release" of the fixation reflex following a unilateral frontal lesion: A case report. *Neuropsychologia, 26*(4), 533–545.

Caplan, L. R., Schmahmann, J. D., Kase, C. S., Feldmann, E., Baquis, G., Greenberg, J. P., . . . Hier, D. B. (1990). Caudate infarcts. *Archives of Neurology, 47*(2), 133–143.

Cairns, H. (1941). Akinetic mutism with an epidermoid cyst of the 3rd ventricle Brain, *64*, 273.

Chainay, H., Louarn, C., & Humphreys, G. W. (2006). Ideational action impairments in Alzheimer's disease. *Brain and Cognition*, *62*(3), 198–205.

Chavis, D. A., & Pandya, D.N. (1976). Further observations on corticofrontal connections in the rhesus monkey. *Brain Research*, *117*(3), 369–386.

Cimino-Knight, A. M., Gonzalez Rothi, L. J., He, Y., & Heilman, K. M. (2017). Callosal ideomotor apraxia in Alzheimer's disease. *Journal of Clinical and Experimental Neuropsychology*, *39*(1), 1–8.

Cohen, M. L., Schwab, N. A., Price, C. C., & Heilman, K. M. (2015). Impaired switching from self-prepared actions in mild Parkinson disease. *Journal of Parkinson's Disease*, *5*(4), 961–970.

Coslett, H. B., & Heilman, K. M. (1989). Hemihypokinesia after right hemisphere stroke. *Brain and Cognition*, *9*(2), 267–278.

Crucian, G. P., Heilman, K., Junco, E., Maraist, M., Owens, W. E., Foote, K. D., & Okun, M. S. (2007). The crossed response inhibition task in Parkinson's disease: Disinhibition hyperkinesia. *Neurocase*, *13*(3), 158–164.

Crutch, S. J., Rossor, M. N., & Warrington, E. K. (2007). The quantitative assessment of apraxic deficits in Alzheimer's disease. *Cortex*, *43*(7), 976–986.

Della Sala, S., Basso, A., Laiacona, M., & Papagno, C. (1992). Subcortical localization of ideomotor apraxia: A review and an experimental study. In G. Vallar, S. F. Cappa, & C-W. Wellesch (Eds.), *Neuropsychological disorders associated with subcortical lesions* (pp. 357–380). Oxford, England: Oxford University Press.

De Renzi, E., Faglioni, P., & Scotti, G. (1970). Hemispheric contribution to exploration of space through the visual and tactile modality. *Cortex*, *6*(2), 191–203.

DeRenzi, E., & Lucchelli, F. (1988). Ideational apraxia. *Brain*, *111*, 1173–1185.

De Renzi, E., Colombo, A., Faglioni, P., & Gibertoni, M. (1982). Conjugate gaze paresis in stroke patients with unilateral damage: An unexpected instance of hemispheric asymmetry. *Archives of Neurology*, *39*(8), 482–486.

DeRenzi, E., Faglioni, P., Scarpa, M., & Crisi, G. (1986). Limb apraxia in patients with damage confined to the left basal ganglia and thalamus. *Journal of Neurology, Neurosurgery, and Psychiatry*, *49*, 1030–1038.

Dubois, B., Slachevsky, A., Pillon, B., Beato, R., Villalponda, J. M., & Litvan, I. (2005). "Applause sign" helps to discriminate PSP from FTD and PD. *Neurology*, *64*(12), 2132–3.

Ebisch, S. J., Babiloni, C., Del Gratta, C., Ferretti, A., Perrucci, M. G., Caulo, M., . . . Romani G. L. (2007). Human neural systems for conceptual knowledge of proper object use: A functional magnetic resonance imaging study. *Cerebral Cortex*, *17*(11), 2744–2751.

Faglioni, P., & Basso, A. (1985). Historical perspective on apraxia. In E. A. Roy (Ed.), *Neuropsychological studies of apraxia and related disorders* (pp. 2–44). New York, NY: North Holland Press.

Finkelburg, F. (1873). Uber aphasie und aysombolie nebst versuch elmer theorie der sprachbildung. *Archiv fur Psychiatrie*, *6*.

Fisher, C. M. (1956). Left hemiplegia and motor impersistence. *Journal of Mental and Nervous System Disease*, *123*, 201–205.

Fogassi, L., Gallese, V., Buccino, G., Craighero, L., Fadiga, L., & Rizzolatti, G. (2001). Cortical mechanism for the visual guidance of hand grasping movements in the monkey: A reversible inactivation study. *Brain*, *124*(Pt 3), 571–586.

Foki, T., Vanbellingen, T., Lungu, C., Pirker, W., Bohlhalter, S., Nyffeler, T., . . . Beisteiner, R. (2016). Limb-kinetic apraxia affects activities of daily living in Parkinson's disease: A multi-center study. *European Journal of Neurology*, 23(8), 1301–1307.
Forde, E. M., & Humphreys, G. W. (2002). Dissociations in routine behaviour across patients and everyday tasks. *Neurocase*, *8*(1–2), 151–167.
Freund, H. J., & Hummelsheim, H. (1985). Lesions of premotor cortex in man. *Brain*, *108*, 697–733.
Gebhardt, A., Vanbellingen, T., Baronti, F., Kersten, B., & Bohlhalter, S. (2008) Poor dopaminergic response of impaired dexterity in Parkinson's disease: Bradykinesia or limb kinetic apraxia? *Movement Disorders*, *23*(12), 1701–1706.
Geschwind, N. (1965). Disconnection syndromes in animals and man. *Brain*, *88*, 237–294, 585–644.
Geschwind, N., & Levitsky, W. (1968). Human brain: left-right asymmetries in temporal speech region. *Science*, *161*(3837), 186–187.
Ghacibeh, G.A., Mirpuri, R., Drago, V., Jeong, Y., Heilman, K. M., & Triggs, W.J. (2007). Ipsilateral motor activation during unimanual and bimanual motor tasks. *Clinical Neurophysiology*, *118*(2), 325–332.
Giovannetti, T., Schmidt, K.S., Gallo, J. L., Sestito, N., & Libon, D. J. (2006). Everyday action in dementia: Evidence for differential deficits in Alzheimer's disease versus subcortical vascular dementia. *Journal of the International Neuropsychological Society*, *12*(1), 45–53.
Goethals, M., & Santens, P.(2001). Posterior cortical atrophy: Two case reports and a review of the literature. *Clinical Neurology and Neurosurgery*, *103*(2), 115–119.
Gold, M., Adair, J. C., Jacobs, D. H., & Heilman, K. M. (1994). Anosognosia for hemiplegia: An electrophysiologic investigation of the feed-forward hypothesis. *Neurology*, 44(10), 1804–1808.
Goldenberg, G., Wimmer, A., & Auff, E. (1986). Schnaberth G Impairment of motor planning in patients with Parkinson's disease: Evidence from ideomotor apraxia testing. *Journal of Neurology, Neurosurgery, and Psychiatry*, *49*(11), 1266–1272.
Goodglass, H., & Kaplan, E. (1963). Disturbance of gesture and pantomime in aphasia. *Brain*, *86*, 703–720.
Haaland, K. Y., Harrington, D. L., & Knight, R. T. (2000). Neural representations of skilled movement. *Brain*, *123*(Pt 11), 2306–2313.
Halsband, U., Schmitt, J., Weyers, M., Binkofski, F., Grutzner, G., & Freund, H. J. (2001). Recognition and imitation of pantomimed motor acts after unilateral parietal and premotor lesions: A perspective on apraxia. *Neuropsychologia*, *39*(2), 200–216.
Hanna-Pladdy, B., Heilman, K. M., & Foundas, A. L. (2001). Cortical and subcortical contributions to ideomotor apraxia: Analysis of task demands and error types. *Brain*, *124*, 2513–2527.
Hanna-Pladdy, B., Mendoza, J. E., Apostolos, G. T., & Heilman, K. M. (2002). Lateralised motor control: Hemispheric damage and the loss of deftness. *Journal of Neurology, Neurosurgery, and Psychiatry*, *73*, 574–577.
Hanna-Pladdy, B., Heilman, K. M., & Foundas, A. L. (2003). Ecological implications of ideomotor apraxia: Evidence from physical activities of daily living. *Neurology*, *60*(3), 487–490.
Heilman, K. M. (1973). Ideational apraxia: A re-definition. *Brain*, *96*, 861–864.
Heilman, K. M. (2004). Intentional neglect. *Frontiers in Bioscience*, *9*, 694–705.

Heilman, K. M., Bowers, D., Coslett, H. B., Whelan, H., & Watson, R. T. (1985). Directional hypokinesia: Prolonged reaction times for leftward movements in patients with right hemisphere lesions and neglect. *Neurology, 35*, 855–860.

Heilman, K. M., Bowers, D., & Watson, R. T. (1983). Intentional neglect. *Neurology, 33*(5), 661–664.

Heilman, K. M., Maher, L. M., Greenwald, M. L., & Rothi, L. J. R. (1997). Conceptual apraxia from lateralized lesions. *Neurology, 49*, 457–464.

Heilman, K. M., Meador, K. J., & Loring, D. W. (2000). Hemispheric asymmetries of limb-kinetic apraxia: A loss of deftness. *Neurology, 55*, 523–526.

Heilman, K. M., Rothi, L. J. G, & Valenstein, E. (1982). Two forms of ideomotor apraxia. *Neurology, 32*, 415–426.

Heilman, K. M., & Rothi, L. J. G. (2012). Apraxia. In K. M. Heilman & E. Valenstein (Eds.), Clinical neuropsychology (5th ed., pp. 214–237). New York, NY: Oxford University Press.

Heilman, K. M., & Watson, R. T. (2008). The disconnection apraxias. *Cortex, 44*(8), 975–982.

Heilman, K. M., Watson, R. T., Valenstein, E., & Goldberg, M. E. (1987). Attention: Behavior and neural mechanisms. In S. R. Geiger (Ed.), *Handbook of physiology: Vol. 5, Higher functions of the brain* (pp. 461–481). Bethesda, MD: American Physiological Society.

Heilman, K. M., Valenstein, E., Day, A., & Watson R. (1995). Frontal lobe neglect in monkeys. *Neurology, 45*(6), 1205–1210.

Heilman, K. M., & Van Den Abell, T. (1979). Right hemispheric dominance for mediating cerebral activation. *Neuropsychologia, 17*(3–4), 315–321.

Herzog, J., Möller, B., Witt, K., Pinsker, M.O, Deuschl, G., & Volkmann, J. (2009). Influence of subthalamic deep brain stimulation versus levodopa on motor perseverations in Parkinson's disease. *Movement Disorders, 24*(8), 1206–1210.

Hödl, A. K., Hödl, E., Otti, D. V., Herranhof, B., Ille, R., & Bonelli, R. M. (2008). Deomotor limb apraxia in Huntington's disease: A case-control study. *Journal of Neurology, 255*(3), 331–339.

Howes, D., & Boller, F. (1975). Simple reaction time: Evidence for focal impairment from lesions of the right hemisphere. *Brain, 98*(2), 317–332.

Humphreys, G. W., & Forde, E. M. E. (1998). Disordered action schema and action disorganization syndrome. *Cognitive Neuropsychology, 15*, 771–811.

Jorge, R. E., Starkstein, S. E., & Robinson, R. G. (2010). Apathy following stroke. *Canadian Journal of Psychiatry, 55*(6), 350–354.

Kertesz, A., & Ferro, J. M. (1984). Lesion size and location in ideomotor apraxia. *Brain, 107*, 921–933.

Kertesz, A., Nicholson, I., Cancelliere, A., Kassa, K., & Black, S. E. (1985). Motor impersistence: A right-hemisphere syndrome. *Neurology, 35*(5), 662–666.

Kim, E. J., Lee, B. H., Park, K. C., Suh, M. K., Ku, B. D., Heilman, K. M., & Na, D. L. (2009). Consecutive versus return motor perseveration during line cancellation task in hemispatial neglect. *Cognitive and Behavioral Neurology, 22*(2), 122–126.

Kim, E. J., Lee, B., Jo, M. K., Jung, K., You, H., Lee, B. H., . . . Na, D. L. (2013). Directional and spatial motor intentional disorders in patients with right versus left hemisphere strokes. *Neuropsychology, 27*(4), 428–437.

Kleist, K. (1907). Kortikale (innervatorische) Apraxie. *Jahrbuch fur Psychiatrie und Neurologie, 28*, 46–112.

Lauritzen, M., Henriksen, L., & Lassen, N. A. (1981). Regional cerebral blood flow during rest and skilled hand movements by Xenon-133 inhalation and emission computerized tomography. *Journal of Cerebral Blood Flow and Metabolism*, *1*, 385–389.

Lawrence, D. G., & Kuypers, H. G. (1968). The functional organization of the motor system in the monkey. II. The effects of lesions of the descending brain-stem pathways. *Brain*, *91*(1), 15–36.

Leiguarda, R. C., Pramstaller, P. P., Merello, M., Starkstein, S., Lees, A. J., & Marsden, C. D. (1997). Apraxia in Parkinson's disease, progressive supranuclear palsy, multiple system atrophy and neuroleptic-induced parkinsonism. *Brain*, *120*(Pt 1), 75–90.

Liepmann, H., & Maas, O. (1907). Fall von linksseitiger agraphie und apraxie bei rechsseitiger lahmung. *Zeitschrift fur Psychologie und Neurologie*, *10*, 214–227.

Liepmann, H. (1920). Apraxia. *Erbgn der ges Med*, *1*, 516–543.

Luria, A. R. (1980). *Higher cortical functions in man*. New York, NY: Basic Books.

Marcuse, H. (1904). Apraktische symptome bei einen falle von seniler demenz. *Zentrlball fur Neurologie*, *15*, 737–751.

Meador, K. J., Watson, R. T., Bowers, D., & Heilman, K. M. (1986). Hypometria with hemispatial and limb motor neglect. *Brain*, *109*(Pt 2), 293–305.

Mills, R. P., & Swanson, P. D. (1978). Vertical oculomotor apraxia and memory loss. *Annals of Neurology*, *4*(2), 149–153. http://doi.org/10.1002/ana.410040209

Mool, J., de Oliveira-Souza, R., Passman, L. J., Cunha, F. C., Souza-Lima, F., & Andreiuolo, P. A. (2000). Functional MRI correlates of real and imagined tool-use pantomimes. *Neurology*, *54*, 1331–1336.

Monza, D., Soliveri, P., Radice, D., Fetoni, V., Testa, D., Caffarra, P., . . . Girotti, F. (1998). Cognitive dysfunction and impaired organization of complex motility in degenerative parkinsonian syndromes. *Archives of Neurology*, *55*(3), 372–378.

Mountcastle, V. B. (1997). The columnar organization of the neocortex. *Brain*, *120*(Pt 4), 701–722.

Mozaz, M., Rothi, L. J., Anderson, J. M., Crucian, G. P., & Heilman, K. M. (2002). Postural knowledge of transitive pantomimes and intransitive gestures. *Journal of the International Neuropsychological Society*, *8*(7), 958–962.

Mozaz, M., Garaigordobil, M., Gonzalez Rothi, L. J., Anderson, J., Crucian, G. P., & Heilman, K. M. (2006). Posture recognition in Alzheimer's disease. *Brain and Cognition*, *62*(3), 241–245.

Nadeau, S. E., Roeltgen, D. P., Sevush, S., Ballinger, W. E., & Watson, R. T. (1994). Apraxia due to a pathologically documented thalamic infarction. *Neurology*, *44*(11), 2133–2137.

Nagaratnam, N., Nagaratnam, K., Ng, K., & Diu, P. (2004). Akinetic mutism following stroke. *Journal of Clinical Neuroscience*, *11*(1), 25–30.

Nielsen, J. M. (1951). The cortical components of akinetic mutism. *Journal of Nervous and Mental Disease*, *114*(5), 459–461.

Niki, C., Maruyama, T., Muragaki, Y., & Kumada, T. (2009). Disinhibition of sequential actions following right frontal lobe damage. *Cognitive Neuropsychology*, *26*(3), 266–285.

Nirkko, A. C., Ozdoba, C., Redmond, S. M., Bürki, M., Schroth, G., Hess, & C. W., Wiesendanger, M. (2001). Different ipsilateral representations for distal and proximal movements in the sensorimotor cortex: Activation and deactivation patterns. *Neuroimage*, *13*(5), 825–835.

Ochipa, C., Rothi, L. J. G., & Heilman, K. M. (1989). Ideational apraxia: A deficit in tool selection and use. *Annals of Neurology*, *25*, 190–193.

Ochipa, C., Rothi, L. J. G., & Heilman, K. M. (1992). Conceptual apraxia in Alzheimers disease. *Brain, 114*, 2593–2603.

Pharr, V., Uttl, B., Stark, M., Litvan, I., Fantie, B., & Grafman, J. C. (2001). Comparison of apraxia in corticobasal degeneration and progressive supranuclear palsy. *Neurology, 56*(7), 957–963.

Pick, A. (1905). *Sudien uber motorische apraxia und ihre mahestenhende erscheinungen.* Leipzig, Germany: Deuticke.

Poeck, K. (1983). Ideational apraxia. *Journal of Neurology, 230*(1), 1–5.

Poizner, H., Mack, L., Verfaellie, M., Rothi, L. J. G, & Heilman, K. M. (1990). Three dimensional computer graphic analysis of apraxia. *Brain, 113*, 85–101.

Pramstaller, P. P., & Marsden, C. D. (1996). The basal ganglia and apraxia. *Brain, 119* (Pt 1), 319–340.

Quencer, K., Okun, M. S., Crucian, G., Fernandez, H. H., Skidmore, F., & Heilman, K. M. (2007). Limb-kinetic apraxia in Parkinson disease. *Neurology, 68*(2), 150–151.

Qureshi, M., Williamson, J. B., & Heilman, K. M. (2011). Ideational apraxia in Parkinson disease. *Cognitive and Behavioral Neurology, 24*(3), 122–127.

Rao, S. M., Binder, J. R., Bandettini, P. A., Hammeke, T. A., Yetkin, F. Z., Jesmanowicz, A, ... Estkowski, L. D. (1993). Functional magnetic resonance imaging of complex human movements. *Neurology, 43*(11), 2311–2318.

Raymer, A. M., Maher, L. M., Foundas, A. L., Heilman, K. M., & Rothi L. J. G. (1997). The significance of body part as tool errors in limb apraxia. *Brain and Cognition, 34*, 287–292.

Rousseaux, M., Rénier, J., Anicet, L., Pasquier, F., & Mackowiak-Cordoliani, M. A. (2012). Gesture comprehension, knowledge and production in Alzheimer's disease. *European Journal of Neurology, 19*(7):1037–1044.

Rothi, L. J. G, Heilman, K. M., & Watson, R. T. (1985). Pantomime comprehension and ideomotor apraxia. *Journal of Neurology, Neurosurgery and Psychiatry, 48*, 207–210.

Rothi, L. J. G., Mack, L., Verfaellie, M., Brown, P., & Heilman, K. M. (1988). Ideomotor apraxia: Error pattern analysis. *Aphasiology, 2*, 381–387.

Saeki, S., & Hachisuka, K. (2004). The association between stroke location and return to work after first stroke. *Journal of Stroke & Cerebrovascular Diseases, 13*(4), 160–163.

Sandson, J., & Albert, M. L. (1987). Perseveration in behavioral neurology. *Neurology, 37*(11), 1736–1741.

Segarra, J. M. (1970). Cerebral vascular disease and behaviour. I. The syndrome of the mesencephalic artery. *Archives of Neurology, 22*, 401–418.

Schwartz, M. F., Buxbaum, L. J., Ferraro, M., Veramonti, T., & Segal, M. (2002). *Naturalistic action test.* Bury St. Edmunds, England: Thames Valley Test Company.

Shuren, J. E., Maher, L. M., & Heilman, K. M. (1994). Role of the pulvinar in ideomotor praxis. *Journal of Neurology, Neurosurgery, and Psychiatry, 57*(10), 1282–1283.

Silveri, M. C., & Ciccarelli, N. (2009). Semantic memory in object use. *Neuropsychologia, 47*(12), 2634–2641.

Steinthal, P. (1871). *Abriss der Sprach wissenschaft.* Berlin, Germany: F. Dümmlers Verlagsbuchh.

Triggs, W. J., Gold, M., Gerstle, G., Adair, J., & Heilman, K. M. (1994). Motor neglect associated with a discrete parietal lesion. *Neurology, 44*(6), 1164–1166.

Uluduz, D., Ertürk, O., Kenangil, G., Ozekmekçi, S., Ertan, S., Apaydin, H., & Erginöz E. (2010). Apraxia in Parkinson's disease and multiple system atrophy. *European Journal of Neurology, 17*(3), 413–418.

Ungerleider, L. G., & Mishkin, M. (1982). Two cortical visual systems. In M. A. Goodale, D. J. Ingle, & R. J. W. Mansfield (Eds.), *Analysis of visual behavior* (pp. 439–586). Cambridge, England: MIT Press.

Von Monakov, C. (1914). Die lokalisation der Aproxie. In *Die lokalisation im grosshirn und der abbau der function durch kortikale herde* (pp. 489–574). Wiesbaden, Germany: Bergmann.

Watson, R. T., & Heilman, K. M. (1983). Callosal apraxia. *Brain, 106*, 391–403.

Watson, R. T., Miller, B. D., & Heilman, K. M. (1978). Nonsensory neglect. *Annals of Neurology, 3*, 505–508.

Williams, S. M., & Goldman-Rakic, P. S. (1998). Widespread origin of the primate mesofrontal dopamine system. *Cerebral Cortex (New York, N.Y. : 1991), 8*(4), 321–345. http://doi.org/10.1093/cercor/8.4.321

PART 2
NEUROIMAGING

8

Cerebral Small Vessel Disease and the Risk of Dementia and Cognition Decline

Emilia Salvadori, Fabio Fierini, and Leonardo Pantoni

1. Introduction

The term "cerebral small vessel disease" (SVD) encompasses a wide range of neurological disorders induced by alterations of small cerebral vessels (ranging from around 5 μm to 2 mm in diameter; Pantoni, 2010). The concept of SVD has evolved over the years. Historically, French physicians, at the beginning of the 19th century made the first pathological descriptions of lacunes (Poirier & Derouesné, 1985). More contemporaneously, SVD was described by C. Miller Fisher in a series of seminal papers where lacunar infarcts were linked with specific clinical syndromes as well as a pathogenic mechanism such as arteriolosclerosis associated with hypertension (Fisher, 1965). The explosion and interest in SVD as related to dementia has been consequences of the introduction of neuroimaging techniques in the 1980s. Despite the fact that SVD as seen on computed tomography (CT) and magnetic resonance imaging (MRI) scans is quite common, there continues to be considerable debate regarding the clinical influence of these changes. Mechanisms linking cerebral SVD with parenchyma damage, either ischemic or hemorrhagic, are heterogeneous and not completely understood (Pantoni, 2010). Vessel wall changes may in fact be responsible for structural restriction of the vessel lumen, leading to a state of chronic hypoperfusion that is responsible for incomplete infarct, acute focal necrosis, or rupture of the vessel causing hemorrhage (Pantoni, 2010). In addition to these mechanisms, blood–brain barrier (BBB) dysfunction and endothelial dysfunction are understood to underlie the occurrence of SVD. Inflammatory and oxidative stress factors also play an important role in the genesis of SVD (Poggesi et al., 2016; Wardlaw, Smith, Dichgans et al., 2013). As outlined next, the nomenclature of SVD based on neuroimaging is diverse (Wardlaw, Smith, Biessels et al., 2013).

White matter hyperintensity of presumed vascular origin: Signal abnormality in the white matter appearing as hyperintensities on T2-weighted images

Emilia Salvadori, Fabio Fierini, and Leonardo Pantoni, *Cerebral Small Vessel Disease and the Risk of Dementia and Cognition Decline* In: *Vascular Disease, Alzheimer's Disease, and Mild Cognitive Impairment.* Edited by: David J. Libon, Melissa Lamar, Rodney A. Swenson, Kenneth M. Heilman, Oxford University Press (2020).
DOI: 10.1093/oso/9780190634230.003.0009

such as fluid-attenuated inversion recovery, without cavitation (signal different from cerebrospinal fluid). The size may be variable from punctate to confluent hyperintensities.

Recent small subcortical infarct: Neuroimaging provides evidence of an infarction in the territory of one perforating arteriole, with imaging features or clinical symptoms consistent with a lesion.

Lacunes of presumed vascular origin: A round or ovoid, subcortical, fluid-filled cavity (signal similar to cerebrospinal fluid) of between 3 mm and about 15 mm in diameter, consistent with a small subcortical infarct in the territory of one perforating arteriole.

Cerebral microbleeds: Small (generally 2–5 mm in diameter, but sometimes up to 10 mm) areas of signal void with associated blooming seen on T2-weighted or susceptibility-weighted MRI.

Perivascular spaces: Fluid-filled spaces that follow the typical course of a vessel as it goes through gray or white matter. The spaces have signal intensity similar to cerebrospinal fluid on all sequences. Because they follow the course of penetrating vessels, they appear linear when imaged parallel to the course of the vessel, and round or ovoid, with a diameter generally smaller than 3 mm, when imaged perpendicular to the course of the vessel.

Using the T2 weighted MRI sequences, *cortical superficial siderosis* describes the well-defined, homogeneous hypointense curvilinear signal intensity on T2-gradient echo in the superficial layers of the cerebral cortex, within the subarachnoid space, or both. If there is corresponding signal hyperintensity in the subarachnoid space on proton density-weighted or fluid-attenuated inversion recovery sequences (or hyperdense on CT, if available), the term *acute cortical subarachnoid hemorrhage* has been recommended (Charidimou et al., 2016). Overall, SVD contributes to up to 45% of dementias and is considered as a major determinant of disability and mortality (Poggesi et al., 2014). In addition, SVD may influence and contribute to the final clinical picture of neurodegenerative processes such as Alzheimer's disease (AD).

2. Methodological Considerations

To establish search terms for pertinent literature, definitions of SVD lesions were critically reassessed according to terminology used in past and present literature. Dementia diagnosis was based on standard criteria while definitions and diagnostic criteria used for the occurrence or progression of "cognitive decline" were quite heterogeneous. In most studies, cognitive decline was defined as worsening performance on repeated neuropsychological tests. The type and number of cognitive tests used to define the occurrence or progression of cognitive decline varied across studies from global cognitive function tests (Mini-Mental State Examination, Cambridge Cognition Examination, Vascular Dementia Assessment Scale, Clinical Dementia Rating Scale) to neuropsychological tests for specific cognitive domains that are used either as single scores or composite measures calculated by computing the average of the scores in each domain.

Many methodological issues hamper studies describing the role of SVD lesions as predictors of cognitive dysfunction. First, a single SVD lesion rarely occur in isolation, as various expressions of SVD frequently co-exist. Second, there is a high degree of heterogeneity in the definition of various SVD lesions. For example, in several studies visual assessments rather than advanced neuroimaging techniques are used. Third, the use of different cognitive tests introduces a wide variability in neuropsychological assessments, possibly reducing the sensibility for finding subtle or focal cognitive deficits. Finally, outcome often depends on specific characteristics of the population under study, such as elderly healthy subjects, populations at risk (e.g., patients with vascular risk factors, transient ischemic attacks, or stroke), and patients with mild cognitive impairment (MCI).

3. White Matter Hyperintensities

Clear evidence exists supporting the relationship between white matter hyperintensities (WMHs) and cognitive impairment in the elderly (Pantoni et al., 2007). The relation between WMH and subsequent neurocognitive decline is based on the hypothesis that WMHs disrupt fronto-subcortical pathways underlying complex networks involved in the regulation of cognitive control and information processing (Cummings, 1998). Thus, WMHs are generally associated with a neurocognitive profile typified by frontal lobe or frontal systems dysfunction with impairments mainly in processing speed, attention, and executive functions (O'Brien & Thomas, 2015). WMHs are often measured using either visual rating scales, such as the Fazekas or Scheltens scales, or with (semi)-automated advanced techniques, such as volumetric segmentation. Advancement in imaging methods also includes diffusion tensor imaging (DTI), a technique that allows the detection and quantification of subtle structural changes in the integrity of in vivo cerebral white matter pathways. Localization of WMHs is another important issue thought to influence neurocognition. Many studies take into consideration WMHs as a whole, while other research analyzes periventricular, deep and subcortical lesions separately.

A wide debate exists within the scientific community about the possibility that the impact of WMHs on cognition could be mediated through other pathological processes including brain atrophy such that WMHs and infarcts are thought to directly induce cortical brain atrophy. This interactive hypotheses suggests that the co-occurrence of vascular and degenerative lesions can induce a synergistic effect that might potentiate and accelerate cognitive decline. The interactive hypothesis is supported in that recent systematic reviews and meta-analysis (Debette & Markus, 2010; Kloppenborg et al., 2014; Mortamais et al., 2013; Prins & Scheltens, 2015) indicate that both cerebrovascular lesions as well as neurodegenerative alterations progress over time.

3.1. WMHs as Predictor of the Diagnosis of Dementia

Among studies that take into consideration WMHs as a main predictor of dementia, large general population studies show a robust predictive value of WMHs (Debette et al., 2010; Kaffashian et al., 2016; Prins et al., 2004). In the Framingham Study, WMHs have been shown to be related to incidence of stroke, dementia, and mortality in a large community-based cohort (Debette et al., 2010). Despite the relatively low rate of incident cases of dementia, WMHs volume was associated with an increased risk of dementia independent of vascular risk factors and incident stroke. The 3-City Dijon Study has focused on the association between WMHs and incidence of stroke and dementia (Kaffashian et al., 2016). Overall WMH volume as well as periventricular lesions were clearly associated with incident dementia. Results from the Rotterdam Study also found that greater periventricular WMHs increased the risk of dementia (Prins et al., 2004).

Another series of studies has examined WMHs as the main predictor of transition from MCI to dementia. Study designs are heterogeneous in terms of diagnostic criteria, time to diagnosis, and percentages of incident MCI. In two studies, WMHs were found to be a good predictor of transition from MCI to dementia (Clerici et al., 2012; Kim et al., 2015). In these studies, WMHs were evaluated according to a visual rating scale, and a distinction was made between deep and periventricular white matter alterations. Clerici and colleagues (2012) observed significant predictive effect for deep lesions together with other clinical expressions of cerebrovascular disease. Kim and colleagues (2015) found that periventricular WMHs predicted incident all-cause dementia, while subcortical vascular dementia (VaD) was predicted by both periventricular and deep WMHs. However, two other studies did not find an effect of WMHs on the transition from MCI to dementia (Defrancesco et al., 2013; Devine et al., 2013).

Among studies that include WMHs as a predictor in multidimensional models of dementia, large general population studies are consistent and show a strong association between WMHs and an increased risk of dementia, independent from other possible predictors (Brickman et al., 2012; Kuller et al., 2003; Meguro et al., 2007). The Cardiovascular Health Study confirmed a predictive power of

WMHs on incident dementia independent of baseline cognitive performances, global cortical atrophy, and apolipoprotein E (Kuller et al., 2003). In the Osaki-Tajiri Project, WMHs predicted progression to VaD together with cognitive performance and other concomitant cerebrovascular diseases, while cognitive performance and generalized atrophy were significant predictors of progression to AD (Meguro et al., 2007). In the Washington Heights/Inwood Columbia Aging Project (WHICAP), a study mainly focused on determining whether regional WMHs volumes (frontal, temporal, parietal, and occipital lobes) and hippocampal volume predict incident AD, the authors found that WMHs volume in the parietal lobes predicted incident AD, while WMHs volume in other brain regions including the hippocampal did not (Brickman et al., 2012). In summary, longitudinal population studies show that WMH is a better predictor of incident dementia than other degenerative features, such as loss of cortical volume.

Results are inconsistent for research studying WMHs with other possible predictors of transition from MCI to dementia. Four studies showed that WMHs increased the risk of progression from MCI to dementia independent from other markers, (Bombois et al., 2008; Lopez et al., 2014; Staekenborg et al., 2009; van Straaten et al., 2008). The studies from Bombois and colleagues (2008) and Staekenborg and colleagues (2009) concluded that MRI markers of cerebrovascular or neurodegenerative diseases predict the development of different types of dementia in MCI patients. However, Bombois and colleagues did not find an association between WMHs and subsequent risk to developing dementia including AD. By contrast, the risk to develop vascular or mixed dementia increased significantly with increasing amounts of WMHs at baseline, especially periventricular hyperintensities, independent of medial temporal lobe atrophy (MTA), vascular risk factors, and cognitive performance. Similarly, Staekenborg and colleagues (2009) found that baseline MTA, but not cerebrovascular lesions, was associated with progression to AD. Deep and periventricular WMHs predicted progression to non-AD. Other studies examining MCI patients confirm the predictive power of cerebrovascular lesions, but results contradict the hypothesis that different MRI features account for different types of dementia. Van Straaten and colleagues (2008) found an association between periventricular WMHs and an increased risk of progression from amnestic MCI to AD even after accounting for MTA or lacunes. Lopez and colleagues (2014) concluded that measures of hippocampal volume, amyloid-beta deposition, and WMHs alone or in combination were all necessary to predict AD. However, other studies regarding MCI did not confirm the predictive power of WMHs on the transition to dementia (DeCarli et al., 2004; Eckerström et al., 2015; Geroldi et al., 2006; Kantarci et al., 2009; Korf et al., 2004; Smith et al., 2008; Tapiola et al., 2008). In this research, medial temporal lobe and hippocampal volumes were the best predictor of transition from MCI to dementia.

Contrasting results come also from studies on high-risk populations. One study on depressed elderly (Steffens et al., 2007) and two on functionally independent elderly with WMHs (Jokinen et al., 2009; Verdelho et al., 2010) found an association between WMHs and the risk of developing dementia independently from other MRI and biological markers of neurodegeneration. The study from Verdelho and colleagues (2010) found that WMHs, measured at baseline using a visual rating scale, were independent predictors of cognitive decline (dementia and cognitive impairment no dementia) even when controlling for MTA. The results further corroborate the hypothesis that different MRI markers predict different types of dementia. Baseline WMH severity and previous stroke were predictors of VaD independent of MTA while MTA only predicted AD. On the other hand, one previous study on depressed elderly (Steffens et al., 2000) and another on stroke survivors (Firbank et al., 2007) confirm the prominence of degenerative features in predicting dementia.

In line with conclusions drawn in recent systematic reviews and meta-analyses on the longitudinal association between WMHs and incident dementia (Debette & Markus, 2010; Kloppenborg et al., 2014; Mortamais et al., 2013; Prins & Scheltens, 2015), WMHs seem to be a significant and robust predictors of dementia in the general population.

3.2. WMHs as Predictor of Cognitive Decline

Taking into consideration WMHs as the main predictor of cognitive decline, large general population studies (Debette et al., 2010; De Groot et al., 2002; Kaffashian et al., 2016; Prins et al., 2005; Silbert et al., 2009) as well as studies on high-risk populations (Appelros et al., 2005; Debette et al., 2007; Dufouil et al., 2009; Jokinen et al., 2009, 2011) show a robust predictive value of WMHs for the emergence of dementia.

The study of De Groot and colleagues (2002) on the general nondemented Dutch population and the 3-City Dijon study (Kaffashian et al., 2016) evaluated the predictive value of periventricular and deep WMHs on longitudinal changes as assessed with a single global cognitive function test. Subjects with periventricular WMHs experienced an accelerated decline in global cognitive functioning. In addition, the Rotterdam Study separately evaluated periventricular and subcortical WMHs with outcome based on neuropsychological tests measuring specific cognitive domains such as information processing speed, executive function, and memory (Prins et al., 2005). Results confirmed that increasing severity of periventricular WMHs was associated with a steeper decline in information processing speed and executive functions. The Oregon Brain Aging Study (Silbert et al., 2009) and the Framingham Offspring Study

(Debette et al., 2010) used a clinically defined diagnosis of cognitive impairment and found a longitudinal association between WMHs and incident or persistent cognitive impairment in the elderly. Silbert and colleagues (2009) further corroborated the strong predictive value of periventricular lesions considered either as baseline burden or as progression of volume of lesions over time. Among studies examining high risk cerebrovascular populations that included patients with a first ever lacunar infarct, patients with a history of cerebrovascular disease, or functionally independent elderly with WMHs of any grade, the presence of WMHs was a good predictor of neurocognitive decline defined either as changes in cognitive single/compound scores or occurrence of cognitive decline (Appelros et al., 2005; Dufouil et al., 2009; Jokinen et al., 2009, 2011). The only study focused on a cohort of MCI memory clinic patients further confirmed that global WMHs, and especially periventricular WMHs, were significantly associated with progression of cognitive decline, particularly in executive functions (Debette et al., 2007).

Taking into consideration WMHs as one of the possible predictors of cognitive decline in multidimensional models as related to co-occurring degenerative mechanisms, studies on general or high-risk populations, as well as studies on MCI patients, provide contrasting results. The Honolulu-Asia Aging Study (Inaba et al., 2011), the National Heart, Lung, and Blood Institute Twin Study (Swan et al., 1998), and the 3-City Dijon MRI study (Godin et al., 2010) found a significant association between WMHs and progressive cognitive decline on neuropsychological tests. These results were in line with the study by Smith and colleagues (2008) where substantial WMHs predicted progression from normal cognition to MCI (operationally defined as Clinical Dementia Rate [CDR] = 0.5 without mandatory objective memory impairment) independently of whole-brain atrophy and cardiovascular risk factors. Two further general population studies, namely the Cardiovascular Health Study (Kuller et al., 2003) and the PATH Through Life Project (Christensen et al., 2009), failed to find an association between changes in neurocognitive test scores and WMHs.

With regard to studies on MCI patients, van der Flier and colleagues (2005) found that whole brain volume and WMHs were associated with annual decline in scores of a global cognitive function test, while Mungas and colleagues (2002) found that cortical gray matter atrophy and hippocampal atrophy, but not small/lacunar infarcts or WMHs, predicted neurocognitive decline defined as change in a global cognition index. Two further studies on high-risk cerebrovascular populations (Firbank et al., 2007; Smith et al., 2004) did not find a significant association between WMHs and incident or progressive cognitive decline.

Finally, interesting evidence comes from studies that evaluate the longitudinal impact of progression of WMHs on incident or progressive cognitive decline. Longitudinal studies on general (Garde et al., 2005; Longstreth et al., 2005;

Marquine et al., 2010; van Dijk et al., 2008; Vannorsdall et al., 2009; Wolfson et al., 2013) or high risk (van den Heuvel et al., 2006) populations evaluating WMHs progression as the main predictor of neurocognitive decline are consistent in confirming the robust impact of these lesions. The Cardiovascular Health Study (Longstreth et al., 2005) showed that worsening WMHs on serial MRI scans were associated with worsening performances on cognitive tests for both global functioning and speed of information processing. In the community-based elderly sample studied by Wolfson and colleagues (2013), progression of WMHs was associated with changes in scores on neuropsychological tests measuring focused and divided attention. In the study by Garde and colleagues (2005) on the "Glostrup cohort 1914" increase in WMHs volume over time significantly correlated with a simultaneous decline in verbal IQ scores.

The studies that evaluate WMHs progression in different brain locations found neurocognitive decline mainly based on composite measures for several cognitive domains (Marquine et al., 2010; van Dijk et al., 2008; Vannorsdall et al., 2009). The study by Marquine and colleagues (2010) focused on patterns of cognitive decline associated with anterior and posterior WMHs progression. Decline in complex processing speed was independently associated with both anterior and total WMHs progression, while decline in visuoconstructional skills was uniquely associated with posterior WMHs progression. The association between progression in periventricular WMHs and decline in mental processing speed was further corroborated in the study by van den Heuvel and colleagues (2006) in a sample of elderly patients with pre-existing vascular disease.

In summary, periventricular WMHs progression has been shown to be associated with decline in general cognitive function, information processing speed, fluency, and crystallized intelligence (van Dijk et al., 2008; Vannorsdall et al., 2009). Evidence coming from longitudinal studies supports the hypothesis of a robust impact of WMHs and increasing the risk of incident or progressive cognitive decline.

4. Small Lacunar Infarcts

While the role of WMHs in cognitive decline has been widely acknowledged, the clinical significance of small/lacunar infarcts, often incidentally found on MRI, has received less attention. A putative mechanism of the effect of small/lacunar infarcts on cognition, similarly to that described for WMHs, is a disruption and disconnection of the fronto-subcortical circuits (Chui, 2007). Moreover, it has been show that subcortical small infarcts cause loss of tissue in corresponding cortical areas (Duering et al., 2012).

4.1. Small/Lacunar Infarcts as Predictors of the Diagnosis of Dementia

Only a few studies have focused on small/lacunar infarcts as main predictors of dementia. In a report from the Leukoaraiosis and Disability (LADIS) Study, the presence of subcortical ischemic vascular disease—defined by MRI evidence of extensive WMHs and multiple small/lacunar infarcts—was investigated as possible predictor of dementia and cognitive decline in a cohort of 639 participants with small vessel lesions (Jokinen et al., 2009). The overall level of neurocognitive performance over a 3-year follow-up period among subjects with subcortical ischemic vascular disease was inferior in multiple cognitive domains including global cognitive function, immediate memory recall, psychomotor speed, attention and executive functions, and working memory. Moreover, patients with subcortical ischemic vascular disease showed a significant steeper decline during follow-up in tests of psychomotor speed, executive control, and global cognitive function. These participants also had a threefold risk of developing dementia during follow-up independently of age, sex, education, and MTA. Dementia was related to more severe progression of WMHs and incidence of several (≥2) new lacunes and cerebral infarcts during follow-up.

Silent brain infarcts are frequently seen on MRI in healthy elderly people without a history of stroke. There is consistent evidence suggesting that SVD has a crucial role in the pathogenesis of small, silent brain infarcts. The association between silent brain infarcts and the risk of dementia and neurocognitive decline was assessed in 1,015 participants of the Rotterdam Study, who were aged 60 to 90 years and free of dementia and stroke at baseline (Vermeer et al., 2003). They underwent MRI scanning and neuropsychological testing at baseline and within a follow-up of 3 to 5 years. The presence of silent brain infarcts at baseline was associated with a steeper decline in cognitive functions (silent infarcts in the thalamus were associated with a greater decline in memory performance, whereas infarcts located elsewhere resulted in a greater decline in psychomotor speed), and more than doubled the risk of dementia even after adjustment for the severity of WMHs and subcortical atrophy.

Opposite results comes from a study in which the role of small/lacunar infarcts was investigated alongside that of other potential predictors of dementia (Yamamoto et al., 2002). One hundred seventy-seven lacunar stroke patients were tracked with neuropsychological testing for a mean 8.9-year follow-up to elucidate how the combination of ambulatory blood pressure values and MRI findings may predict long-term outcome. Male sex, cognitive impairment, and confluent deep WMHs resulted to be independent predictors of dementia. Multiple small/lacunar infarcts, together with diabetes mellitus and high

24-hour systolic blood pressure, emerged as independent predictors of vascular events after multivariate analysis.

4.2. Small/Lacunar Infarcts as Predictors of Cognitive Decline

In the LADIS Study (Jokinen et al., 2011), 387 functionally independent elderly subjects with WMHs of any degree were evaluated with repeated MRI and neuropsychological testing at baseline and after 3 years to explore the potential impact of new incident small/lacunar infarcts on global cognitive functioning and specific cognitive domains irrespective of baseline lacunar and WMHs load and progression. Small/lacunar infarcts were evaluated as potential main predictors of cognitive decline. At follow-up, the number of new small/lacunar infarcts was related to subtle decrease in compound scores for executive functions, speed, and motor control, but not for memory or global cognitive function. Locations of small/lacunar infarcts in basal ganglia or in subcortical white matter of the frontal lobes played no significant role in determining a cognitive change incremental to that of the overall lesion load. The results of this study suggest that small/lacunar infarcts moderately contribute to longitudinal cognitive impairment in SVD, affecting executive functioning and mental and motor speed with preserved global cognitive functioning and memory.

Other studies have taken into consideration the relationship between small/lacunar infarcts and cognitive decline in a set of clinical, biological, and neuroimaging predictors. The relationship between volumetric MRI correlates and the rate of cognitive decline was assessed in the already cited study by Mungas and colleagues (2002) in a cohort of 120 mixed patients (including cognitively normal, mildly impaired, and demented cases) with and without small/lacunar infarcts. All had brain MRI and neuropsychological testing at baseline and after a 3-year follow-up. MRI measures included hippocampal volume, cortical gray matter volume, total small/lacunar infarcts volume, and WMHs volume. As previously stated, neither small/lacunar infarcts nor WMHs independently predicted cognitive decline. Cortical gray matter atrophy predicted neurocognitive decline regardless of whether small/lacunar infarcts were present, while hippocampal atrophy predicted decline only in those without small/lacunar infarcts.

In a prospective study based on an identical cohort of 103 mixed patients with and without small/lacunar infarcts, Mungas and colleagues (2005) sought to examine how baseline and longitudinal volumetric change in MRI relate to longitudinal change in cognition. All patients had neuropsychological testing with a mean 4.8-year follow-up and two or more MRI scans at least 1 year apart with a mean 3.4-year follow-up. Change in executive functions was predicted by baseline small/lacunar infarcts. Change in memory was predicted by baseline hippocampal volume and was associated with change in hippocampal volume. When demented cases were excluded, change in small/lacunar infarcts had a stronger effect on executive function decline.

In a study on MCI patients (amnestic and subcortical vascular type), the relative impact of small/lacunar infarcts, amyloid-beta, and their associated downstream imaging markers on cognitive trajectories were assessed over a 3-year follow-up (Kim et al., 2016). Eighty-three patients from this cohort received annual follow-up with neuropsychological testing and brain MRI for 3 years. Structural networks based on DTI and cortical thickness were analyzed. The results suggested that small/lacunar infarcts were associated with the degree of frontoparietal network disruption or cortical thinning, which appeared to induce a decline in frontal-executive functions. Furthermore, small/lacunar infarct number showed the strongest effect on digit span backward and Stroop tests scores. The effect of amyloid-beta was also assessed in 87 patients who underwent a positron emission tomography at baseline and after a variable follow-up revealed that Pittsburgh compound B uptake was associated with temporoparietal thinning and correlated with memory decline.

Pavlovic and colleagues (2014) investigated predictors of neurocognitive decline (assessed by neuropsychological testing at baseline and after 3–5 years of follow-up) in 294 patients with SVD who initially presented with first-ever small subcortical stroke of lacunar type but had normal cognitive status. At follow-up, total number of small/lacunar infarcts and the severity of WMHs at baseline were identified as independent predictors of vascular cognitive impairment. Similar results came from another population-based sample of elderly people (aged 60–90 years) who underwent repeated MRI scanning and neuropsychological testing within 3-year follow-up (van Dijk et al., 2008). Periventricular WMHs progression and incident small/lacunar infarcts were associated with a decline in general cognitive function and in particular information processing speed, whereas no relationship between lesion progression and change in memory function was observed.

In another study, 50 healthy elderly subjects underwent MRI scanning and cognitive testing at baseline and again at follow-up, with a mean follow-up interval of 45 months (Kramer et al., 2007). Volumetric MRI measures were hippocampus, cortical gray matter, WMHs, and small/lacunar infarcts. Neuropsychological measures were psychometrically robust composite scores of episodic memory and executive functioning. Hierarchical multiple regression analyses showed that a decrease in hippocampal volume was associated with a decline in memory, whereas decreased cortical gray matter and increased WMHs were independently associated with a decline in executive functions. The decline in memory and executive functions was not predicted by the increase in small/lacunar infarcts.

In summary, the longitudinal studies described above show an inconsistent association between small/lacunar infarcts and cognitive functioning. One of the limitations of this conclusion is that most of the available evidence has focused on only a small number of cognitive domains (notably executive functions) and evaluating transition to dementia.

4.3. Cerebral Microbleeds as Predictors of a Diagnosis of Dementia

In recent years, cerebral microbleeds have received much attention as SVD markers carrying prognostic information, particularly in the sense of hemorrhagic risk. However, their impact on neurocognition, especially in longitudinal sense, remains to be further elucidated. Longitudinal studies regarding microbleeds and their implications on dementia are scarce. In the Rotterdam Study, the presence, number, and location of microbleeds at baseline was assessed on brain MRI in healthy participants who underwent baseline and follow-up neuropsychological testing with a mean interval of 5.9 years (Akoudad et al., 2016). In total, the association of microbleeds with cognitive decline and dementia was studied in 3,257 individuals. The presence of microbleeds was associated with an increased risk for dementia (including AD) after adjustment for age, sex, and educational level. The presence of lobar microbleeds were associated with a decline in executive functions, information processing, and memory function, whereas microbleeds in other brain regions were associated with a decline in information processing and motor speed.

Two studies investigated the role of microbleeds in predicting progression from MCI to dementia. In a sample of 152 MCI patients followed for a mean duration of 2 years, 80 patients remained stable during follow-up, 56 progressed to AD, and 16 progressed to another type of dementia (Staekenborg et al., 2009). At baseline, patients who progressed to non-AD showed a higher prevalence of microbleeds compared to nonconverters. Furthermore, the presence of microbleeds conferred an equal to or greater than twofold increase, although nonsignificant, risk of non-AD. In another study, baseline microbleeds load detected on susceptibility-weighted sequences was found to predict progression to dementia in 73 MCI patients followed up to 5 years (Kirsch et al., 2009).

4.4. Cerebral Microbleeds as Predictors of Cognitive Decline Without Dementia

Similar data came from studies focusing on microbleeds as main predictors of cognitive decline without dementia. In a 5-year follow-up study based on patients with suspected ischemic stroke or transient ischemic attack, 25 patients with microbleeds and a control group of 30 patients without any microbleeds but otherwise similar in vascular risk factors were selected (Gregoire et al., 2012). Patients with microbleeds more often showed problems in executive functioning than patients without any microbleeds. Furthermore, baseline microbleeds were associated with executive dysfunction at follow-up. In a prospective multicenter cohort of 350 patients with a transient ischemic attack or minor ischemic stroke who underwent brain MRI within 3 months after their ischemic event and were cognitively assessed after a mean 3.8-year follow-up, the presence of microbleeds did not correlate with global cognitive performances (Brundel et al., 2014). Another study analyzed the relationship between microbleeds and the rate of cognitive decline in 221 AD patients with baseline MRI scans and repeated neuropsychological testing obtained more than 1 year apart (van der Vlies et al., 2012). No association was found between the presence of microbleeds and baseline or change in cognitive performances, even after adjustment for atrophy, WMHs, lacunes, or vascular risk factors, after stratification for microbleeds location, apolipoprotein E ε4 carriers, or age at onset.

In conclusion, despite the previously discussed limitations, it can be stated that cerebral microbleeds may predict cognitive decline and dementia. However, contrasting results have been reported. An association between microbleeds and executive and attention dysfunction does emerge from healthy and cerebrovascular cohorts. Despite the recognized importance of microbleeds (especially lobar) in the context of AD, at the present time there not enough convincing evidence that their presence may significantly accelerate cognitive failure and modify the course of the disease over time.

5. Perivascular Spaces

Enlargement of perivascular spaces (PVS), also referred to as Virchow–Robin spaces, is considered one of morphological features of SVD (Wardlaw, Smith, Biessels et al., 2013). The clinical significance of enlarged PVS is still somewhat controversial. Several cross-sectional studies have associated more prominent enlarged PVS with worse cognitive function (Chen et al., 2011; Hansen et al., 2015; Maclullich et al., 2004; Patankar et al., 2005; Ramirez et al., 2015, 2016; Riba-Llena et al., 2016). To the best of our knowledge, only two longitudinal studies

(Yao et al., 2014; Zhu et al., 2010) from the same population cohort assessed the association between severity of PVS dilatation and risk of incident dementia and cognitive decline. Zhu and colleagues (2010) found that the highest degree of PVS dilatation, both in white matter and in basal ganglia, was associated with an increased risk of incident dementia independently of other standard risk factors. In additional analyses, the location of PVS seemed to have a differential impact. In one study, after adjustment for WMHs volume and infarcts, the association between PVS dilatation and increased risk of dementia remained significant only for PVS dilatation in the white matter. In another study, a higher rate of cognitive decline was related to high degree of PVS dilatation in basal ganglia but not in white matter. Yao and colleagues (2014) evaluated in the same population the impact of hippocampal dilated PVS on incident dementia. Despite a significant association between hippocampal dilated PVS and the extent of WMHs and the presence of small/lacunar infarcts, the load of hippocampal dilated PVS was not associated with the occurrence of dementia.

Whereas both cross-sectional and longitudinal studies provide some preliminary evidence for an association between enlarged PVS and cognitive

Table 8.1 Main Findings Concerning the Relationship Between Cerebral Small Vessel Disease (MRI Lesions) and the Risk of Dementia and Cognitive Decline

Cognitive outcome	MRI lesion	Finding	Strength of the Association
Dementia	WMH burden	Moderately increased risk	+ +
	Small/lacunar infarcts	Moderately increased risk	+ +
	Cerebral microbleeds	Potentially increased risk	+
	Perivascular spaces	Potentially increased risk	+
Cognitive decline	WMH burden	Highly increased risk	+ + +
	WMH progression	Highly increased risk	+ + +
	Small/lacunar infarcts	Highly increased risk	+ + +
	Cerebral microbleeds	Contrasting results	+/−
	Perivascular spaces	Potentially increased risk	+

Notes: MRI, magnetic resonance imaging; WMH, white matter hyperintensity.

impairment or dementia, additional studies examining the longitudinal predictive power of enlarged PVS in different locations on incident cognitive decline are needed to clarify the clinical significance.

6. Conclusions

In this chapter, we have reviewed research that has dealt with the prognostic role of MRI-based SVD features on cognition, subdividing research between studies that assessed for dementia versus studies that assessed cognitive decline short of dementia (Table 8.1). The bulk of this research points to a rather clear role of SVD as a marker and determinant of neurocognitive impairment. Some features of SVD, such as WMH and small lacunar infarcts, have been studied for many years. The evidence supporting the relationship between these pathological states and a decline of cognitive abilities is quite strong. In contrast, for other types of SVD lesions, such as microbleeds and PVS, the evidence is more limited, and further studies are needed.

References

Akoudad, S., Wolters, F. J., Viswanathan, A., de Bruijn, R. F., van der Lugt, A., Hofman, A., . . . Vernooij, M. W. (2016). Association of cerebral microbleeds with cognitive decline and dementia. *JAMA Neurology*, 73, 934–943.

Appelros, P., Samuelsson, M., & Lindell, D. (2005). Lacunar infarcts: Functional and cognitive outcomes at five years in relation to MRI findings. *Cerebrovascular Diseases, 20*, 34–40.

Bombois, S., Debette, S., Bruandet, A., Delbeuck, X., Delmaire, C., Leys, D., & Pasquier, F. (2008). Vascular subcortical hyperintensities predict conversion to vascular and mixed dementia in MCI patients. *Stroke, 39*, 2046–2051.

Brickman, A. M., Provenzano, F. A., Muraskin, J., Manly, J. J., Blum, S., Apa, Z., . . . Mayeux, R. (2012). Regional white matter hyperintensity volume, not hippocampal atrophy, predicts incident Alzheimer disease in the community. *Archives of Neurology, 69*, 1621–1627.

Brundel, M., Kwa, V. I., Bouvy, W. H., Algra, A., Kappelle, L. J., & Biessels, G. J.; MICRO Study Group. (2014). Cerebral microbleeds are not associated with long-term cognitive outcome in patients with transient ischemic attack or minor stroke. *Cerebrovascular Diseases, 37*, 195–202.

Charidimou, A., Pantoni, L., & Love, S. (2016). The concept of sporadic cerebral small vessel disease: A road map on key definitions and current concepts. *International Journal of Stroke, 11*, 6–18.

Chen, W., Song, X., & Zhang, Y., for the Alzheimer's Disease Neuroimaging Initiative. (2011). Assessment of the Virchow-Robin spaces in Alzheimer disease, mild cognitive impairment, and normal aging, using high-field MR imaging. *American Journal of Neuroradiology, 32*, 1490–1495.

Christensen, H., Batterham, P. J., Mackinnon, A. J., Anstey, K. J., Wen, W., & Sachdev, P. S. (2009). Education, atrophy, and cognitive change in an epidemiological sample in early old age. *American Journal of Geriatric Psychiatry, 17*, 218–226.

Chui, H. C. (2007). Subcortical ischemic vascular dementia. *Neurologic Clinics, 25*, 717–740.

Clerici, F., Caracciolo, B., Cova, I., Fusari Imperatori, S., Maggiore, L., Galimberti, D., . . . Fratiglioni, L. (2012). Does vascular burden contribute to the progression of mild cognitive impairment to dementia? *Dementia and Geriatric Cognitive Disorders, 34*, 235–243.

Cummings, J. L. (1998). Frontal-subcortical circuits and human behavior. *Journal of Psychosomatic Research, 44*, 627–628.

De Groot, J. C., De Leeuw, F. E., Oudkerk, M., Van Gijn, J., Hofman, A., Jolles, J., & Breteler, M. M. (2002). Periventricular cerebral white matter lesions predict rate of cognitive decline. *Annals of Neurology, 52*, 335–341.

Debette, S., Beiser, A., DeCarli, C., Au, R., Himali, J. J., Kelly-Hayes, M., . . . Seshadri, S. (2010). Association of MRI markers of vascular brain injury with incident stroke, mild cognitive impairment, dementia, and mortality: The Framingham Offspring Study. *Stroke, 41*, 600–606.

Debette, S., Bombois, S., Bruandet, A., Delbeuck, X., Lepoittevin, S., Delmaire, C., . . . Pasquier, F. (2007). Subcortical hyperintensities are associated with cognitive decline in patients with mild cognitive impairment. *Stroke, 38*, 2924–2930.

Debette, S., & Markus, H. S. (2010). The clinical importance of white matter hyperintensities on brain magnetic resonance imaging: Systematic review and meta-analysis. *BMJ, 341*, c3666.

DeCarli, C., Mungas, D., Harvey, D., Reed, B., Weiner, M., Chui, H., & Jagust, W. (2004). Memory impairment, but not cerebrovascular disease, predicts progression of MCI to dementia. *Neurology, 63*, 220–227.

Defrancesco, M., Marksteiner, J., Deisenhammer, E., Kemmler, G., Djurdjevic, T., & Schocke, M. (2013). Impact of white matter lesions and cognitive deficits on conversion from mild cognitive impairment to Alzheimer's disease. *Journal of Alzheimer's Disease, 34*, 665–672.

Devine, M. E., Fonseca, J. A., Walker, Z. (2013). Do cerebral white matter lesions influence the rate of progression from mild cognitive impairment to dementia? *International Psychogeriatrics, 25*, 120–127.

Duering, M., Righart, R., Csanadi, E., Jouvent, E., Hervé, D., Chabriat, H., & Dichgans, M. (2012). Incident subcortical infarcts induce focal thinning in connected cortical regions. *Neurology, 79*, 2025–2028.

Dufouil, C., Godin, O., Chalmers, J., Coskun, O., MacMahon, S., Tzourio-Mazoyer, N., . . . Tzourio, C; PROGRESS MRI Substudy Investigators. (2009). Severe cerebral white matter hyperintensities predict severe cognitive decline in patients with cerebrovascular disease history. *Stroke, 40*, 2219–2221.

Eckerström, C., Olsson, E., Klasson, N., Berge, J., Nordlund, A., Bjerke, M., & Wallin, A. (2015). Multimodal prediction of dementia with up to 10 years follow up: The Gothenburg MCI study. *Journal of Alzheimer's Disease, 44*, 205–214.

Firbank, M. J., Burton, E. J., Barber, R., Stephens, S., Kenny, R. A., Ballard, C., . . . O'Brien, J. T. (2007). Medial temporal atrophy rather than white matter hyperintensities predict cognitive decline in stroke survivors. *Neurobiology of Aging, 28*, 1664–1669.

Fisher, C. M. (1965). Lacunes: Small, deep cerebral infarcts. *Neurology, 15*, 774–784.

Garde, E., Lykke Mortensen, E., Rostrup, E., & Paulson, O. B. (2005). Decline in intelligence is associated with progression in white matter hyperintensity volume. *Journal of Neurology, Neurosurgery, and Psychiatry, 76*, 1289–1291.

Geroldi, C., Rossi, R., Calvagna, C., Testa, C., Bresciani, L., Binetti, G., . . . Frisoni, G. B. (2006). Medial temporal atrophy but not memory deficit predicts progression to dementia in patients with mild cognitive impairment. *Journal of Neurology, Neurosurgery, and Psychiatry, 77*, 1219–1222.

Godin, O., Tzourio, C., Rouaud, O., Zhu, Y., Maillard, P., Pasquier, F., . . . Dufouil C. (2010). Joint effect of white matter lesions and hippocampal volumes on severity of cognitive decline: The 3C-Dijon MRI study. *Journal of Alzheimer's Disease, 20*, 453–463.

Gregoire, S. M., Smith, K., Jäger, H. R., Benjamin, M., Kallis, C., Brown, M. M., . . . Werring, D. J. (2012). Cerebral microbleeds and long-term cognitive outcome: Longitudinal cohort study of stroke clinic patients. *Cerebrovascular Diseases, 33*, 430–435.

Hansen, T. P., Cain, J., Thomas, O., & Jackson, A. (2015). Dilated perivascular spaces in the Basal Ganglia are a biomarker of small-vessel disease in a very elderly population with dementia. *American Journal of Neuroradiology, 36*, 893–898.

Inaba, M., White, L., Bell, C., Chen, R., Petrovitch, H., Launer, L., . . . Masaki, K. (2011). White matter lesions on brain magnetic resonance imaging scan and 5-year cognitive decline: The Honolulu-Asia aging study. *Journal of the American Geriatrics Society, 59*, 1484–1489.

Jokinen, H., Gouw, A. A., Madureira, S., Ylikoski, R., van Straaten, E. C., van der Flier, W. M., . . . Erkinjuntti, T.; LADIS Study Group. (2011). Incident lacunes influence cognitive decline: The LADIS study. *Neurology, 76*, 1872–1878.

Jokinen, H., Kalska, H., Ylikoski, R., Madureira, S., Verdelho, A., van der Flier, W. M., . . . Erkinjuntti, T.; LADIS group. (2009). Longitudinal cognitive decline in subcortical ischemic vascular disease—The LADIS Study. *Cerebrovascular Diseases, 27*, 384–391.

Kaffashian, S., Soumaré, A., Zhu, Y. C., Mazoyer, B., Debette, S., & Tzourio, C. (2016). Long-term clinical impact of vascular brain lesions on magnetic resonance imaging in older adults in the population. *Stroke, 47*, 2865–2869.

Kantarci, K., Weigand, S. D., Przybelski, S. A., Shiung, M. M., Whitwell, J. L., Negash, S., . . . Jack, C. R., Jr. (2009). Risk of dementia in MCI: Combined effect of cerebrovascular disease, volumetric MRI, and 1H MRS. *Neurology, 72*, 1519–1525.

Kim, H. J., Yang, J. J., Kwon, H., Kim, C., Lee, J. M., Chun, P., . . . Seo, S. W. (2016). Relative impact of amyloid-β, lacunes, and downstream imaging markers on cognitive trajectories. *Brain, 139*, 2516–2527.

Kim, S., Choi, S. H., Lee, Y. M., Kim, M. J., Kim, Y. D., Kim, J. Y., . . . Kim, D. K. (2015). Periventricular white matter hyperintensities and the risk of dementia: A CREDOS study. *International Psychogeriatric, 27*, 2069–2077.

Kirsch, W., McAuley, G., Holshouser, B., Petersen, F., Ayaz, M., Vinters, H. V., . . . Kido, D. (2009). Serial susceptibility weighted MRI measures brain iron and microbleeds in dementia. *Journal of Alzheimer's Disease, 17*, 599–609.

Kloppenborg, R. P., Nederkoorn, P. J., Geerlings, M. I., & van den Berg, E. (2014). Presence and progression of white matter hyperintensities and cognition: A meta-analysis. *Neurology, 82*, 2127–2138.

Korf, E. S., Wahlund, L. O., Visser, P. J., & Scheltens, P. (2004). Medial temporal lobe atrophy on MRI predicts dementia in patients with mild cognitive impairment. *Neurology, 63,* 94–100.

Kramer, J. H., Mungas, D., Reed, B. R., Wetzel, M. E., Burnett, M. M., Miller, B. L., . . . Chui, H. C. (2007). Longitudinal MRI and cognitive change in healthy elderly. *Neuropsychology, 21,* 412–418.

Kuller, L. H., Lopez, O. L., Newman, A., Beauchamp, N. J., Burke, G., Dulberg, C., . . . Haan M. N. (2003). Risk factors for dementia in the cardiovascular health cognition study. *Neuroepidemiology, 22,* 13–22.

Longstreth, W. T., Jr, Arnold, A. M., Beauchamp, N. J., Jr., Manolio, T. A., Lefkowitz, D., Jungreis, C., . . . Furberg, C. D. (2005). Incidence, manifestations, and predictors of worsening white matter on serial cranial magnetic resonance imaging in the elderly: The Cardiovascular Health Study. *Stroke, 36,* 56–61.

Lopez, O. L., Klunk, W. E., Mathis, C., Coleman, R. L., Price, J., Becker, J. T., . . . Kuller, L. H. (2014). Amyloid, neurodegeneration, and small vessel disease as predictors of dementia in the oldest-old. *Neurology, 83,* 1804–1811.

Maclullich, A. M., Wardlaw, J. M., Ferguson, K. J., Starr, J. M., Seckl, J. R., & Deary, I. J. (2004). Enlarged perivascular spaces are associated with cognitive function in healthy elderly men. *Journal of Neurology, Neurosurgery, and Psychiatry, 75,* 1519–1523.

Marquine, M. J., Attix, D. K., Goldstein, L. B., Samsa, G. P., Payne, M. E., Chelune, G. J., & Steffens D. C. (2010). Differential patterns of cognitive decline in anterior and posterior white matter hyperintensity progression. *Stroke, 41,* 1946–1950.

Meguro, K., Ishii, H., Kasuya, M., Akanuma, K., Meguro, M., Kasai, M., . . . Asada T. (2007). Incidence of dementia and associated risk factors in Japan: The Osaki-Tajiri Project. *Journal of the Neurological Sciences, 260,* 175–182.

Mortamais, M., Artero, S., & Ritchie, K. (2013). Cerebral white matter hyperintensities in the prediction of cognitive decline and incident dementia. *International Review of Psychiatry, 25,* 686–698.

Mungas, D., Harvey, D., Reed, B. R., Jagust, W. J., DeCarli, C., Beckett, L., . . . Chui, H. C. (2005). Longitudinal volumetric MRI change and rate of cognitive decline. *Neurology, 65,* 565–571.

Mungas, D., Reed, B. R., Jagust, W. J., DeCarli, C., Mack, W. J., Kramer, J. H., . . . Chui, H. C. (2002). Volumetric MRI predicts rate of cognitive decline related to AD and cerebrovascular disease. *Neurology, 59,* 867–873.

O'Brien, J. T., & Thomas, A. (2015). Vascular dementia. *Lancet, 24*(386), 1698–1706.

Pantoni, L., Poggesi, A., & Inzitari, D. (2007). The relation between white-matter lesions and cognition. *Current Opinion in Neurology, 20,* 390–397.

Pantoni, L. (2010). Cerebral small vessel disease: From pathogenesis and clinical characteristics to therapeutic challenges. *Lancet Neurology, 9,* 689–701.

Patankar, T. F., Mitra, D., Varma, A., Snowden, J., Neary, D., & Jackson, A. (2005). Dilatation of the Virchow-Robin space is a sensitive indicator of cerebral microvascular disease: Study in elderly patients with dementia. *American Journal of Neuroradiology, 26,* 1512–1520.

Pavlovic, A. M., Pekmezovic, T., Tomic, G., Trajkovic, J. Z., & Sternic, N. (2014). Baseline predictors of cognitive decline in patients with cerebral small vessel disease. *Journal of Alzheimer's Disease, 42*(Suppl 3), S37–S43.

Poggesi, A., Pantoni, L., & Inzitari, D. (2014). Consequences of cerebral small vessel disease: Disability, mortality, and prognosis. In L. Pantoni & P. B. Gorelick (Eds.), *Cerebral small vessel disease* (pp. 273–282). Cambridge, England: Cambridge University Press, 2014.

Poggesi, A., Pasi, M., Pescini, F., Pantoni, L., & Inzitari, D. (2016). Circulating biologic markers of endothelial dysfunction in cerebral small vessel disease: A review. *Journal of Cerebral Blood Flow & Metabolism, 36*, 72–94.

Poirier, J., & Derouesné, C. (1985). The concept of cerebral lacunae from 1838 to the present. *Revue Neurologique, 141*, 3–17.

Prins, N. D., & Scheltens, P. (2015). White matter hyperintensities, cognitive impairment and dementia: An update. *Nature Reviews Neurology, 11*, 157–165.

Prins, N. D., van Dijk, E. J., den Heijer, T., Vermeer, S. E., Jolles, J., Koudstaal, P. J., . . . Breteler, M. M. (2005). Cerebral small-vessel disease and decline in information processing speed, executive function and memory. *Brain, 128*, 2034–2041.

Prins, N. D., van Dijk, E. J., den Heijer, T., Vermeer, S. E., Koudstaal, P. J., Oudkerk, M., . . . Breteler, M. M. (2004). Cerebral white matter lesions and the risk of dementia. *Archives of Neurology, 61*, 1531–1534.

Ramirez, J., Berezuk, C., McNeely, A. A., Gao, F., McLaurin, J., & Black, S. E. (2016). Imaging the perivascular space as a potential biomarker of neurovascular and neurodegenerative diseases. *Cellular and Molecular Neurobiology, 36*, 289–299.

Ramirez, J., Berezuk, C., McNeely, A. A., Scott, C. J., Gao, F., & Black, S. E. (2015). Visible Virchow-Robin spaces on magnetic resonance imaging of Alzheimer's disease patients and normal elderly from the Sunnybrook Dementia study. *Journal of Alzheimer's Disease, 43*, 415–424.

Riba-Llena, I., Nafría, C., Mundet, X., López-Rueda, A., Fernández-Cortiñas, I., Jarca, C. I., . . . Delgado, P. (2016). Assessment of enlarged perivascular spaces and their relation to target organ damage and mild cognitive impairment in patients with hypertension. *European Journal of Neurology, 23*, 1044–1050.

Silbert, L. C., Howieson, D. B., Dodge, H., & Kaye, J. A. (2009). Cognitive impairment risk: White matter hyperintensity progression matters. *Neurology, 73*, 120–125.

Smith, E. E., Egorova, S., Blacker, D., Killiany, R. J., Muzikansky, A., Dickerson, B. C., . . . Guttmann, C. R. (2008). Magnetic resonance imaging white matter hyperintensities and brain volume in the prediction of mild cognitive impairment and dementia. *Archives of Neurology, 65*, 94–100.

Smith, E. E., Gurol, M. E., Eng, J. A., Engel, C. R., Nguyen, T. N., Rosand, J., & Greenberg, S. M. (2004). White matter lesions, cognition, and recurrent hemorrhage in lobar intracerebral hemorrhage. *Neurology, 63*, 1606–1612.

Staekenborg, S. S., Koedam, E. L., Henneman, W. J., Stokman, P., Barkhof, F., Scheltens, P., & van der Flier, W. M. (2009). Progression of mild cognitive impairment to dementia: Contribution of cerebrovascular disease compared with medial temporal lobe atrophy. *Stroke, 40*, 1269–1274.

Steffens, D. C., MacFall, J. R., Payne, M. E., Welsh-Bohmer, K. A., & Krishnan, K. R. (2000). Grey-matter lesions and dementia. *Lancet, 356*, 1686–1687.

Steffens, D. C., Potter, G. G., McQuoid, D. R., MacFall, J. R., Payne, M. E., Burke, J. R., . . . Welsh-Bohmer, K. A. (2007). Longitudinal magnetic resonance imaging vascular changes, apolipoprotein E genotype, and development of dementia in the neurocognitive outcomes of depression in the elderly study. *American Journal of Geriatric Psychiatry, 15*, 839–849.

Swan, G. E., DeCarli, C., Miller, B. L., Reed, T., Wolf, P. A., Jack, L. M., & Carmelli, D. (1998). Association of midlife blood pressure to late-life cognitive decline and brain morphology. *Neurology, 51*, 986–993.

Tapiola, T., Pennanen, C., Tapiola, M., Tervo, S., Kivipelto, M., Hänninen, T., . . . Soininen, H. (2008). MRI of hippocampus and entorhinal cortex in mild cognitive impairment: A follow-up study. *Neurobiology of Aging, 29*, 31–38.

van den Heuvel, D. M., ten Dam, V. H., de Craen, A. J., Admiraal-Behloul, F., Olofsen, H., Bollen, E. L., . . . van Buchem, M. A. (2006). Increase in periventricular white matter hyperintensities parallels decline in mental processing speed in a non-demented elderly population. *Journal of Neurology, Neurosurgery, and Psychiatry, 77*, 149–153.

van der Flier, W. M., van der Vlies, A. E., Weverling-Rijnsburger, A. W., de Boer, N. L., Admiraal-Behloul, F., Bollen, E. L., . . . Middelkoop, H. A. (2005). MRI measures and progression of cognitive decline in nondemented elderly attending a memory clinic. *International Journal of Geriatric Psychiatry, 20*, 1060–1066.

van der Vlies, A. E., Goos, J. D., Barkhof, F., Scheltens, P., & van der Flier, W. M. (2012). Microbleeds do not affect rate of cognitive decline in Alzheimer disease. *Neurology, 79*, 763–769.

van Dijk, E. J., Prins, N. D., Vrooman, H. A., Hofman, A., Koudstaal, P. J., & Breteler, M. M. (2008). Progression of cerebral small vessel disease in relation to risk factors and cognitive consequences: Rotterdam Scan study. *Stroke, 39*, 2712–2719.

van Straaten, E. C., Harvey, D., Scheltens, P., Barkhof, F., Petersen, R. C., Thal, L. J., . . . DeCarli, C.; Alzheimer's Disease Cooperative Study Group. (2008). Periventricular white matter hyperintensities increase the likelihood of progression from amnestic mild cognitive impairment to dementia. *Journal of Neurology, 255*, 1302–1308.

Vannorsdall, T. D., Waldstein, S. R., Kraut, M., Pearlson, G. D., & Schretlen, D. J. (2009). White matter abnormalities and cognition in a community sample. *Archives of Clinical Neuropsychology, 24*, 209–217.

Verdelho, A., Madureira, S., Moleiro, C., Ferro, J. M., Santos, C. O., Erkinjuntti, T., . . . Inzitari, D.; LADIS Study. (2010). White matter changes and diabetes predict cognitive decline in the elderly: The LADIS study. *Neurology, 75*, 160–167.

Vermeer, S. E., Prins, N. D., den Heijer, T., Hofman, A., Koudstaal, P. J., & Breteler, M. M. (2003). Silent brain infarcts and the risk of dementia and cognitive decline. *New England Journal of Medicine, 348*, 1215–1222.

Wardlaw, J. M., Smith, C., & Dichgans, M. (2013). Mechanisms of sporadic cerebral small vessel disease: Insights from neuroimaging. *Lancet Neurology, 12*, 483–497.

Wardlaw, J. M., Smith, E. E., Biessels, G. J., Cordonnier, C., Fazekas, F., Frayne, R., . . . Dichgans, M. (2013). Standards for reporting vascular changes on neuroimaging (STRIVE v1): Neuroimaging standards for research into small vessel disease and its contribution to ageing and neurodegeneration. *Lancet Neurology, 12*, 822–838.

Wolfson, L., Wakefield, D. B., Moscufo, N., Kaplan, R. F., Hall, C. B., Schmidt, J. A., . . . White, W. B. (2013). Rapid buildup of brain white matter hyperintensities over 4 years linked to ambulatory blood pressure, mobility, cognition, and depression in old persons. *Journals of Gerontology: Series A, Biological Sciences and Medical Sciences, 68*, 1387–1394.

Yamamoto, Y., Akiguchi, I., Oiwa, K., Hayashi, M., Kasai, T., & Ozasa, K. (2002). Twenty-four-hour blood pressure and MRI as predictive factors for different outcomes in patients with lacunar infarct. *Stroke, 33*, 297–305.

Yao, M., Zhu, Y. C., Soumaré, A., Dufouil, C., Mazoyer, B., Tzourio, C., & Chabriat, H. (2014). Hippocampal perivascular spaces are related to aging and blood pressure but not to cognition. *Neurobiology of Aging, 35*, 2118–2125.

Zhu, Y. C., Dufouil, C., Soumaré, A., Mazoyer, B., Chabriat, H., & Tzourio, C. (2010). High degree of dilated Virchow-Robin spaces on MRI is associated with increased risk of dementia. *Journal of Alzheimer's Disease, 22*, 663–672.

9

Structural MRI in Alzheimer's Disease

Are We Measuring the Right Stuff?

Briana S. Last, Batool Rizvi, and Adam M. Brickman

1. Introduction

Alzheimer's disease (AD) is a progressive neurodegenerative disease that leads to deterioration of cognitive, functional, and behavioral abilities. It accounts for the overwhelming majority of dementia cases and has become increasingly clinically relevant as the aging population grows. Hypothetical models (Jack et al., 2010, 2013) emphasize a single-pathway pathogenic cascade of events that begins with the deposition of beta amyloid followed by tau pathology that manifests as neurodegeneration and cognitive decline. These changes can be operationally defined with neuroimaging and fluid biological markers, which have been incorporated formally into newly formulated research framework and set of diagnostic criteria for AD (Jack et al., 2016, 2018). Within this framework, biomarkers for amyloid, tau, and neurodegeneration (i.e., A/T/N) but not measures of cognition are used for diagnosis and cognitive status is incorporated for clinical staging after a diagnosis of AD is established (Jack et al., 2016, 2018). Single-pathway models of AD pathogenesis have not gone unchallenged (Drachman, 2014; Le Couteur, Hunter, & Brayne, 2016; Morris, Clark, & Vissel, 2018; Sweeney et al., 2019), and recent research suggests that other biological changes and pathological features not historically associated with AD play a critical role in the etiology, clinical expression, or progression of the disease. This chapter focuses on brain structural changes in AD and its antecedent conditions both in terms of "traditional" biomarkers that are thought to represent core features of the disease and markers not traditionally associated with AD that might provide additional insight into disease etiology or clinical expression.

Identifying the biological changes that induce AD is vital to predicting its onset, strategizing appropriate interventions, tracking disease progression, assessing drug efficacy and or other treatments, and, ultimately, developing a cure. Due to advances in acquisition and analytic protocols, magnetic resonance imaging (MRI) has emerged as a powerful noninvasive tool to characterize brain structure and function in vivo. By applying varying pulse sequences

Briana S. Last, Batool Rizvi, and Adam M. Brickman, *Structural MRI in Alzheimer's Disease* In: *Vascular Disease, Alzheimer's Disease, and Mild Cognitive Impairment*. Edited by: David J. Libon, Melissa Lamar, Rodney A. Swenson, Kenneth M. Heilman, Oxford University Press (2020). © Oxford University Press. DOI: 10.1093/oso/9780190634230.003.0010 during scan acquisition, MRI technology can exploit differences in tissue properties to recreate images that approximate the morphology or structure of the underlying tissue. Qualitative or quantitative analyses of these images provide operationalized assessments of individual or group differences in morphology or of pathological changes associated with development or disease. When discussing structural MRI in the context of AD and its antecedent conditions, most authors focus on the neurodegenerative aspects of the disease, with particular regard to macrostructural global and regional atrophy (Jack et al., 2010). However, structural MRI scans can also be used to identify and quantify vascular abnormalities and white matter microstructure, which have emerged as important elements in our understanding of AD. In the following discussion, we review some of the most common observations related to AD risk and progression that come from MRI studies of macrostructure (i.e., volume and cortical thickness), vascular abnormalities, and microstructure.

2. Structural Morphology

2.1. Brain Volumetry

Before turning to AD and its antecedent conditions, it is important to emphasize that normal aging—that is, aging in the absence of major neurodegenerative conditions—is associated with macrostructural change. A challenge that has emerged in the neuroimaging literature is how to disambiguate these two constructs. While some variability across studies exists, likely due to differences in methodology and sample characteristics, there is a general consensus on the pattern of macrostructural changes that occur across the healthy lifespan. Earlier cross-sectional lifespan studies demonstrated that total brain volume among adults aged 71 to 80 years was smaller than the brain volume of 2- and 3-year-old participants (Courchesne et al., 2000). Findings from both research samples and population cohorts (DeCarli et al., 2005; Good et al., 2001; Resnick et al., 2000) generally support the view that total brain volume begins to decline as early as age 30 continuing gradually until about age 60, continuing precipitously after that point. In terms of the regional pattern of aging-associated volumetric loss, there is general support for the "frontal aging hypothesis" (West, 1996), which stipulates a relatively greater age-related decline in frontal lobe volume and associated neuropsychological functions compared with more posterior brain systems. The anterior weighting of age-related structural changes is also consistent with hypotheses about normal aging that evoke "retrogenesis" (Rathi et al., 2014; Salat et al., 2004)—that is, the phenomenon in which brain structures that are the last to mature fully during development are the most vulnerable to decline in later life. Indeed, volumetric studies of normal aging (DeCarli et al., 1994; N. Raz et al., 1997; Resnick, Pham, Kraut, Zonderman, & Davatzikos, 2003; Salat, Kaye, & Janowsky, 1999; Tisserand et al., 2002) generally support the idea that frontal lobe volume declines disproportionately with aging. It is important to note, however, that much of our knowledge base regarding normal aging— not just regarding brain imaging but also behavioral and cognitive studies— has been generated without the incorporation of disease-specific biomarkers to large-scale studies. That is, as noted in other chapters in this volume, up to 30% of older adults without frank cognitive impairment have the underlying pathological stigmata of AD (Karlawish, Jack, Rocca, Snyder, & Carrillo, 2017) and were likely included in studies of "normal" aging.

Similar to research examining volumetric changes in normal aging, the earliest MRI studies of AD focused on global volumetry, including total absolute brain volume or relative brain volume (i.e., the ratio of total volume to the volume of the intracranial cavity). Global volumetric measures provide some insight into overall brain health or staging of overall neurodegenerative effects, but speak little to regional selectivity or neurobiological specificity of disease. Early cross-sectional and longitudinal MRI studies of patients with prevalent AD showed consistent reduction in total brain volume and/or expansion of the ventricular system (a marker of global or regional tissue loss) that track with the severity of disease symptomatology (Chan et al., 2001, 2003; Fox, Freeborough, & Rossor, 1996; Fox, Scahill, Crum, & Rossor, 1999; Murphy et al., 1993; Ohnishi, Matsuda, Tabira, Asada, & Uno, 2001; Seab et al., 1988; Tanabe et al., 1997). Consistent with observations from postmortem pathological analysis of brain volume in AD (Kaur et al., 2014), MRI studies of patients with AD demonstrated that the rate of whole volume reduction is 2.5% per year as compared with healthy controls whose brain volume shrinks at 0.4 to 0.9% per year (Hampel et al., 2008). Whole brain volumetric measurements are not specific enough to discriminate between AD patients and normal controls, making it a limited heuristic for researchers and clinicians. Nonetheless, the degree of atrophy observed in individuals with frank AD documents the extent of neurodegeneration that is a defining feature of the disease.

The pathological progression of AD, however, follows a circumscribed pattern (Braak & Braak, 1991, 1996), and regional volumetric studies of AD are generally in line with histopathological observations. Pathological studies confirm that tau-related neurodegenerative changes in AD begin in the medial temporal lobe, with a particular predilection for the hippocampal formation and entorhinal cortex in particular (Serrano-Pozo, Frosch, Masliah, & Hyman, 2011). Pathological or degenerative changes in the medial temporal lobe are thought to mediate the earliest cognitive symptoms of AD (Small, Schobel, Buxton, Witter, & Barnes, 2011). The majority of regional volumetry studies in

AD has therefore focused on these regions. In the hippocampus proper, early studies suggested reductions in volume ranging from 10% to 60% depending on disease stage (Bobinski et al., 1995; Jack et al., 1997; Killiany et al., 2002; Seab et al., 1988). Most studies that have examined hippocampal volume in AD have indeed shown significant reduction in volume compared with controls (Bobinski et al., 1999; Csernansky et al., 2000; Du et al., 2001; Krasuski et al., 1998). Killiany and colleagues (2002) observed a 10% reduction in hippocampal volumes among patients with AD compared with controls but about a 60% reduction in entorhinal cortex volume (Figure 9.1).

Other reports showed more subtle differences, but usually in the same direction, with relatively greater entorhinal volume reduction than hippocampal volume reduction in AD (Bobinski et al., 1999; Du et al., 2001; Whitwell et al., 2007). Moreover, entorhinal volume reduction appears to be correlated with severity of neurofibrillary tangles, one of the defining pathological markers of AD (Bobinski et al., 1999; Josephs et al., 2013).

After the spread of tau according to neuropathological staging (Braak & Braak, 1991) there is subsequent atrophy progressing from the medial temporal lobe to other areas of the cortex following a temporal-parietal-frontal trajectory (Pini et al., 2016) with AD-related volume loss observed in the parietal lobes, throughout the cortical mantle (with sparing of primary sensory and motor cortices), occipital lobes, and frontal lobes (DeCarli et al., 1995; Foundas, Leonard, Mahoney, Agee, & Heilman, 1997; Hampel et al., 2008; Kidron et al., 1997;

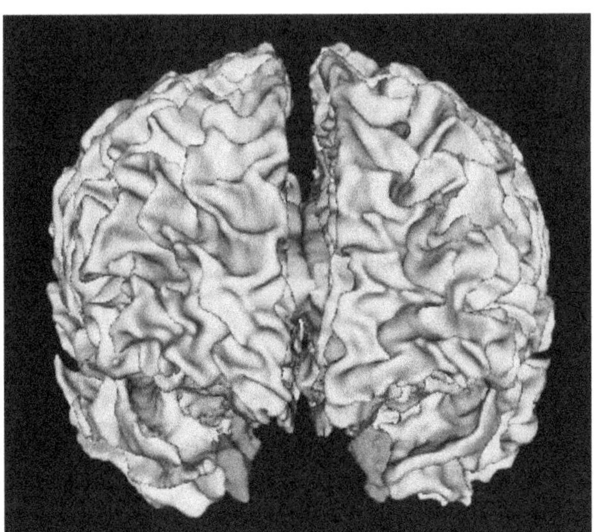

Figure 9.1. Bilateral entorhinal cortex labeled in red.

Laakso et al., 1998; McDonald et al., 2009; Rusinek et al., 1991; Sepulcre et al., 2016; Weiler et al., 2015; Whitwell et al.). Among individuals with prevalent AD, atrophy rates also appear to vary across region, with the medial temporal lobe progressing with the greatest rapidity. In one study, hippocampal atrophy rate was 3% to 7% per year in AD patients compared with 0.9% for controls (Hampel et al., 2008). Consistent with the cross-sectional findings mentioned previously, entorhinal cortex volumetric reductions occur at an accelerated pace compared to the hippocampal atrophy rate (Du et al., 2004).

Researchers have attempted to leverage this volumetric knowledge and evaluate its ability to predict conversion from neurologically healthy older adults to either mild cognitive impairment (MCI), a prodromal phase of the disease, or to frank clinical AD. Several studies showed that lower hippocampal and, specifically, entorhinal cortex volumes predict conversion from MCI to AD within 3 to 5 years (Apostolova et al., 2006; Devanand et al., 2007; Ewers et al., 2012).

Although the examination of regional volume reduction has provided insight into the neurobiology of AD by confirming neurodegenerative changes and providing quantitative measures of degree of regional atrophy, it is important to contemplate the diagnostic or clinical utility of MRI volumetric analysis. Among individuals with dementia, it is sometimes useful to evaluate the regional pattern of atrophy when trying to differentiate one subtype of dementia from another. For example, compared with controls, AD is characterized by medial temporal and parietal lobe atrophy whereas cortical frontal and temporal atrophy are prominent features of individuals with frontotemporal dementia (Du et al., 2007); the pattern of regional atrophy can provide supportive information for diagnostic decision-making. There has been an effort to standardize acquisition and analysis streams that can be deployed on a large-scale basis for clinical purposes (e.g., Brewer, 2009); these efforts have resulted in the generation of normative data sets and population metrics against which an individual's brain volumes can be compared. While not diagnostic per se, normative data allow clinicians to determine the degree of deviation in volume from expected values and track changes longitudinally. Clinically, volumetric data should only be interpreted in the context of a detailed neuropsychological and clinical examination.

2.2. Cortical Thickness

There is a growing recognition that cortical thickness, the distance between the external layer of cortex and the junction between gray and white matter in the cortical ribbon, captures important information about neuronal integrity that complements or is more relevant than volumetric measures. The cytoarchitectural layers that comprise the human cerebral cortex are differentially involved in AD (Pearson, Esiri, Hiorns, Wilcock, & Powell, 1985; Rogers & Morrison, 1985) and evaluation of cortical thickness may yield more specific data on changes relevant to disease and associated clinical outcomes. Automated methods of measuring cortical thickness have been developed and applied to T1-weighted MRI scans (Fischl & Dale, 2000). The cerebral cortex, the folded outer layer of neural tissue, is not uniformly distributed over all areas in the brain. Longitudinal studies found that the cortex thins globally as adults age normally and that thinning differentially spares some areas such as the temporal and parahippocampal cortex (Salat et al., 2004; Thambisetty et al., 2010). There has been a growing interest in assessing patterns of cortical thickness and their utility as a biological marker for AD. As a result of these efforts, Dickerson and colleagues (Bakkour, Morris, & Dickerson, 2009; Dickerson et al., 2009, 2011; Dickerson & Wolk, 2012) identified a cortical thinning "signature" of AD, which includes regionally specific cortical thinning (in largely the temporal and parietal cortices) associated with the disease. This *AD cortical signature* differentiates AD patients from normal controls, is associated with disease severity and AD cerebrospinal biomarkers, and predicts progression to AD in both normal healthy controls and those in preclinical stages of the disease. Thinning of the medial temporal lobe cortex is the best predictor of poorer episodic memory performance in AD. However, we have shown that among neurologically healthy younger and older adults, cortical thinning in AD signature regions (Figure 9.2) is similarly associated with episodic memory, a cognitive domain affected by AD (Busovaca et al., 2016). The observation suggests that the AD cortical thickness signature might be a biomarker for individual differences in episodic memory and not for AD per se.

3. Contribution of Cerebrovascular Disease

Despite the pervasiveness of single-pathway models of AD pathogenesis, which emphasize the precipitating role of amyloid pathology, there is overwhelming evidence that other factors are relevant for risk and clinical expression of AD. Years of observations from the epidemiological literature implicate vascular health factors, including hypertension, diabetes, insulin resistance, hyperlipidemia, and midlife overweight/obesity as risk factors for the emergence and progression of AD (Castellani & Perry, 2012; Elkins et al., 2004; Helzner et al., 2009; Kilander, Nyman, Boberg, Hansson, & Lithell, 1998; Kivipelto, Helkala, Hanninen, et al., 2001; Kivipelto, Helkala, Laakso, et al., 2001; Knopman et al., 2001; Luchsinger, Patel, Tang, Schupf, & Mayeux, 2007; Luchsinger et al., 2005; Luchsinger, Tang, Shea, & Mayeux, 2004; Luchsinger, Tang, Stern, Shea, & Mayeux, 2001; Swan, Carmelli, & Larue, 1998; Swan et al., 1998; Toledo et al., 2013).

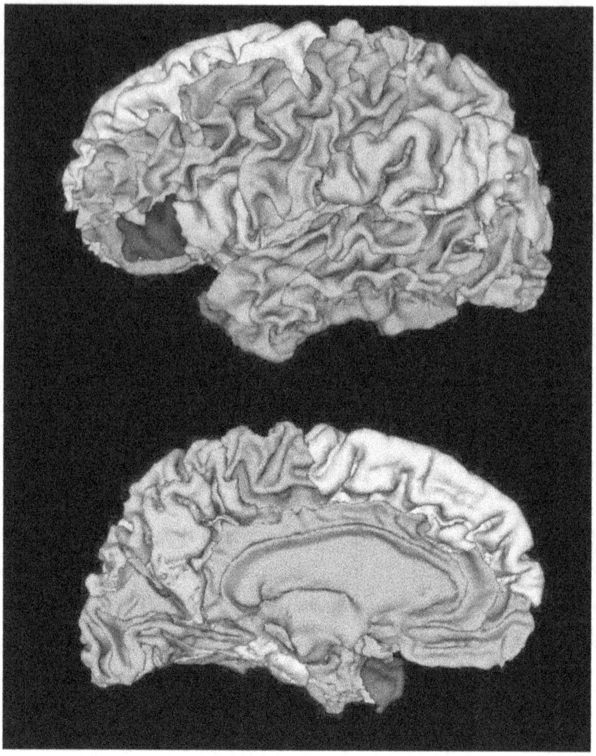

Figure 9.2. In differently labeled colors, are areas related to the Alzheimer's disease "cortical signature."

There is much debate about the role that cerebrovascular factors play in AD, and three conceptual nonmutually exclusive possibilities exist. Vascular risk factors may have a direct impact on primary AD pathology, or, more likely, via small and large vessel cerebrovascular disease that causes "end-organ" damage. Small vessel cerebrovascular disease itself may contribute independently but additively to symptom onset or severity and/or could interact mechanistically with primary AD pathology. Autopsy studies (e.g., Boyle et al., 2017; Kapasi, DeCarli, & Schneider, 2017; Schneider, Arvanitakis, Bang, & Bennett, 2007) consistently show increased small vessel cerebrovascular disease among patients with AD relative to controls. We have also showed that MRI markers of small vessel disease are associated with more severe symptomatology among individuals with amyloid pathology and MCI (Provenzano et al., 2013; Tosto, Zimmerman, Carmichael, & Brickman, 2014). But there is also emerging evidence that cerebrovascular disease may disrupt amyloid clearance or promote

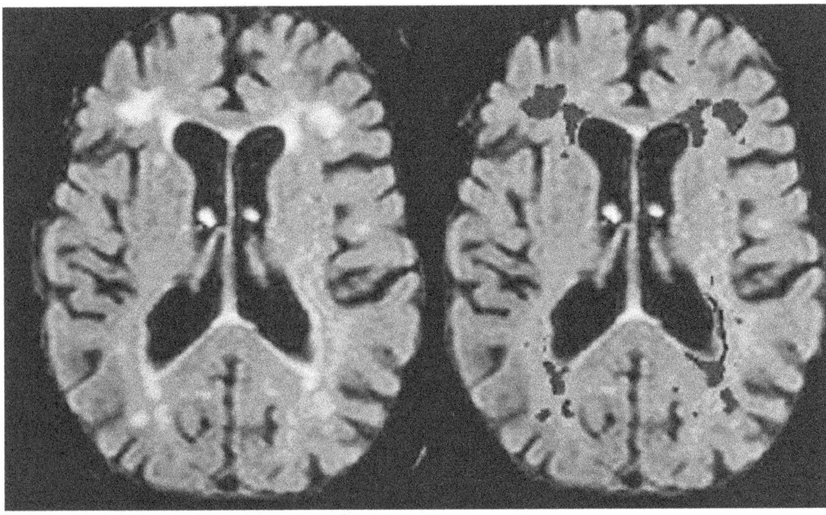

Figure 9.3. White matter hyperintensities (WMH) are displayed unlabeled on the left; WMH labeled with our previously developed labeling technique is presented on the right.

its deposition via venous collagenosis and arteriolar morphological damage (Keith et al., 2017; Mawuenyega et al., 2010) and proposed models that incorporate cerebrovascular disease into AD pathogenesis (Zlokovic, 2005, 2011). Further, emerging data from animal models show that experimental models of hypoperfusion injury induce tau pathology in the affected cerebral hemisphere (Gordon-Krajcer, Kozniewska, Lazarewicz, & Ksiezak-Reding, 2007; Koike, Green, Blurton-Jones, & Laferla, 2010; Raz et al., 2018). It is also important to note that the APOE-ε4 allele, the strongest genetic risk factor for late onset AD, disrupts neurovascular regulation and promotes white matter damage and small vessel disease (Brickman et al., 2014; Koizumi et al., 2018).

Cerebrovascular disease typically manifests on MRI scans in one of four ways. First, white matter hyperintensities (WMH; see Figures 9.3 and 9.4) are restricted areas of increased signal visualized on T2-weighted, including fluid-attenuated inversion recovery (FLAIR) scans. WHM can be conceptualized as markers of the severity of small vessel cerebrovascular disease and have been linked pathologically to arteriosclerosis, demyelination and axonal loss due to ischemia, and microglia activation (Wardlaw, Valdes Hernandez, & Munoz-Maniega, 2015).

Second, microbleeds (Figure 9.5) are discrete collections of hemosiderin that manifest radiologically as focal signal loss on T2*-weighted gradient echo or susceptibility weighted MRI scans. When distributed in deep nuclei, such as the

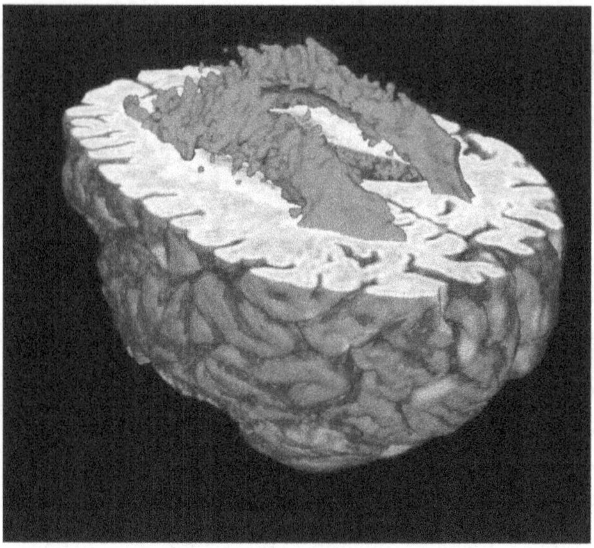

Figure 9.4. Three-dimensional rendering of labeled white matter hyperintensities (WMH) with an axial cut of a T2-weighted scan.

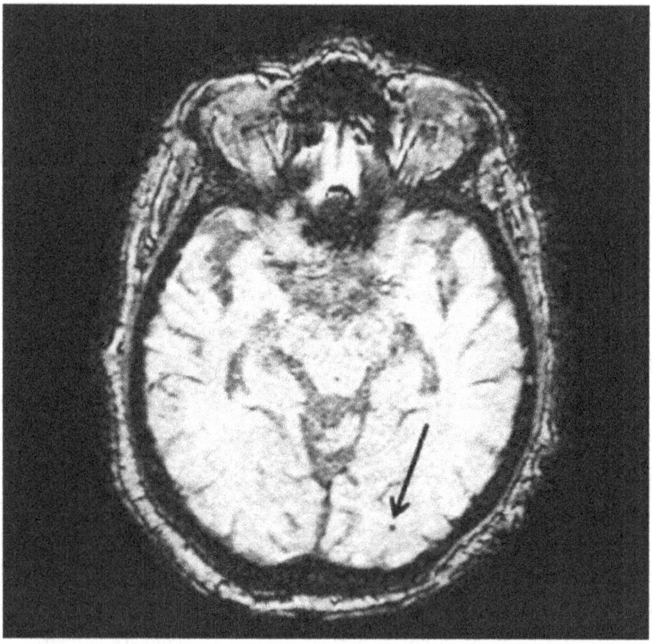

Figure 9.5. An example of a microbleed in a posterior region.

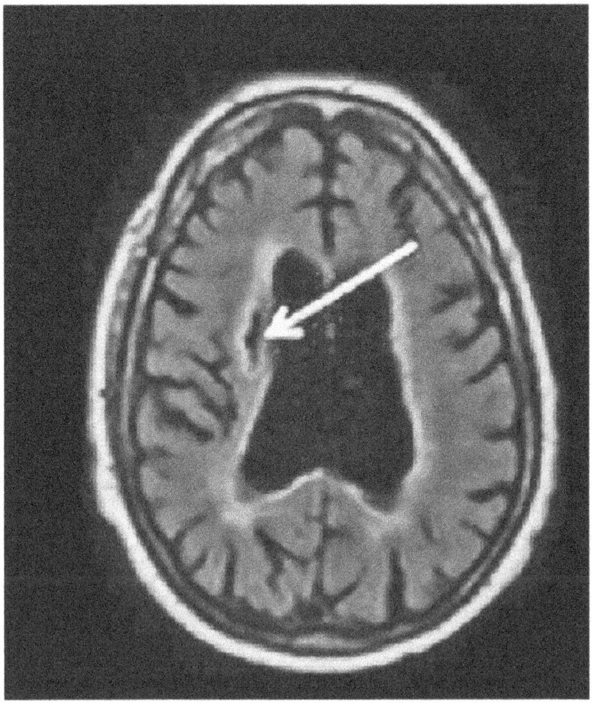

Figure 9.6. This hypointense lesion surrounded by a hyperintense ring on the T2-weighted scan is a frontal-subcortical infarct.

basal ganglia, they are thought to reflect hemorrhagic lesions due to hypertensive injury; when distributed in lobar regions, particularly in posterior regions, they are thought to be secondary to the vascular deposition of beta amyloid (i.e., amyloid angiopathy; van Rooden et al., 2009).

Third, infarctions (Figure 9.6) are visualized on T1-weighted and MRI scans as signal void with a hyperintense ring on T2-weighted MRI scans. Finally, although not specific to cerebrovascular disease, microstructural white matter abnormalities can be appreciated by quantifying the diffusion properties of water via diffusion tensor imaging (DTI; Figures 9.7 and 9.8). Common metrics of derived from DTI include fractional anisotropy, radial diffusivity, and axial diffusivity (for review, see Alexander, Lee, Lazar, & Field, 2007; Mascalchi et al., 2005). These MRI markers are not considered to be specific to AD, but mounting evidence suggests that they may play a unique role in AD.

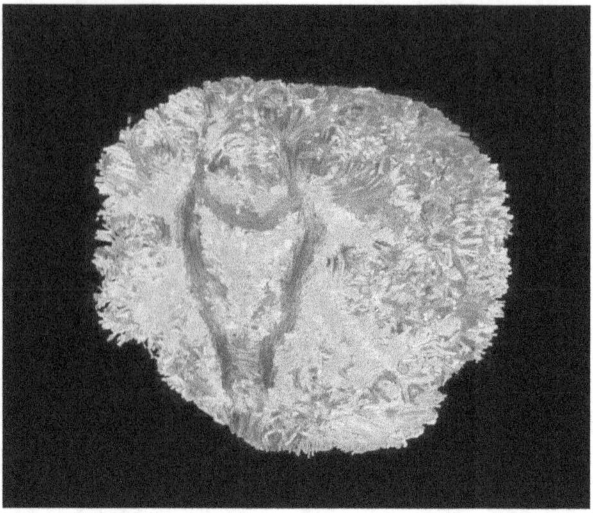

Figure 9.7. Coronal cut of a diffusion tensor imaging scan analyzed by whole brain tractography.

4. White Matter Hyperintensities

We have been studying the contribution of WMH to cognitive aging and AD for several years (Brickman, 2013). Since the 1990s, there have been myriad studies linking the WMH burden (severity or volume) to suboptimal cognition and decline among older adults. While WMH have traditionally been linked to executive dysfunction and deficits in speed of processing (Gunning-Dixon & Raz, 2000, 2003), increasing evidence suggests that they are implicated in other cognitive domains, in particular memory function (Price et al., 2009). For example, in our previous work, we demonstrated that increased WMH volume is associated with worse memory and with diagnosis of AD and MCI, which are characterized primarily by an amnestic syndrome (Meier et al., 2012) and a recent study by Holz and colleagues (2017) found that WMH were related most strongly with performance on tests of episodic memory compared with other cognitive domains.

Inspired by early observations that showed reliably increased WMH among patients with AD (Kalaria, 2000; Rezek, Morris, Fulling, & Gado, 1987; Scheltens et al., 1992), our lab has been interested in determining the extent to which WMH represent a core feature of AD. Among community-dwelling older adults, we first compared WMH burden across individuals classified as amnestic MCI, nonamnestic MCI, and controls. Contrary to our expectations the amnestic MCI group displayed elevated and white matter burden compared with nonamnestic

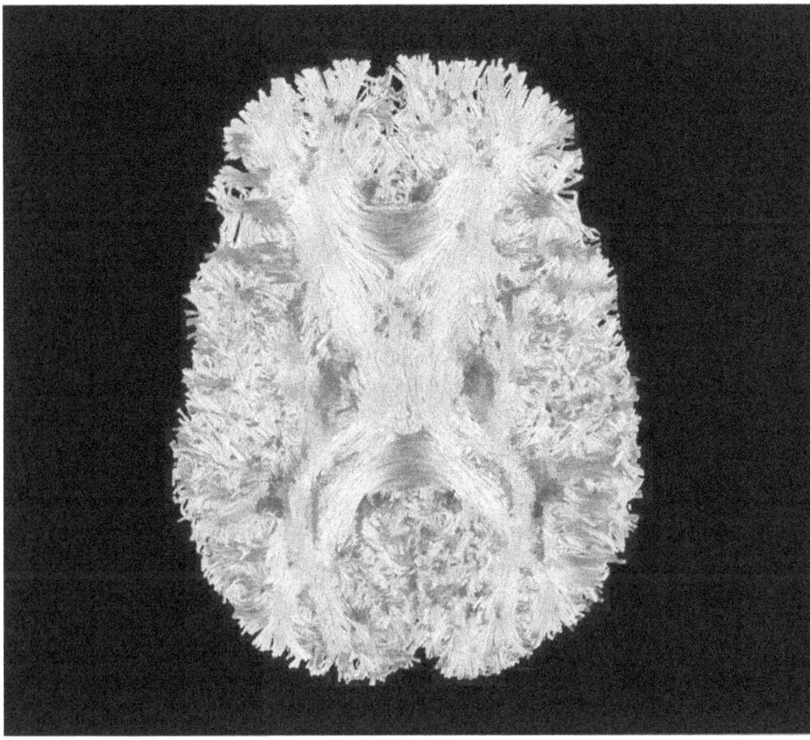

Figure 9.8. Axial slice of a diffusion tensor imaging scan analyzed by whole brain tractography.

MCI participants and controls (Luchsinger et al., 2009). When we compared regional distribution of WMH among groups and patients with AD, we first noted an increased distribution white matter burden in frontal and parietal regions lobes, which is consistent with previous reports (Gootjes et al., 2004). Next, all groups (i.e., amnestic MCI, nonamnestic MCI, and AD patients) displayed increased WMH volume in the frontal lobes relative to controls, but those with amnestic MCI and AD had selectively increased parietal lobe WMH distribution (Brickman et al., 2010). We replicated these findings (Meier et al., 2012), which joins a growing body of work that documents the elevated posterior WMH in AD (Leys et al., 1991; Yoshita et al., 2006). Moreover, baseline parietal lobe WMH severity and longitudinal change in parietal WMH severity specifically predicted incident clinical AD in a large community-based study (Brickman et al., 2012; Brickman, Zahodne, et al., 2015). Our work, together along with the efforts from other laboratories, support the idea that WMH represent a co-morbidity that, at a minimum, contributes additively to the clinical presentation of AD.

More recently, we established a more definitive link between WMH and AD (Lee et al., 2016) We examined the severity and distribution of WMH among participants in the Dominantly Inherited Alzheimer's Network (Bateman et al., 2012). These are individuals with a parent who has a verified autosomal dominant, fully penetrant, and mutation for AD and therefore have about a 50% probability of inheriting the mutation and developing AD. Among the 299 participants studied, 184 (61.5%) had a mutation for AD. We calculated the estimated years until expected symptom onset by subtracting the affected parent's symptom onset age (a reliable predictor of affected offspring age of onset) from the participant's age and then modeled the severity and distribution of WMH as a function of this value and the presence of the mutation. Mutation carriers had reliably greater total WMH volumes, which appeared to manifest approximately 6 years prior to estimated symptom onset.

When examined regionally WMH volumes were particularly elevated among mutation carriers in parietal and occipital lobes, an effect that appeared to emerge about 20 years prior to anticipated symptom onset. To the extent that autosomal dominant forms of AD can be conceptualized as a model system of late onset "sporadic" AD, these findings clearly establish that WMH represent a core feature of AD, which should be incorporated into models of disease pathogenesis (Jack et al., 2016). This research suggests that further investigation is needed to learn the potential interactive and additive role of WMH with traditional AD biomarkers including amyloid accumulation, tau deposition, neurodegeneration, and functional changes in metabolism and networks is needed. WMH may not only be acting independently of these AD-related markers to increase AD risk, but also may potentiate them or interact with them to have a synergistic effect on clinical symptoms. The time-course of these events is not clearly defined thus far, as WMH may help initiate these distinct pathologies separately or act as the propagator of the cascade or may interact with these pathologies at different stages of the disease.

As amyloid alone is not sufficient to account for the clinical symptoms of AD, there is accumulating evidence that WMH may be interacting with and perhaps predisposing deposition of amyloid itself to increase risk of developing clinical features of AD. Our earlier findings suggested that WMH severity interacts with amyloidosis, as individuals deemed "amyloid positive" on the basis of molecular positron emission tomography (PET) imaging were more likely to be diagnosed with AD clinically when presenting with increased WMH volume (Provenzano et al., 2013). We further examined the complex relationship among vascular health, cerebrovascular disease, and amyloid pathology in a study that measured cerebral autoregulation together with WMH and amyloid burden on PET (Brickman, Guzman, et al., 2015). Cerebral autoregulation is a process in which blood flow to the brain is maintained at a relatively constant level across varying blood pressure levels. We showed a three-way relationship—decreased cerebral autoregulation was associated with increased amyloid levels and WMH, which, in turn were associated with each other. Cerebral autoregulation dysfunction may promote amyloid accumulation or impair clearance either through its effects on cerebral small vessels or directly.

As previously noted, the prevailing hypothesis of AD pathogenesis stipulates that amyloid pathology *causes* tau deposition or propagation of tau pathology that ultimately results in cognitive impairment. However, recent work that has incorporated amyloid and tau PET scanning shows, in some cases, that the relationship between tau pathology and cognitive functioning is not amyloid dependent (Bejanin et al., 2017; Maass et al., 2018). By contrast, other research shows tau and cognition are related but only in individuals with amyloid pathology (Jacobs et al., 2018). We hypothesize that other factors, apart from amyloid pathology, including cerebrovascular disease are involved with the deposition and propagation of tau pathology. Indeed, cerebrovascular disease may cause or potentiate tangle formation and neurodegeneration (Erten-Lyons et al., 2013; Zlokovic, 2011) leading to tau hyperphosphorylation and aggregation (Erten-Lyons et al., 2013) as seen in patients with traumatic brain injury (Ojo et al., 2016). Animal models, which clearly show increased tau phosphorylation due to ischemic damage and hypoperfusion (Gordon-Krajcer et al., 2007; Koike et al., 2010), support this possibility. Neuroimaging data, including data from our laboratory, are beginning to emerge that demonstrate a relationship between markers of small vessel disease, including WMH, and increased markers of tau pathology (Erten-Lyons et al., 2013; Gabel et al., 2017; Marnane et al., 2016; McAleese et al., 2015).

In our previous work, WMH severity predicted accumulating tau pathology in the cerebrospinal fluid (CSF; Tosto et al., 2015), suggesting that WMH promotes neurodegenerative changes. However, other researchers have not found a cross-sectional relationship between WMH and CSF-derived tau (Kester et al., 2014) or interpreted similar findings as evidence that tau pathology promotes WMH through Wallerian-like processes (McAleese et al., 2015). As we found that higher WMH volume predicts future CSF increases in tau protein, but not vice versa (Tosto et al., 2015), our hypothesis is that WMH are part of a process that promotes tau-mediated neurodegeneration. These observations are consistent with observations that WMH are associated with rates of cortical atrophy (Lambert et al., 2016). These data are further supported by recent observations that the relationship between WMH volume and cognition is mediated by cortical thickness in AD-related areas (Rizvi et al., 2018).

5. Microbleeds

The apparent involvement of a posterior distribution of WMH in AD (Brickman et al., 2011; Lee et al., 2016) raises the question of whether the underlying pathology of WMH varies by region. WMH in the context of AD tend to localize in areas with the greatest amount of AD pathology and metabolic dysfunction (Braak & Braak, 1991). While current pathogenic models of AD implicate parenchymal deposition of Aβ protein and declining peripheral levels of Aβ42 that are associated with increased AD risk, presumably due to oligomerization and deposition of Aβ peptides in senile plaques (Schupf et al., 2008), it is also possible that *vascular* deposition of Aβ may play a significant role in disease pathogenesis (Miwa et al., 2014). Vascular forms of Aβ may interfere with the ability of blood vessels to shunt deposited Aβ peptides through the periarterial spaces and the white matter of AD (Niwa, Carlson, & Iadecola, 2000; Preston, Steart, Wilkinson, Nicoll, & Weller, 2003; Thomas, Thomas, McLendon, Sutton, & Mullan, 1996; Weller, Cohen, & Nicoll, 2004). There may also be direct toxicity from vascular or parenchymal forms of Aβ in AD. Autopsy studies have revealed that cerebral amyloid angiopathy (CAA), which reflects vessel damage secondary to the deposition of Aβ in cerebral arterioles, is present in the vast majority of individuals with AD.

Using T2*-weighted gradient echo MRI, CAA manifests radiologically as cerebral microbleeds distributed in lobar regions (Greenberg et al., 2009; van Rooden et al., 2009). Microbleeds located in subcortical nuclei are more associated with traditional vascular risk factors, such as hypertension, than with amyloid pathology per se. Presence of one or more microbleeds in lobar, cortical, or cortico-subcortical regions among older individuals provides evidence for possible or probable CAA, respectively, according to the Boston criteria for CAA (Knudsen, Rosand, Karluk, & Greenberg, 2001). WMH are more severe in the presence of clinical CAA or microbleeds and individuals with microbleeds are more likely to have progressive WMH (Chen et al., 2006; Holland et al., 2008; Maia, Vasconcelos, Seixas, Magalhaes, & Correia, 2006). In patients with AD, microbleeds are distributed mostly in posterior regions, similar to the distribution of WMH (Pettersen et al., 2008), and more posterior distribution of WMH independently predicts CAA (Thanprasertsuk et al., 2014).

Microbleeds are very small hemorrhages that typically do not have obvious clinical sequelae, although they have been associated with cognitive decline and risk for future ischemia or hemorrhage (Gao, Wang, & Zhang, 2008; Greenberg, Eng, Ning, Smith, & Rosand, 2004; Jeon et al., 2007; Meier et al., 2014; Werring, Gregoire, & Cipolotti, 2010; Yates et al., 2014). They are detectable on MRI because of the paramagnetic properties of iron in the blood; when vessel walls rupture, the surrounding hemosiderin pool creates a susceptibility effect that is detected by T2*-weighted gradient recalled echo images and, with greater sensitivity, by susceptibility-weighted imaging. Microbleed prevalence is age-dependent and has been reported to be as high as 36% among individuals 80-years-old and older in population-based studies (Poels et al., 2010; Wiegman et al., 2014).

Detection of microbleeds is highly dependent on magnet field strength and resolution, including slice thickness, of the acquired MRI scan, so reported prevalence rates are likely to underestimate the prevalence of underlying CAA pathology in older adults and those with AD (Brundel et al., 2012). Nonetheless, several studies have reported a reliable and dramatic relationship of the number of microbleeds with cognitive impairment and AD-related biological markers (Goos et al., 2009, 2012; Shams, Granberg, Martola, Charidimou, et al., 2016; Shams, Granberg, Martola, Li, et al., 2016; Shams et al., 2015), including a two-fold risk of developing dementia in the context of having cerebral microbleeds (Akoudad et al., 2016).

We view cerebral microbleeds as important vascular markers that bridge amyloid-focused models for AD with vascular-oriented models of AD pathogenesis. Lobar-distributed microbleeds are an example of direct biological interaction between AD pathology (i.e., amyloid) and cerebrovascular lesions (i.e., small hemorrhages).

Microbleeds have also emerged as important phenomena related to amyloid-focused pharmacological treatment for AD. Amyloid-related imaging abnormalities (ARIA) were observed in early Aβ monoclonal antibody treatment trials (Black et al., 2010; Salloway et al., 2009; Sperling et al., 2012) and can be divided into two categories. ARIA-E refers to presumably amyloid-related changes on FLAIR images that suggest vasogenic edema and/or sulcal effusion; whereas ARIA-H refers to the amyloid-related hemosiderin deposits associated with small hemorrhagic lesions on T2*-weighted gradient echo or susceptibility weighted images (i.e., microbleeds; DiFrancesco, Longoni, & Piazza, 2015; Sperling, Jack, et al., 2011). These lesions are considered an important side effect in immunotherapeutic approaches to AD (DiFrancesco et al., 2015).

6. Stroke

It is important to review basic terminology when contemplating the contribution of stroke to AD. "Stroke" refers to the clinical syndrome that accompanies a cerebral infarction or hemorrhage with sudden onset, although it is often used interchangeably to refer to the lesion itself in the absence of clinical signs or symptoms. When cerebral infarction occurs without obvious clinical correlates, it is often referred to as a "silent stroke." However, emerging literature (e.g.,

Blum et al., 2012) suggests that even in the absence of a clinical syndrome, brain infarcts are associated with relative neuropsychological decline; thus, we prefer the terms "quiet stroke" or "covert brain infarct" over "silent stroke."

On pathological examination the co-occurrence of brain infarction and AD pathology is extremely common (Kalaria & Ballard, 1999; Schneider, Arvanitakis, Leurgans, & Bennett, 2009; Schneider & Bennett, 2010; White et al., 2002). Also, a direct relationship between the presence of atherothrombotic injury and amyloid pathology has been reported (Neuropathology Group of the Medical Research Council Cognitive Function and Ageing Study, 2001; Petrovitch et al., 2005; Roher et al., 2003; Zhou et al., 2015). There appears to be specificity in the relationship between vascular lesions and AD compared with other causes of dementia, as cerebrovascular disease was more commonly observed among AD patients at autopsy than among those with frontotemporal lobar degeneration due to tau pathology, TDP-43 immunoreactive deposits, hippocampal sclerosis, and prion disease (Toledo et al., 2013).

Clinical studies have generally paralleled these pathological observations. For example, history of stroke is associated with late onset AD (Tosto et al., 2016) and stroke risk factors interact with biomarkers of AD to predict cognitive functioning and cognitive decline (Hohman et al., 2015). Among large, community-based cohorts, individuals with silent infarct identified with MRI were more than two times more likely to develop dementia than those who had no infarcts (Vermeer et al., 2003). On the other hand, while cerebral infarction is more common among patients with AD, neuroimaging studies suggest that the two processes are independent of each other. That is, there does not appear to be increased fibrillar amyloid pathology in infarcted areas and brain infarction does not appear to increase the risk of future amyloid accumulation (Sahathevan et al., 2016). It should be noted, although, that with the implementation of higher field strength magnets and better protocols for the acquisition of structural data, there is an increasing recognition that cortical microinfarcts—infarcts of submillimeter size—may be particularly ubiquitous among older adults, particularly in those with AD (van Dalen et al., 2015; van Rooden et al., 2014; van Veluw et al., 2013; Yassi, Desmond, & Masters, 2016).

Our view is that large vessel cerebrovascular disease, which manifests as infarct or clinical stroke, is a process that contributes independently to the clinical presentation of AD, whereas small vessel pathology, which manifests as WMH, microbleeds, and cortical microinfarction, is more mechanistically related to AD and interacts synergistically with AD pathology. Future studies that systematically combine structural MRI markers of cerebrovascular disease with specific biological markers of AD pathology will result in a deeper understanding of the relative independent and interactive contributions of each.

7. White Matter Microstructure

While individual or group differences in white matter microstructure does not necessarily reflect the influence of cerebrovascular disease per se, we review some of this literature in the context of non-traditional structural MRI makers that are relevant to AD. White matter microstructure is typically estimated with DTI. This modality allows for in vivo characterization and quantification of differential diffusion of molecules on a cellular level (Medina & Gaviria, 2008). Because white matter is strictly organized into fibrous tracts composed of myelinated axons, water moves anisotropically in this tissue. DTI quantifies this anisotropic movement by ascribing a fractional anisotropy or a related metric value to each voxel (Basser & Pierpaoli, 1996). Fractional anisotropy is the most commonly utilized DTI measures, particularly when characterizing microstructural changes. Mean diffusivity, radial diffusivity, and axial diffusivity are also useful when multiple measures are used synchronously (Alexander, Lee, Lazar, & Field; 2007). DTI tractography offers measures of white matter integrity along the entire tract, a method that allows for 3D reconstruction of fiber tracts (for an explanation, see Basser, Pajevic, Pierpaoli, Duda, & Aldroubi, 2000). Several studies showed DTI abnormalities, primarily in posterior brain regions, among individuals with MCI and AD (Bozzali et al., 2002; Duan et al., 2006; Fellgiebel et al., 2004, 2008; Head et al., 2004; Huang & Auchus, 2007; Huang, Friedland, & Auchus, 2007; Naggara et al., 2006; Rose et al., 2000; Sydykova et al., 2007; Takahashi et al., 2002; Yoshiura et al., 2002). Of note, DTI abnormalities have also been found in MCI and AD patients involving the parahippocampus, hippocampus, posterior cingulum, and splenium (Chua, Wen, Slavin, & Sachdev, 2008; Ewers et al., 2011; Zhang et al., 2007, 2010). Other research has suggested that DTI indices of white matter changes in normal aging brains occur more extensively in the frontal lobe and the anterior corpus callosum (Head et al., 2004).

8. Conclusion

MRI provides tremendous insight into structural changes associated with aging and AD. While single-pathway models of disease pathogenesis emphasize atrophic changes as most proximal to the clinical and neuropsychological onset and course of AD, neuroimaging studies suggests far greater complexity regarding underlying biological changes associated with AD and underscore the importance of wide number of cerebrovascular alterations. Neuroimaging is a powerful tool to visualize and quantitate structural, molecular, and functional aspects of the aging brain, but it is important to emphasize the importance of the behavioral and neuropsychological characterization of participants as our ultimate goal is to understand the sources of suboptimal cognitive aging and to provide appropriate treatment.

Despite the incredible advances the burgeoning technology related to neuroimaging confers, this technology has limitations. For instance, while findings comparing healthy adults with AD patients and cross-sectional studies have overwhelmingly informed scientists of structural brain differences between AD patients and the healthy young and old, they are not sufficient to characterize the disease fully. Cross-sectional studies are important; however, following older adults over time will enable researchers to establish and better understand mechanistic changes that occur well before symptoms arise. Despite the rate at which we are developing tools to understand the brain's structural changes over time, there is a dearth of studies that have the resources to fund such large-scale work over such long periods with regular imaging follow-ups. Moreover, even with infinite resources and time, it remains unknown whether mechanistic changes can be fully identified radiologically. Given these practical and methodological considerations, it is essential to delineate what our current neuroimaging studies can claim about AD and what they cannot.

References

Akoudad, S., Wolters, F. J., Viswanathan, A., de Bruijn, R. F., van der Lugt, A., Hofman, A., . . . Vernooij, M. W. (2016). Association of cerebral microbleeds with cognitive decline and dementia. *JAMA Neurology, 73*(8), 934–943. doi:10.1001/jamaneurol.2016.1017

Alexander, A. L., Lee, J. E., Lazar, M., & Field, A. S. (2007). Diffusion tensor imaging of the brain. *Neurotherapeutics, 4*(3), 316–329. doi:10.1016/j.nurt.2007.05.011

Apostolova, L. G., Dinov, I. D., Dutton, R. A., Hayashi, K. M., Toga, A. W., Cummings, J. L., & Thompson, P. M. (2006). 3D comparison of hippocampal atrophy in amnestic mild cognitive impairment and Alzheimer's disease. *Brain, 129*(Pt 11), 2867–2873. doi:10.1093/brain/awl274

Bakkour, A., Morris, J. C., & Dickerson, B. C. (2009). The cortical signature of prodromal AD: Regional thinning predicts mild AD dementia. *Neurology, 72*(12), 1048–1055. doi:10.1212/01.wnl.0000340981.97664.2f

Basser, P. J., & Pierpaoli, C. (1996). Microstructural and physiological features of tissues elucidated by quantitative-diffusion-tensor MRI. *Journal of Magnetic Resonance. Series B, 111*(3), 209–219. http://doi.org/10.1006/jmrb.1996.0086

Basser, P. J., Pajevic, S., Pierpaoli, C., Duda, J., & Aldroubi, A. (2000). In vivo fiber tractography using DT-MRI data. *Magnetic Resonance in Medicine, 44*(4), 625–632.

Bateman, R. J., Xiong, C., Benzinger, T. L., Fagan, A. M., Goate, A., Fox, N. C., . . . Morris, J. C. (2012). Clinical and biomarker changes in dominantly inherited Alzheimer's disease. *New England Journal of Medicine, 367*(9), 795–804. doi:10.1056/NEJMoa1202753

Bejanin, A., Schonhaut, D. R., La Joie, R., Kramer, J. H., Baker, S. L., Sosa, N., . . . Rabinovici, G. D. (2017). Tau pathology and neurodegeneration contribute to cognitive impairment in Alzheimer's disease. *Brain, 140*(12), 3286–3300. doi:10.1093/brain/awx243

Black, R. S., Sperling, R. A., Safirstein, B., Motter, R. N., Pallay, A., Nichols, A., & Grundman, M. (2010). A single ascending dose study of bapineuzumab in patients with Alzheimer disease. *Alzheimer Disease and Associated Disorders*, *24*(2), 198–203. doi:10.1097/WAD.0b013e3181c53b00

Blum, S., Luchsinger, J. A., Manly, J. J., Schupf, N., Stern, Y., Brown, T. R., . . . Brickman, A. M. (2012). Memory after silent stroke: Hippocampus and infarcts both matter. *Neurology*, *78*(1), 38–46. doi:10.1212/WNL.0b013e31823ed0cc

Bobinski, M., de Leon, M. J., Convit, A., De Santi, S., Wegiel, J., Tarshish, C. Y., . . . Wisniewski, H. M. (1999). MRI of entorhinal cortex in mild Alzheimer's disease. *Lancet*, *353*(9146), 38–40.

Bobinski, M., Wegiel, J., Wisniewski, H. M., Tarnawski, M., Reisberg, B., Mlodzik, B., . . . Miller, D. C. (1995). Atrophy of hippocampal formation subdivisions correlates with stage and duration of Alzheimer disease. *Dementia*, *6*(4), 205–210.

Boyle, P. A., Yu, L., Wilson, R. S., Leurgans, S. E., Schneider, J. A., & Bennett, D. A. (2017). Person-specific contribution of neuropathologies to cognitive loss in old age. *Annals of Neurology*, 83(1), 74–83. doi:10.1002/ana.25123

Bozzali, M., Falini, A., Franceschi, M., Cercignani, M., Zuffi, M., Scotti, G., . . . Filippi, M. (2002). White matter damage in Alzheimer's disease assessed in vivo using diffusion tensor magnetic resonance imaging. *Journal of Neurology, Neurosurgery, and Psychiatry*, *72*(6), 742–746.

Braak, H., & Braak, E. (1991). Neuropathological stageing of Alzheimer-related changes. *Acta Neuropathologica*, *82*(4), 239–259.

Braak, H., & Braak, E. (1996). Evolution of the neuropathology of Alzheimer's disease. *Acta Acta Neurologica Scandinavica*, *165*, 3–12.

Brewer, J. B. (2009). Fully-automated volumetric MRI with normative ranges: Translation to clinical practice. *Behavioural Neurology*, *21*(1), 21–28. doi:10.3233/ben-2009-0226

Brickman, A. M. (2013). Contemplating Alzheimer's disease and the contribution of white matter hyperintensities. *Current Neurology and Neuroscience Reports*, *13*(12), 415. doi:10.1007/s11910-013-0415-7

Brickman, A. M., Guzman, V. A., Gonzalez-Castellon, M., Razlighi, Q., Gu, Y., Narkhede, A., . . . Marshall, R. S. (2015). Cerebral autoregulation, beta amyloid, and white matter hyperintensities are interrelated. *Neuroscience Letters*, *592*, 54–58. doi:10.1016/j.neulet.2015.03.005S0304-3940(15)00182-2 [pii]

Brickman, A. M., Muraskin, J., Provenzano, F. A., Luchsinger, J. A., Manly, J. J., Apa, Z. L., . . . Mayeux, R. (July, 2010). *Regional distribution of white matter hyperintensities in mild cognitive impairment*. Paper presented at the International Conference on Alzheimer's Disease, Honolulu, HI.

Brickman, A. M., Provenzano, F. A., Muraskin, J., Manly, J. J., Blum, S., Apa, Z., . . . Mayeux, R. (2012). Regional white matter hyperintensity volume, not hippocampal atrophy, predicts incident Alzheimer disease in the community. *Archives of Neurology*, *69*(12), 1621–1627. doi:10.1001/archneurol.2012.15271356498 [pii]

Brickman, A. M., Provenzano, F. A., Richards, C., Wasserman, B. T., Manly, J. J., Blum, S., . . . Mayeux, R. (July, 2011). *Parietal lobe white matter hyperintensities, but not hippocampal volume, predict incident dementia*. Paper presented at the International Congress on Alzheimer's Disease, Paris, France.

Brickman, A. M., Schupf, N., Manly, J. J., Stern, Y., Luchsinger, J. A., Provenzano, F. A., . . . Portet, F. (2014). APOE epsilon4 and risk for Alzheimer's disease: Do regionally distributed white matter hyperintensities play a role? *Alzheimer's & Dementia, 10*(6), 619–629. doi:10.1016/j.jalz.2014.07.155

Brundel, M., Heringa, S. M., de Bresser, J., Koek, H. L., Zwanenburg, J. J., Jaap Kappelle, L., . . . Biessels, G. J. (2012). High prevalence of cerebral microbleeds at 7Tesla MRI in patients with early Alzheimer's disease. *Journal of Alzheimer's Disease, 31*(2), 259–263. doi:10.3233/jad-2012-120364

Busovaca, E., Zimmerman, M. E., Meier, I. B., Griffith, E. Y., Grieve, S. M., Korgaonkar, M. S., . . . Brickman, A. M. (2016). Is the Alzheimer's disease cortical thickness signature a biological marker for memory? *Brain Imaging and Behavior, 10*(2), 517–523. doi:10.1007/s11682-015-9413-5

Castellani, R. J., & Perry, G. (2012). Pathogenesis and disease-modifying therapy in Alzheimer's disease: The flat line of progress. *Archives of Medical Research, 43*(8), 694–698. doi:10.1016/j.arcmed.2012.09.009S0188-4409(12)00278-0

Chan, D., Fox, N. C., Jenkins, R., Scahill, R. I., Crum, W. R., & Rossor, M. N. (2001). Rates of global and regional cerebral atrophy in AD and frontotemporal dementia. *Neurology, 57*(10), 1756–1763.

Chan, D., Janssen, J. C., Whitwell, J. L., Watt, H. C., Jenkins, R., Frost, C., . . . Fox, N. C. (2003). Change in rates of cerebral atrophy over time in early-onset Alzheimer's disease: Longitudinal MRI study. *Lancet, 362*(9390), 1121–1122.

Chen, Y. W., Gurol, M. E., Rosand, J., Viswanathan, A., Rakich, S. M., Groover, T. R., . . . Smith, E. E. (2006). Progression of white matter lesions and hemorrhages in cerebral amyloid angiopathy. *Neurology, 67*(1), 83–87. doi:10.1212/01.wnl.0000223613.57229.24

Chua, T. C., Wen, W., Slavin, M. J., & Sachdev, P. S. (2008). Diffusion tensor imaging in mild cognitive impairment and Alzheimer's disease: A review. *Current Opinion in Neurology, 21*(1), 83–92. doi:10.1097/WCO.0b013e3282f4594b

Courchesne, E., Chisum, H. J., Townsend, J., Cowles, A., Covington, J., Egaas, B., . . . Press, G. A. (2000). Normal brain development and aging: Quantitative analysis at in vivo MR imaging in healthy volunteers. *Radiology, 216*(3), 672–682.

Csernansky, J. G., Wang, L., Joshi, S., Miller, J. P., Gado, M., Kido, D., . . . Miller, M. I. (2000). Early DAT is distinguished from aging by high-dimensional mapping of the hippocampus: Dementia of the Alzheimer type. *Neurology, 55*(11), 1636–1643.

DeCarli, C., Massaro, J., Harvey, D., Hald, J., Tullberg, M., Au, R., . . . Wolf, P. A. (2005). Measures of brain morphology and infarction in the Framingham Heart Study: Establishing what is normal. *Neurobiology of Aging, 26*(4), 491–510.

DeCarli, C., Murphy, D. G., Gillette, J. A., Haxby, J. V., Teichberg, D., Schapiro, M. B., & Horwitz, B. (1994). Lack of age-related differences in temporal lobe volume of very healthy adults. *American Journal of Neuroradiology, 15*(4), 689–696.

DeCarli, C., Murphy, D. G., McIntosh, A. R., Teichberg, D., Schapiro, M. B., & Horwitz, B. (1995). Discriminant analysis of MRI measures as a method to determine the presence of dementia of the Alzheimer type. *Psychiatry Research 57*(2), 119–130.

Devanand, D. P., Pradhaban, G., Liu, X., Khandji, A., De Santi, S., Segal, S., . . . de Leon, M. J. (2007). Hippocampal and entorhinal atrophy in mild cognitive impairment: Prediction of Alzheimer disease. *Neurology, 68*(11), 828–836. doi:10.1212/01.wnl.0000256697.20968.d7

Dickerson, B. C., Bakkour, A., Salat, D. H., Feczko, E., Pacheco, J., Greve, D. N., . . . Buckner, R. L. (2009). The cortical signature of Alzheimer's disease: Regionally specific cortical thinning relates to symptom severity in very mild to mild AD dementia and is detectable in asymptomatic amyloid-positive individuals. *Cerebral Cortex, 19*(3), 497–510. doi:10.1093/cercor/bhn113

Dickerson, B. C., Stoub, T. R., Shah, R. C., Sperling, R. A., Killiany, R. J., Albert, M. S., . . . Detoledo-Morrell, L. (2011). Alzheimer-signature MRI biomarker predicts AD dementia in cognitively normal adults. *Neurology, 76*(16), 1395–1402. doi:10.1212/WNL.0b013e3182166e96

Dickerson, B. C., & Wolk, D. A. (2012). MRI cortical thickness biomarker predicts AD-like CSF and cognitive decline in normal adults. *Neurology, 78*(2), 84–90. doi:10.1212/WNL.0b013e31823efc6c

DiFrancesco, J. C., Longoni, M., & Piazza, F. (2015). Anti-Aβ autoantibodies in amyloid related imaging abnormalities (ARIA): Candidate biomarker for immunotherapy in Alzheimer's disease and cerebral amyloid angiopathy. *Frontiers in Neurology, 6*, 207. doi:10.3389/fneur.2015.00207

Drachman, D. A. (2014). The amyloid hypothesis, time to move on: Amyloid is the downstream result, not cause, of Alzheimer's disease. *Alzheimer's & Dementia, 10*(3), 372–380. doi:10.1016/j.jalz.2013.11.003S1552-5260(13)02914-2

Du, A. T., Schuff, N., Amend, D., Laakso, M. P., Hsu, Y. Y., Jagust, W. J., . . . Weiner, M. W. (2001). Magnetic resonance imaging of the entorhinal cortex and hippocampus in mild cognitive impairment and Alzheimer's disease. *Journal of Neurology, Neurosurgery, and Psychiatry, 71*(4), 441–447.

Du, A. T., Schuff, N., Kramer, J. H., Ganzer, S., Zhu, X. P., Jagust, W. J., . . . Weiner, M. W. (2004). Higher atrophy rate of entorhinal cortex than hippocampus in AD. *Neurology, 62*(3), 422–427.

Du, A. T., Schuff, N., Kramer, J. H., Rosen, H. J., Gorno-Tempini, M. L., Rankin, K., . . . Weiner, M. W. (2007). Different regional patterns of cortical thinning in Alzheimer's disease and frontotemporal dementia. *Brain, 130*(Pt 4), 1159–1166. doi:10.1093/brain/awm016

Duan, J. H., Wang, H. Q., Xu, J., Lin, X., Chen, S. Q., Kang, Z., & Yao, Z. B. (2006). White matter damage of patients with Alzheimer's disease correlated with the decreased cognitive function. *Surgical and Radiologic Anatomy, 28*(2), 150–156. doi:10.1007/s00276-006-0111-2

Elkins, J. S., O'Meara, E. S., Longstreth, W. T., Jr., Carlson, M. C., Manolio, T. A., & Johnston, S. C. (2004). Stroke risk factors and loss of high cognitive function. *Neurology, 63*(5), 793–799.

Erten-Lyons, D., Woltjer, R., Kaye, J., Mattek, N., Dodge, H. H., Green, S., . . . Silbert, L. C. (2013). Neuropathologic basis of white matter hyperintensity accumulation with advanced age. *Neurology, 81*(11), 977–983. doi:10.1212/WNL.0b013e3182a43e45WNL.0b013e3182a43e45

Ewers, M., Frisoni, G. B., Teipel, S. J., Grinberg, L. T., Amaro, E., Jr., Heinsen, H., . . . Hampel, H. (2011). Staging Alzheimer's disease progression with multimodality neuroimaging. *Progress in Neurobiology, 95*(4), 535–546. doi:10.1016/j.pneurobio.2011.06.004

Ewers, M., Walsh, C., Trojanowski, J. Q., Shaw, L. M., Petersen, R. C., Jack, C. R., Jr., . . . Hampel, H. (2012). Prediction of conversion from mild cognitive impairment to Alzheimer's disease dementia based upon biomarkers and neuropsychological test performance. *Neurobiology of Aging, 33*(7), 1203–1214. doi:10.1016/j.neurobiolaging.2010.10.019

Fellgiebel, A., Schermuly, I., Gerhard, A., Keller, I., Albrecht, J., Weibrich, C., . . . Stoeter, P. (2008). Functional relevant loss of long association fibre tracts integrity in early Alzheimer's disease. *Neuropsychologia, 46*(6), 1698–1706. doi:10.1016/j.neuropsychologia.2007.12.010

Fellgiebel, A., Wille, P., Muller, M. J., Winterer, G., Scheurich, A., Vucurevic, G., . . . Stoeter, P. (2004). Ultrastructural hippocampal and white matter alterations in mild cognitive impairment: A diffusion tensor imaging study. *Dementia and Geriatric Cognitive Disorders, 18*(1), 101–108. doi:10.1159/000077817

Fischl, B., & Dale, A. M. (2000). Measuring the thickness of the human cerebral cortex from magnetic resonance images. *Proceedings of the National Academy of Sciences of the United States of America, 97*(20), 11050–11055. doi:10.1073/pnas.200033797

Foundas, A. L., Leonard, C. M., Mahoney, S. M., Agee, O. F., & Heilman, K. M. (1997). Atrophy of the hippocampus, parietal cortex, and insula in Alzheimer's disease: A volumetric magnetic resonance imaging study. *Neuropsychiatry, Neuropsychology and Behavioral Neurology, 10*(2), 81–89.

Fox, N. C., Freeborough, P. A., & Rossor, M. N. (1996). Visualisation and quantification of rates of atrophy in Alzheimer's disease. *Lancet, 348*(9020), 94–97.

Fox, N. C., Scahill, R. I., Crum, W. R., & Rossor, M. N. (1999). Correlation between rates of brain atrophy and cognitive decline in AD. *Neurology, 52*(8), 1687–1689.

Gabel, S., Mak, E., Cervenka, S., Jones, P. S., Surendranathan, A., Bevan-Jones, W. R., . . . O'Brien, J. T. (2017, July). *[18F]AV-1451 PET imaging of tau pathology predicts white matter hyperintensities in healthy aging, mild cognitive impairment, and Alzheimer's disease: The NIMROD study.* Paper presented at the Alzheimer's Association International Conference, London, England.

Gao, T., Wang, Y., & Zhang, Z. (2008). Silent cerebral microbleeds on susceptibility-weighted imaging of patients with ischemic stroke and leukoaraiosis. *Neurological Research, 30*(3), 272–276. doi:10.1179/016164107x251556

Good, C. D., Johnsrude, I. S., Ashburner, J., Henson, R. N., Friston, K. J., & Frackowiak, R. S. (2001). A voxel-based morphometric study of ageing in 465 normal adult human brains. *Neuroimage, 14*(1 Pt 1), 21–36.

Goos, J. D., Kester, M. I., Barkhof, F., Klein, M., Blankenstein, M. A., Scheltens, P., & van der Flier, W. M. (2009). Patients with Alzheimer disease with multiple microbleeds: Relation with cerebrospinal fluid biomarkers and cognition. *Stroke, 40*(11), 3455–3460. doi:10.1161/strokeaha.109.558197

Goos, J. D., Teunissen, C. E., Veerhuis, R., Verwey, N. A., Barkhof, F., Blankenstein, M. A., . . . van der Flier, W. M. (2012). Microbleeds relate to altered amyloid-beta metabolism in Alzheimer's disease. *Neurobiology of Aging, 33*(5), 1011.e1011–1019. doi:10.1016/j.neurobiolaging.2011.10.026

Gootjes, L., Teipel, S. J., Zebuhr, Y., Schwarz, R., Leinsinger, G., Scheltens, P., . . . Hampel, H. (2004). Regional distribution of white matter hyperintensities in vascular dementia, Alzheimer's disease and healthy aging. *Dementia and Geriatric Cognitive Disorder, 18*(2), 180–188.

Gordon-Krajcer, W., Kozniewska, E., Lazarewicz, J. W., & Ksiezak-Reding, H. (2007). Differential changes in phosphorylation of tau at PHF-1 and 12E8 epitopes during brain ischemia and reperfusion in gerbils. *Neurochemical Research, 32*(4-5), 729–737. doi:10.1007/s11064-006-9199-3

Greenberg, S. M., Eng, J. A., Ning, M., Smith, E. E., & Rosand, J. (2004). Hemorrhage burden predicts recurrent intracerebral hemorrhage after lobar hemorrhage. *Stroke, 35*(6), 1415–1420. doi:10.1161/01.STR.0000126807.69758.0e01.STR.0000126807.69758.0e

Greenberg, S. M., Vernooij, M. W., Cordonnier, C., Viswanathan, A., Al-Shahi Salman, R., Warach, S., . . . Breteler, M. M. (2009). Cerebral microbleeds: A guide to detection and interpretation. *Lancet Neurology*, *8*(2), 165–174. doi:S1474-4422(09)70013-4

Gunning-Dixon, F. M., & Raz, N. (2000). The cognitive correlates of white matter abnormalities in normal aging: A quantitative review. *Neuropsychology*, *14*(2), 224–232.

Gunning-Dixon, F. M., & Raz, N. (2003). Neuroanatomical correlates of selected executive functions in middle-aged and older adults: A prospective MRI study. *Neuropsychologia*, *41*(14), 1929–1941.

Hampel, H., Burger, K., Teipel, S. J., Bokde, A. L., Zetterberg, H., & Blennow, K. (2008). Core candidate neurochemical and imaging biomarkers of Alzheimer's disease. *Alzheimer's & Dementia*, *4*(1), 38–48. doi:10.1016/j.jalz.2007.08.006

Head, D., Buckner, R. L., Shimony, J. S., Williams, L. E., Akbudak, E., Conturo, T. E., . . . Snyder, A. Z. (2004). Differential vulnerability of anterior white matter in nondemented aging with minimal acceleration in dementia of the Alzheimer type: Evidence from diffusion tensor imaging. *Cerebral Cortex*, *14*(4), 410–423.

Helzner, E. P., Luchsinger, J. A., Scarmeas, N., Cosentino, S., Brickman, A. M., Glymour, M. M., & Stern, Y. (2009). Contribution of vascular risk factors to the progression in Alzheimer disease. *Archives of Neurology*, *66*(3), 343–348. doi:10.1001/archneur.66.3.34366/3/343

Hohman, T. J., Samuels, L. R., Liu, D., Gifford, K. A., Mukherjee, S., Benson, E. M., . . . Jefferson, A. L. (2015). Stroke risk interacts with Alzheimer's disease biomarkers on brain aging outcomes. *Neurobiology of Aging*, *36*(9), 2501–2508. doi:10.1016/j.neurobiolaging.2015.05.021

Holland, C. M., Smith, E. E., Csapo, I., Gurol, M. E., Brylka, D. A., Killiany, R. J., . . . Greenberg, S. M. (2008). Spatial distribution of white-matter hyperintensities in Alzheimer disease, cerebral amyloid angiopathy, and healthy aging. *Stroke*, *39*(4), 1127–1133.

Holz, M. R., Kochhann, R., Ferreira, P., Tarrasconi, M., Chaves, M. L. F., & Fonseca, R. P. (2017). Cognitive performance in patients with mild cognitive impairment and Alzheimer's disease with white matter hyperintensities: An exploratory analysis. *Dementia & Neuropsychologia*, *11*(4), 426–433. doi:10.1590/1980-57642016dn11-040013

Huang, J., & Auchus, A. P. (2007). Diffusion tensor imaging of normal appearing white matter and its correlation with cognitive functioning in mild cognitive impairment and Alzheimer's disease. *Annals of the New York Academy of Sciences*, *1097*, 259–264. doi:10.1196/annals.1379.021

Huang, J., Friedland, R. P., & Auchus, A. P. (2007). Diffusion tensor imaging of normal-appearing white matter in mild cognitive impairment and early Alzheimer disease: Preliminary evidence of axonal degeneration in the temporal lobe. *American Journal of Neuroradiology*, *28*(10), 1943–1948. doi:10.3174/ajnr.A0700

Jack, C. R., Jr., Bennett, D. A., Blennow, K., Carrillo, M. C., Dunn, B., Haeberlein, S. B., . . . Sperling, R. (2018). NIA-AA research framework: Toward a biological definition of Alzheimer's disease. *Alzheimer's & Dementia*, *14*(4), 535–562. doi:10.1016/j.jalz.2018.02.018

Jack, C. R., Jr., Bennett, D. A., Blennow, K., Carrillo, M. C., Feldman, H. H., Frisoni, G. B., . . . Dubois, B. (2016). A/T/N: An unbiased descriptive classification scheme for Alzheimer disease biomarkers. *Neurology*, *87*(5), 539–547. doi:10.1212/wnl.0000000000002923

Jack, C. R., Jr., Knopman, D. S., Jagust, W. J., Petersen, R. C., Weiner, M. W., Aisen, P. S., . . . Trojanowski, J. Q. (2013). Tracking pathophysiological processes in Alzheimer's disease: An updated hypothetical model of dynamic biomarkers. *Lancet Neurology, 12*(2), 207–216. doi:10.1016/S1474-4422(12)70291-0S1474-4422(12)70291-0

Jack, C. R., Jr., Knopman, D. S., Jagust, W. J., Shaw, L. M., Aisen, P. S., Weiner, M. W., . . . Trojanowski, J. Q. (2010). Hypothetical model of dynamic biomarkers of the Alzheimer's pathological cascade. *Lancet Neurology, 9*(1), 119–128.

Jack, C. R., Jr., Petersen, R. C., Xu, Y. C., Waring, S. C., O'Brien, P. C., Tangalos, E. G., . . . Kokmen, E. (1997). Medial temporal atrophy on MRI in normal aging and very mild Alzheimer's disease. *Neurology, 49*(3), 786–794.

Jacobs, H. I. L., Hedden, T., Schultz, A. P., Sepulcre, J., Perea, R. D., Amariglio, R. E., . . . Johnson, K. A. (2018). Structural tract alterations predict downstream tau accumulation in amyloid-positive older individuals. *Nature Neuroscience, 21*(3), 424–431. doi:10.1038/s41593-018-0070-z

Jeon, S. B., Kang, D. W., Cho, A. H., Lee, E. M., Choi, C. G., Kwon, S. U., & Kim, J. S. (2007). Initial microbleeds at MR imaging can predict recurrent intracerebral hemorrhage. *Journal of Neurology, 254*(4), 508–512. doi:10.1007/s00415-006-0406-6

Josephs, K. A., Dickson, D. W., Murray, M. E., Senjem, M. L., Parisi, J. E., Petersen, R. C., . . . Whitwell, J. L. (2013). Quantitative neurofibrillary tangle density and brain volumetric MRI analyses in Alzheimer's disease presenting as logopenic progressive aphasia. *Brain and Language, 127*(2), 127–134. doi:10.1016/j.bandl.2013.02.003

Kalaria, R. N. (2000). The role of cerebral ischemia in Alzheimer's disease. *Neurobiology of Aging, 21*(2), 321–330.

Kalaria, R. N., & Ballard, C. (1999). Overlap between pathology of Alzheimer disease and vascular dementia. *Alzheimer Disease and Associated Disorders, 13*(Suppl 3), S115–S123.

Kapasi, A., DeCarli, C., & Schneider, J. A. (2017). Impact of multiple pathologies on the threshold for clinically overt dementia. *Acta Neuropathologica, 134*(2), 171–186. doi:10.1007/s00401-017-1717-7

Karlawish, J., Jack, C. R., Jr., Rocca, W. A., Snyder, H. M., & Carrillo, M. C. (2017). Alzheimer's disease: The next frontier-Special Report 2017. *Alzheimer's & Dementia, 13*(4), 374–380. doi:10.1016/j.jalz.2017.02.006

Kaur, B., Himali, J. J., Seshadri, S., Beiser, A. S., Au, R., McKee, A. C., . . . DeCarli, C. S. (2014). Association between neuropathology and brain volume in the Framingham Heart Study. *Alzheimer Disease and Associated Disorders, 28*(3), 219–225. doi:10.1097/wad.0000000000000032

Keith, J., Gao, F. Q., Noor, R., Kiss, A., Balasubramaniam, G., Au, K., . . . Black, S. E. (2017). Collagenosis of the deep medullary veins: An underrecognized pathologic correlate of white matter hyperintensities and periventricular infarction? *Journal of Neuropathology and Experimental Neurology, 76*(4), 299–312. doi:10.1093/jnen/nlx009

Kester, M. I., Goos, J. C., Teunissen, C. E., Benedictus, M. R., Bouwman, F. H., Wattjes, M. P., . . . van der Flier, W. M. (2014). Associations between cerebral small-vessel disease and Alzheimer disease pathology as measured by cerebrospinal fluid biomarkers. *JAMA Neurology, 71*(7), 855–862. doi:10.1001/jamaneurol.2014.754

Kidron, D., Black, S. E., Stanchev, P., Buck, B., Szalai, J. P., Parker, J., . . . Bronskill, M. J. (1997). Quantitative MR volumetry in Alzheimer's disease: Topographic markers and the effects of sex and education. *Neurology, 49*(6), 1504–1512.

Kilander, L., Nyman, H., Boberg, M., Hansson, L., & Lithell, H. (1998). Hypertension is related to cognitive impairment: A 20-year follow-up of 999 men. *Hypertension*, *31*(3), 780–786.

Killiany, R. J., Hyman, B. T., Gomez-Isla, T., Moss, M. B., Kikinis, R., Jolesz, F., . . . Albert, M. S. (2002). MRI measures of entorhinal cortex vs hippocampus in preclinical AD. *Neurology*, *58*(8), 1188–1196.

Kivipelto, M., Helkala, E. L., Hanninen, T., Laakso, M. P., Hallikainen, M., Alhainen, K., . . . Nissinen, A. (2001). Midlife vascular risk factors and late-life mild cognitive impairment: A population-based study. *Neurology*, *56*(12), 1683–1689.

Kivipelto, M., Helkala, E. L., Laakso, M. P., Hanninen, T., Hallikainen, M., Alhainen, K., . . . Nissinen, A. (2001). Midlife vascular risk factors and Alzheimer's disease in later life: Longitudinal, population based study. *BMJ*, *322*(7300), 1447–1451.

Knopman, D., Boland, L. L., Mosley, T., Howard, G., Liao, D., Szklo, M., . . . Folsom, A. R. (2001). Cardiovascular risk factors and cognitive decline in middle-aged adults. *Neurology*, *56*(1), 42–48.

Knudsen, K. A., Rosand, J., Karluk, D., & Greenberg, S. M. (2001). Clinical diagnosis of cerebral amyloid angiopathy: Validation of the Boston criteria. *Neurology*, *56*(4), 537–539.

Koike, M. A., Green, K. N., Blurton-Jones, M., & Laferla, F. M. (2010). Oligemic hypoperfusion differentially affects tau and amyloid-β. *American Journal of Pathology*, *177*(1), 300–310. doi:10.2353/ajpath.2010.090750

Koizumi, K., Hattori, Y., Ahn, S. J., Buendia, I., Ciacciarelli, A., Uekawa, K., . . . Iadecola, C. (2018). Apoepsilon4 disrupts neurovascular regulation and undermines white matter integrity and cognitive function. *Nature Communions*, *9*(1), 3816. doi:10.1038/s41467-018-06301-2

Krasuski, J. S., Alexander, G. E., Horwitz, B., Daly, E. M., Murphy, D. G., Rapoport, S. I., & Schapiro, M. B. (1998). Volumes of medial temporal lobe structures in patients with Alzheimer's disease and mild cognitive impairment (and in healthy controls). *Biolology Psychiatry*, *43*(1), 60–68.

Laakso, M. P., Soininen, H., Partanen, K., Lehtovirta, M., Hallikainen, M., Hanninen, T., . . . Riekkinen, P. J., Sr. (1998). MRI of the hippocampus in Alzheimer's disease: Sensitivity, specificity, and analysis of the incorrectly classified subjects. *Neurobiology of Aging*, *19*(1), 23–31.

Lambert, C., Benjamin, P., Zeestraten, E., Lawrence, A. J., Barrick, T. R., & Markus, H. S. (2016). Longitudinal patterns of leukoaraiosis and brain atrophy in symptomatic small vessel disease. *Brain*, 139(Pt 4), 1136–1151. doi:10.1093/brain/aww009

Le Couteur, D. G., Hunter, S., & Brayne, C. (2016). Solanezumab and the amyloid hypothesis for Alzheimer's disease. *BMJ*, *355*, i6771. doi:10.1136/bmj.i6771

Lee, S., Viqar, F., Zimmerman, M. E., Narkhede, A., Tosto, G., Benzinger, T. L., . . . Brickman, A. M. (2016). White matter hyperintensities are a core feature of Alzheimer's disease: Evidence from the dominantly inherited Alzheimer network. *Annals of Neurology*, *79*(6), 929–939. doi:10.1002/ana.24647

Leys, D., Pruvo, J. P., Parent, M., Vermersch, P., Soetaert, G., Steinling, M., . . . Clarisse, J. (1991). Could Wallerian degeneration contribute to "leuko-araiosis" in subjects free of any vascular disorder? *Journal of Neurology, Neurosurgery & Psychiatry*, *54*(1), 46–50.

Luchsinger, J. A., Brickman, A. M., Reitz, C., Cho, S. J., Schupf, N., Manly, J. J., . . . Brown, T. R. (2009). Subclinical cerebrovascular disease in mild cognitive impairment. *Neurology*, *73*(6), 450–456. doi:10.1212/WNL.0b013e3181b1636a73/6/450

Luchsinger, J. A., Patel, B., Tang, M. X., Schupf, N., & Mayeux, R. (2007). Measures of adiposity and dementia risk in elderly persons. *Archives of Neurology, 64*(3), 392–398.

Luchsinger, J. A., Reitz, C., Honig, L. S., Tang, M. X., Shea, S., & Mayeux, R. (2005). Aggregation of vascular risk factors and risk of incident Alzheimer disease. *Neurology, 65*(4), 545–551.

Luchsinger, J. A., Tang, M. X., Shea, S., & Mayeux, R. (2004). Hyperinsulinemia and risk of Alzheimer disease. *Neurology, 63*(7), 1187–1192.

Luchsinger, J. A., Tang, M. X., Stern, Y., Shea, S., & Mayeux, R. (2001). Diabetes mellitus and risk of Alzheimer's disease and dementia with stroke in a multiethnic cohort. *American Journal of Epidemiology, 154*(7), 635–641.

Maass, A., Lockhart, S. N., Harrison, T. M., Bell, R. K., Mellinger, T., Swinnerton, K., . . . Jagust, W. J. (2018). Entorhinal tau pathology, episodic memory decline, and neurodegeneration in aging. *Journal of Neuroscience, 38*(3), 530–543. doi:10.1523/jneurosci.2028-17.2017

Maia, L. F., Vasconcelos, C., Seixas, S., Magalhaes, R., & Correia, M. (2006). Lobar brain hemorrhages and white matter changes: Clinical, radiological and laboratorial profiles. *Cerebrovascular Diseases, 22*(2–3), 155–161.

Marnane, M., Al-Jawadi, O. O., Mortazavi, S., Pogorzelec, K. J., Wang, B. W., Feldman, H. H., & Hsiung, G. Y. (2016). Periventricular hyperintensities are associated with elevated cerebral amyloid. *Neurology, 86*(6), 535–543. doi:10.1212/wnl.0000000000002352

Mascalchi, M., Filippi, M., Floris, R., Fonda, C., Gasparotti, R., & Villari, N. (2005). Diffusion-weighted MR of the brain: Methodology and clinical application. *La Radiologia Medica, 109*(3), 155–197.

Mawuenyega, K. G., Sigurdson, W., Ovod, V., Munsell, L., Kasten, T., Morris, J. C., . . . Bateman, R. J. (2010). Decreased clearance of CNS beta-amyloid in Alzheimer's disease. *Science, 330*(6012), 1774. doi:10.1126/science.1197623

McAleese, K. E., Firbank, M., Dey, M., Colloby, S. J., Walker, L., Johnson, M., . . . Attems, J. (2015). Cortical tau load is associated with white matter hyperintensities. *Acta Neuropathologica Communications, 3*, 60. doi:10.1186/s40478-015-0240-0

McDonald, C. R., McEvoy, L. K., Gharapetian, L., Fennema-Notestine, C., Hagler, D. J., Jr., Holland, D., . . . Dale, A. M. (2009). Regional rates of neocortical atrophy from normal aging to early Alzheimer disease. *Neurology, 73*(6), 457–465. doi:10.1212/WNL.0b013e3181b16431

Medina, D. A., & Gaviria, M. (2008). Diffusion tensor imaging investigations in Alzheimer's disease: the resurgence of white matter compromise in the cortical dysfunction of the aging brain. *Neuropsychiatric Disease and Treatment, 4*(4), 737–742. http://doi.org/10.2147/ndt.s3381

Meier, I. B., Gu, Y., Guzaman, V. A., Wiegman, A. F., Schupf, N., Manly, J. J., . . . Brickman, A. M. (2014). Lobar microbleeds are associated with a decline in executive functioning in older adults. *Cerebrovascular Diseases, 38*(5), 377–383.

Meier, I. B., Manly, J. J., Provenzano, F. A., Louie, K. S., Wasserman, B. T., Griffith, E. Y., . . . Brickman, A. M. (2012). White matter predictors of cognitive functioning in older adults. *Journal of the International Neuropsychological Society, 18*(3), 414–427. doi:10.1017/s1355617712000227

Meier, I. B., Narkhede, A., Provenzano, F. A., Luchsinger, J. A., Manly, J. J., Willey, J. Z., . . . Brickman, A. M. (2012). Lobar microbleeds are associated with white matter hyperintensities and memory in older adults [abstract]. *Journal of the International Neuropsychological Society*, 18(3), 414–427.

Miwa, K., Tanaka, M., Okazaki, S., Yagita, Y., Sakaguchi, M., Mochizuki, H., & Kitagawa, K. (2014). Multiple or mixed cerebral microbleeds and dementia in patients with vascular risk factors. *Neurology, 83*(7), 646–653. doi:10.1212/wnl.0000000000000692

Morris, G. P., Clark, I. A., & Vissel, B. (2018). Questions concerning the role of amyloid-beta in the definition, aetiology and diagnosis of Alzheimer's disease. *Acta Neuropathologica, 136*(5), 663–689. doi:10.1007/s00401-018-1918-8

Murphy, D. G., DeCarli, C. D., Daly, E., Gillette, J. A., McIntosh, A. R., Haxby, J. V., . . . Horwitz, B. (1993). Volumetric magnetic resonance imaging in men with dementia of the Alzheimer type: Correlations with disease severity. *Biological Psychiatry, 34*(9), 612–621.

Naggara, O., Oppenheim, C., Rieu, D., Raoux, N., Rodrigo, S., Dalla Barba, G., & Meder, J. F. (2006). Diffusion tensor imaging in early Alzheimer's disease. *Psychiatry Research, 146*(3), 243–249. doi:10.1016/j.pscychresns.2006.01.005

Neuropathology Group of the Medical Research Council Cognitive Function and Ageing Study. (2001). Pathological correlates of late-onset dementia in a multicentre, community-based population in England and Wales. *Lancet, 357*(9251), 169–175.

Niwa, K., Carlson, G. A., & Iadecola, C. (2000). Exogenous A beta1-40 reproduces cerebrovascular alterations resulting from amyloid precursor protein overexpression in mice. *Journal of Cerebral Blood Flow & Metabolism, 20*(12), 1659–1668.

Ohnishi, T., Matsuda, H., Tabira, T., Asada, T., & Uno, M. (2001). Changes in brain morphology in Alzheimer disease and normal aging: Is Alzheimer disease an exaggerated aging process? *American Journal of Neuroradiology, 22*(9), 1680–1685.

Ojo, J. O., Mouzon, B., Algamal, M., Leary, P., Lynch, C., Abdullah, L., . . . Crawford, F. (2016). Chronic repetitive mild traumatic brain injury results in reduced cerebral blood flow, axonal injury, gliosis, and increased T-tau and tau oligomers. *Journal of Neuropathology & Experimental Neurology*, 75(7), 636–655. doi:10.1093/jnen/nlw035

Pearson, R. C., Esiri, M. M., Hiorns, R. W., Wilcock, G. K., & Powell, T. P. (1985). Anatomical correlates of the distribution of the pathological changes in the neocortex in Alzheimer disease. *Proceedings of the National Academy of Sciences of the United States of America, 82*(13), 4531–4534.

Petrovitch, H., Ross, G. W., Steinhorn, S. C., Abbott, R. D., Markesbery, W., Davis, D., . . . White, L. R. (2005). AD lesions and infarcts in demented and non-demented Japanese-American men. *Annals of Neurology, 57*(1), 98–103.

Pettersen, J. A., Sathiyamoorthy, G., Gao, F. Q., Szilagyi, G., Nadkarni, N. K., St George-Hyslop, P., . . . Black, S. E. (2008). Microbleed topography, leukoaraiosis, and cognition in probable Alzheimer disease from the Sunnybrook dementia study. *Archives of Neurology, 65*(6), 790–795. doi:10.1001/archneur.65.6.79065/6/790

Pini, L., Pievani, M., Bocchetta, M., Altomare, D., Bosco, P., Cavedo, E., . . . Frisoni, G. B. (2016). Brain atrophy in Alzheimer's disease and aging. *Ageing Research Reviews, 30*, 25–48. doi:10.1016/j.arr.2016.01.002

Poels, M. M., Vernooij, M. W., Ikram, M. A., Hofman, A., Krestin, G. P., van der Lugt, A., & Breteler, M. M. (2010). Prevalence and risk factors of cerebral microbleeds: An update of the Rotterdam scan study. *Stroke, 41*(10 Suppl), S103–S106. doi:10.1161/strokeaha.110.595181

Preston, S. D., Steart, P. V., Wilkinson, A., Nicoll, J. A., & Weller, R. O. (2003). Capillary and arterial cerebral amyloid angiopathy in Alzheimer's disease: Defining the perivascular route for the elimination of amyloid beta from the human brain. *Neuropathology and Applied Neurobiology, 29*(2), 106–117.

Price, C. C., Garrett, K. D., Jefferson, A. L., Cosentino, S., Tanner, J. J., Penney, D. L., . . . Libon, D. J. (2009). Leukoaraiosis severity and list-learning in dementia. *Clinical Neuropsychologist, 23*(6), 944–961. http://doi.org/10.1080/13854040802681664

Provenzano, F. A., Muraskin, J., Tosto, G., Narkhede, A., Wasserman, B. T., Griffith, E. Y., . . . Brickman, A. M. (2013). White matter hyperintensities and cerebral amyloidosis: Necessary and sufficient for clinical expression of Alzheimer disease? *JAMA Neurology*, 70(4), 455–461. doi:10.1001/jamaneurol.2013.13211653648

Rathi, Y., Pasternak, O., Savadjiev, P., Michailovich, O., Bouix, S., Kubicki, M., . . . Shenton, M. E. (2014). Gray matter alterations in early aging: A diffusion magnetic resonance imaging study. *Human Brain Mapping, 35*(8), 3841–3856. doi:10.1002/hbm.22441

Raz, L., Bhaskar, K., Weaver, J., Marini, S., Zhang, Q., Thompson, J. F., . . . Rosenberg, G. A. (2018). Hypoxia promotes tau hyperphosphorylation with associated neuropathology in vascular dysfunction. *Neurobiology of Disease, 126*, 124–136. doi:10.1016/j.nbd.2018.07.009

Raz, N., Gunning, F. M., Head, D., Dupuis, J. H., McQuain, J., Briggs, S. D., . . . Acker, J. D. (1997). Selective aging of the human cerebral cortex observed in vivo: Differential vulnerability of the prefrontal gray matter. *Cerebral Cortex, 7*(3), 268–282.

Resnick, S. M., Goldszal, A. F., Davatzikos, C., Golski, S., Kraut, M. A., Metter, E. J., . . . Zonderman, A. B. (2000). One-year age changes in MRI brain volumes in older adults. *Cerebral Cortex, 10*(5), 464–472.

Resnick, S. M., Pham, D. L., Kraut, M. A., Zonderman, A. B., & Davatzikos, C. (2003). Longitudinal magnetic resonance imaging studies of older adults: A shrinking brain. *Journal of Neuroscience, 23*(8), 3295–3301.

Rezek, D. L., Morris, J. C., Fulling, K. H., & Gado, M. H. (1987). Periventricular white matter lucencies in senile dementia of the Alzheimer type and in normal aging. *Neurology, 37*(8), 1365–1368.

Rizvi, B., Narkhede, A., Last, B. S., Budge, M., Tosto, G., Manly, J. J., . . . Brickman, A. M. (2018). The effect of white matter hyperintensities on cognition is mediated by cortical atrophy. *Neurobiology of Aging, 64*, 25–32. doi:10.1016/j.neurobiolaging.2017.12.006

Rogers, J., & Morrison, J. H. (1985). Quantitative morphology and regional and laminar distributions of senile plaques in Alzheimer's disease. *Journal of Neurosciene, 5*(10), 2801–2808.

Roher, A. E., Esh, C., Kokjohn, T. A., Kalback, W., Luehrs, D. C., Seward, J. D., . . . Beach, T. G. (2003). Circle of Willis atherosclerosis is a risk factor for sporadic Alzheimer's disease. *Arteriosclerosis, Thrombosis, and Vascular Biology, 23*(11), 2055–2062. doi:10.1161/01.atv.0000095973.42032.44

Rose, S. E., Chen, F., Chalk, J. B., Zelaya, F. O., Strugnell, W. E., Benson, M., . . . Doddrell, D. M. (2000). Loss of connectivity in Alzheimer's disease: An evaluation of white matter tract integrity with colour coded MR diffusion tensor imaging. *Journal of Neurology, Neurosurgery, and Psychiatry, 69*(4), 528–530.

Rusinek, H., de Leon, M. J., George, A. E., Stylopoulos, L. A., Chandra, R., Smith, G., . . . Kowalski, H. (1991). Alzheimer disease: Measuring loss of cerebral gray matter with MR imaging. *Radiology, 178*(1), 109–114.

Sahathevan, R., Linden, T., Villemagne, V. L., Churilov, L., Ly, J. V., Rowe, C., . . . Brodtmann, A. (2016). Positron emission tomographic imaging in stroke: Cross-sectional and follow-up assessment of amyloid in ischemic stroke. *Stroke, 47*(1), 113–119. doi:10.1161/strokeaha.115.010528

Salat, D. H., Buckner, R. L., Snyder, A. Z., Greve, D. N., Desikan, R. S., Busa, E., . . . Fischl, B. (2004). Thinning of the cerebral cortex in aging. *Cerebral Cortex, 14*(7), 721–730.

Salat, D. H., Kaye, J. A., & Janowsky, J. S. (1999). Prefrontal gray and white matter volumes in healthy aging and Alzheimer disease. *Archives of Neurology, 56*(3), 338–344.

Salloway, S., Sperling, R., Gilman, S., Fox, N. C., Blennow, K., Raskind, M., . . . Grundman, M. (2009). A phase 2 multiple ascending dose trial of bapineuzumab in mild to moderate Alzheimer disease. *Neurology, 73*(24), 2061–2070. doi:10.1212/WNL.0b013e3181c67808

Scheltens, P., Barkhof, F., Valk, J., Algra, P. R., van der Hoop, R. G., Nauta, J., & Wolters, E. C. (1992). White matter lesions on magnetic resonance imaging in clinically diagnosed Alzheimer's disease: Evidence for heterogeneity. *Brain, 115*(Pt 3), 735–748.

Schneider, J. A., Arvanitakis, Z., Bang, W., & Bennett, D. A. (2007). Mixed brain pathologies account for most dementia cases in community-dwelling older persons. *Neurology, 69*(24), 2197–2204. doi:01.wnl.0000271090.28148.24

Schneider, J. A., Arvanitakis, Z., Leurgans, S. E., & Bennett, D. A. (2009). The neuropathology of probable Alzheimer disease and mild cognitive impairment. *Annals of Neurology, 66*(2), 200–208. doi:10.1002/ana.21706

Schneider, J. A., & Bennett, D. A. (2010). Where vascular meets neurodegenerative disease. *Stroke, 41*(10 Suppl), S144–146. doi:10.1161/strokeaha.110.598326

Schupf, N., Tang, M. X., Fukuyama, H., Manly, J., Andrews, H., Mehta, P., . . . Mayeux, R. (2008). Peripheral Aβ subspecies as risk biomarkers of Alzheimer's disease. *Proceedings of the National Academy of Sciences of the United States of America, 105*(37), 14052–14057.

Seab, J. P., Jagust, W. J., Wong, S. T., Roos, M. S., Reed, B. R., & Budinger, T. F. (1988). Quantitative NMR measurements of hippocampal atrophy in Alzheimer's disease. *Magnetic Resonance in Medicine, 8*(2), 200–208.

Sepulcre, J., Schultz, A. P., Sabuncu, M., Gomez-Isla, T., Chhatwal, J., Becker, A., . . . Johnson, K. A. (2016). In vivo tau, amyloid, and gray matter profiles in the aging brain. *Journal of Neuroscience, 36*(28), 7364–7374. doi:10.1523/jneurosci.0639-16.2016

Serrano-Pozo, A., Frosch, M. P., Masliah, E., & Hyman, B. T. (2011). Neuropathological alterations in Alzheimer disease. *Cold Spring Harbor Perspectives in Medicine, 1*(1), a006189.

Shams, S., Granberg, T., Martola, J., Charidimou, A., Li, X., Shams, M., . . . Wahlund, L. O. (2016). Cerebral microbleeds topography and cerebrospinal fluid biomarkers in cognitive impairment. *Journal of Cerebral Blood Flow and Metabolism*. doi:10.1177/0271678x16649401

Shams, S., Granberg, T., Martola, J., Li, X., Shams, M., Fereshtehnejad, S. M., . . . Wahlund, L. O. (2016). Cerebrospinal fluid profiles with increasing number of cerebral microbleeds in a continuum of cognitive impairment. *Journal of Cerebral Blood Flow and Metabolism, 36*(3), 621–628. doi:10.1177/0271678x15606141

Shams, S., Martola, J., Granberg, T., Li, X., Shams, M., Fereshtehnejad, S. M., . . . Wahlund, L. O. (2015). Cerebral microbleeds: Different prevalence, topography, and risk factors depending on dementia diagnosis: The Karolinska Imaging Dementia Study. *American Journal of Neuroradiology, 36*(4), 661–666. doi:10.3174/ajnr.A4176

Small, S. A., Schobel, S. A., Buxton, R. B., Witter, M. P., & Barnes, C. A. (2011). A pathophysiological framework of hippocampal dysfunction in ageing and disease. *Nature Reviews Neuroscience, 12*(10), 585–601.

Sperling, R. A., Aisen, P. S., Beckett, L. A., Bennett, D. A., Craft, S., Fagan, A. M., . . . Phelps, C. H. (2011). Toward defining the preclinical stages of Alzheimer's disease: Recommendations from the National Institute on Aging–Alzheimer's Association workgroups on diagnostic guidelines for Alzheimer's disease. *Alzheimer's & Dementia*, *7*(3), 280–292. doi:10.1016/j.jalz.2011.03.003S1552-5260(11)00099-9

Sperling, R. A., Salloway, S., Brooks, D. J., Tampieri, D., Barakos, J., Fox, N. C., . . . Grundman, M. (2012). Amyloid-related imaging abnormalities in patients with Alzheimer's disease treated with bapineuzumab: A retrospective analysis. *Lancet Neurology*, *11*(3), 241–249. doi:10.1016/s1474-4422(12)70015-7

Sperling, R. A., Jack, C. R., Jr., Black, S. E., Frosch, M. P., Greenberg, S. M., Hyman, B. T., . . . Schindler, R. J. (2011). Amyloid-related imaging abnormalities in amyloid-modifying therapeutic trials: Recommendations from the Alzheimer's Association Research Roundtable Workgroup. *Alzheimer's & Dementia*, *7*(4), 367–385. doi:10.1016/j.jalz.2011.05.2351

Swan, G. E., Carmelli, D., & Larue, A. (1998). Systolic blood pressure tracking over 25 to 30 years and cognitive performance in older adults. *Stroke*, *29*, 2334–2340.

Swan, G. E., DeCarli, C., Miller, B. L., Reed, T., Wolf, P. A., Jack, L. M., & Carmelli, D. (1998). Association of midlife blood pressure to late-life cognitive decline and brain morphology. *Neurology*, *51*(4), 986–993.

Sweeney, M. D., Montagne, A., Sagare, A. P., Nation, D. A., Schneider, L. S., Chui, H. C., . . . Zlokovic, B. V. (2019). Vascular dysfunction: The disregarded partner of Alzheimer's disease. *Alzheimer's & Dementia*, *15*(1), 158–167. doi:10.1016/j.jalz.2018.07.222

Sydykova, D., Stahl, R., Dietrich, O., Ewers, M., Reiser, M. F., Schoenberg, S. O., . . . Teipel, S. J. (2007). Fiber connections between the cerebral cortex and the corpus callosum in Alzheimer's disease: A diffusion tensor imaging and voxel-based morphometry study. *Cerebral Cortex*, *17*(10), 2276–2282. doi:10.1093/cercor/bhl136

Takahashi, S., Yonezawa, H., Takahashi, J., Kudo, M., Inoue, T., & Tohgi, H. (2002). Selective reduction of diffusion anisotropy in white matter of Alzheimer disease brains measured by 3.0 Tesla magnetic resonance imaging. *Neuroscience Letters*, *332*(1), 45–48.

Tanabe, J. L., Amend, D., Schuff, N., DiSclafani, V., Ezekiel, F., Norman, D., . . . Weiner, M. W. (1997). Tissue segmentation of the brain in Alzheimer disease. *American Journal of Neuroradiology*, *18*(1), 115–123.

Thambisetty, M., Wan, J., Carass, A., An, Y., Prince, J. L., & Resnick, S. M. (2010). Longitudinal changes in cortical thickness associated with normal aging. *Neuroimage*, *52*(4), 1215–1223. doi:10.1016/j.neuroimage.2010.04.258

Thanprasertsuk, S., Martinez-Ramirez, S., Pontes-Neto, O. M., Ni, J., Ayres, A., Reed, A., . . . Viswanathan, A. (2014). Posterior white matter disease distribution as a predictor of amyloid angiopathy. *Neurology*, *83*(9), 794–800. doi:10.1212/wnl.0000000000000732

Thomas, T., Thomas, G., McLendon, C., Sutton, T., & Mullan, M. (1996). β-Amyloid-mediated vasoactivity and vascular endothelial damage. *Nature*, *380*(6570), 168–171.

Tisserand, D. J., Pruessner, J. C., Sanz Arigita, E. J., van Boxtel, M. P., Evans, A. C., Jolles, J., & Uylings, H. B. (2002). Regional frontal cortical volumes decrease differentially in aging: An MRI study to compare volumetric approaches and voxel-based morphometry. *Neuroimage*, *17*(2), 657–669.

Toledo, J. B., Arnold, S. E., Raible, K., Brettschneider, J., Xie, S. X., Grossman, M., . . . Trojanowski, J. Q. (2013). Contribution of cerebrovascular disease in autopsy confirmed neurodegenerative disease cases in the National Alzheimer's Coordinating Centre. *Brain, 136*(Pt 9), 2697–2706. doi:10.1093/brain/awt188awt188 [pii]

Tosto, G., Bird, T. D., Bennett, D. A., Boeve, B. F., Brickman, A. M., Cruchaga, C., . . . Mayeux, R.; National Institute on Aging Late-Onset Alzheimer Disease/National Cell Repository for Alzheimer Disease (NIA-LOAD/NCRAD) Family Study Group. (2016). The role of cardiovascular risk factors and stroke in familial Alzheimer disease. *JAMA Neurology, 73*(10), 1231–1237. doi:10.1001/jamaneurol.2016.2539

Tosto, G., Zimmerman, M. E., Carmichael, O. T., & Brickman, A. M. (2014). Predicting aggressive decline in mild cognitive impairment: The importance of white matter hyperintensities. *JAMA Neurology, 71*(7), 872–877. doi:10.1001/jamaneurol.2014.6671867509

Tosto, G., Zimmerman, M. E., Hamilton, J. L., Carmichael, O. T., & Brickman, A. M.; Alzheimer's Disease Neuroimaging Initiative. (2015). The effect of white matter hyperintensities on neurodegeneration in mild cognitive impairment. *Alzheimer's & Dementia, 11*(12), 1510–1519. doi:10.1016/j.jalz.2015.05.014

van Dalen, J. W., Scuric, E. E., van Veluw, S. J., Caan, M. W., Nederveen, A. J., Biessels, G. J., . . . Richard, E. (2015). Cortical microinfarcts detected in vivo on 3 Tesla MRI: Clinical and radiological correlates. *Stroke, 46*(1), 255–257. doi:10.1161/strokeaha.114.007568

van Rooden, S., Goos, J. D., van Opstal, A. M., Versluis, M. J., Webb, A. G., Blauw, G. J., . . . van der Grond, J. (2014). Increased number of microinfarcts in Alzheimer disease at 7-T MR imaging. *Radiology, 270*(1), 205–211. doi:10.1148/radiol.13130743radiol.13130743 [pii]

van Rooden, S., van der Grond, J., van den Boom, R., Haan, J., Linn, J., Greenberg, S. M., & van Buchem, M. A. (2009). Descriptive analysis of the Boston criteria applied to a Dutch-type cerebral amyloid angiopathy population. *Stroke, 40*(9), 3022–3027. doi:10.1161/STROKEAHA.109.554378STROKEAHA.109.554378

van Veluw, S. J., Zwanenburg, J. J., Engelen-Lee, J., Spliet, W. G., Hendrikse, J., Luijten, P. R., & Biessels, G. J. (2013). In vivo detection of cerebral cortical microinfarcts with high-resolution 7T MRI. *Journal of Cerebral Blood Flow and Metabolism, 33*(3), 322–329. doi:10.1038/jcbfm.2012.196

Vermeer, S. E., Prins, N. D., den Heijer, T., Hofman, A., Koudstaal, P. J., & Breteler, M. M. (2003). Silent brain infarcts and the risk of dementia and cognitive decline. *New England Journal of Medicine, 348*(13), 1215–1222.

Wardlaw, J. M., Valdes Hernandez, M. C., & Munoz-Maniega, S. (2015). What are white matter hyperintensities made of? Relevance to vascular cognitive impairment. *Journal of the American Heart Association, 4*(6), 001140. doi:10.1161/jaha.114.001140

Weiler, M., Agosta, F., Canu, E., Copetti, M., Magnani, G., Marcone, A., . . . Falini, A. (2015). Following the spreading of brain structural changes in Alzheimer's disease: A longitudinal, multimodal MRI study. *Journal of Alzheimer's Disease, 47*(4), 995–1007.

Weller, R. O., Cohen, N. R., & Nicoll, J. A. (2004). Cerebrovascular disease and the pathophysiology of Alzheimer's disease. Implications for therapy. *Panminerva Medica, 46*(4), 239–251.

Werring, D. J., Gregoire, S. M., & Cipolotti, L. (2010). Cerebral microbleeds and vascular cognitive impairment. *Journal of the Neurological Sciences, 299*(1–2), 131–135. doi:10.1016/j.jns.2010.08.034

West, R. L. (1996). An application of prefrontal cortex function theory to cognitive aging. *Psychology Bulletin, 120*(2), 272–292.

White, L., Petrovitch, H., Hardman, J., Nelson, J., Davis, D. G., Ross, G. W., . . . Markesbery, W. R. (2002). Cerebrovascular pathology and dementia in autopsied Honolulu-Asia Aging Study participants. *Annals of the New York Academy of Sciences, 977*, 9–23.

Whitwell, J., Dickson, D., Murray, M., Senjem, M., Gunter, J., Spychalla, A., . . . Josephs, K. (2013). Rates of atrophy differ across pathologically defined subtypes of Alzheimer's disease: A longitudinal MRI study. *Alzheimer's & Dementia, 9*(4), P600. doi:10.1016/j.jalz.2013.05.1196

Whitwell, J. L., Przybelski, S. A., Weigand, S. D., Knopman, D. S., Boeve, B. F., Petersen, R. C., & Jack, C. R., Jr. (2007). 3D maps from multiple MRI illustrate changing atrophy patterns as subjects progress from mild cognitive impairment to Alzheimer's disease. *Brain, 130*(Pt 7), 1777–1786. doi:awm112 [pii]10.1093/brain/awm112

Wiegman, A. F., Meier, I. B., Schupf, N., Manly, J. J., Guzman, V. A., Narkhede, A., . . . Brickman, A. M. (2014). Cerebral microbleeds in a multiethnic elderly community: Demographic and clinical correlates. *Journal of Neurological Sciences, 345*, 125–130.

Yassi, N., Desmond, P. M., & Masters, C. L. (2016). Magnetic resonance imaging of vascular contributions to cognitive impairment and dementia. *Journal of Molecular Neuroscience*, 60(3), 349–353. doi:10.1007/s12031-016-0799-3

Yates, P. A., Villemagne, V. L., Ellis, K. A., Desmond, P. M., Masters, C. L., & Rowe, C. C. (2014). Cerebral microbleeds: A review of clinical, genetic, and neuroimaging associations. *Frontiers in Neurology, 4*, 205. doi:10.3389/fneur.2013.00205

Yoshita, M., Fletcher, E., Harvey, D., Ortega, M., Martinez, O., Mungas, D. M., . . . DeCarli, C. S. (2006). Extent and distribution of white matter hyperintensities in normal aging, MCI, and AD. *Neurology, 67*(12), 2192–2198.

Yoshiura, T., Mihara, F., Ogomori, K., Tanaka, A., Kaneko, K., & Masuda, K. (2002). Diffusion tensor in posterior cingulate gyrus: Correlation with cognitive decline in Alzheimer's disease. *Neuroreport, 13*(17), 2299–2302. doi:10.1097/01.wnr.0000044991.13025.e6

Zhang, Y., Schuff, N., Jahng, G. H., Bayne, W., Mori, S., Schad, L., . . . Weiner, M. W. (2007). Diffusion tensor imaging of cingulum fibers in mild cognitive impairment and Alzheimer disease. *Neurology, 68*(1), 13–19. doi:10.1212/01.wnl.0000250326.77323.01

Zhou, J., Yu, J. T., Wang, H. F., Meng, X. F., Tan, C. C., Wang, J., . . . Tan, L. (2015). Association between stroke and Alzheimer's disease: Systematic review and meta-analysis. *Journal of Alzheimer's Disease, 43*(2), 479–489. doi:10.3233/JAD-140666

Zhuang, L., Wen, W., Zhu, W., Trollor, J., Kochan, N., Crawford, J., . . . Sachdev, P. (2010). White matter integrity in mild cognitive impairment: A tract-based spatial statistics study. *Neuroimage, 53*(1), 16–25. doi:10.1016/j.neuroimage.2010.05.068

Zlokovic, B. V. (2005). Neurovascular mechanisms of Alzheimer's neurodegeneration. *Trends in Neuroscience, 28*(4), 202–208. doi:10.1016/j.tins.2005.02.001

Zlokovic, B. V. (2011). Neurovascular pathways to neurodegeneration in Alzheimer's disease and other disorders. *Nature Reviews Neuroscience, 12*(12), 723–738. doi:10.1038/nrn3114

10

Brain Structural Alterations Common to Cardiovascular Disease Risk Factors and Alzheimer's Dementia

Implications for Connectomics and Cognition

Melissa Lamar, Elizabeth A. Boots, Konstantinos Arfanakis, Lisa L. Barnes, and Julie A. Schneider

1. Introduction

Over 3,000 publications exist demonstrating that cardiovascular disease risk factors (CVD-RFs) are associated with alterations of brain structure that increase the risk for developing dementia including Alzheimer's dementia. Yet clinical trials and research criteria for Alzheimer's dementia continue to focus on the central biomarkers of disease (Jack et al., 2018) that, while key to Alzheimer's disease (AD), may not reflect the complete picture of neuropathological alterations that are present in individuals with Alzheimer's dementia at death (i.e., over 230 different combinations of neuropathologies have been reported to date; Boyle et al., 2018). Thus, considering the potential overlap of brain structural alterations associated with CVD-RFs *and* Alzheimer's dementia in vivo and the role that such overlap may play in brain–behavior relationships may offer potential (and modifiable) targets for more encompassing interventions. In this chapter, we will present evidence of the overlap between gray matter and subcortical structural alterations associated with CVD-RFs and gray matter and subcortical structural alterations associated with Alzheimer's dementia. We will argue that white matter integrity, also vulnerable to CVD-RFs and Alzheimer's dementia, needs to be integrated with gray matter and subcortical structural alterations for a more holistic approach to understanding brain aging and dementia. Examples from the literature directly focused on the interplay of regional vulnerabilities associated with CVD-RFs and Alzheimer's dementia using tract-based structural connectomics in nondemented older adults will be reviewed and used as a call for future studies continuing in this vein. Only with a more integrated approach to brain aging that (a) considers commonalities in brain structural alterations

Melissa Lamar, Elizabeth A. Boots, Konstantinos Arfanakis, Lisa L. Barnes, and Julie A. Schneider, *Brain Structural Alterations Common to Cardiovascular Disease Risk Factors and Alzheimer's Dementia* In: *Vascular Disease, Alzheimer's Disease, and Mild Cognitive Impairment.* Edited by: David J. Libon, Melissa Lamar, Rodney A. Swenson, Kenneth M. Heilman, Oxford University Press (2020). © Oxford University Press.
DOI: 10.1093/oso/9780190634230.003.0011

between CVD-RFs and Alzheimer's dementia, (b) uses advances in neuroimaging analytics to detect more subtle metrics of disease in vivo, and (c) translates these findings to real-world cognitive outcomes will we be able to move beyond increasingly isolated and unsuccessful clinical trials to slow and ultimately stop risk for and development of dementia.

2. Neuroimaging of Gray Matter and Subcortical Structures

2.1. Cardiovascular Disease Risk

Mid-life CVD-RFs including hypertension and diabetes have been linked to late-life alterations in whole brain as well as regional gray matter and subcortical structures, with less albeit still robust evidence suggesting late-life CVD-RFs are also associated with late-life structural alterations. For example, hypertension has been associated with cross-sectional differences and increased rates of change in whole brain atrophy in older adults (Firbank et al., 2007; Wiseman et al., 2004) as well as specific hippocampal vulnerability (Firbank et al., 2007; Wiseman et al., 2004). In a qualitative review of 29 studies conducted in mid- to late-life adults (i.e., 45–80 years of age), hypertension as well as higher blood pressure in individuals without hypertension were associated with reductions in frontal, parietal, and temporal lobe volumes as well as the hippocampus (Beauchet et al., 2013). More recently, an analysis of 9,722 mid- to late-life participants in the U.K. Biobank revealed that hypertension was linked to alterations in global brain outcomes as well as regionally specific alterations within the frontal and temporal lobes and subcortical structures including the pallidum, accumbens, thalamus, putamen, hippocampus, and amygdala (Cox et al., 2019).

Many of these same results have been reported for in mid- and late-life adults with Type 2 diabetes. Type 2 diabetes mellitus (DM) has been associated with decreased whole brain, particularly gray matter volumes in a recent systematic review (Wu, Lin, Zhang, & Wu, 2017). Additionally, work detailing cerebral localization of DM associates has reported reductions within frontal and temporal regions in the presence of mid- (e.g., Bruehl et al., 2009) and late-life DM (e.g., Kumar et al., 2008). There are also multiple reports of associations between mid- and/or late-life DM and structural reductions in the limbic system including the hippocampus (Roberts et al., 2014; Zhang et al., 2015), the amygdala, and subcortical structures including the putamen (Cox et al., 2019; Cui et al., 2019), caudate, thalamus, and nucleus accumbens (Chen et al., 2017; Cox et al., 2019). While the separate contributions of DM and hypertension are significant and the focus of much research, investigations of CVD-RFs also take the form of overall burden scores that include additional CVD-RFS.

Several comprehensive empirical studies examining composite CVD-RF burden scores that incorporate multiple risk factors such as hypertension, DM, smoking, hypercholesterolemia, and obesity report relationships between increased CVD-RF burden and decreased regional gray matter and subcortical structures. For example, increased CVD-RF burden was associated with decreased frontal and more posterior regional brain volumes as well as the hippocampus across participants ranging in age between 43 and 89 (Debette et al., 2011; Gonzales et al., 2017; Lamar et al., 2015; Leritz et al., 2011). A 2014 review further confirmed that in individuals without a history of overt cardiovascular disease, the presence of CVD-RFs was associated with these same structural brain changes (Friedman et al., 2014). Lastly, cumulative CVD-RF burden has also been shown to be associated with a reduction of subcortical volumes in the hippocampus, and several subcortical structures including the nucleus accumbens, caudate, putamen, pallidum, and thalamus (Cox et al., 2019). Thus, CVD-RFs combined or in isolation have been associated with reductions in the same brain regions (Table 10.1); brain regions often implicated in risk for and development of Alzheimer's dementia as outlined in the following discussion.

2.2. Alzheimer's Dementia Risk and Development

Initial studies as well as more recent work investigating risk for developing Alzheimer's dementia point to the importance of key brain regions to cognitive decline and incident dementia (Table 10.2). For example, countless studies report that volume loss in the hippocampus is either associated with or predictive of risk for and development of Alzheimer's dementia (Apostolova et al., 2010; den Heijer et al., 2010; Fox et al., 1996). Furthermore, longitudinal staging of brain structural alterations suggest that early in the development of the disease, there is atrophy of the hippocampus and then atrophy of the amygdala (Eskildsen et al., 2013). In fact, loss of hippocampal and amygdala volumes, along with volume loss within the posterior cingulate gyrus and the inferior parietal and superior frontal lobes, show better prognostic accuracy for conversion from an at-risk state to Alzheimer's dementia than clinical ratings scores used in the Alzheimer's Disease Neuroimaging Initiative (ADNI; Aksu, Miller, Kesidis, Bigler, & Yang, 2011). These results are consistent with the cortical signature of Alzheimer's dementia put forth by Dickerson and colleagues (2009). These investigators reported a structural phenotype of Alzheimer's dementia, including alterations in the medial and inferior temporal lobes, the posterior cingulate/precuneus, the superior parietal, and superior and inferior frontal cortices. This structural phenotype not only correlates with disease severity antemortem (Dickerson et al., 2009) but also mirrors the topography of neuropathology found postmortem.

Table 10.1 Gray Matter and Subcortical Regions Associated With Cardiovascular Disease Risk Factors Based on a Sampling of Papers When Referencing This Subject Matter

Literature	*Regions of Interest*
Beauchet, O., Celle, S., Roche, F., Bartha, R., Montero-Odasso, M., Allali, G., & Annweiler, C. (2013). Blood pressure levels and brain volume reduction: A systematic review and meta-analysis. *Journal of Hypertension, 31*(8), 1502–1516.	• Superior frontal gyrus • Middle frontal gyrus • Orbitofrontal cortex • Anterior cingulate • Precentral gyrus • Supplementary motor areas • Middle temporal gyrus • Inferior temporal gyrus • Supramarginal gyrus • Cuneus • Hippocampus • Entorhinal cortex • Amygdala • Thalamus
Gianaros, P. J., Greer, P. J., Ryan, C. M., & Jennings, J. R. (2006). Higher blood pressure predicts lower regional gray matter volume: Consequences on short-term information processing. *NeuroImage*, 31(2), 754–765.	• Superior frontal gyrus • Anterior cingulate cortex • Supplementary motor areas • Middle temporal gyrus
Glodzik, L., Mosconi, L., Tsui, W., de Santi, S., Zinkowski, R., Pirraglia, E., . . . Ali, F. (2012). Alzheimer's disease markers, hypertension, and gray matter damage in normal elderly. *Neurobiology of Aging, 33*(7), 1215–1227.	• Superior frontal gyrus • Inferior frontal gyrus • Lingual gyrus • Cerebellum
Moran, C., Phan, T. G., Chen, J., Blizzard, L., Beare, R., Venn, A., . . . Pearson, S. (2013). Brain Atrophy in Type 2 Diabetes. *Diabetes Care, 36*(12), 4036–4042.	• Middle frontal gyrus • Inferior frontal gyrus • Medial frontal gyrus • Precentral gyrus • Anterior cingulate • Middle temporal gyrus • Inferior temporal gyrus • Transverse temporal gyrus • Insula • Precuneus • Hippocampus • Parahippocampal gyrus • Caudate • Putamen
Moulton, C. D., Costafreda, S. G., Horton, P., Ismail, K., & Fu, C. H. (2015). Meta-analyses of structural regional cerebral effects in type 1 and type 2 diabetes. *Brain Imaging and Behavior, 9*(4), 651–662.	• Orbitofrontal cortex • Hippocampus • Basal ganglia

Table 10.1 *Continued*

Literature	*Regions of Interest*
Raji, C. A., Ho, A. J., Parikshak, N. N., Becker, J. T., Lopez, O. L., Kuller, L. H., . . . Thompson, P. M. (2010). Brain structure and obesity. *Human Brain Mapping, 31*(3), 353–364.	• Orbitofrontal cortex • Anterior cingulate • Medial temporal lobe • Hippocampus • Thalamus • Basal ganglia
Zhang, Y., Zhang, X., Zhang, J., Liu, C., Yuan, Q., Yin, X., . . . Wang, J. (2014). Gray matter volume abnormalities in type 2 diabetes mellitus with and without mild cognitive impairment. *Neuroscience Letters, 562*, 1–6.	• Superior frontal gyrus • Medial frontal gyrus • Anterior cingulate • Superior temporal gyrus • Middle temporal gyrus • Fusiform gyrus • Posterior cingulate • Middle occipital gyrus • Precuneus

Note: Given the expansive research conducted to date on this topic, we provide reviews and/or meta-analyses where possible or cite examples as opposed to an exhaustive list of citations.

Table 10.2 Gray Matter and Subcortical Regions Associated with Alzheimer's Dementia Based on a Sampling of Papers When Referencing This Subject Matter

Literature	*Regions of Interest*
Dickerson, B. C., Bakkour, A., Salat, D. H., Feczko, E., Pacheco, J., Greve, D. N., . . . Sperling, R. A. (2008). The cortical signature of Alzheimer's disease: Regionally specific cortical thinning relates to symptom severity in very mild to mild AD dementia and is detectable in asymptomatic amyloid-positive individuals. *Cerebral Cortex, 19*(3), 497–510.	• Superior frontal gyrus • Inferior frontal gyrus • Supramarginal Gyrus • Medial temporal cortex • Inferior temporal gyrus • Temporal pole • Angular gyrus • Superior parietal lobule • Precuneus
Kiuchi, K., Kitamura, S., Taoka, T., Yasuno, F., Tanimura, M., Matsuoka, K., . . . Kosaka, J. (2014). Gray and white matter changes in subjective cognitive impairment, amnestic mild cognitive impairment and Alzheimer's disease: A voxel-based analysis study. *PloS One, 9*(8), e104007.	• Superior frontal gyrus • Middle frontal gyrus • Interior frontal gyrus • Anterior cingulate • Supramarginal gyrus • Precentral gyrus • Postcentral gyrus • Superior temporal gyrus • Middle temporal gyrus • Transverse temporal gyrus • Inferior temporal gyrus

(*continued*)

Table 10.2 *Continued*

Literature	*Regions of Interest*
	• Insula • Posterior cingulate • Middle occipital gyrus • Precuneus • Parahippocampal gyrus
Möller, C., Vrenken, H., Jiskoot, L., Versteeg, A., Barkhof, F., Scheltens, P., & van der Flier, W. M. (2013). Different patterns of gray matter atrophy in early-and late-onset Alzheimer's disease. *Neurobiology of Aging, 34*(8), 2014–2022.	• Inferior frontal cortex • Anterior cingulate • Superior temporal gyrus • Middle temporal gyrus • Inferior parietal lobule • Posterior cingulate • Angular gyrus • Precuneus • Hippocampus • Parahippocampal gyrus
Pini, L., Pievani, M., Bocchetta, M., Altomare, D., Bosco, P., Cavedo, E., . . . Frisoni, G. B. (2016). Brain atrophy in Alzheimer's disease and aging. *Ageing Research Reviews, 30*, 25–48.	• Superior frontal gyrus • Middle frontal gyrus • Orbitofrontal cortex • Medial and lateral temporal lobes • Posterior cingulate • Hippocampus • Entorhinal cortex • Amygdala • Thalamus • Caudate nucleus • Putamen • Nucleus accumbens • Globus pallidus • Basal forebrain
Wang, W. Y., Yu, J. T., Liu, Y., Yin, R. H., Wang, H. F., Wang, J., . . . Tan, L. (2015). Voxel-based meta-analysis of gray matter changes in Alzheimer's disease. *Translational Neurodegeneration, 4*(1), 6.	• Superior frontal gyrus • Posterior cingulate gyrus • Fusiform gyrus • Parahippocampal gyrus
Whitwell, J. L., Tosakulwong, N., Weigand, S. D., Senjem, M. L., Lowe, V. J., Gunter, J. L., . . . Jack, C. R. (2013). Does amyloid deposition produce a specific atrophic signature in cognitively normal subjects?. *NeuroImage: Clinical, 2*, 249–257.	• Middle temporal gyrus • Inferior temporal gyrus • Inferior parietal lobe • Hippocampus • Entorhinal cortex

Note: Given the expansive research conducted to date on this topic, we provide reviews and/or meta-analyses where possible or cite examples as opposed to an exhaustive list of citations.

Despite the anatomic similarities, relatively less work has been done comparing the neuroimaging phenotype of Alzheimer's dementia with the neuroimaging phenotype of CVD-RFs in older adults.

2.3. Commonalities Across CVD-RFs and Alzheimer's Dementia

By reviewing the previously cited work and other sources outlined in Tables 10.1 and 10.2 (e.g., (Cardenas et al., 2012; Glodzik et al., 2012; Moulton, Costafreda, Horton, Ismail, & Fu, 2015; Pini et al., 2016), we noted several gray matter and cortical and subcortical structures that are consistently associated with both CVD-RFs and Alzheimer's dementia (Figure 10.1). In addition to the previously mentioned anatomic similarity, there are a total of 23 brain areas that are

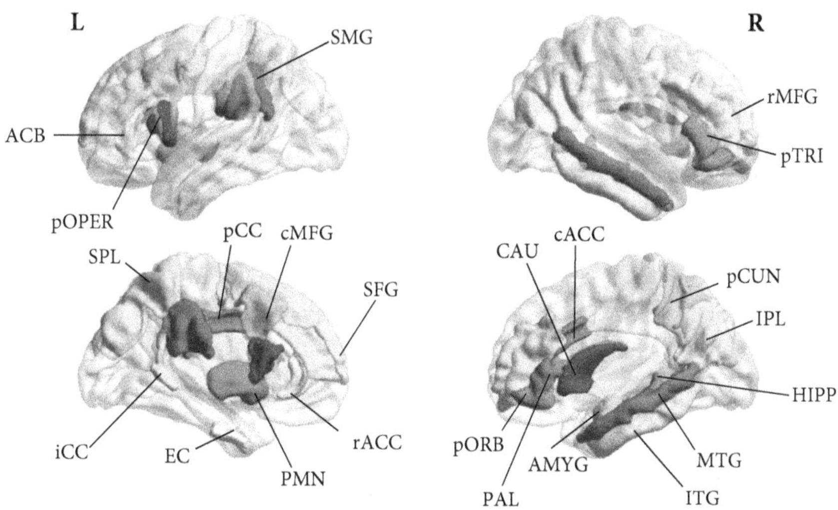

Figure 10.1. Grey matter and subcortical regions associated with both cardiovascular disease risk factor burden and Alzheimer's dementia.

Notes: Colors do not delineate specific brain regions as some colors are used more than once to highlight regions of interest. cACC = caudal anterior cingulate; rACC = rostral anterior cingulate; iCC = isthmus cingulate; pCC = posterior cingulate; CAU = caudate; cMFG = caudal middle frontal gyrus; rMFG = rostral middle frontal gyrus; pORB = pars orbitalis; pOPER = pars opercularis; pTRI = pars triangularis; SMG = supramarginal gyrus; EC = entorhinal cortex; HIPP = hippocampus; AMYG = amygdala; ACB = accumbens; IPL = inferior parietal cortex; ITG = inferior temporal gyrus; MTG = middle temporal gyrus; PAL = pallidum; PMN = putamen; SFG = superior frontal gyrus; SPL = superior parietal cortex; pCUN = precuneus.

commonly congruently associated with CVD-RF and Alzheimer's dementia; these areas include the superior frontal gyrus; inferior frontal gyrus (pars opercularis, pars triangularis, pars orbitalis); rostral and caudal middle frontal gyrus; caudal and rostral anterior, posterior, and isthmus cingulate cortex; entorhinal cortex; supramarginal gyrus; middle and inferior temporal gyrus; hippocampus; amygdala; superior and inferior parietal cortex; the basal ganglia (caudate, putamen, pallidum, and accumbens); and precuneus. Although other regions showed overlap, the congruence of these areas was not as high and consistent as these 23 regions.

To confirm the congruence of injury to these regions as it relates to CVD-RFs and Alzheimer's dementia in vivo, we investigated the association between our identified regions of interest with autopsy-confirmed cerebrovascular-related neuropathologies including microinfarcts and small vessel disease that have been related to CVD-RFs including hypertension (L. Y. Wang et al., 2009) and diabetes (Abner et al., 2016) and AD-related neuropathologies of senile plaques and neurofibrillary tangles. We leveraged existing neuropathologic data from a sample of 41 decedents (~70 years of age at death) who had received an in vivo 3T magnetic resonance imaging (MRI) as part of their participation in the Rush Alzheimer's Disease Center Memory and Aging Project (MAP; Bennett et al., 2012, 2018) and were nondemented at the time of their scan. Results of these analyses revealed inverse associations between bilateral inferior parietal gray matter volumes and severity of atherosclerosis (beta =-13.3, SE = 7.0, p = 0.05) as well as total amyloid burden (beta = −4.8, SE = 1.9, p = 0.01) after adjusting for age at death, sex, education, and total white matter hyperintensity burden at the time of in vivo MRI. While these data are preliminary, they do provide an example of possible relationships between key gray matter regions, outside of the hippocampus (Neltner et al., 2014) associated with CVD-RFs and Alzheimer's dementia.

3. Neuroimaging of White Matter: Implications for CVD-RFs and Alzheimer's Dementia

Although alterations of white matter are not the focus of this chapter, we recognize the importance of these pathological changes as they relate both to CVD-RFs and Alzheimer's dementia. Briefly, CVD-RFs have long been associated with white matter alterations, and there is increasing evidence suggesting that white matter alterations may manifest earlier than originally thought (i.e., in 30–40 year old adults with elevated blood pressure; Weinstein et al., 2015) or blood glucose (Maillard et al., 2012). Hypertension and DM are associated with increased white matter hyperintensities (Debette et al., 2011; Iadecola et al.,

2016; Meusel et al., 2014) also called leukoaraiosis (Hachinski, Potter, & Merskey, 1986). In addition, diffusion-tensor imaging (DTI) measures of fractional anisotropy (FA) also reveals a loss of white matter integrity associated with these same CVD-RFs (Gonzales et al., 2017; Hoogenboom et al., 2014; Jacobs et al., 2013). In a large study of older adults, severe hypertension, current smoking, and DM were all associated with worse white matter tract integrity within both association and commissural fibers (de Groot et al., 2015). Further, research done in a cross-sectional study of late-middle-aged men found that individuals reporting a longer duration of hypertension showed lower DTI-derived measures of white matter integrity within several long association fibers connecting anterior to posterior regions of brain including the inferior and superior longitudinal fasciculi (McEvoy et al., 2015). Similar findings have been noted in more diverse samples both cross-sectionally (Gonzales et al., 2017; Kennedy & Raz, 2009) and longitudinally (R. Wang et al., 2015). Findings relating CVD-RFs to alterations in white matter integrity, once thought to influence vascular forms of dementia only, have increasingly been seen as a key contributor to risk for and development of Alzheimer's dementia, regardless of etiology.

Over the past two decades, a literature has emerged citing the importance of white matter alterations to risk for and development of Alzheimer's dementia (Delano-Wood et al., 2009; Libon et al., 2008; Price et al., 2012). In fact, the companion chapter by Brickman and colleagues (see Chapter 9 of this volume) presents a compelling argument for the role of white matter hyperintensities as an important cause of many of the signs and symptoms associated with Alzheimer's dementia. Given the in-depth nature of that chapter, we will not repeat that information here. Suffice it to say, the alterations of white matter that are observed in both CVD-RFs and Alzheimer's dementia, when combined with congruent alterations in the cortical and subcortical gray matter as previously discussed, suggest the need for a more integrated approach to neuroimaging that includes multimodal capture and analytic integration of these distinct areas of brain tissue. Although historically speaking, much of the work to date on brain aging, CVD-RFs and Alzheimer's dementia has focused on a single neuroimaging modality approach, recent advances in the inclusion of white matter morphometrics into studies of more subtle neuroimaging biomarkers as well as more integrated tract-based structural connectivity approaches are beginning to alter the landscape of brain aging research.

This increase in interest in white matter hyperintensities is due, in part, to the role of these white matter changes in producing injury to white matter tracks thereby causing disconnections. Figure 10.2 outlines results of tract-based spatial statistics in 467 nondemented older adults (~80 years old; average Mini-Mental State Examination score ~28) that assessed the relationship of white matter hyperintensity burden measured via total volume with DTI-derived FA

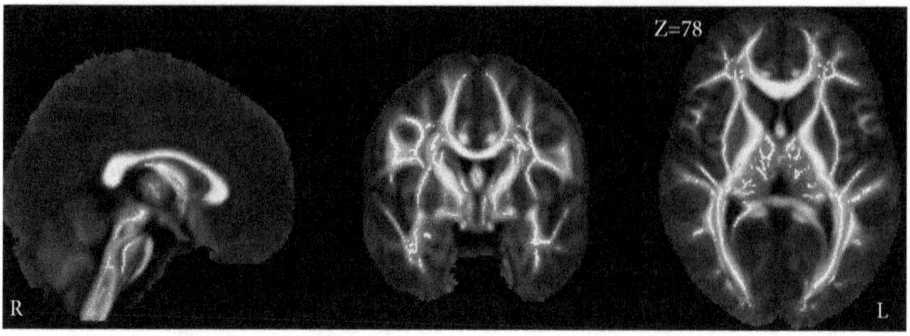

Figure 10.2. Results of tract-based spatial statistics investigating the association of white matter hyperintensity burden—more specifically, total volume in warm colors with diffusion tensor imaging–derived fractional anisotropy (mean skeletonized white matter tracts in green) using linear regression models adjusted for age, sex, race, education, intracranial volume, and white matter hyperintensity burden measured voxelwise ($p \leq 0.01$ familwise error correction corrected).

adjusting for age, sex, race, education, intracranial volume, and white matter hyperintensity measured voxelwise. Results suggest that the total volume of white matter hyperintensity burden was inversely associated with FA ($p \leq 0.01$ familywise error-corrected for multiple comparisons). Thus, higher white matter hyperintensity volumes (Figure 10.2) were associated with lower FA within the majority of white matter tracts of the brain. This suggests that overall white matter hyperintensity burden (as represented by white matter hyperintensity volume) is detrimental to overall brain health regardless of whether any given voxel contains or does not contain white matter damage. This, in conjunction with results from other investigators (de Groot et al., 2015; Langen et al., 2017, 2018; Seiler et al., 2018) signals the importance of including white matter hyperintensity burden as a consideration in applying advances in multimodal integration to evaluate white matter tractography and brain network connectivity in older adults.

4. Multimodal Neuroimaging Integration of Connectomics and Cognition

While we have cited examples of commonalities in brain structural alterations between CVD-RF exposure and Alzheimer's dementia, we still do not understand how the common cortical gray matter, subcortical structures, and white matter alterations come together to impact patterns of connectivity *between* cortical gray matter, subcortical structures, and white matter morphometry.

Gaining a better understanding of the connectivity between gray matter, subcortical structures, and white matter regions commonly affected by CVD-RF and Alzheimer's dementia through a more integrated approach would allow for the identification of a more holistic brain structural phenotype associated with alterations in cognition that are more subtle and may be detected earlier than the currently used signs and symptoms that, to date, have proven too late in the process of pathological aging for disease modification.

Advances in image analytics, through the application of graph theory, have made possible the ability to examine the structural connectivity of gray matter, subcortical structures, and white matter as it relates to indices of interest (Rubinov & Sporns, 2010). These advanced neuroimaging methods allow analysis of brain structure in a more integrated form, including but not limited to, system properties of how the brain exchanges information (efficiency), how strong connections are between brain regions (strength), how important regions are to effective network communication (hubness), and how groups of brain regions preferentially interact to form communities (modularity). Information on these metrics of brain network integrity will fill gaps in the literature related to the interplay of cortical gray matter, subcortical structures, and white matter brain structures common to CVD-RF exposure and risk for and development of Alzheimer's dementia in older adults.

Whole brain studies of tract-based structural connectomics (i.e., studies that use cortical gray matter and subcortical volumetrics to determine white matter tract-based streamlines connecting these brain regions) exist and span normal aging and risk for and development of Alzheimer's dementia; however, less work has used this technique in investigations of CVD-RF burden. Within the normal aging literature, tract-based structural connectomics have been used to predict brain age (Lin et al., 2016), investigate regional importance for brain network efficiency as well as age-related reductions in network strength between frontal and temporal regions (e.g., Zhao et al., 2015). Other studies have used this analytic approach to outline key network hubs (i.e., regions critically important for efficient network communication) and the changes associated with normal aging (Betzel et al., 2014; Perry et al., 2015; Sun et al., 2015). Many of these regions including temporal and prefrontal, precentral, and precuneus, and superior and inferior parietal gray matter regions, as well as limbic and basal ganglia structures, including the anterior cingulate, striatum, and insula, have also been identified in distinct modularity structures (Perry et al., 2015). These same gray matter and subcortical structures have been consistently identified in tract-based structural connectomics as applied to risk for and development of Alzheimer's dementia suggesting alterations in network efficiency and strength as well as hub modularity exist across normal aging, mild cognitive impairment, and Alzheimer's dementia (Daianu et al., 2013, 2015; Jacquemont et al., 2017; Mallio et al., 2015; Nir et al., 2015; Yan et al., 2018). While several tract-based structural connectome studies of individuals with cerebral small vessel disease have been reported in the literature (e.g., Lawrence, Tozer, Stamatakis, & Markus, 2018; Tuladhar et al., 2017), less work has focused on antecedents to cerebrovascular disease including CVD-RFs or the relationship between a common CVD-RF/Alzheimer's dementia structural phenotype and cognition.

We recently investigated tract-based structural connectomics of the 23 identified regions of interests common to both CVD-RFs and Alzheimer's dementia in a community-based cohort of 94 nondemented older adults (~68 years of age, ~29 on the Mini-Mental State Examination). Our investigation (Boots et al., 2019) revealed that CVD-RFs differentially impact the efficiency and nodal strength of the tract-based structural connectome within AD-associated regions in fully adjusted models that included a term for white matter hyperintensity burden (i.e., total volume). More specifically, higher CVD-RF burden was associated with lower efficiency within the left hippocampus and right pars opercularis, and higher efficiency in the right supramarginal gyrus as well as lower nodal strength in bilateral rostral middle frontal gyri, bilateral hippocampi, the thalamus bilaterally, right pars triangularis, and left amygdala (Boots et al., 2019). Furthermore, the tract-based structural connectome metric of nodal strength for left and right hippocampi mediated the association between CVD-RF burden and cognition, specifically attention and information processing, while this same metric for the left middle frontal gyrus mediated the association between CVD-RF burden and attention and information processing, as well as executive function (Boots et al., 2019). This work highlights the usefulness of tract-based structural connectomics to provide insight into the associations between CVD-RFs and brain–behavior relationships when focused on gray matter and subcortical structural vulnerabilities common to CVD-RFs and Alzheimer's dementia.

5. Conclusion

This chapter presents compelling evidence of the overlap between gray matter and subcortical structural alterations reportedly associated with CVD-RFs as well as Alzheimer's dementia. It further advocates that white matter integrity, also vulnerable to CVD-RFs and Alzheimer's dementia, needs to be integrated with gray matter and subcortical structural alterations for a more holistic approach to understanding brain aging and dementia. In the first instance, white matter hyperintensity burden should be included as a covariate in analyses of more subtle alterations in white matter integrity (e.g., DTI-derived FA and tract-based spatial statistics). When considering multimodal neuroimaging integration, advances in brain network connectomics, particularly tract-based structural connectomics, is increasingly being used to understand the interplay between gray, subcortical, and white matter structural integrity across the spectrum of normal aging to dementia. Furthermore, examples now exist in the literature directly focused on the interplay of regional vulnerabilities associated with CVD-RFs and Alzheimer's dementia using tract-based structural connectomics in nondemented older adults; however, more work is needed. Only with a more integrated approach will we be able to move beyond increasingly isolated and unsuccessful clinical trials to slow and ultimately stop risk for and development of Alzheimer's dementia.

Acknowledgements and Funding Sources

The authors would like to thank the participants of the Rush Alzheimer's Disease Center (RADC) cohort studies. RADC research presented in this chapter was supported by the National Institute on Aging (P30 AG010161; R01 AG056405; R01 AG052200) and the National Institute of Neurological Disorders and Stroke (UH3 NS100599).

References

Abner, E. L., Nelson, P. T., Kryscio, R. J., Schmitt, F. A., Fardo, D. W., Woltjer, R. L., . . .0 Arvanitakis, Z. (2016). Diabetes is associated with cerebrovascular but not Alzheimer's disease neuropathology. *Alzheimers & Dementia*, *12*(8), 882–889. doi:10.1016/j.jalz.2015.12.006

Aksu, Y., Miller, D. J., Kesidis, G., Bigler, D. C., & Yang, Q. X. (2011). An MRI-derived definition of MCI-to-AD conversion for long-term, automatic prognosis of MCI patients. *PLoS One*, *6*(10), e25074. doi:10.1371/journal.pone.0025074

Apostolova, L. G., Mosconi, L., Thompson, P. M., Green, A. E., Hwang, K. S., Ramirez, A., . . . de Leon, M. J. (2010). Subregional hippocampal atrophy predicts Alzheimer's dementia in the cognitively normal. *Neurobiology of Aging*, *31*(7), 1077–1088. doi:10.1016/j.neurobiolaging.2008.08.008

Beauchet, O., Celle, S., Roche, F., Bartha, R., Montero-Odasso, M., Allali, G., & Annweiler, C. (2013). Blood pressure levels and brain volume reduction: A systematic review and meta-analysis. *Journal of Hypertension*, *31*(8), 1502–1516. doi:10.1097/HJH.0b013e32836184b5

Bennett, D. A., Buchman, A. S., Boyle, P. A., Barnes, L. L., Wilson, R. S., & Schneider, J. A. (2018). Religious Orders Study and Rush Memory and Aging Project. *Journal of Alzheimer's Disease*, *64*(Suppl 1), S161–S189. doi:10.3233/JAD-179939

Bennett, D. A., Schneider, J. A., Buchman, A. S., Barnes, L. L., Boyle, P. A., & Wilson, R. S. (2012). Overview and findings from the Rush Memory and Aging Project. *Current Alzheimer's Research*, *9*(6), 646–663.

Betzel, R. F., Byrge, L., He, Y., Goni, J., Zuo, X. N., & Sporns, O. (2014). Changes in structural and functional connectivity among resting-state networks across the human lifespan. *NeuroImage, 102*(Pt 2), 345–357. doi:10.1016/j.neuroimage.2014.07.067

Boots, E. A., Zhan, L., Dion, C., Karstens, A. J., Peven, J. C., Ajilore, O., & Lamar, M. (2019). Cardiovascular disease risk factors, tract-based structural connectomics, and cognition in older adults. *NeuroImage, 96*, 152–160. doi:10.1016/j.neuroimage.2019.04.024

Boyle, P. A., Yu, L., Wilson, R. S., Leurgans, S. E., Schneider, J. A., & Bennett, D. A. (2018). Person-specific contribution of neuropathologies to cognitive loss in old age. *Annals of Neurology, 83*(1), 74–83. doi:10.1002/ana.25123

Bruehl, H., Wolf, O. T., Sweat, V., Tirsi, A., Richardson, S., & Convit, A. (2009). Modifiers of cognitive function and brain structure in middle-aged and elderly individuals with type 2 diabetes mellitus. *Brain Research, 1280*, 186–194. doi:10.1016/j.brainres.2009.05.032

Cardenas, V. A., Reed, B., Chao, L. L., Chui, H., Sanossian, N., DeCarli, C. C., . . . Weiner, M. W. (2012). Associations among vascular risk factors, carotid atherosclerosis, and cortical volume and thickness in older adults. *Stroke, 43*(11), 2865–2870. doi:10.1161/STROKEAHA.112.659722

Chen, J., Zhang, J., Liu, X., Wang, X., Xu, X., Li, H., . . . Chen, Z. (2017). Abnormal subcortical nuclei shapes in patients with type 2 diabetes mellitus. *European Radiology, 27*(10), 4247–4256. doi:10.1007/s00330-017-4790-3

Cox, S. R., Lyall, D. M., Ritchie, S. J., Bastin, M. E., Harris, M. A., Buchanan, C. R., . . . Deary, I. J. (2019). Associations between vascular risk factors and brain MRI indices in UK Biobank. *European Heart Journal, 40*(28), 2290–2300. doi:10.1093/eurheartj/ehz100

Cui, D., Liu, X., Liu, M., Cao, W., Xue, Y., Guo, Y., . . . Jiao, Q. (2019). Subcortical gray matter structural alterations in prediabetes and type 2 diabetes. *Neuroreport, 30*(6), 441–445. doi:10.1097/WNR.0000000000001224

Daianu, M., Jahanshad, N., Nir, T. M., Jack, C. R., Jr., Weiner, M. W., Bernstein, M. A., & Thompson, P. M.; Alzheimer's Disease Neuroimaging Initiative. (2015). Rich club analysis in the Alzheimer's disease connectome reveals a relatively undisturbed structural core network. *Human Brain Mapping, 36*(8), 3087–3103. doi:10.1002/hbm.22830

Daianu, M., Jahanshad, N., Nir, T. M., Toga, A. W., Jack, C. R., Jr., Weiner, M. W., . . . Thompson, P. M.; Alzheimer's Disease Neuroimaging Iniatative. (2013). Breakdown of brain connectivity between normal aging and Alzheimer's disease: A structural k-core network analysis. *Brain Connectivity, 3*(4), 407–422. doi:10.1089/brain.2012.0137

de Groot, M., Ikram, M. A., Akoudad, S., Krestin, G. P., Hofman, A., van der Lugt, A., . . . Vernooij, M. W. (2015). Tract-specific white matter degeneration in aging: The Rotterdam Study. *Alzheimers & Dementia, 11*(3), 321–330. doi:10.1016/j.jalz.2014.06.011

Debette, S., Seshadri, S., Beiser, A., Au, R., Himali, J. J., Palumbo, C., . . . DeCarli, C. (2011). Midlife vascular risk factor exposure accelerates structural brain aging and cognitive decline. *Neurology, 77*(5), 461–468. doi:10.1212/WNL.0b013e318227b227

Delano-Wood, L., Bondi, M. W., Sacco, J., Abeles, N., Jak, A. J., Libon, D. J., & Bozoki, A. (2009). Heterogeneity in mild cognitive impairment: Differences in neuropsychological profile and associated white matter lesion pathology. *Journal of the International Neuropsychology Society, 15*(6), 906–914. doi:10.1017/S1355617709990257

den Heijer, T., van der Lijn, F., Koudstaal, P. J., Hofman, A., van der Lugt, A., Krestin, G. P., . . . Breteler, M. M. (2010). A 10-year follow-up of hippocampal volume on magnetic resonance imaging in early dementia and cognitive decline. *Brain, 133*(Pt 4), 1163–1172. doi:10.1093/brain/awq048

Dickerson, B. C., Bakkour, A., Salat, D. H., Feczko, E., Pacheco, J., Greve, D. N., . . . Buckner, R. L. (2009). The cortical signature of Alzheimer's disease: Regionally specific cortical thinning relates to symptom severity in very mild to mild AD dementia and is detectable in asymptomatic amyloid-positive individuals. *Cerebral Cortex, 19*(3), 497–510. doi:10.1093/cercor/bhn113

Eskildsen, S. F., Coupe, P., Garcia-Lorenzo, D., Fonov, V., Pruessner, J. C., & Collins, D. L.; Alzheimer's Disease Neuroimaging Initiative. (2013). Prediction of Alzheimer's disease in subjects with mild cognitive impairment from the ADNI cohort using patterns of cortical thinning. *NeuroImage, 65*, 511–521. doi:10.1016/j.neuroimage.2012.09.058

Firbank, M. J., Wiseman, R. M., Burton, E. J., Saxby, B. K., O'Brien, J. T., & Ford, G. A. (2007). Brain atrophy and white matter hyperintensity change in older adults and relationship to blood pressure. Brain atrophy, WMH change and blood pressure. *Journal of Neurology, 254*(6), 713–721. doi:10.1007/s00415-006-0238-4

Fox, N. C., Warrington, E. K., Freeborough, P. A., Hartikainen, P., Kennedy, A. M., Stevens, J. M., & Rossor, M. N. (1996). Presymptomatic hippocampal atrophy in Alzheimer's disease: A longitudinal MRI study. *Brain, 119*(Pt 6), 2001–2007.

Friedman, J. I., Tang, C. Y., de Haas, H. J., Changchien, L., Goliasch, G., Dabas, P., . . . Narula, J. (2014). Brain imaging changes associated with risk factors for cardiovascular and cerebrovascular disease in asymptomatic patients. *JACC Cardiovasc Imaging, 7*(10), 1039–1053. doi:10.1016/j.jcmg.2014.06.014

Glodzik, L., Mosconi, L., Tsui, W., de Santi, S., Zinkowski, R., Pirraglia, E., . . . de Leon, M. J. (2012). Alzheimer's disease markers, hypertension, and gray matter damage in normal elderly. *Neurobiology of Aging, 33*(7), 1215–1227. doi:10.1016/j.neurobiolaging.2011.02.012

Gonzales, M. M., Ajilore, O., Charlton, R. C., Cohen, J., Yang, S., Sieg, E., . . . Lamar, M. (2017). Divergent influences of cardiovascular disease risk factor domains on cognition and gray and white matter morphology. *Psychosomatic Medicine, 79*(5), 541–548. doi:10.1097/PSY.0000000000000448

Hachinski, V. C., Potter, P., & Merskey, H. (1986). Leuko-araiosis: An ancient term for a new problem. *Canadian Journal of Neurological Sciences, 13*(4 Suppl), 533–534.

Hoogenboom, W. S., Marder, T. J., Flores, V. L., Huisman, S., Eaton, H. P., Schneiderman, J. S., . . . Musen, G. (2014). Cerebral white matter integrity and resting-state functional connectivity in middle-aged patients with type 2 diabetes. *Diabetes, 63*(2), 728–738. doi:10.2337/db13-1219

Iadecola, C., Yaffe, K., Biller, J., Bratzke, L. C., Faraci, F. M., Gorelick, P. B., . . . Zeki Al Hazzouri, A; American Heart Association Council on Hypertension; Council on Clinical Cardiology; Council on Cardiovascular Disease in the Young; Council on Cardiovascular and Stroke Nursing; Council on Quality of Care and Outcomes Research; and Stroke Council. (2016). Impact of hypertension on cognitive function: A scientific statement from the American Heart Association. *Hypertension, 68*(6), e67–e94. doi:10.1161/HYP.0000000000000053

Jack, C. R., Jr., Bennett, D. A., Blennow, K., Carrillo, M. C., Dunn, B., Haeberlein, S. B., . . . Contributors. (2018). NIA-AA Research Framework: Toward a biological definition of Alzheimer's disease. *Alzheimers & Dementia, 14*(4), 535–562. doi:10.1016/j.jalz.2018.02.018

Jacobs, H. I., Leritz, E. C., Williams, V. J., Van Boxtel, M. P., van der Elst, W., Jolles, J., . . . Salat, D. H. (2013). Association between white matter microstructure, executive functions, and processing speed in older adults: The impact of vascular health. *Human Brain Mapping, 34*(1), 77–95. doi:10.1002/hbm.21412

Jacquemont, T., De Vico Fallani, F., Bertrand, A., Epelbaum, S., Routier, A., Dubois, B., . . . Alzheimer's Disease Neuroimaging, I. (2017). Amyloidosis and neurodegeneration result in distinct structural connectivity patterns in mild cognitive impairment. *Neurobiology of Aging, 55*, 177–189. doi:10.1016/j.neurobiolaging.2017.03.023

Kennedy, K. M., & Raz, N. (2009). Pattern of normal age-related regional differences in white matter microstructure is modified by vascular risk. *Brain Research, 1297*, 41–56. doi:10.1016/j.brainres.2009.08.058

Kumar, A., Haroon, E., Darwin, C., Pham, D., Ajilore, O., Rodriguez, G., & Mintz, J. (2008). Gray matter prefrontal changes in type 2 diabetes detected using MRI. *Journal of Magnetic Resonance Imaging, 27*(1), 14–19. doi:10.1002/jmri.21224

Lamar, M., Rubin, L. H., Ajilore, O., Charlton, R., Zhang, A., Yang, S., . . . Kumar, A. (2015). What metabolic syndrome contributes to brain outcomes in African American and Caucasian cohorts. *Current Alzheimer's Research, 12*(7), 640–647.

Langen, C. D., Cremers, L. G. M., de Groot, M., White, T., Ikram, M. A., Niessen, W. J., & Vernooij, M. W. (2018). Disconnection due to white matter hyperintensities is associated with lower cognitive scores. *NeuroImage, 183*, 745–756. doi:10.1016/j.neuroimage.2018.08.037

Langen, C. D., Zonneveld, H. I., White, T., Huizinga, W., Cremers, L. G. M., de Groot, M., . . . Vernooij, M. W. (2017). White matter lesions relate to tract-specific reductions in functional connectivity. *Neurobiology of Aging, 51*, 97–103. doi:10.1016/j.neurobiolaging.2016.12.004

Lawrence, A. J., Tozer, D. J., Stamatakis, E. A., & Markus, H. S. (2018). A comparison of functional and tractography based networks in cerebral small vessel disease. *NeuroImage: Clinical, 18*, 425–432. doi:10.1016/j.nicl.2018.02.013

Leritz, E. C., Salat, D. H., Williams, V. J., Schnyer, D. M., Rudolph, J. L., Lipsitz, L., . . . Milberg, W. P. (2011). Thickness of the human cerebral cortex is associated with metrics of cerebrovascular health in a normative sample of community dwelling older adults. *NeuroImage, 54*(4), 2659–2671. doi:10.1016/j.neuroimage.2010.10.050

Libon, D. J., Price, C. C., Giovannetti, T., Swenson, R., Bettcher, B. M., Heilman, K. M., & Pennisi, A. (2008). Linking MRI hyperintensities with patterns of neuropsychological impairment: Evidence for a threshold effect. *Stroke, 39*(3), 806–813. doi:10.1161/STROKEAHA.107.489997

Lin, L., Jin, C., Fu, Z., Zhang, B., Bin, G., & Wu, S. (2016). Predicting healthy older adult's brain age based on structural connectivity networks using artificial neural networks. *Computer Methods and Programs in Biomedicine, 125*, 8–17. doi:10.1016/j.cmpb.2015.11.012

Maillard, P., Seshadri, S., Beiser, A., Himali, J. J., Au, R., Fletcher, E., . . . DeCarli, C. (2012). Effects of systolic blood pressure on white-matter integrity in young adults in the Framingham Heart Study: A cross-sectional study. *Lancet Neurology, 11*(12), 1039–1047. doi:10.1016/S1474-4422(12)70241-7

Mallio, C. A., Schmidt, R., de Reus, M. A., Vernieri, F., Quintiliani, L., Curcio, G., . . . van den Heuvel, M. P. (2015). Epicentral disruption of structural connectivity in Alzheimer's disease. *CNS Neuroscience & Therapeutics, 21*(10), 837–845. doi:10.1111/cns.12397

McEvoy, L. K., Fennema-Notestine, C., Eyler, L. T., Franz, C. E., Hagler, D. J., Jr., Lyons, M. J., . . . Kremen, W. S. (2015). Hypertension-related alterations in white matter microstructure detectable in middle age. *Hypertension, 66*(2), 317–323. doi:10.1161/HYPERTENSIONAHA.115.05336

Meusel, L. A., Kansal, N., Tchistiakova, E., Yuen, W., MacIntosh, B. J., Greenwood, C. E., & Anderson, N. D. (2014). A systematic review of type 2 diabetes mellitus and hypertension in imaging studies of cognitive aging: Time to establish new norms. *Frontiers in Aging Neuroscience, 6*, 148. doi:10.3389/fnagi.2014.00148

Moulton, C. D., Costafreda, S. G., Horton, P., Ismail, K., & Fu, C. H. (2015). Meta-analyses of structural regional cerebral effects in type 1 and type 2 diabetes. *Brain Imaging & Behavior, 9*(4), 651–662. doi:10.1007/s11682-014-9348-2

Neltner, J. H., Abner, E. L., Baker, S., Schmitt, F. A., Kryscio, R. J., Jicha, G. A., . . . Nelson, P. T. (2014). Arteriolosclerosis that affects multiple brain regions is linked to hippocampal sclerosis of ageing. *Brain, 137*(Pt 1), 255–267. doi:10.1093/brain/awt318

Nir, T. M., Jahanshad, N., Toga, A. W., Bernstein, M. A., Jack, C. R., Jr., Weiner, M. W., & Thompson, P. M.; Alzheimer's Disease Neuroimaging Initiative. (2015). Connectivity network measures predict volumetric atrophy in mild cognitive impairment. *Neurobiology of Aging, 36 Suppl 1*, S113–120. doi:10.1016/j.neurobiolaging.2014.04.038

Perry, A., Wen, W., Lord, A., Thalamuthu, A., Roberts, G., Mitchell, P. B., . . . Breakspear, M. (2015). The organisation of the elderly connectome. *NeuroImage, 114*, 414–426. doi:10.1016/j.neuroimage.2015.04.009

Pini, L., Pievani, M., Bocchetta, M., Altomare, D., Bosco, P., Cavedo, E., . . . Frisoni, G. B. (2016). Brain atrophy in Alzheimer's disease and aging. *Ageing Research Reviews, 30*, 25–48. doi:10.1016/j.arr.2016.01.002

Price, C. C., Mitchell, S. M., Brumback, B., Tanner, J. J., Schmalfuss, I., Lamar, M., . . . Libon, D. J. (2012). MRI-leukoaraiosis thresholds and the phenotypic expression of dementia. *Neurology, 79*(8), 734–740. doi:10.1212/WNL.0b013e3182661ef6

Roberts, R. O., Knopman, D. S., Przybelski, S. A., Mielke, M. M., Kantarci, K., Preboske, G. M., . . . Jack, C. R., Jr. (2014). Association of type 2 diabetes with brain atrophy and cognitive impairment. *Neurology, 82*(13), 1132–1141. doi:10.1212/WNL.0000000000000269

Rubinov, M., & Sporns, O. (2010). Complex network measures of brain connectivity: Uses and interpretations. *NeuroImage, 52*(3), 1059–1069. doi:10.1016/j.neuroimage.2009.10.003

Seiler, S., Fletcher, E., Hassan-Ali, K., Weinstein, M., Beiser, A., Himali, J. J., . . . Maillard, P. (2018). Cerebral tract integrity relates to white matter hyperintensities, cortex volume, and cognition. *Neurobiology of Aging, 72*, 14–22. doi:10.1016/j.neurobiolaging.2018.08.005

Sun, Y., Lee, R., Chen, Y., Collinson, S., Thakor, N., Bezerianos, A., & Sim, K. (2015). Progressive gender differences of structural brain networks in healthy adults: A longitudinal, diffusion tensor imaging study. *PLoS One, 10*(3), e0118857. doi:10.1371/journal.pone.0118857

Tuladhar, A. M., Lawrence, A., Norris, D. G., Barrick, T. R., Markus, H. S., & de Leeuw, F. E. (2017). Disruption of rich club organisation in cerebral small vessel disease. *Human Brain Mapping, 38*(4), 1751–1766. doi:10.1002/hbm.23479

Wang, L. Y., Larson, E. B., Sonnen, J. A., Shofer, J. B., McCormick, W., Bowen, J. D., . . . Li, G. (2009). Blood pressure and brain injury in older adults: Findings from a community-based autopsy study. *Journal of the Am Geriatrics Society, 57*(11), 1975–1981. doi:10.1111/j.1532-5415.2009.02493.x

Wang, R., Fratiglioni, L., Laukka, E. J., Lovden, M., Kalpouzos, G., Keller, L., . . . Qiu, C. (2015). Effects of vascular risk factors and APOE epsilon4 on white matter integrity and cognitive decline. *Neurology, 84*(11), 1128–1135. doi:10.1212/WNL.0000000000001379

Weinstein, G., Maillard, P., Himali, J. J., Beiser, A. S., Au, R., Wolf, P. A., . . . DeCarli, C. (2015). Glucose indices are associated with cognitive and structural brain measures in young adults. *Neurology, 84*(23), 2329–2337. doi:10.1212/WNL.0000000000001655

Wiseman, R. M., Saxby, B. K., Burton, E. J., Barber, R., Ford, G. A., & O'Brien, J. T. (2004). Hippocampal atrophy, whole brain volume, and white matter lesions in older hypertensive subjects. *Neurology, 63*(10), 1892–1897.

Wu, G., Lin, L., Zhang, Q., & Wu, J. (2017). Brain gray matter changes in type 2 diabetes mellitus: A meta-analysis of whole-brain voxel-based morphometry study. *Journal of Diabetes and Its Complications, 31*(12), 1698–1703. doi:10.1016/j.jdiacomp.2017.09.001

Yan, T., Wang, W., Yang, L., Chen, K., Chen, R., & Han, Y. (2018). Rich club disturbances of the human connectome from subjective cognitive decline to Alzheimer's disease. *Theranostics, 8*(12), 3237–3255. doi:10.7150/thno.23772

Zhang, Y. W., Zhang, J. Q., Liu, C., Wei, P., Zhang, X., Yuan, Q. Y., . . . Wang, J. (2015). Memory dysfunction in type 2 diabetes mellitus correlates with reduced hippocampal CA1 and subiculum volumes. *Chinese Medical Journal (England), 128*(4), 465–471. doi:10.4103/0366-6999.151082

Zhao, T., Cao, M., Niu, H., Zuo, X. N., Evans, A., He, Y., . . . Shu, N. (2015). Age-related changes in the topological organization of the white matter structural connectome across the human lifespan. *Human Brain Mapping, 36*(10), 3777–3792. doi:10.1002/hbm.22877

PART 3

BLOOD–BRAIN BARRIER AND CARDIOGENIC MECHANISMS

11

The Blood–Brain Barrier in Cognitive Decline and Alzheimer's Disease

Daniel A. Nation and Elissa McIntosh

1. The Vascular Hypothesis of Alzheimer's Disease

The brain contains over 400 miles of blood vessels, 85% of which are capillary microvessels (Kisler, Nelson, Montagne, & Zlokovic, 2017). Despite representing only 2% of the body mass, the brain receives approximately 20% of whole body glucose and oxygen (Cipolla, 2009; Kisler et al., 2017). The torrential blood flow required to meet brain metabolic demands relies heavily on autoregulation of the brain microvascular bed (Iadecola, 2004). If this rich and delicate microvascular network is not healthy, the brain networks underpinning cognitive, affective, and behavioral processes cannot normally function (Iadecola, 2013).

The microvascular endothelium of the brain capillary network is distinguished from other organ systems in several important ways. Brain capillary endothelial cells form just one part of a neurovascular unit, which is comprised of the coordinated anatomy and function of several cell subtypes at the interface between the vascular compartment and the brain parenchyma (Cipolla, 2009). The neurovascular unit also involves astrocytes, pericytes, and neurons (Sweeney, Ayyadurai, & Zlokovic, 2016), and all of these cell-types play key roles in the two neurovascular unit functions: (a) regulation of cerebral perfusion and (b) maintaining blood–brain barrier (BBB) integrity (Zlokovic, 2008).

The neurovascular unit works to ensure that metabolic supply in the form of capillary perfusion meets metabolic demand for local brain activity (Iadecola, 2017). Any mismatch in this supply–demand relationship may lead to oligemia (i.e., hypoperfusion), ischemia with brain tissue dysfunction or injury and eventual infarction (Toth, Tarantini, Csiszar, & Ungvari, 2017). In addition to this role in modulating tissue perfusion, the neurovascular unit also ensures the integrity of the BBB. Blood contains a host of neurotoxic factors, including toxic proteins like albumin and fibrinogen, but also toxic ions, metabolites, and cells, all of which cause neuronal dysfunction or death if they enter the brain parenchyma (Zlokovic, 2011). To keep these toxic blood products from entering the brain, the neurovascular unit forms the BBB through the coordinated structure

Daniel A. Nation and Elissa McIntosh, *The Blood–Brain Barrier in Cognitive Decline and Alzheimer's Disease*
In: *Vascular Disease, Alzheimer's Disease, and Mild Cognitive Impairment.* Edited by: David J. Libon, Melissa Lamar, Rodney A. Swenson, Kenneth M. Heilman, Oxford University Press (2020).
DOI: 10.1093/oso/9780190634230.003.0012

and function of its constituent cell-types. Brain microvascular endothelial cells are joined by special proteins that form tight junctions, minimizing the space between endothelial cells. These spaces are so small that very few blood products other than water and oxygen may pass. Glucose and other nutrients must be actively transported across the endothelial layer by specialized transporter proteins (e.g., glucose transporter-1 [GLUT-1]). Similarly, potentially neurotoxic brain waste products (e.g., amyloid-beta [Aβ] protein species) must be actively transported across the capillary endothelial layer to be directly excreted into circulation by transporters (e.g., low-density lipoprotein receptor-related protein [LRP-1]; Donahue et al., 2006).

The brain capillary endothelium is also surrounded by pericytes, capillary mural cells that play a key role in regulating endothelial layer permeability and vessel caliber by means of several recently described signaling pathways and contractile proteins (Attwell, Mishra, Hall, O'Farrell, & Dalkara, 2016; Sweeney et al., 2016), and the *glia limitans*, a wall of astrocytic end-feet that forms a barrier between the vessel and the brain parenchyma (Cipolla, 2009). Thus, dysfunction of the BBB, characterized by increased permeability, is a major consequence of neurovascular unit injury that may lead to brain damage and dysfunction. Despite the importance of these neurovascular units for brain function, surprisingly little has been known about its complex functions until recently (Iadecola, 2017). Cerebral blood flow (CBF) and its regulatory mechanisms have been intensively investigated for decades in healthy humans and in both sporadic Alzheimer's disease (AD; de la Torre, 2017) and autosomal dominant AD (Yan et al., 2018), but BBB function has been more difficult to study in humans.

Technical advancements have steadily improved our ability to study neurovascular unit function in clinical studies (Heye, Culling, Valdes Hernandez Mdel, Thrippleton, & Wardlaw, 2014; Montagne et al., 2016). Findings from transgenic animal models of AD and patients with sporadic AD have led to the hypothesis that neurovascular unit dysfunction is a primary initiating event in AD (Sweeney, Sagare, & Zlokovic, 2018; Zlokovic, 2011). Perhaps the strongest evidence to date comes from a comprehensive analysis of longitudinal biomarker data collected as part of the Alzheimer's Disease Neuroimaging Initiative (ADNI), showing that the earliest biofluid and neuroimaging markers to exhibit abnormalities are vascular markers (Iturria-Medina et al., 2016). Specifically, arterial spin-labeling magnetic resonance imaging (MRI) markers indicating reduced CBF were the first abnormalities observed, followed by neuropsychological markers of memory dysfunction. Unfortunately, biomarkers of BBB permeability were not included in the ADNI study as these are still in the early stages of investigation. To date, at least three independent studies have identified BBB breakdown during the early stages of AD (Montagne et al., 2015; Nation et al., 2019; van de Haar, Burgmans, et al., 2016b). Ongoing studies are focusing on whether these markers may show even earlier changes. In what follows, we review some of these markers and the extant research on their role in neuropsychological impairment in AD.

2. CSF Albumin Index (Q_{alb})

Albumin is a very large protein produced by the liver and found in the blood. Early studies on aging and cerebral permeability found albumin in the cerebrospinal fluid (CSF), demonstrating that albumin can be transported across the blood–CSF barrier (Rosenberg, 2014). Because albumin is a large protein that cannot cross the BBB, albumin quotient (Q_{alb}) calculated as the ratio of CSF to plasma or serum albumin has been used to assess BBB disruption. Early studies of Q_{alb} as an indicator of BBB breakdown in AD and vascular dementia were mixed. One early study investigated CSF albumin concentrations and Q_{alb} in AD and multi-infarct vascular dementia and found that both patient groups had significantly higher CSF albumin concentrations than controls. In addition, the multi-infarct group had significantly higher CSF albumin compared to the AD group. In another study, increased Q_{alb} was only observed in the multi-infarct dementia group relative to the AD and control groups, with no significant differences observed between the AD and control groups (Alafuzoff, Adolfsson, Bucht, & Winblad, 1983). Elovaara, Icen, Palo, and Erkinjuntti (1985) showed Q_{alb} elevation in both ambulatory AD and institutionalized AD patients compared to controls. Several years later, another study did not detect any differences in Q_{alb} among early-onset AD patients, late-onset AD patients, patients with major depression, and age-matched controls. However, Elovaara et al. noted that a subset of patients in the major depression (29%) and AD (16%) groups were more likely to show pathological Q_{alb} levels compared to controls (Hampel, Kotter, & Moller, 1997). Another study found increased Q_{alb} in both AD and vascular dementia patients compared to non-demented controls (Wada, 1998).

In one of the new longitudinal studies of BBB in the very elderly, Skoog and colleagues (1998) reported that both AD and vascular dementia patients exhibited increased Q_{alb} compared to nondemented individuals, but the ratio was not associated with dementia severity. Women who were dementia-free at baseline but later developed dementia had significantly higher baseline Q_{alb} than those who did not develop dementia. In a study of incident AD, Algottson and Winblad (2007) reported 42% of men and 13% of women with AD had pathologically elevated Q_{alb} (set at Q_{alb} >9.2), demonstrating significant gender differences in Q_{alb} ($p < 0.001$). In patients with mild to moderate AD, Bowman and colleagues found 22% of patients had elevated Q_{alb}. Age, sex, and apolipoprotein (APOE)-ε4 were not associated with the Q_{alb}. Vascular risk factors explained about 31% of the variance in Q_{alb} values ($p = 0.066$). Notably, Q_{alb} was correlated with annual change on cognitive tests (Mini-Mental State Examination [MMSE], Clinical Dementia Rating sum-of-boxes), and ventricular volume change (Bowman et al., 2007).

Despite some cross-sectional and longitudinal evidence for increased Q_{alb} in AD (as previously reviewed), it is critical to note that several studies have reported no evidence of increased Q_{alb}. Mecocci and colleagues (1991) found CSF albumin and Q_{alb} were significantly higher in multi-infarct dementia patients, but not in patients with early-onset AD or senile dementia of the Alzheimer's type. Additional studies from other groups also did not find increased Q_{alb} in patients with probable AD when compared to healthy controls and found no association with cerebral atrophy (Frolich et al., 1991; Kay et al., 1987).

The mixed findings relating Q_{alb} to AD may be explained by issues in differentiating AD and vascular dementia. It is now recognized that the majority of AD patients exhibited some cerebrovascular pathologies, blurring the lines between vascular and AD dementia (Arvanitakis, Capuano, Leurgans, Bennett, & Schneider, 2016; Toledo et al., 2013). In an attempt to disentangle the role of Q_{alb} in these different pathologies, Blennow and colleagues (1990) reported that although AD patients had a higher Q_{alb} compared to healthy controls, it was vascular factors that accounted for this relationship. In another study of dementia with both AD and vascular dementia patients, those with white matter changes had significantly higher Q_{alb}, and patients with the most severe white-matter changes had the highest Q_{alb}, suggesting that cerebrovascular damage is most closely related to increases in BBB permeability (Wallin, Sjogren, Edman, Blennow, & Regland, 2000).

Other studies have noted relationships between vascular risk factors and BBB breakdown. For example, Bowman Kaye, and Quinn (2012) showed that patients with mild to moderate AD with BBB impairment (elevated Q_{alb}) had significantly higher plasma triglycerides and lower high density lipoprotein (HDL) cholesterol. Plasma triglycerides explained 22% of the variance in BBB integrity. The relationship between dyslipidemia and Q_{alb} remained significant after controlling for age, gender, APOE-ε4 carrier status, blood pressure, and statin medication use. Thus, the study showed dyslipidemia was more common in AD subjects with BBB dysfunction as measured by the Q_{alb}. In Farrall and Wardlaw's (2009) review of 21 Q_{alb} studies in AD, only 9 of these studies performed separate analyses for vascular disease. Of these studies, six studies reported significantly more BBB disruption in vascular dementia compared to AD (Alafuzoff et al., 1983; Blennow, Wallin, & Chong, 1995; Elovaara et al., 1985; Leonardi, Gandolfo, Caponnetto, Arata, & Vecchia, 1985; Shindo, Haruo, Shimizu, Iwamoto, & Tokyo Medical Univ., 2005; Skoog et al., 1998; Wada, 1998), while three found no differences (Bronge & Wahlund, 2000; Hampel et al., 1997; Mecocci et al., 1991).

These studies point to the importance of vascular factors in understanding BBB dysfunction in age-related dementias.

One limitation of these early studies was the quality of control groups. Control groups that are younger and healthier than patient groups could overestimate differences between healthy and patient groups. On the contrary, control groups that may have BBB disruption due to other causes (e.g., vascular risk factors) could underestimate differences between healthy and patient groups. Since other factors, such as CSF turnover rate, can affect CSF albumin levels, measurements of only Q_{alb} have many limitations as an index of BBB permeability. More recent work has shown that aging and AD can slow CSF turnover (Erickson & Banks, 2013).

In summary, the existing literature suggests that BBB breakdown, as measured by Q_{alb}, is increased with aging, vascular risk factor burden, cerebrovascular disease, and possibly AD (Erickson & Banks, 2013; Farrall & Wardlaw, 2009). Future Q_{alb} studies should investigate the role of BBB breakdown in the context of AD biomarkers (amyloid and tau pathology), independent of other vascular risk factors (e.g., dyslipidemia, obesity, type 2 diabetes) and cerebrovascular pathologies (e.g., white matter lesions) to better understand the etiology of BBB impairment in AD, vascular dementia, and normal aging.

3. Dynamic Contrast-Enhanced Magnetic Resonance Imaging

Dynamic contrast-enhanced MRI (DCE-MRI) is an in vivo neuroimaging tool that can measure BBB leakage volume, leakage rates, and kinetics of contrast agents (e.g., gadolinium) to quantity BBB integrity. Gadolinium, a popular contrast agent, leaks passively through cellular tight junctions (Zlokovic, 2008). Quantitative analysis of an individual's arterial input function during dynamic MRI with contrast allows for calculation of the blood-to-brain transfer constant, k_{trans}, which can be imaged as an index of brain microvascular permeability (Montagne et al., 2015; Taheri, Gasparovic, Huisa, et al., 2011; Taheri, Gasparovic, Shah, & Rosenberg, 2011; van de Haar et al., 2015; van de Haar, Burgmans, et al., 2016a; van de Haar, Jansen, et al., 2016).

Recent DCE-MRI studies have investigated BBB permeability using both mild cognitive impairment (MCI) and AD patient groups. In an initial study, Wang Golob, and Su (2006) studied cerebrovascular volume and BBB permeability indices using DCE-MRI in 11 MCI subjects and 11 healthy controls. Findings indicated significantly smaller right hippocampal vascular volume in MCI, but there were no significant differences between MCI patients and controls in the BBB permeability index in the bilateral hippocampi or cerebellum. In another small study, DCE-MRI studied BBB permeability in 15 AD participants and 15 healthy controls with regions of interest in the deep gray matter, cortical gray matter, white matter, CSF, and the basilar and internal carotid arteries. AD patients did not differ from normal controls in the extent of leakage, but there was a significant time-by-AD interaction suggesting altered blood–brain–CSF compartmental kinetics in AD (Starr, Farrall, Armitage, McGurn, & Wardlaw, 2009).

In a larger, more recent study of MCI and normal aging, Montagne and colleagues (2015) found a progressive loss of BBB integrity that was age-dependent and specific to the hippocampus, including the CA1 and dentate gyrus (DG) subfields. These age-related BBB changes in the hippocampus were observed in individuals free from dementia but did not occur in other brain regions. The study also found that MCI patients had increased BBB permeability in the hippocampus and medial temporal lobes when compared to age-matched cognitively normal controls, but not in other cortical, subcortical, and white matter regions. Consistent with the hippocampal differences noted between MCI and age-matched controls, MCI individuals also had a 30% increase in the Q_{alb}. Increased Q_{alb} was also correlated with DCE-MRI indexed BBB permeability values in the hippocampus. These individuals with MCI did not have smaller hippocampal volumes compared to cognitively normal adults, indicating that findings were not due solely to volumetric changes and further raising the possibility that changes in BBB permeability precede AD-related hippocampal atrophy.

In an independent replication, van de Haar, Burgman, et al. (2016a) also reported higher BBB leakage rates in MCI and AD patients compared to healthy controls, which involved the total gray matter and cerebral cortex. In addition, patients had significantly greater volume leaked in the gray matter, normal-appearing white matter, deep gray matter, and cortex. Across all subjects, leakage volume was negatively correlated with MMSE scores. After controlling for vascular factors, the findings remained significant, suggesting that BBB impairment was not explained by other traditional vascular factors. Since regions with high BBB leakage were not contained within specific areas but were diffusely distributed, Van de Haar, Jansen, et al. (2016) suggested that global tight junction impairment may be present. In the same patient cohort, the authors reported reduced CBF was correlated with increased leakage rate.

As previously reviewed, the early DCE-MRI studies in AD were null but were likely underpowered to detect significant differences. More recent studies with larger sample sizes demonstrate increased BBB permeability within the medial temporal lobe and perhaps other cortical regions in patients with MCI or mild AD dementia. Imaging studies of vascular dementia have also shown evidence of increased BBB permeability, particularly in people with white matter lesions (Rosenberg, 2014). In a study of BBB permeability in patients with vascular cognitive impairment, characterized by subcortical ischemic vascular disease, multiple and lacunar infarcts, and leukoaraiosis, both DCE-MRI and Q_{alb} were significantly increased in patients compared to controls. Using MRI fluid-attenuated inversion recovery (FLAIR) images of white matter hyperintensities (WMHs), regions of increased permeability were determined to be within the WMHs, specifically in the center. Thus, the study provided evidence of a relationship between BBB damage and WMHs (Taheri, Gasparovic, Huisa, et al., 2011). Similar studies of BBB permeability in Binswanger's disease, a condition characterized by severe white matter lesion pathology, examined periventricular WMHs with contrast-enhanced MRI (Hanyu et al., 2002). The study investigated differences between Binswanger's disease patients with periventricular WMHs, nondemented patients with ischemic cerebrovascular events and periventricular WMHs, and age-matched controls with periventricular WMHs. The authors reported significantly greater BBB disruption in Binswanger's disease patients compared to nondemented patients and controls, but no significant change between nondemented patients and controls. MMSE score was significantly correlated with BBB permeability in periventricular WMHs in Binswanger's patients. The results of this study suggest that there is BBB dysfunction in periventricular WMHs in Binswanger's disease, and that BBB dysfunction is related to dementia (Hanyu et al., 2002). Skoog and colleagues (1998) reported that the Q_{alb} was higher in subjects with moderate or severe white matter lesions compared to subjects with mild or no lesions. Additionally, they reported vascular dementia patients had higher Q_{alb} than AD patients.

Other studies using nondemented populations have also found relationships between white matter damage and BBB dysfunction. Starr and colleagues (2003) found BBB permeability was higher in patients with type II diabetes mellitus compared to controls. Further, in all subjects, BBB permeability was higher in subjects with more WMHs (Starr et al., 2003). In elderly patients, a relationship was observed between Q_{alb} and degree of periventricular high intensity signal on MRI, suggesting that white matter damage is related to BBB dysfunction (Yamaguchi et al., 1989).

Thus, a clear connection between vascular contributions to cognitive impairment and BBB breakdown has been established by Q_{alb} and DCE-MRI studies, but it has remained unclear whether any BBB breakdown occurs in AD patients, independent of traditional vascular comorbidities. It has also been unclear whether there is any relationship between BBB breakdown and either amyloid or tau pathologies in AD patients. Studies identifying associations between vascular dysfunction and AD pathology have frequently cited the vasculotoxic effects of amyloid and tau, an interpretation consistent with a causal directionality of AD pathology causing vascular pathology. To determine whether DCE-MRI BBB permeability markers are independent of traditional vascular factors and AD pathologies, Nation and colleagues (2019)conducted a study in over 160 older adults along the cognitively normal MCI AD dementia clinical spectrum, wherein BBB permeability was measured by DCE-MRI concurrently with markers of amyloid and tau. Findings indicated increased medial temporal and subcortical BBB permeability in older adults with cognitive impairment, regardless of traditional vascular risk profiles, amyloid levels or tau levels. These results indicate that BBB breakdown is an independent biomarker of cognitive impairment in older adults, distinct from commonly employed vascular and AD markers. Further studies are needed to establish the timeline of BBB breakdown in relation to the course of amyloid, tau and cognitive derangements in AD.

4. Soluble Platelet-Derived Growth Factor Receptor–Beta

Indicators of BBB breakdown and reduced CBF are useful for evaluating neurovascular unit integrity but tell us little about the cell types involved and even less about the molecular mechanism that is responsible. Pericytes are critical for maintaining BBB integrity (Armulik et al., 2010), and pericyte injury has been implicated in animal models of neurodegeneration (Sagare et al., 2013). Although there have been few molecular markers specific to pericytes, increased CSF soluble platelet-derived growth factor receptor beta (sPDGFRβ) has been linked to pericyte injury in animal models (Sagare, Sweeney, Makshanoff, & Zlokovic, 2015). A recent study attempted to disentangle the various cell-types involved by using molecular markers in CSF that index astrocytic, inflammatory, neuronal, and vascular-endothelial cell injury, with a particular emphasis on a marker of pericyte injury (sPDGFRβ). Findings indicated that CSF sPDGFRβ levels were elevated in patients with MCI and mild AD dementia and that sPDGFRβ correlated with BBB breakdown indexed by DCE-MRI (Montagne et al., 2015). Thus, evidence from both animal and human clinical studies suggest that pericyte loss may be an early cellular event leading to BBB breakdown and neurodegeneration in aging adults.

In the same DCE-MRI BBB permeability study reviewed in the previously section, Nation and colleagues (2019) also included CSF sPDGFRβ, and provided in vitro data linking this biomarker to injury-related pericyte shedding via a disintegrin and metalloproteinase domain-containing protein 10 (ADAM-10). Examination of this marker in the same patients indicated increased CSF sPDGFRβ in older adults with cognitive impairment, regardless of traditional vascular factors, amyloid, or tau. Levels of CSF sPDGFRβ also correlated positively with BBB permeability on DCE-MRI. Findings indicate that pericyte injury may be an early and independent pathological process related to BBB breakdown and cognitive impairment in AD patients. Future studies are focused on establishing the timeline of pericyte injury and BBB breakdown in relation to amyloid and tau pathologies and cognitive decline in older adults.

5. The Role of Apolipoprotein-ε4

The APOE-ε4 allele is the most important genetic risk factor for sporadic AD, accounting for up to 7-fold increased risk in heterozygotes and 14-fold risk for homozygotes (Bu, 2009). Although APOE-ε4 may impact AD pathophysiology through a variety of mechanisms, mounting evidence indicates extensive cerebrovascular effects that may implicate APOE-ε4 in neurovascular unit injury (Tai et al., 2016). Careful animal studies have provided powerful evidence that APOE-ε4 may lead to neurovascular unit dysfunction and BBB breakdown through signaling pathways involving cyclophilin A and matrix metalloproteinase 9 (MMP-9)-mediated degradation of the capillary basement membrane (Bell et al., 2012). Support for a similar mechanism in aging humans comes from a study demonstrating increased Q_{alb} in older adult APOE-ε4 carriers relative to younger APOE-ε4 carriers and age-matched APOE-ε4 noncarriers (Halliday et al., 2013). These results could suggest that an age-dependent increase in BBB breakdown but only in APOE-ε4 carriers. Given this information, future studies should also investigate the role of APOE genotype in BBB integrity using DCE-MRI.

6. Summary

Recent appreciation for the neurovascular unit as a critical organ of the brain microvasculature regulating CBF and BBB integrity has led to interest in its potential role in neuropsychological decline and AD. The advent of new neuroimaging and biomarker technologies has allowed renewed investigation into BBB function in AD. Studies to date implicate early pericyte injury and resulting loss of BBB integrity in the early stages of AD, particularly among older APOE-ε4 carriers.

References

Alafuzoff, I., Adolfsson, R., Bucht, G., & Winblad, B. (1983). Albumin and immunoglobulin in plasma and cerebrospinal fluid, and blood-cerebrospinal fluid barrier function in patients with dementia of Alzheimer type and multi-infarct dementia. *Journal of the Neurological Sciences*, *60*(3), 465–472.

Algotsson, A., & Winblad, B. (2007). The integrity of the blood–brain barrier in Alzheimer's disease. *Acta Neurologica Scandinavica, 115*(6), 403–408. doi:10.1111/j.1600-0404.2007.00823.x

Armulik, A., Genove, G., Mae, M., Nisancioglu, M. H., Wallgard, E., Niaudet, C., . . . Betsholtz, C. (2010). Pericytes regulate the blood–brain barrier. *Nature, 468*(7323), 557–561. doi:10.1038/nature09522

Arvanitakis, Z., Capuano, A. W., Leurgans, S. E., Bennett, D. A., & Schneider, J. A. (2016). Relation of cerebral vessel disease to Alzheimer's disease dementia and cognitive function in elderly people: A cross-sectional study. *Lancet Neurology, 15*(9), 934–943. doi:10.1016/S1474-4422(16)30029-1

Attwell, D., Mishra, A., Hall, C. N., O'Farrell, F. M., & Dalkara, T. (2016). What is a pericyte? *Journal of Cerebral Blood Flow & Metabolism, 36*(2), 451–455. doi:10.1177/0271678X15610340

Bell, R. D., Winkler, E. A., Singh, I., Sagare, A. P., Deane, R., Wu, Z., . . . Zlokovic, B. V. (2012). Apolipoprotein E controls cerebrovascular integrity via cyclophilin A. *Nature, 485*(7399), 512–516. doi:10.1038/nature11087

Blennow, K., Wallin, A., & Chong, J. K. (1995). Cerebrospinal fluid "neuronal thread protein" comes from serum by passage over the blood–brain barrier. *Neurodegeneration, 4*(2), 187–193.

Blennow, K., Wallin, A., Fredman, P., Karlsson, I., Gottfries, C. G., & Svennerholm, L. (1990). Blood-brain barrier disturbance in patients with Alzheimer's disease is related to vascular factors. *Acta Neurologica Scandinavica, 81*(4), 323–326.

Bowman, G. L., Kaye, J. A., Moore, M., Waichunas, D., Carlson, N. E., & Quinn, J. F. (2007). Blood-brain barrier impairment in Alzheimer disease: Stability and functional significance. *Neurology, 68*(21), 1809–1814. doi:10.1212/01.wnl.0000262031.18018.1a

Bowman, G. L., Kaye, J. A., & Quinn, J. F. (2012). Dyslipidemia and blood–brain barrier integrity in Alzheimer's disease. *Current Gerontology and Geriatrics Research, 2012*. doi:doi:10.1155/2012/184042

Bronge, L., & Wahlund, L. O. (2000). White matter lesions in dementia: An MRI study on blood–brain barrier dysfunction. *Dementia and Geriatric Cognitive Disorders, 11*(5), 263–267. doi:17248

Bu, G. (2009). Apolipoprotein E and its receptors in Alzheimer's disease: Pathways, pathogenesis and therapy. *Nature Reviews Neuroscience, 10*(5), 333–344. doi:10.1038/nrn2620

Cipolla, M. J. (2009). *The cerebral circulation*. San Rafael, CA: Morgan & Claypool.

de la Torre, J. C. (2017). Are major dementias triggered by poor blood flow to the brain? Theoretical considerations. *Journal of Alzheimer's Disease, 57*(2), 353–371. doi:10.3233/JAD-161266

Donahue, J. E., Flaherty, S. L., Johanson, C. E., Duncan, J. A., 3rd, Silverberg, G. D., Miller, M. C., . . . Stopa, E. G. (2006). RAGE, LRP-1, and amyloid-beta protein in Alzheimer's disease. *Acta Neuropathologica, 112*(4), 405–415. doi:10.1007/s00401-006-0115-3

Elovaara, I., Icen, A., Palo, J., & Erkinjuntti, T. (1985). CSF in Alzheimer's disease: Studies on blood–brain barrier function and intrathecal protein synthesis. *Journal of the Neurological Sciences, 70*(1), 73–80.

Erickson, M. A., & Banks, W. A. (2013). Blood–brain barrier dysfunction as a cause and consequence of Alzheimer's disease. *Journal of Cerebral Blood Flow & Metabolism, 33*(10), 1500–1513. doi:10.1038/jcbfm.2013.135

Farrall, A. J., & Wardlaw, J. M. (2009). Blood-brain barrier: ageing and microvascular disease: Systematic review and meta-analysis. *Neurobiology of Aging*, *30*(3), 337–352. doi:10.1016/j.neurobiolaging.2007.07.015

Frolich, L., Kornhuber, J., Ihl, R., Fritze, J., Maurer, K., & Riederer, P. (1991). Integrity of the blood-CSF barrier in dementia of Alzheimer type: CSF/serum ratios of albumin and IgG. *European Archives of Psychiatry and Clinical Neuroscience*, *240*(6), 363–366.

Halliday, M. R., Pomara, N., Sagare, A. P., Mack, W. J., Frangione, B., & Zlokovic, B. V. (2013). Relationship between cyclophilin a levels and matrix metalloproteinase 9 activity in cerebrospinal fluid of cognitively normal apolipoprotein e4 carriers and blood–brain barrier breakdown. *JAMA Neurology*, *70*(9), 1198–1200. doi:10.1001/jamaneurol.2013.3841

Hampel, H., Kotter, H. U., & Moller, H. J. (1997). Blood–cerebrospinal fluid barrier dysfunction for high molecular weight proteins in Alzheimer disease and major depression: Indication for disease subsets. *Alzheimer Disease and Associated Disorders*, *11*(2), 78–87.

Hanyu, H., Asano, T., Tanaka, Y., Iwamoto, T., Takasaki, M., & Abe, K. (2002). Increased blood–brain barrier permeability in white matter lesions of Binswanger's disease evaluated by contrast-enhanced MRI. *Dementia and Geriatric Cognitive Disorders*, *14*(1), 1–6. doi:58326

Heye, A. K., Culling, R. D., Valdes Hernandez Mdel, C., Thrippleton, M. J., & Wardlaw, J. M. (2014). Assessment of blood–brain barrier disruption using dynamic contrast-enhanced MRI: A systematic review. *NeuroImage Clinical*, *6*, 262–274. doi:10.1016/j.nicl.2014.09.002

Iadecola, C. (2004). Neurovascular regulation in the normal brain and in Alzheimer's disease. *Nature Reviews Neuroscience*, *5*(5), 347–360. doi:10.1038/nrn1387

Iadecola, C. (2013). The pathobiology of vascular dementia. *Neuron*, *80*(4), 844–866. doi:10.1016/j.neuron.2013.10.008

Iadecola, C. (2017). The neurovascular unit coming of age: a journey through neurovascular coupling in health and disease. *Neuron*, *96*(1), 17–42. doi:10.1016/j.neuron.2017.07.030

Iturria-Medina, Y., Sotero, R. C., Toussaint, P. J., Mateos-Perez, J. M., &Evans, A. C.; Alzheimer's Disease Neuroimaging Initiative. (2016). Early role of vascular dysregulation on late-onset Alzheimer's disease based on multifactorial data-driven analysis. *Nature Communications*, *7*, 11934. doi:10.1038/ncomms11934

Kay, A. D., May, C., Papadopoulos, N. M., Costello, R., Atack, J. R., Luxenberg, J. S., . . . Rapoport, S. I. (1987). CSF and serum concentrations of albumin and IgG in Alzheimer's disease. *Neurobiology of Aging*, *8*(1), 21–25.

Kisler, K., Nelson, A. R., Montagne, A., & Zlokovic, B. V. (2017). Cerebral blood flow regulation and neurovascular dysfunction in Alzheimer disease. *Nature Reviews Neuroscience*, *18*(7), 419–434. doi:10.1038/nrn.2017.48

Leonardi, A., Gandolfo, C., Caponnetto, C., Arata, L., & Vecchia, R. (1985). The integrity of the blood–brain barrier in Alzheimer's type and multi-infarct dementia evaluated by the study of albumin and IgG in serum and cerebrospinal fluid. *Journal of the Neurological Sciences*, *67*(2), 253–261.

Mecocci, P., Parnetti, L., Reboldi, G. P., Santucci, C., Gaiti, A., Ferri, C., . . . Senin, U. (1991). Blood-brain-barrier in a geriatric population: Barrier function in degenerative and vascular dementias. *Acta Neurologica Scandinavica*, *84*(3), 210–213.

Montagne, A., Barnes, S. R., Sweeney, M. D., Halliday, M. R., Sagare, A. P., Zhao, Z., . . . Zlokovic, B. V. (2015). Blood–brain barrier breakdown in the aging human hippocampus. *Neuron, 85*(2), 296–302. doi:10.1016/j.neuron.2014.12.032

Montagne, A., Nation, D. A., Pa, J., Sweeney, M. D., Toga, A. W., & Zlokovic, B. V. (2016). Brain imaging of neurovascular dysfunction in Alzheimer's disease. *Acta Neuropathologica, 131*(5), 687–707. doi:10.1007/s00401-016-1570-0

Nation, D. A., Sweeney, M. D., Montagne, A., Sagare, A. P., D'Orazio, L. M., Pachicano, M. . . . Zlokovic, B. V. (2019). Blood–brain barrier breakdown is an early biomarker of human cognitive dysfunction. *Nature Medicine*. 25(2), 270–276. doi:10.1038/s41591-018-0297-y

Rosenberg, G. A. (2014). Blood–brain barrier permeability in aging and Alzheimer's disease. *Journal of Prevention of Alzheimer's Disease, 1*(3), 138–139. doi:10.14283/jpad.2014.25

Sagare, A. P., Bell, R. D., Zhao, Z., Ma, Q., Winkler, E. A., Ramanathan, A., & Zlokovic, B. V. (2013). Pericyte loss influences Alzheimer-like neurodegeneration in mice. *Nature Commununication, 4*, 2932. doi:10.1038/ncomms3932

Sagare, A. P., Sweeney, M. D., Makshanoff, J., & Zlokovic, B. V. (2015). Shedding of soluble platelet-derived growth factor receptor-beta from human brain pericytes. *Neuroscience Letters, 607*, 97–101. doi:10.1016/j.neulet.2015.09.025

Shindo, H., Haruo, H., Shimizu, S. &, Iwamoto, T. (2005). Blood–brain barrier dysfunction in white matter lesions of elderly patients with dementia. *Tokyo Ika Daigaku Zasshi, 63*(5), 395–400.

Skoog, I., Wallin, A., Fredman, P., Hesse, C., Aevarsson, O., Karlsson, I., . . . Blennow, K. (1998). A population study on blood–brain barrier function in 85-year-olds: relation to Alzheimer's disease and vascular dementia. *Neurology, 50*(4), 966–971.

Starr, J. M., Farrall, A. J., Armitage, P., McGurn, B., & Wardlaw, J. (2009). Blood–brain barrier permeability in Alzheimer's disease: A case-control MRI study. *Psychiatry Research, 171*(3), 232–241. doi:10.1016/j.pscychresns.2008.04.003

Starr, J. M., Wardlaw, J., Ferguson, K., MacLullich, A., Deary, I. J., & Marshall, I. (2003). Increased blood–brain barrier permeability in type II diabetes demonstrated by gadolinium magnetic resonance imaging. *Journal of Neurology, Neurosurgery, and Psychiatry, 74*(1), 70–76.

Sweeney, M. D., Ayyadurai, S., & Zlokovic, B. V. (2016). Pericytes of the neurovascular unit: key functions and signaling pathways. *Nature Neuroscience, 19*(6), 771–783. doi:10.1038/nn.4288

Sweeney, M. D., Sagare, A. P., & Zlokovic, B. V. (2018). Blood–brain barrier breakdown in Alzheimer disease and other neurodegenerative disorders. *Nature Reviews Neurology, 14*(3), 133–150. doi:10.1038/nrneurol.2017.188

Taheri, S., Gasparovic, C., Huisa, B. N., Adair, J. C., Edmonds, E., Prestopnik, J., . . . Rosenberg, G. A. (2011). Blood–brain barrier permeability abnormalities in vascular cognitive impairment. *Stroke, 42*(8), 2158–2163. doi:10.1161/strokeaha.110.611731

Taheri, S., Gasparovic, C., Shah, N. J., & Rosenberg, G. A. (2011). Quantitative measurement of blood–brain barrier permeability in human using dynamic contrast-enhanced MRI with fast T1 mapping. *Magnetic Resonance Medicine, 65*(4), 1036–1042. doi:10.1002/mrm.22686

Tai, L. M., Thomas, R., Marottoli, F. M., Koster, K. P., Kanekiyo, T., Morris, A. W., & Bu, G. (2016). The role of APOE in cerebrovascular dysfunction. *Acta Neuropathologica, 131*(5), 709–723. doi:10.1007/s00401-016-1547-z

Toledo, J. B., Arnold, S. E., Raible, K., Brettschneider, J., Xie, S. X., Grossman, M., . . . Trojanowski, J. Q. (2013). Contribution of cerebrovascular disease in autopsy confirmed neurodegenerative disease cases in the National Alzheimer's Coordinating Centre. *Brain, 136*(Pt 9), 2697–2706. doi:10.1093/brain/awt188

Toth, P., Tarantini, S., Csiszar, A., & Ungvari, Z. (2017). Functional vascular contributions to cognitive impairment and dementia: mechanisms and consequences of cerebral autoregulatory dysfunction, endothelial impairment, and neurovascular uncoupling in aging. *American Journal of Physiology-Heart and Circulatory Physiology, 312*(1), H1–H20. doi:10.1152/ajpheart.00581.2016

van de Haar, H. J., Burgmans, S., Hofman, P. A., Verhey, F. R., Jansen, J. F., & Backes, W. H. (2015). Blood–brain barrier impairment in dementia: current and future in vivo assessments. *Neuroscience and Biobehavioral Revews, 49*, 71–81. doi:10.1016/j.neubiorev.2014.11.022

van de Haar, H. J., Burgmans, S., Jansen, J. F., van Osch, M. J., van Buchem, M. A., Muller, M., . . . Backes, W. H. (2016a). Blood-Brain Barrier Leakage in Patients with Early Alzheimer Disease. *Radiology, 281*(2), 527–535. doi:10.1148/radiol.2016152244

van de Haar, H. J., Burgmans, S., Jansen, J. F., van Osch, M. J., van Buchem, M. A., Muller, M., . . . Backes, W. H. (2016b). Blood–brain barrier leakage in patients with early Alzheimer disease. *Radiology*, 152244. doi:10.1148/radiol.2016152244

van de Haar, H. J., Jansen, J. F., van Osch, M. J., van Buchem, M. A., Muller, M., Wong, S. M., . . . Backes, W. H. (2016). Neurovascular unit impairment in early Alzheimer's disease measured with magnetic resonance imaging. *Neurobiology of Aging, 45*, 190–196. doi:10.1016/j.neurobiolaging.2016.06.006

Wada, H. (1998). Blood–brain barrier permeability of the demented elderly as studied by cerebrospinal fluid-serum albumin ratio. *Internal Medicine, 37*(6), 509–513.

Wallin, A., Sjogren, M., Edman, A., Blennow, K., & Regland, B. (2000). Symptoms, vascular risk factors and blood–brain barrier function in relation to CT white-matter changes in dementia. *European Neurology, 44*(4), 229–235.

Wang, H., Golob, E. J., & Su, M. Y. (2006). Vascular volume and blood–brain barrier permeability measured by dynamic contrast enhanced MRI in hippocampus and cerebellum of patients with MCI and normal controls. *Journal of Magnetic Resonance Imaging, 24*(3), 695–700. doi:10.1002/jmri.20669

Yamaguchi, K., Tanaka, Y., Kubo, H., Takagi, Y., Tachikawa, S., & Katsunuma, H. (1989). [Comparison between PVHIS on the MRI and the permeability of brain blood vessels in elderly patients]. *Nihon Ronen Igakkai Zasshi, 26*(6), 624–629.

Yan, L., Liu, C. Y., Wong, K. P., Huang, S. C., Mack, W. J., Jann, K., . . . Wang, D. J. J. (2018). Regional association of pCASL-MRI with FDG-PET and PiB-PET in people at risk for autosomal dominant Alzheimer's disease. *Neuroimage Clinical, 17*, 751–760. doi:10.1016/j.nicl.2017.12.003

Zlokovic, B. V. (2008). The blood–brain barrier in health and chronic neurodegenerative disorders. *Neuron, 57*(2), 178–201. doi:10.1016/j.neuron.2008.01.003

Zlokovic, B. V. (2011). Neurovascular pathways to neurodegeneration in Alzheimer's disease and other disorders. *Nature Reviews Neuroscience, 12*(12), 723–738. doi:10.1038/nrn3114

12

Arterial Stiffening and Cerebrovascular Resistance in Cognitive Decline and Alzheimer's Disease

Belinda Yew, Anna Blanken, and Daniel A. Nation

1. Overlap and Synergy of Alzheimer's and Vascular Pathologies

Alzheimer's disease (AD) is a progressive neurodegenerative disorder characterized by cerebral accumulation of amyloid β plaques and neurofibrillary tangles, which are thought to produce the neurodegeneration underlying deficits in memory, executive function, language, and ultimately other cognitive and behavioral domains (Ballard et al., 2011; Bondi et al., 2008). Vascular cognitive impairment, previously termed "vascular dementia" (VaD), entails cognitive decline due to discrete vascular brain injuries observed on clinical or radiological exams (Gorelick et al., 2011). In these cases, cognitive decline is often stepwise and must be temporally linked to onset and progression of cognitive impairment. Vascular cognitive impairment may be due to single or multiple strokes, as in strategic or multi-infarct dementias. Vascular cognitive impairment may also be due to more insidious progression of white matter lesions and/or progressive accumulation of cortical microinfarcts, subcortical microbleeds, and/or lacunar infarcts. In these cases, the corresponding damage to subcortical white and gray matter structures, along with the predisposition of the perforating arteries perfusing these subcortical regions to occult hypoperfusion events, often leads to frontal-subcortical impairment profiles characterized by slowed speed of processing, inattention, and executive dysfunction (Libon et al., 2014; Libon, Price, Davis Garrett, & Giovannetti, 2004; Reed et al., 2004).

Notably, cognitive decline with aging is often associated with both AD pathology and microvascular brain damage, the combination of which may increase risk for cognitive impairment (Arvanitakis, Capuano, Leurgans, Bennett, & Schneider, 2016; Chui et al., 2006; Gorelick et al., 2011; Toledo et al., 2013b). This overlap reflects ongoing ambiguity surrounding clinical distinction

Belinda Yew, Anna Blanken, and Daniel A. Nation, *Arterial Stiffening and Cerebrovascular Resistance in Cognitive Decline and Alzheimer's Disease* In: *Vascular Disease, Alzheimer's Disease, and Mild Cognitive Impairment.* Edited by: David J. Libon, Melissa Lamar, Rodney A. Swenson, Kenneth M. Heilman, Oxford University Press (2020).
DOI: 10.1093/oso/9780190634230.003.0013

between AD and vascular cognitive impairment. The latter is both clinically and neuropathologically heterogeneous, in that it may involve various forms of vascular brain injury, impacting a wide range of neuroanatomical regions and cognitive functions. Although patients with vascular brain injury exhibit a predilection for injury to frontal-subcortical structures that mediate executive functions, cortical and subcortical vascular lesions may disturb a variety of brain networks depending on the location of the injury. Vascular factors and cerebrovascular disease have been shown to increase risk and severity of symptoms of cognitive decline and dementia (Breteler, 2000; Hughes, Craft, & Lopez, 2015). Moreover, research has increasingly implicated vascular dysfunction in AD pathogenesis (Arvanitakis et al., 2016; Li et al., 2011).

Although AD is thought to be the most common cause of dementia in older adults, vascular lesions also occur at high rates in AD dementia, and there is increasing recognition of vascular contributions to both cognitive decline and the pathophysiological process underlying AD (Snyder et al., 2015; Toledo et al., 2013a; Zlokovic, 2011). In support of the importance of vascular factors, the risk for AD dementia is increased by the presence of cardiovascular risk factors, such as hypertension, diabetes, and dyslipidemia (Breteler, 2000; de la Torre, 2002; Schmidt, Schmidt, & Fazekas, 2000). Furthermore, midlife vascular risk factors predict the emergence of AD pathology decades later (Gottesman et al., 2017), and the presence of vascular risk factors has been linked to increased AD pathophysiology in older adults (Villeneuve et al., 2014).

The vast majority of AD cases are sporadic or late-onset AD variety but rarer genetic forms of AD, which show earlier age of onset, have been associated with autosomal dominant mutations in the presenilin-1 (*PSEN1*), amyloid precursor protein (*APP*) or presenilin-2 (*PSEN2*) genes (Bateman et al., 2012). Greatly increased rates of AD with early onset are also observed in Down's syndrome caused by trisomy 21 gene mutation (Cork, 1990). The dominant view has been that these genes cause AD through their well-established effects on cerebral amyloid production and cleavage. This is consistent with the amyloid cascade hypothesis of AD (Hardy & Higgins, 1992; Selkoe & Hardy, 2016). More recent findings, however, suggest that vascular lesions may predate the emergence of cerebral amyloidosis, even in autosomal dominant forms of the disease (Lee et al., 2016) and that previously unrecognized vascular lesions also occur in trisomy 21 (Drachman, Smith, Alkamachi, & Kane, 2017). The most potent genetic risk factor for the sporadic form of AD, the apolipoprotein (APOE)-ε4 allele, plays a key role in a wide variety of physiological processes relevant to brain function. Mounting research suggests, however, that it may also cause cognitive decline, at least in part, through cerebrovascular mechanisms (Bu, 2009; Tai et al., 2016). Finally, dramatic evidence from biomarker studies in late-onset AD indicates that markers of vascular dysfunction from magnetic resonance imaging (MRI) and biofluids are the earliest markers to show abnormality in older adults who ultimately progress to AD dementia (Iturria-Medina et al., 2016).

Despite these convergent findings implicating vascular factors in AD, it is well known that many AD patients appear to exhibit remarkable systemic health and show no evidence of traditional vascular risk factors or known vascular disease. Aging itself may be the most important risk factor for AD, as even the genetic forms of the disease are age-dependent, and the more common sporadic form shows increasing prevalence with each successive decade in late life. Thus, recent work has sought to investigate age-related changes in vascular function beyond traditional vascular risk factors, in an attempt to better understand how aging causes AD. Specifically, age-related changes in arterial stiffness and cerebral hemodynamics have emerged as potentially interesting contributing factors in cognitive aging and AD.

2. Pathophysiology of Arterial Stiffening

As we age there is a convergence of biomechanical and physiological processes that ultimately promote the loss of elastin fibers and their replacement with stiffer collagen fibers within the elastic lamina of the arterial wall (Zieman, Melenovsky, & Kass, 2005). These age-related changes in arterial elasticity predominantly affect the larger arteries, such as the aorta and carotid arteries, which are more compliant and contain relatively more elastin fibers than other arterial compartments. The stiffening of these larger arteries has a cascading effect on hemodynamic processes with far reaching implications for not only vascular health, but the health of other organs that depend on torrential blood flow for normal functioning (e.g., the kidneys and brain). These hemodynamic abnormalities can be sensitively measured and serve as surrogates of the arterial stiffening process.

With normally functioning vasculature, the compliance of larger vessels facilitates the steady perfusion of distal capillary beds through the so-called Windkessel effect (Nichols, O'Rourke, & Vlachopoulos, 2011). Cardiac contractions drive blood flow in pulse waves that must propagate through the arterial tree, but tissues require continuous and steady flow to function properly. The ability of the aorta and other large vessels to stretch and recoil with the passing of each pulse wave facilitates this transition by slowing and elongating the pulse wave, decreasing the amplitude of the wave when it reaches the microvasculature (Mitchell, 2004; Mitchell et al., 2011). Pulse waves are also reflected back to the heart by vessel walls. In a compliant aorta, this reflected wave dampens the amplitude of the subsequent wave, further facilitating a decrease in pulse wave amplitude while also allowing for improved filling of the coronary arteries, altogether aiding cardiac perfusion (Nichols et al., 2011).

Age-related degradation of elastin fibers within the aorta and its replacement with stiffer collagen fibers leads to an overall stiffening of larger vessels. This begins with the most elastic components of the proximal aorta before progressing distally through the aorta to other large arteries (e.g., carotid). The fluid mechanical result of large artery stiffening is decreased pulse wave buffering (i.e., Windkessel effect) and increased velocity of the pulse wave. The resulting change in pulse wave timing leads to several undesirable hemodynamic effects, including early return of the reflected waves. This causes augmentation rather than reduction of the subsequent pulse wave, impairing rather than facilitating filling of the coronary arteries (Mitchell, 2008; O'Rourke & Safar, 2005). Together these effects are thought to contribute to systolic hypertension and cardiac dysfunction, respectively, in older adults. Beyond the exacerbation of these traditional cardiovascular risk factors, increased pulse wave velocity (PWV) is thought to increase the risk of end organ damage, particularly in the highly perfused microvasculature of the kidneys and brain, by increasing the downstream amplitude of arterial pulsation (Mitchell, 2004; Mitchell et al., 2011).

The brain is also highly dependent upon local cerebrovascular autoregulation for adjustment of cerebral perfusion to meet neuronal metabolic needs (i.e., functional hyperemia). Dysfunction of these regulatory functions can lead to a mismatch between neuronal supply and demand, analogous to that observed in chronic heart disease, potentially causing neuronal dysfunction and subsequent cognitive decline. The brain receives up to 20% of cardiac output despite comprising only 2% of the body mass (Kisler, Nelson, Montagne, & Zlokovic, 2017; Zlokovic, 2011). The torrential blood flow required to support brain metabolic function and fill its estimated 400 miles of vascular territory suggests that it may be particularly vulnerable to hemodynamic abnormalities caused by arterial stiffening. In particular, increased PWV, amplitude, and oscillation may place undue stress on the brain's arteriolar network, which provides the majority of the resistance to blood flow and protects the delicate capillary beds from potentially disruptive hemodynamic forces. This suggests that arterial stiffening may play a causal role in the observed increases in cerebral small vessel disease in older adults.

3. Markers of Arterial Stiffening

Arterial stiffening can be measured noninvasively via various indices of pulse wave timing and velocity. PWV measures the speed at which the pressure wave travels across a specified distance, ideally between two points along the same artery. This approach relies upon proximity of the target artery to the body's surface, making it difficult to directly measure the pulse wave in larger, deeper vessels such as the aorta. Aortic stiffness is thus estimated using pulse wave measurement obtained at branching arteries. Carotid-femoral PWV (cfPWV), for example, is determined by measuring pulse wave transit time from the carotid artery branch to the femoral artery, via the aorta. More specifically, time is measured from the end of diastole when the "foot" of the pulse wave departs the carotid artery to the time at which the wave foot reaches the femoral artery. PWV is then calculated by dividing the distance between the carotid and femoral sampling points by this transit time. Brachial-ankle PWV (baPWV) is similarly calculated by measuring the time taken for the pulse wave to propagate from the brachial artery branch to the tibial artery. The distance between these arteries is then divided by the recorded transit time to calculate baPWV. Currently, cfPWV represents the "gold standard" for measuring arterial stiffness (Gorelick et al., 2011; Laurent et al., 2006) and has been shown to predict cardiovascular events (Boutouyrie et al., 2002; Laurent et al., 2001; Sutton-Tyrrell et al., 2005), particularly in older adults (McEniery et al., 2005). Differences between PWV assessment sites (e.g., carotid-femoral vs. brachial-ankle) may influence relationships between arterial stiffening and cognitive impairment (van Sloten et al., 2015). For example, cfPWV appears to index central artery stiffening, where baPWV may be more indicative of peripheral artery resistance (Pase, Herbert, Grima, Pipingas, & O'Rourke, 2012).

4. Arterial Stiffening and Cognitive Decline

Given prior links between arterial stiffening and cerebrovascular disease (Mitchell, 2008; Mitchell et al., 2011; O'Rourke & Safar, 2005; Tzourio, Laurent, & Debette, 2014; van Sloten et al., 2015), the contribution of arterial stiffening to cognitive decline, cardiac and cerebrovascular events, and dementia has been increasingly studied. For example, arterial stiffening appears to be involved in cerebral small vessel disease, as evidenced by greater incidence of white matter hyperintensities, cerebral microbleeds, and lacunar infarcts in individuals with higher pulse pressure (Poels et al., 2010; Tsao et al., 2013; Verhaaren et al., 2013). Furthermore, microvascular damage seems to play a role in development of cognitive impairment (Mitchell et al., 2011). Pulse pressure also influences cerebral perfusion (Qiu, Winblad, Viitanen, & Fratiglioni, 2003), abnormalities in which have been linked to incipient and later-stage AD (Bangen et al., 2012; Mattson et al., 2014).

Both measures of arterial stiffening (i.e., elevated pulse pressure and increased PWV) have been related to cognitive decline and risk of dementia (Fujiwara et al.,

2005; Mitchell et al., 2011; Poels et al., 2007; Waldstein et al., 2008). However, it remains unclear whether arterial stiffening directly causes cognitive impairment or exacerbates existing neurodegenerative processes. It is also possible that dementia and arterial stiffening share a common etiology. Research exploring relationships between pulse pressure and cognitive decline in older adults has yielded mixed results. Cross-sectional studies reveal significant negative association between pulse pressure and global measures of cognitive dysfunction (Davis, Massman, & Doody, 2003; Fujiwara et al., 2005; Robbins, Elias, Elias, & Budge, 2005), memory (Davis et al., 2003; Mitchell et al., 2011; Pase et al., 2013; Robbins et al., 2005; Tsao et al., 2013), processing speed (Pase et al., 2013; Robbins et al., 2005), attention, and executive functions (Davis et al., 2003; Pase et al., 2013) in nonclinical middle aged populations. In contrast, a number of studies report superior global and domain-specific cognitive functioning in AD or very old (i.e., >85 years of age) subjects with higher pulse pressure. This may reflect the ameliorative effect of higher blood pressure in individuals with incomplete white matter infarctions that would otherwise impede cerebral blood flow (CBF) and, in turn, cognition. Alternatively, cases with worse cognitive performance may experience abnormally low blood pressure (Davis et al., 2003; Molander, Gustafson, & Lovheim, 2010; van Bruchem-Visser, Mattace-Raso, & van der Cammen, 2009). Certainly, it has been suggested that neural structures compromised in AD are also involved in blood pressure regulation (Skoog, 2003).

Support for links between arterial stiffening and cognitive decline is also evident in longitudinal studies. Waldstein and colleagues (2008), for example, found higher pulse pressure to be associated with greater cognitive decline over time. More specifically, individuals with elevated baseline pulse pressure experienced declines in performance on verbal and nonverbal learning and memory tests, as well as a screening test for memory and concentration impairment (Blessed information–memory–concentration test). Furthermore, pulse pressure increases over time were accompanied by decreases in working memory performance. McFall et al. (2014) and Yasar, Ko, Nothelle, et al. (2011) reported consistent results, with worse executive function observed for older adults exhibiting higher pulse pressure. As in the cross-sectional findings, however, some studies revealed positive associations between pulse pressure and cognitive performance in very old individuals (i.e., age 85 and older; Sabayan et al., 2012). One community-based study also reported a U-shaped association between pulse pressure and cognitive decline in older adult subjects without dementia, suggesting that subjects with very low or very high pulse pressure had increased risk of AD and dementia (Qiu et al., 2003).

Although peripheral pulse pressure represents a useful estimate of arterial stiffness, it is difficult to obtain such blood pressure measurements at central sites, including the aorta (Lehmann, 2000), where the earliest stages of arterial stiffening are observed (O'Rourke, Safar, & Dzau, 2010). PWV, however, offers a noninvasive means of indexing stiffening in these regions, and has been shown to predict coronary blood flow (Lehmann, 1999). Higher PWV has been observed in patients with cardiovascular risk (Boutouyrie et al., 2002; Laurent et al., 2001) or preclinical cardiovascular disease (Mattace-Raso et al., 2006; Sutton-Tyrrell et al., 2005). Several studies investigating links between arterial stiffening and cognitive decline have indicated that PWV but not pulse pressure correlates with cross-sectional or longitudinal cognitive function after adjusting for mean arterial pressure (MAP), heart rate, and cardiovascular risk factors (Poels et al., 2007). Similarly, cases with higher PWV but not pulse pressure exhibited greater white matter hyperintensity volume and presence of lacunar infarcts (Henskens et al., 2008). Moreover, consistent associations between both baPWV and cfPWV with white matter lesion burden have been shown by several other research groups in healthy and hypertensive adults (Coutinho, Turner, & Kullo, 2011; Hatanaka et al., 2011; Mitchell et al., 2011).

Associations between PWV and cognition have been investigated in a number of populations. Hanon and colleagues (2005) demonstrated higher PWV in individuals with MCI than non-impaired subjects, and higher PWV in VaD and AD participants than individuals without cognitive impairment. Likewise, Rabkin and Jarvie's (2011) meta-analysis revealed higher PWV in VaD patients compared to AD and cognitively normal participants. Finally, one study detected no significant PWV differences between VaD, AD, and controls but found greater vascular stiffening in VaD relative to other groups when different measures (i.e., reduced central arterial compliance, increased augmentation index) were employed (Dhoat, Ali, Bulpitt, & Rajkumar, 2008).

In cross-sectional studies, increased PWV was related to poorer cognitive functioning on a test of global cognition in cognitively impaired and cognitively normal older adults (Fukuhara et al., 2006; Hanon et al., 2005; Zhong et al., 2014). Likewise, Nilsson and colleagues (2014) showed a significant non-linear relationship between PWV and longitudinal global cognition, largely driven by individuals with high (i.e., 90th percentile) PWV (Nilsson et al., 2014). Higher PWV in both cognitively impaired and cognitively normal individuals has also been associated with worse verbal learning (Zhong et al., 2014), memory (Elias et al., 2009; Mitchell et al., 2011; Tarumi & Zhang, 2014), executive functioning (Elias et al., 2009; Lim et al., 2016; Tarumi & Zhang, 2014; Zhong et al., 2014), and processing speed (Elias et al., 2009; Mitchell et al., 2011). Furthermore, higher PWV was also linked to worse memory impairment in hypertensive older adults with subjective memory complaints (Kearney-Schwartz et al., 2009).

Building upon cross-sectional findings, PWV has been investigated as a predictor of cognitive decline over time. Benetos et al. (2012), for example, identified increased PWV as a predictor of global cognitive decline in older adults over a 1-year period, independent of age, education, and blood pressure. Two additional studies reported that adults free of dementia and cardiovascular disease but with higher baseline PWV showed progressive cognitive decline in domains of verbal learning, recall, nonverbal memory, and a global cognitive screening measure (Scuteri et al., 2013; Waldstein et al., 2008). Watson and colleagues (2011) reported a longitudinal association of higher PWV with declines in global functioning and psychomotor speed over 6 years. Similarly, Scuteri et al. (2013) indicated that subjects with elevated PWV, white matter lesions, and hypotension showed significantly worse declines in global cognition. In a prospective study over 9 years, individuals with greater PWV-indexed arterial stiffening demonstrated worse declines in global cognition. Furthermore, subjects in the highest PWV tertile exhibited faster declines than those with lower PWV (Zeki Al Hazzouri et al., 2013). Poels and colleagues (2007), however, did not find significant associations between PWV and cognitive decline, possibly due to their employment of a younger sample with superior cardiovascular health.

5. Arterial Stiffening and Alzheimer's Pathology

The in vivo markers of AD pathophysiological process include (a) cerebrospinal fluid (CSF) assays for amyloid β ($A\beta_{1\text{-}42}$) and phosphorylated tau (p-tau), (b) positron emission tomography (PET) with amyloid and tau ligands (e.g., florbetapir, Pittsburgh compound B [PiB]), or ^{18}F-AV-1451). Although definitive diagnosis awaits postmortem neuropathological confirmation of amyloid plaques and neurofibrillary tangles, the most recent research recommendations for AD diagnosis have emphasized the equivalence of in vivo biomarkers and postmortem findings (Jack et al., 2016).

Greater arterial stiffening, as measured by PWV, predicted greater PET PiB-indexed cerebral amyloidosis, both concurrently (Hughes et al., 2013) and 2 years later in older adults (Hughes et al., 2014). These relationships were independent of blood pressure and apolipoprotein (APOE)-ε4 status, and demonstrated an additive effect of PWV on both amyloid deposition and white matter lesion burden (Hughes et al., 2013, 2014). A related study in younger adults found higher PWV correlated with diminished white and gray matter integrity, in areas previously linked to AD (Maillard et al., 2016). There is thus a growing body of PWV research linking arterial stiffening to AD pathology.

Additional support is provided by studies employing brachial artery pulse pressure. Nation, Edland et al. (2013) detected positive associations between pulse pressure and CSF p-tau, as well as negative associations between pulse pressure and CSF $A\beta_{1\text{-}42}$ in older adults. In a later study using a separate sample from the Alzheimer's Disease Neuroimaging Initiative (ADNI), pulse pressure was found to be elevated in older adults across the normal aging MCI spectrum who were biomarker positive for CSF p-tau. Interestingly, among the very old participants (i.e., aged 80–91), those exhibiting positive biomarker status for both CSF $A\beta_{1\text{-}42}$ and p-tau had dramatically higher pulse pressure levels (>10 mmHg). Among the very old, those with pulse pressure elevation (>63 mmHg) progressed to dementia more rapidly. Importantly, these relationships remained significant after controlling for age, sex, APOE-ε4 status, body mass index, vascular risk factors, and use of antihypertensive medications (Nation et al., 2015). PET studies have also detected greater cerebral amyloidosis in individuals with higher pulse pressure (Langbaum et al., 2012; Rodrigue et al., 2013). Collectively, these results suggest that arterial stiffening may contribute to amyloid retention in the brain, possibly due to impaired facilitation of amyloid clearance by arterial pulsation (Weller, Subash, Preston, Mazanti, & Carare, 2008).

6. Cerebral Blood Flow and Alzheimer's Disease

The contributions of arterial stiffening to AD may operate through hemodynamic consequences for CBF, neurovascular coupling and their regulatory mechanisms. Notably, the evolution of CBF research in AD has been hugely influenced by available methods for assessing CBF in humans.

6.1. Transcranial Doppler Ultrasound

Earlier studies of CBF primarily employed transcranial Doppler (TCD) ultrasonography, a noninvasive technique wherein high frequency sound waves are applied to the areas of skull presenting least distortion (e.g., temples). Ultrasound wave echoes (i.e., reverberation as signals bounce off blood cells) were then measured to determine speed and direction of blood flow through large intracranial arteries. Differences between emitted and echo frequencies are proportionate to velocity of CBF (Aaslid, Markwalder, & Nornes, 1982). Thus, by applying fast Fourier transformation to the signal, data can be presented graphically. Specifically, velocity (i.e., frequency) is plotted against time, with signal magnitude (i.e., amplitude) expressed as brightness. The maximum velocity for a given cardiac cycle can then be identified and averaged across cardiac cycles to determine mean CBF velocity (Stroobant & Vingerhoets, 2000).

Earlier work indicated that older adults exhibiting lower CBF velocity, experienced greater cognitive decline over a proceeding 6.5 year period, as well as greater amygdala and hippocampal atrophy (Ruitenberg et al., 2005). Similarly, individuals with VaD or AD demonstrated reduced CBF relative to cognitively normal controls, consistent with vessel narrowing and increased vascular resistance (Schreiber, Doepp, Spruth, Kopp, & Valdueza, 2005). A later study of individuals with cerebral amyloid angiopathy revealed direct associations between Alzheimer's pathology and impaired cerebrovascular function. Specifically, cerebral amyloid angiopathy patients demonstrated delayed onset and slower velocity of CBF response compared to healthy controls during a visual task (Smith et al., 2008). TCD research has thus implicated reductions of CBF in cognitive decline and neurodegenerative disease.

Although TCD is an affordable, noninvasive method of CBF monitoring with high temporal resolution, a major limitation is the need for an appropriate bone window through which the vessel of interest can be insonated. This precludes a significant portion of individuals from study. Beyond this reduction in potential study participants, the main weakness of TCD is its relatively low spatial resolution. Frequency differences between emitted and reflected ultrasound signal are not determined by CBF velocity alone; blood flow direction relative to ultrasound signal also influences frequency differences. Since this angle can only be loosely approximated, TCD-estimated CBF velocity is generally inexact (Naqvi, Yap, Ahmad, & Ghosh, 2013). More recent TCD variants (e.g., those incorporating angle-independent dual-beam flow) have significantly improved accuracy (Wintermark et al., 2005), but spatial resolution is still further compromised by restriction of TCD to accessible parts of larger intracranial vessels. Blood flow through smaller arterioles often fails to produce detectable velocity increases in the larger vessels to which TCD is applied. Detection of CBF to vessels and regions beyond larger arteries is thus unfeasible, preventing assessment of small vessel disease (Duschek & Schandry, 2003; Stroobant & Vingerhoets, 2000). Importantly, sites of highest blood pressure variation across vascular compartments, and therefore highest vascular resistance, lie at the transition of arterioles into capillaries (Nichols, O' Rourke, & Vlachopoulos, 2011). The improved spatial resolution of magnetic resonance imaging (MRI) methods is thus necessary for comprehensive evaluation of cerebrovascular changes.

6.2. Arterial Spin Labeling Magnetic Resonance Imaging

Arterial spin labeling (ASL) MRI offers a more direct gauge of CBF through measurement of magnetized arterial blood water. By applying a radiofrequency pulse to a volume of arterial blood proximal to, yet earlier in the arterial tree than, the region of interest, net magnetization of the blood water is inverted and water molecules are "labeled." When labeled blood enters the brain region of interest, it is exchanged with tissue water, altering overall tissue magnetization, and resulting in reduced magnetic resonance signal. At this point, a "tag" image is taken and compared to a control image in which blood is not labeled. The resulting perfusion image therefore reflects the amount of arterial blood delivered to each voxel of interest within a specified time period (Wang, 2014).

In recent years ASL has been increasingly applied to aging research. Several studies have reported CBF abnormalities in patients with AD and MCI (Alsop, Dai, Grossman, & Detre, 2010; Wang, 2014), beyond reductions merely attributable to the decreased need for CBF accompanying neurodegeneration (Niedermeyer, 2006). Decreased CBF in AD patients relative to healthy controls, for example, has been observed in brain regions implicated in AD (e.g., inferior temporal cortex, precuneus, and posterior cingulate; Alsop, Detre, & Grossman, 2000; Asllani et al., 2008; Yoshiura et al., 2009). Regional hypoperfusion also correlates with global cognition (Alsop et al., 2010), cerebral amyloidosis, and brain atrophy (Mattson et al., 2014). Furthermore, CBF decreases in inferior parietal, posterior cingulate, and precuneus areas are exhibited by individuals with MCI (Chao et al., 2009; Dai et al., 2009; Johnson et al., 2005), implicating CBF changes in early disease processes.

Interestingly, CBF *increases* have also been identified in AD cases, predominantly in medial temporal regions (Alsop, Casement, de Bazelaire, Fong, & Press, 2008; Dai et al., 2009). Some MCI samples have shown hyperperfusion in similar brain areas, as well as the striatum (Dai et al., 2009; Fleisher et al., 2009). Such hyperperfusion may reflect compensatory increases in neural activity, inflammation, and/or vasodilator production in response to AD disease processes. Indeed, CBF increases for both AD and preclinical AD cases have been primarily reported (Alsop et al., 2008) for regions associated with sites of earliest tissue loss in AD (Matsuda et al., 2002). Alternatively, brain hyperperfusion may drive AD pathogenesis (Cohen et al., 2009). In any case, hyperperfusion sites overlap with major cerebrovasculature (Alsop et al., 2008), consistent with proposed vascular origins of AD (Iadecola & Davisson, 2008).

7. Cerebrovascular Resistance and Alzheimer's Disease

As previously reviewed, changes in both blood pressure and CBF have been implicated in AD. Specifically, midlife hypertension has been linked to elevated AD risk in later life (Qiu, Winblad, & Fratiglioni, 2005), highlighting the importance of chronic hypertension in disease development. There is, however, also evidence that low later-life blood pressure may increase risk of dementia in the very old (i.e., individuals over 80), suggesting that the influence of blood pressure on AD may be dependent upon other physiological and health-related factors (Qiu et al., 2005). Contributions of CBF to AD are similarly ambiguous, with both hypoperfusion and hyperperfusion implicated in AD pathogenesis.

Despite the importance of blood pressure in determining CBF, as well as the clear links between AD pathology and both blood pressure and CBF (Mattsson et al., 2014; Nation, Wierenga et al., 2013; Nation et al., 2015; Rodrigue et al., 2013), the vast majority of studies examining CBF in AD have ignored the contribution of blood pressure. Interactions between blood pressure and CBF have received only cursory attention, with one study connecting baseline blood pressure to later declines in CBF (Deverdun et al., 2016) and another indicating that combined low blood pressure and low CBF may increase risk for cortical atrophy (den Heijer et al., 2003). No comprehensive model, however, has been proposed to explain why both high and low blood pressure, or high and low CBF, would be related to AD risk, nor how blood pressure and CBF alterations in AD may be connected.

The tendency within the field to ignore contributions of blood pressure to CBF may be partly attributable to the fact that cerebral autoregulation enables constant CBF across a wide range of blood pressure values (e.g., arterial pressures from 60–150 mmHg), even in pathological aging (Paulson, Strandgaard, & Edvinsson, 1990). Although it is known that chronic hypertension may shift this autoregulatory curve "rightward," potentially placing the brain at increased risk for cerebral hypoperfusion during dips in blood pressure, Alzheimer's research has focused largely on CBF without consideration of blood pressure. Indeed, the stability facilitated by these autoregulatory processes has led some investigators to conclude that blood pressure does not meaningfully influence CBF in typical older adults. More recently, however, the concept of cerebrovascular resistance (CVR) has sparked interest in blood pressure as an important agent in cerebrovascular function. As shown in Box 12.1, CVR is the ratio of cerebral perfusion pressure (P_α) to CBF, where P_α is MAP—intracranial pressure. The relationship between blood vessel diameter (i.e., vessel radius, *r*), and CBF is also influenced by vessel length (θ) and blood viscosity (η), as described by Poiseuille's law (see Equation 12.2). Notably, CBF is proportional to the radius of the vessel to the fourth power, reflecting the profound changes in CBF that accompany even

Box 12.1 Cerebrovascular Resistance and Regulation of Blood Flow

[1] Cerebral perfusion pressure (P_α) $= \text{MAP} - \text{ICP}$

(Reger et al.) Cerebrovascular resistance $= \frac{P_\alpha}{\text{CBF}} \approx \frac{\text{MAP}}{\text{CBF}}$

The relationship between blood vessel diameter (or radius, r) and CBF is also influenced by vessel length (θ) and blood viscosity (η)

[3] Blood flow $= \frac{\Delta BP \times \pi \times r^4}{8 \times \eta \times \theta}$

modest changes in vessel diameter. Combined with the fact that θ and η are of a relatively stable nature, CBF changes are thus largely determined by vessel radius (Buxton, 2009).

The relationship between blood vessel diameter (or radius, *r*) and CBF is also influenced by vessel length (θ) and blood viscosity (η).

As can be observed by examining Equation 12.2 and Figure 12.1, CBF is maintained across wide fluctuations in blood pressure through dynamic changes in CVR. Blood pressure increases elicit vasoconstriction, reducing vessel diameter. Conversely, blood pressure decreases trigger vasodilation and subsequent enlargement of vessel diameter (Buxton, 2009). Examination of CBF and blood pressure separately may therefore mask dramatic changes in CVR needed to maintain steady CBF in the face of dramatic blood pressure changes.

Although cerebral perfusion is influenced by a number of highly complex mechanisms, animal studies indicate that vascular resistance in the brain is

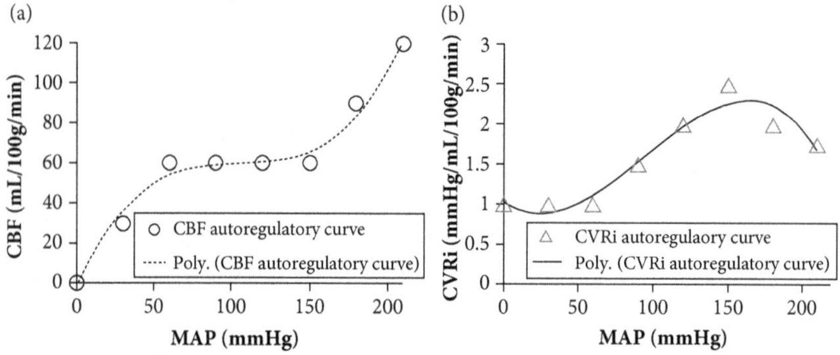

Figure 12.1. (A) A mathematical model is displayed for the standard cerebral autoregulatory curve (dashed black line with open circles), which is flat (set at cerebral blood flow [CBF] of roughly 50 mL/100g/minute) across a broad blood pressure range (roughly between mean arterial pressure [MAP] of 60 and 150 mmHg). This lack of correlation between blood pressure and CBF within a broad blood pressure range has led some investigators to ignore blood pressure and focus exclusively on CBF. (B) A superimposed model of the Cardiovascular Risk Index curve (between MAP of 60 to 150 mmHg) from the same hypothetical data set is shown (solid black line with open triangles). It can be seen that resistance is dynamic across the 60 to 150 mmHg range, increasing with increased blood pressure as CBF remains static, and dropping precipitously above this range due to autoregulatory "breakthrough." The models illustrate how focusing only on CBF and ignoring blood pressure actually masks dynamic cerebrovascular changes. These changes in vascular resistance represent the primary mechanism by which the cerebrovasculature is able to maintain constant flow across such a broad blood pressure range.

predominantly generated by the cerebral arterioles (Cox, Woolsey, & Rovainen, 1993; Ngai, Ko, Morii, & Winn, 1988). Arteriolar vessels are ideally situated for this task as they project between medium- to large-sized arteries and the rich microvascular network of delicate capillary beds. These small but muscular arterioles are capable of stemming CBF at a set point through constriction and dilation of vascular smooth muscle cells during blood pressure increases and decreases, respectively. Vasoconstriction and vasodilation of vascular smooth muscle cells are influenced by local flow as well as various moderating factors such as extrinsic autonomic innervation, carbon dioxide pressure, and perivascular macrophages, the product of which is steady downstream perfusion at safe pressure (Iadecola, 2004; Nichols et al., 2011). Downstream of arterioles, the capillary neurovascular unit also contributes to modulation of resistance. Specifically, capillary vasodilation instigates increases in flow velocity, prompting upstream sheer stress elevation, which in turn triggers endothelial and eventual arteriolar dilation for further increases in blood flow to the capillary network (Iadecola, 2004; Kisler, Nelson, Montagne, & Zlokovic, 2017). Notably, regional increases in blood supply may supplement resting CBF to meet the metabolic demand of local neuronal activation. Homeostatic CBF is primarily, however, controlled by cerebrovascular mechanisms.

These autoregulatory processes are largely resistant to effects of aging and AD (Zazulia, Videen, Morris, & Powers, 2010). However, a "rightward shift" in the autoregulatory curve is often observed in older adults, such that the range of blood pressure values across which CBF can be maintained now encompasses higher pressures. This adaptive response fundamentally entails an increase in cerebrovascular resistance to offset the chronic hypertension and the risk of mechanical injury to the cerebrovasculature. An undesirable consequence is the diminished capacity for CBF regulation at lower pressures, which can leave the brain more vulnerable to hypoperfusion when hypotension occurs (Paulson et al., 1990; van Beek, Claassen, Rikkert, & Jansen, 2008). Consistent with this, cerebrovascular autoregulation in response to more acute changes appears impaired in AD despite relatively intact static autoregulation (Meel-van den Abeelen, Lagro, van Beek, & Claassen, 2014; Niwa et al., 2002). Deficits in acute cerebrovascular autoregulation may reflect subtle changes to cerebrovasculature through which pathological aging occurs. Examination of CVR may thus be imperative to understanding of mechanisms through which AD arises.

7.1. Transcranial Doppler and Cerebrovascular Resistance in AD

More recent work employing TCD has highlighted the influence of blood pressure on reported CBF changes (Roher et al., 2011). Several studies have detected elevated CVR estimates in AD patients compared to those of cognitively normal adults, across various cerebral arteries (Claassen, Levine, & Zhang, 2009; Gommer et al., 2012; Rivera-Rivera et al., 2016; van Beek, Sijbesma, Jansen, Olde Rikkert, & Claassen, 2010, 2012). AD-associated impairments in cerebrovascular autoregulation have also been observed in MCI samples, with higher CVR estimates observed in MCI cases who later converted to AD relative to nonconverters (Gommer et al., 2012). Gommer et al. (2016) also linked higher CVR to increased whole-brain and medial temporal atrophy, linking CVR elevation to neurodegeneration. Some TCD investigations have failed to detect AD differences in CVR, possibly due to "over-filtering" of vascular dysfunction from samples (Meel-van den Abeelen et al., 2014; Shim et al., 2015). Nevertheless, TCD research has identified repeated, albeit nondefinitive, increases in CVR. This is consistent with suggested disruption to vascular autoregulatory mechanisms.

7.2. Arterial Spin Labeling and Cerebrovascular Resistance in AD

As with TCD, ASL-based research has increasingly recognized the contribution of blood pressure to blood flow, as well as its role in broader cerebrovascular autoregulation. ASL research in healthy older adults has identified increased CVR in very old versus young old individuals, using CVR as well as pulse pressure-based estimates of CVR. In regions typically affected by AD (e.g., middle temporal and parietal areas), very old participants demonstrated higher CVR than their younger counterparts. Furthermore, higher regional CVR was also accompanied by poorer cognitive performance and greater white matter lesion volume (Clark et al., 2015; Nation, Wierenga et al., 2013). More recent work has evaluated cerebrovascular compliance, which indexes vessel elasticity and is therefore inversely related to cerebrovascular resistance. Compliance is the change in blood volume divided by the change in pressure (see Equation 12.4). Yan and colleagues (2016) found that greater compliance predicted increased CBF but decreased with vessel size. Similar findings have been reported using an alternative method to index vascular compliance by measuring the change in cerebral vessel diameter over a cardiac cycle (Warnert, Murphy, Hall, & Wise, 2015). The observed changes in arterial compliance are consistent with known increases in resistance—the opposite of compliance—as larger arteries transition to smaller arterioles (Nichols et al., 2011). Resistance (R), shown in Equation 12.5, is calculated as the change in pressure as blood moves from larger to smaller blood 0vessels (ΔP), divided by blood flow per unit of time (Q).

[4]
$$C = \frac{\Delta V}{\Delta P}$$

[5]
$$\mathrm{R} = \frac{\Delta \mathrm{P}}{\mathrm{Q}}$$

ASL-indexed CVR has been increasingly explored in AD patients, with CVR elevations in AD exceeding CBF in magnitude and sensitivity. Higher CVR has been detected in AD relative to cognitively normal and MCI cases, across frontal, parietal, and medial temporal brain regions (Nation, Wierenga et al., 2013; Yew & Nation, 2017). Evidence for cerebrovascular dysfunction in AD has also been found in studies of CVR in conditions commonly regarded as precursors to dementia. Individuals diagnosed with MCI exhibited increased CVR compared to cognitively normal older adults for various neural regions (Liu et al., 2014; Nation, Wierenga et al., 2013), with elevations in subcortical areas proportionate to deficits in global cognition and greater white matter disease (Nation, Wierenga et al., 2013). Increased CVR was also observed in individuals exhibiting early pathological changes (i.e., elevated amyloid load) relative to amyloid-negative controls. Furthermore, even in nondemented cases, higher CVR across various brain regions predicted greater and faster-declining global cognition over a 2-year period. In the same study, elevated hippocampal and prefrontal lobe CVR predicted worse declines in memory and executive function, respectively. Moreover, individuals exhibiting elevated baseline inferior temporal CVR were characterized by greater amyloid load 4 years later and worse brain atrophy 2 years later. CVR in a number of brain regions also predicted elevated likelihood of later dementia above and beyond cerebral amyloid load (Yew & Nation, 2017). CVR elevations in preclinical and early-stage AD cases appear to be intermediate (i.e., higher than that of controls but lower than that of AD patients), consistent with suggestions that CVR increases parallel and contribute to disease progression (Nation, Wierenga et al., 2013; Yew & Nation, 2017). Crucially, observed CVR differences were observed in more regions and at earlier disease stages than CBF itself (Nation, Wierenga et al., 2013; Yew & Nation, 2017), suggesting that resistance increases represent more sensitive markers of early pathological change than blood flow alone. It remains unclear whether the observed changes in cerebrovascular stiffness and resistance are purely due to downstream hemodynamic effects from central artery stiffening or whether there is an actual primary change in the cerebrovasculature itself. It is also difficult to know from MRI studies alone whether the changes in cerebrovascular resistance and compliance represent functional changes in terms of vessel contractility or whether there is an actual change in the stiffness of the intracranial vessels or perhaps even cerebral arterioles. At least one neuropathological study did identify age-related changes to the internal elastic lamina of intracranial vessels in autopsy material from patients with AD dementia, and these changes were linked to regional amyloid deposition (Gutierrez et al., 2016). Further studies are needed to characterize the molecular and structural events in the cerebrovasculature that lead to increased vessel resistance and compliance so that potential therapeutic targets may be identified.

8. Cerebrovascular Resistance in the Pathogenesis of Alzheimer's Disease

Given mounting evidence for cerebrovascular contributions to Alzheimer's pathogenesis, various mechanisms through which AD may arise have been proposed. Greater resistance of vessels can, for example, decrease pulsation amplitude and consequently capacity for amyloid drainage (Weller et al., 2008). Disruption of autoregulatory processes may similarly impede brain lymphatic function, further impairing clearance capacity (Iliff, Goldman, & Nedergaard, 2015; Nedergaard, 2013). With increasing amyloid accumulation, plaque formation and white matter disease are more likely, further promoting Alzheimer's symptomatology (Bell et al., 2009; Qiu et al., 2005; Weller, Boche, & Nicoll, 2009). Amyloidosis beyond a certain severity can also give rise to structural changes in vessel walls (e.g., loss of smooth muscle cells) and neurotoxicity caused by amyloid oligomers, further obstructing blood and perivascular fluid flow (Weller et al., 2008; Zlokovic, 2011). In addition, amyloid-driven vasotoxicity itself may induce further vasoconstriction (Han et al., 2015).

Amid even mild CBF declines, protein synthesis is disrupted, impeding synaptic plasticity crucial for memory formation (Mies, Ishimaru, Xie, Seo, & Hossmann, 1991). More substantial CBF declines may instigate hypoxia, hampering enzymatic activity necessary for initiation of action potentials and disturbing brain pH, electrolyte, and water gradient homeostasis. With prolonged disturbance, the brain is rendered vulnerable to white matter lesion and neurotoxicity, including pathophysiological hallmarks of AD (i.e., accumulation of amyloid-β and hyperphosphorylated tau; Zlokovic, 2011). Ischemic hypoxia, for example, promotes activation of amyloid-β producing enzymes (Guglielmotto et al., 2009), while decreasing amyloid-β degrading enzyme neprilysin (Wang et al., 2011). These enzymatic changes may be exacerbated by hypoxia-driven alterations to genes underlying maintenance of cerebrovascular endothelium. This can, in turn, trigger deterioration of cerebral blood vessels and CBF deregulation (Chow et al., 2007; Wu et al., 2005). As cerebrovascular function is increasingly disrupted, cognitive deficits arise, followed and exacerbated by the neuronal loss that characterizes later-stage AD (Iadecola & Davisson, 2008).

There is growing evidence to suggest that cerebral amyloidosis may represent only part of the AD picture, alongside sizeable contributions from vascular dysfunction (de la Torre, 2002; Zlokovic, 2011). The outlined research reveals deficient cerebrovascular autoregulation (Meel-van den Abeelen et al., 2014; Niwa et al., 2002) and consequent CBF (Bangen et al., 2012; Mattson et al., 2014) in both AD and conditions associated with elevated risk for AD. These changes appear to be the result of arterial stiffening, the onset of which may predate and/or operate in conjunction with amyloid retention (Hughes et al., 2014; Nation, Wierenga et al., 2013; Yew & Nation, 2017). Taken together, these findings implicate arterial stiffening in the changes (e.g., cerebral amyloidosis, tau hyperphosphorylation, and hypoperfusion) that characterize early stages of AD pathogenesis (Montagne et al., 2016; Weller et al., 2008; Zlokovic, 2011). Future research and therapeutic efforts may therefore benefit from further investigation of these areas.

References

Aaslid, R., Markwalder, T.-M., & Nornes, H. (1982). Noninvasive transcranial Doppler ultrasound recording of flow velocity in basal cerebral arteries. *Journal of Neurosurgery*, *57*(6), 769–774. doi:10.3171/jns.1982.57.6.0769

Alsop, D. C., Casement, M., de Bazelaire, C., Fong, T., & Press, D. Z. (2008). Hippocampal hyperperfusion in Alzheimer's disease. *NeuroImage*, *42*(4), 1267–1274.

Alsop, D. C., Dai, W., Grossman, M., & Detre, J. A. (2010). Arterial spin labeling blood flow MRI: Its role in the early characterization of Alzheimer's disease. *Journal of Alzheimer's Disease*, *20*(3), 871–880.

Alsop, D. C., Detre, J. A., & Grossman, M. (2000). Assessment of cerebral blood flow in Alzheimer's disease by spin-labeled magnetic resonance imaging. *Annals of Neurology*, *47*(1), 93–100. doi:10.1002/1531-8249(200001)47:1<93::aid-ana15>3.0.co;2-8

Arvanitakis, Z., Capuano, A. W., Leurgans, S. E., Bennett, D. A., & Schneider, J. A. (2016). Relation of cerebral vessel disease to Alzheimer's disease dementia and cognitive function in elderly people: A cross-sectional study. *Lancet Neurology*, *15*(9), 934–943. doi:10.1016/s1474-4422(16)30029-1

Asllani, I., Habeck, C., Scarmeas, N., Borogovac, A., Brown, T. R., & Stern, Y. (2008). Multivariate and univariate analysis of continuous arterial spin labeling perfusion MRI in Alzheimer's disease. *Journal of Cerebral Blood Flow & Metabolism*, *28*, 725–736.

Ballard, C., Gauthier, S., Corbett, A., Brayne, C., Aarsland, D., & Jones, E. (2011). Alzheimer's disease. *Lancet*, *377*(9770), 1019–1031.

Bangen, K. J., Restom, K., Liu, T. T. T., Wierenga, C. E., Jak, A. J., Salmon, D. P., & Bondi, M. W. (2012). Assessment of Alzheimer's disease risk with functional magnetic resonance imaging: An arterial spin labeling study. *Journal of Alzheimer's Disease*, *31*(0), S59–S74.

Bateman, R. J., Xiong, C., Benzinger, T. L., Fagan, A. M., Goate, A., Fox, N. C., . . . Morris, J. C.; Dominantly Inherited Alzheimer Network. (2012). Clinical and biomarker changes in dominantly inherited Alzheimer's disease. *New England Journal of Medicine, 367*(9), 795–804. doi:10.1056/NEJMoa1202753

Bell, R. D., Deane, R., Chow, N., Long, X., Sagare, A., Singh, I., . . . Zlokovic, B. V. (2009). SRF and myocardin regulate LRP-mediated amyloid-beta clearance in brain vascular cells. *Nature Cell Biology, 11*(2), 143.

Benetos, A., Watfa, G., Hanon, O., Salvi, P., Fantin, F., Toulza, O., . . . Gautier, S. (2012). Pulse wave velocity is associated with 1-year cognitive decline in the elderly older than 80 years: The PARTAGE study. *Journal of the American Medical Directors Association, 13*(3), 239–243. doi:10.1016/j.jamda.2010.08.014

Bondi, M. W., Jak, A. J., Delano-Wood, L., Jacobson, M. W., Delis, D. C., & Salmon, D. P. (2008). Neuropsychological contributions to the early identification of Alzheimer's disease. *Neuropsychology Review, 18*(1), 73–90. doi:10.1007/s11065-008-9054-1

Boutouyrie, P., Tropeano, A. I., Asmar, R., Gautier, I., Benetos, A., Lacolley, P., & Laurent, S. (2002). Aortic stiffness is an independent predictor of primary coronary events in hypertensive patients: A longitudinal study. *Hypertension, 39*(1), 10–15.

Breteler, M. M. B. (2000). Vascular risk factors for Alzheimer's disease: An epidemiologic perspective. *Neurobiology of Aging, 21*(2), 153–160.

Bu, G. (2009). Apolipoprotein E and its receptors in Alzheimer's disease: Pathways, pathogenesis, and therapy. *Nature Reviews Neuroscience, 10*, 333–344.

Buxton, R. (2009). *An introduction to functional magnetic resonance imaging: Principles and techniques* (2nd ed.). New York, NY: Cambridge University Press.

Chao, L. L., Pa, J., Duarte, A., Schuff, N., Weiner, M. W., Kramer, J. H., . . . Johnson, J. K. (2009). Patterns of cerebral hypoperfusion in amnestic and dysexecutive MCI. *Alzheimer's Disease and Associated Disorders, 23*, 245–252.

Chow, N., Bell, R. D., Deane, R., Streb, J. W., Chen, J., Brooks, A., . . . Zlokovic, B. V. (2007). Serum response factor and myocardin mediate arterial hypercontractility and cerebral blood flow dysregulation in Alzheimer's phenotype. *Proceedings of the National Academy of Sciences of the United States of America, 104*(3), 823–828. doi:10.1073/pnas.0608251104

Chui, H. C., Zarow, C., Mack, W. J., Ellis, W. G., Zheng, L., Jagust, W. J., . . . Vinters, H. V. (2006). Cognitive impact of subcortical vascular and Alzheimer's disease pathology. *Annals of Neurology, 60*(6), 677–687.

Claassen, J. A. H. R., Levine, B. D., & Zhang, R. (2009). Dynamic cerebral autoregulation during repeated squat-stand maneuvers. *Journal of Applied Physiology, 106*(1), 153–160.

Clark, L. R., Nation, D. A., Wierenga, C. E., Bangen, K. J., Dev, S. I., Shin, D. D., . . . Bondi, M. W. (2015). Elevated cerebrovascular resistance index is associated with cognitive dysfunction in the very-old. *Alzheimer's Research & Therapy, 7*(1), 1–9. doi:10.1186/s13195-014-0080-3

Cohen, A. D., Price, J. C., Weissfeld, L. A., James, J., Rosario, B. L., Bi, W., . . . Klunk, W. E. (2009). Basal cerebral metabolism may modulate the cognitive effects of Abeta in mild cognitive impairment: An example of brain reserve. *Journal of Neuroscience, 29*(47), 14770. doi:10.1523/jneurosci.3669-09.2009

Cork, L. C. (1990). Neuropathology of Down syndrome and Alzheimer disease. *American Journal of Medical Genetics–Part A, 7*, 282–286.

Coutinho, T., Turner, S. T., & Kullo, I. J. (2011). Aortic pulse wave velocity is associated with measures of subclinical target organ damage. *JACC Cardiovasc Imaging, 4*(7), 754–761. doi:10.1016/j.jcmg.2011.04.011

Cox, S. B., Woolsey, T. A., & Rovainen, C. M. (1993). Localized dynamic changes in cortical blood flow with whisker stimulation corresponds to matched vascular and neuronal architecture of rat barrels. *Journal of Cerebral Blood Flow & Metabolism*, *13*(6), 899–913.

Dai, W. Y., Lopez, O. L., Carmichael, O. T., Becker, J. T., Kuller, L. H., & Gachm, H. M. (2009). Mild cognitive impairment and Alzheimer disease: Patterns of altered cerebral blood flow at MR imaging. *Radiology*, *250*, 856–866.

Davis, R. N., Massman, P. J., & Doody, R. S. (2003). Effects of blood pressure on neuropsychological functioning in Alzheimer's disease. *Archives of Clinical Neuropsychology*, *18*(1), 19–32.

de la Torre, J. C. (2002). Alzheimer disease as a vascular disorder: Nosological evidence. *Stroke*, *33*, (9), 2147–2148.

den Heijer, T., Skoog, I., Oudkerk, M., de Leeuw, F., de Groot, J. C., Hofman, A., & Breteler, M. M. (2003). Association between blood pressure levels over time and brain atrophy in the elderly. *Neurobiology of Aging*, *24*(2), 307–313.

Deverdun, J., Akbaraly, T. N., Charroud, C., Abdennour, M., Brickman, A. M., Chemouny, S., . . . Menjot de Champfleur, N. (2016). Mean arterial pressure change associated with cerebral blood flow in healthy older adults. *Neurobiology of Aging*, *46*, 49–57. doi:10.1016/j.neurobiolaging.2016.05.012

Dhoat, S., Ali, K., Bulpitt, C. J., & Rajkumar, C. (2008). Vascular compliance is reduced in vascular dementia and not in Alzheimer's disease. *Age & Ageing*, *37*(6), 653–659. doi:10.1093/ageing/afn158

Drachman, D. A., Smith, T. W., Alkamachi, B., & Kane, K. (2017). Microvascular changes in Down syndrome with Alzheimer-type pathology: Insights into a potential vascular mechanism for Down syndrome and Alzheimer's disease. *Alzheimer's & Dementia*, *13*(12), 1389–1396. doi:10.1016/j.jalz.2017.05.003

Duschek, S., & Schandry, R. (2003). Functional transcranial Doppler sonography as a tool in psychophysiological research. *Psychophysiology*, *40*(3), 436–454. doi:10.1111/1469-8986.00046

Elias, M. F., Robbins, M. A., Budge, M. M., Abhayaratna, W. P., Dore, G. A., & Elias, P. K. (2009). Arterial pulse wave velocity and cognition with advancing age. *Hypertension*, *53*(4), 668–673. doi:10.1161/HYPERTENSIONAHA.108.126342

Fleisher, A. S., Podraza, K. M., Bangen, K. J., Taylor, C., Sherzai, A., Sidhar, K., . . . Buxton, R. B. (2009). Cerebral perfusion and oxygenation differences in Alzheimer's disease risk. *Neurobiology of Aging*, *30*(11), 1737–1748.

Fujiwara, Y., Chaves, P. H., Takahashi, R., Amano, H., Yoshida, H., Kumagai, S., . . . Shinkai, S. (2005). Arterial pulse wave velocity as a marker of poor cognitive function in an elderly community-dwelling population. *Journals of Gerontology. Series A, Biological Sciences and Medical Sciences*, *60*(5), 607–612.

Fukuhara, M., Matsumura, K., Ansai, T., Takata, Y., Sonoki, K., Akifusa, S., . . . Takehara, T. (2006). Prediction of cognitive function by arterial stiffness in the very elderly. *Circulation Journal*, *70*(6), 756–761.

Gommer, E. D., Martens, E. G., Aalten, P., Shijaku, E., Verhey, F. R., Mess, W. H., . . . Reulen, J. P. (2012). Dynamic cerebral autoregulation in subjects with Alzheimer's disease, mild cognitive impairment, and controls: Evidence for increased peripheral vascular resistance with possible predictive value. *Journal of Alzheimer's Disease*, *30*, 805–813.

Gorelick, P. B., Scuteri, A., Black, S. E., Decarli, C., Greenberg, S. M., Iadecola, C., . . . Seshadri, S. (2011). Vascular contributions to cognitive impairment and dementia: A statement for healthcare professionals from the American Heart Association/American Stroke Association. *Stroke, 42*(9), 2672–2713.

Gorelick, P. B., Scuteri, A., Black, S. E., Decarli, C., Greenberg, S. M., Iadecola, C., . . . Seshadri, S.; American Heart Association Stroke Council, Council on Epidemiology and Prevention, Council on Cardiovascular Nursing, Council on Cardiovascular Radiology and Intervention, and Council on Cardiovascular Surgery and Anesthesia. (2011). Vascular contributions to cognitive impairment and dementia: A statement for healthcare professionals from the American Heart Association/American Stroke Association. *Stroke, 42*(9), 2672–2713. doi:10.1161/STR.0b013e3182299496

Gottesman, R. F., Schneider, A. L., Zhou, Y., Coresh, J., Green, E., Gupta, N., . . . Mosley, T. H. (2017). Association between midlife vascular risk factors and estimated brain amyloid deposition. *JAMA, 317*(14), 1443–1450. doi:10.1001/jama.2017.3090

Guglielmotto, M., Aragno, M., Autelli, R., Giliberto, L., Novo, E., Colombatto, S., . . . Tabaton, M. (2009). The up-regulation of BACE1 mediated by hypoxia and ischemic injury: Role of oxidative stress and HIF1α. *Journal of Neurochemistry, 108*(4), 1045–1056. doi:10.1111/j.1471-4159.2008.05858.x

Gutierrez, J., Honig, L., Elkind, M. S., Mohr, J. P., Goldman, J., Dwork, A. J., . . . Marshall, R. S. (2016). Brain arterial aging and its relationship to Alzheimer dementia. *Neurology, 86*(16), 1507–1515. doi:10.1212/WNL.0000000000002590

Han, B. H., Zhou, M.-l., Johnson, A. W., Singh, I., Liao, F., Vellimana, A. K., . . . Zipfel, G. J. (2015). Contribution of reactive oxygen species to cerebral amyloid angiopathy, vasomotor dysfunction, and microhemorrhage in aged Tg2576 mice. *Proceedings of the National Academy of Sciences, 112*(8), E881–E890.

Hanon, O., Haulon, S., Lenoir, H., Seux, M.-L., Rigaud, A.-S., Safar, M., . . . Forette, F. (2005). Relationship between arterial stiffness and cognitive function in elderly subjects with complaints of memory loss. *Stroke, 36*(10), 2193–2197. doi:10.1161/01.STR.0000181771.82518.1c

Hardy, J. A., & Higgins, G. A. (1992). Alzheimer's disease: The amyloid cascade hypothesis. *Science, 256*(5054), 184–185.

Hatanaka, R., Obara, T., Watabe, D., Ishikawa, T., Kondo, T., Ishikura, K., . . . Imai, Y. (2011). Association of arterial stiffness with silent cerebrovascular lesions: The Ohasama Study. *Cerebrovascular Diseases, 31*(4), 329–337. doi:10.1159/000322599

Henskens, L. H., Kroon, A. A., van Oostenbrugge, R. J., Gronenschild, E. H., Fuss-Lejeune, M. M., Hofman, P. A., . . . de Leeuw, P. W. (2008). Increased aortic pulse wave velocity is associated with silent cerebral small-vessel disease in hypertensive patients. *Hypertension, 52*(6), 1120–1126. doi:10.1161/HYPERTENSIONAHA.108.119024

Hughes, T. M., Craft, S., & Lopez, O. L. (2015). Review of "The potential role of arterial stiffness in the pathogenesis of Alzheimer's disease." *Neurodegenerative Disease Management, 5*(2), 121–135. doi:10.2217/nmt.14.53

Hughes, T. M., Kuller, L. H., Barinas-Mitchell, E. J., Mackey, R. H., McDade, E. M., Klunk, W. E., . . . Lopez, O. L. (2013). Pulse wave velocity is associated with beta-amyloid deposition in the brains of very elderly adults. *Neurology, 81*(19), 1711–1718. doi:10.1212/01.wnl.0000435301.64776.37

Hughes, T. M., Kuller, L. H., Barinas-Mitchell, E. M., McDade, E. M., Klunk, W. E., Cohen, A. D., . . . Lopez, O. L. (2014). Arterial stiffness and β-amyloid progression in nondemented elderly adults. *JAMA Neurology, 71*(5), 562–568. doi:10.1001/jamaneurol.2014.186

Iadecola, C. (2004). Neurovascular regulation in the normal brain and in Alzheimer's disease. *Nature Reviews Neuroscience, 5*, 347–360.

Iadecola, C., & Davisson, R. L. (2008). Hypertension and cerebrovascular dysfunction. *Cell Metabolism, 7*, 476–484.

Iliff, J. J., Goldman, S. A., & Nedergaard, M. (2015). Implications of the discovery of brain lymphatic pathways. *Lancet. Neurology, 14*(10), 977–979. doi:10.1016/s1474-4422(15)00221-5

Iturria-Medina, Y., Sotero, R. C., Toussaint, P. J., Mateos-Perez, J. M., & Evans, A. C.; Alzheimer's Disease Neuroimaging Initiative. (2016). Early role of vascular dysregulation on late-onset Alzheimer's disease based on multifactorial data-driven analysis. *Nature Communications, 7*, 11934. doi:10.1038/ncomms11934

Jack, C. R., Jr., Bennett, D. A., Blennow, K., Carrillo, M. C., Feldman, H. H., Frisoni, G. B., . . . Dubois, B. (2016). A/T/N: An unbiased descriptive classification scheme for Alzheimer disease biomarkers. *Neurology, 87*(5), 539–547.

Johnson, N. A., Jahng, G., Weiner, M. W., Miller, B. L., Chui, H. C., Jagust, W. J., . . . Schuff, N. (2005). Pattern of cerebral hypoperfusion in Alzheimer disease and mild cognitive impairment measured with arterial spin-labeling MR imaging: Initial experience. *Radiology, 234*(3), 851–859.

Kearney-Schwartz, A., Rossignol, P., Bracard, S., Felblinger, J., Fay, R., Boivin, J. M., . . . Zannad, F. (2009). Vascular structure and function is correlated to cognitive performance and white matter hyperintensities in older hypertensive patients with subjective memory complaints. *Stroke, 40*(4), 1229–1236. doi:10.1161/strokeaha.108.532853

Kisler, K., Nelson, A. R., Montagne, A., & Zlokovic, B. V. (2017). Cerebral blood flow regulation and neurovascular dysfunction in Alzheimer disease. *Nature Reviews Neuroscience, 18*(7), 419–434. doi:10.1038/nrn.2017.48

Langbaum, J. B. S., Chen, K., Launer, L. J., Fleisher, A. S., Lee, W., Liu, X., . . . Reiman, E. M. (2012). Blood pressure is associated with higher brain amyloid burden and lower glucose metabolism in healthy late middle-age persons. *Neurobiology of Aging, 33*(4), 827.e811–827.e819.

Laurent, S., Boutouyrie, P., Asmar, R., Gautier, I., Laloux, B., Guize, L., . . . Benetos, A. (2001). Aortic stiffness is an independent predictor of all-cause and cardiovascular mortality in hypertensive patients. *Hypertension, 37*(5), 1236–1241.

Laurent, S., Cockcroft, J., Bortel, L. V., Boutouyrie, P., Giannattasio, C., Hayoz, D., . . . Struijker-Boudier, H.; European Network for Non-Invasive Investigation of Large Arteries. (2006). Expert consensus document on arterial stiffness: Methodological issues and clinical applications. *European Heart Journal*, 27(21), 2588–2605. doi:10.1093/eurheartj/ehl254

Lee, S., Viqar, F., Zimmerman, M. E., Narkhede, A., Tosto, G., Benzinger, T. L., . . . Brickman, A. M.; Dominantly Inherited Alzheimer Network. (2016). White matter hyperintensities are a core feature of Alzheimer's disease: Evidence from the dominantly inherited Alzheimer network. *Annals of Neurology, 79*(6), 929–939. doi:10.1002/ana.24647

Lehmann, E. D. (1999). Clinical value of aortic pulse-wave velocity measurement. *Lancet, 354*, 528–529.

Lehmann, E. D. (2000). Aortic pulse-wave velocity versus pulse pressure and pulse-wave analysis. *Lancet, 355*(9201), 412. doi:10.1016/S0140-6736(05)74040-X

Li, J., Wang, Y. J., Zhang, M., Xu, Z. Q., Gao, C. Y., Fang, C. Q., . . . Zhou, H.D.; Chongqing Ageing Study Group. (2011). Vascular risk factors promote conversion from mild cognitive impairment to Alzheimer disease. *Neurology, 76*(17), 1485–1491.

Libon, D. J., Drabick, D. A. G., Giovannetti, T., Price, C. C., Bondi, M. W., Eppig, J., . . . Swenson, R. (2014). Neuropsychological syndromes associated with Alzheimer's/vascular dementia: A latent class analysis. *Journal of Alzheimer's Disease, 42*(3), 999–1014. doi:10.3233/JAD-132147

Libon, D. J., Price, C. C., Davis Garrett, K., & Giovannetti, T. (2004). From Binswanger's disease to leuokoaraiosis: What we have learned about subcortical vascular dementia. *Clinical Neuropsychologist, 18*(1), 83–100. doi:10.1080/13854040490507181

Lim, S. L., Gao, Q., Nyunt, M. S., Gong, L., Lunaria, J. B., Lim, M. L., . . . Ng, T. P. (2016). Vascular health indices and cognitive domain function: Singapore Longitudinal Ageing Studies. *Journal of Alzheimer's Disease, 50*(1), 27–40. doi:10.3233/jad-150516

Liu, J., Zhu, Y.-S., Khan, M. A., Brunk, E., Martin-Cook, K., Weiner, M. F., . . . Zhang, R. (2014). Global brain hypoperfusion and oxygenation in amnestic mild cognitive impairment. *Alzheimer's & Dementia, 10*(2), 162–170.

Maillard, P., Mitchell, G. F., Himali, J. J., Beiser, A., Tsao, C. W., Pase, M. P., . . . DeCarli, C. (2016). Effects of arterial stiffness on brain integrity in young adults from the Framingham Heart Study. *Stroke, 47*(4), 1030–1036. doi:10.1161/strokeaha.116.012949

Matsuda, H., Kitayama, N., Ohnishi, T., Asada, T., Nakano, S., Sakamoto, S., . . . Katoh, A. (2002). Longitudinal evaluation of both morphologic and functional changes in the same individuals with Alzheimer's disease. *Journal of Nuclear Medicine, 43*, 304–311.

Mattace-Raso, F. U., van der Cammen, T. J., Hofman, A., van Popele, N. M., Bos, M. L., Schalekamp, M. A., . . . Witteman, J. C. (2006). Arterial stiffness and risk of coronary heart disease and stroke. *Circulation, 113*(5), 657–663. doi:10.1161/CIRCULATIONAHA.105.555235

Mattson, N., Tosun, D., Insel, P. S., Simonson, A., Jack, C. R., Beckett, L. A., . . . Weiner, M. W. (2014). Association of brain amyloid-ß with cerebral perfusion and structure in Alzheimer's disease and mild cognitive impairment. *Brain, 137*, 1550–1561.

Mattsson, N., Tosun, D., Insel, P. S., Simonson, A., Jack, C. R., Jr., Beckett, L. A., . . . Weiner, M. W.; Alzheimer's Disease Neuroimaging Initiative. (2014). Association of brain amyloid-beta with cerebral perfusion and structure in Alzheimer's disease and mild cognitive impairment. *Brain, 137*(Pt 5), 1550–1561. doi:10.1093/brain/awu043

McEniery, C. M., Yasmin, Hall, I. R., Qasem, A., Wilkinson, I. B., & Cockcroft, J. R. (2005). Normal vascular aging: differential effects on wave reflection and aortic pulse wave velocity: The Anglo-Cardiff Collaborative Trial (ACCT). *Journal of the American College of Cardiology, 46*(9), 1753–1760. doi:10.1016/j.jacc.2005.07.037

McFall, G. P., Wiebe, S. A., Vergote, D., Jhamandas, J., Westaway, D., & Dixon, R. A. (2014). IDE (rs6583817) polymorphism and pulse pressure are independently and interactively associated with level and change in executive function in older adults. *Psychology and Aging, 29*(2), 418. doi:10.1037/a0034656

Meel-van den Abeelen, A. S., Lagro, J., van Beek, A. H., & Claassen, J. A. (2014). Impaired cerebral autoregulation and vasomotor reactiity in sporadic Alzheimer's disease. *Current Alzheimer Research, 11*, 11–17.

Mies, G., Ishimaru, S., Xie, Y., Seo, K., & Hossmann, K. A. (1991). Ischemic thresholds of cerebral protein synthesis and energy state following middle cerebral artery occlusion in rat. *Journal of Cerebral Blood Flow & Metabolism, 11*(5), 753–761.

Mitchell, G. F. (2004). Changes in arterial stiffness and wave reflection with advancing age in healthy men and women. *Hypertension, 43*(6), 1239–1245.

Mitchell, G. F. (2008). Effects of central arterial aging on the structure and function of the peripheral vasculature: Implications for end-organ damage. *Journal of Applied Physiology, 105*(5), 1652–1660.

Mitchell, G. F., Buchem, M. A. v., Sigurdsson, S., Gotal, J. D., Jonsdottir, M. K., Kjartansson, Ó., . . . Launer, L. J. (2011). Arterial stiffness, pressure and flow pulsatility and brain structure and function: The Age, Gene/Environment Susceptibility—Reykjavik Study. *Brain, 134*(Pt 11): 3398–3407. doi:10.1093/brain/awr253

Molander, L., Gustafson, Y., & Lovheim, H. (2010). Low blood pressure is associated with cognitive impairment in very old people. *Dementia and Geriatric Cognitive Disorders, 29*(4), 335–341. doi:10.1159/000289821

Montagne, A., Nation, D. A., Pa, J., Sweeney, M. D., Toga, A. W., & Zlokovic, B. V. (2016). Brain imaging of neurovascular dysfunction in Alzheimer's disease. *Acta Neuropathology, 131*(5), 687–707. doi:10.1007/s00401-016-1570-0

Naqvi, J., Yap, K. H., Ahmad, G., & Ghosh, J. (2013). Transcranial Doppler ultrasound: A review of the physical principles and major applications in critical care. *International Journal of Vascular Medicine, 2013*, 1–13.

Nation, D. A., Edland, S. D., Bondi, M. W., Salmon, D. P., Delano-Wood, L., Peskind, E. R., . . . Galasko, D. R. (2013). Pulse pressure is associated with Alzheimer biomarkers in cognitively normal older adults. *Neurology, 81*, 2024–2027.

Nation, D. A., Edmonds, E. C., Bangen, K. J., Delano-Wood, L., Scanlon, B. K., Han, S. D., . . . Bondi, M. W. Alzheimer's Disease Neuroimaging Initiative. (2015). Pulse pressure in relation to tau-mediated neurodegeneration, cerebral amyloidosis, and progression to dementia in very old adults. *JAMA Neurology, 72*(5), 546–553. doi:10.1001/jamaneurol.2014.4477

Nation, D. A., Wierenga, C. E., Clark, L. R., Dev, S. I., Stricker, N. H., Jak, A. J., . . . Bondi, M. W. (2013). Cortical and subcortical cerebrovascular resistance index in mild cognitive impairment and Alzheimer's disease. *Journal of Alzheimer's Disease, 36*, 689–698.

Nedergaard, M. (2013). Garbage truck of the brain. *Science, 340*(6140), 1529.

Ngai, A. C., Ko, K. R., Morii, S., & Winn, H. R. (1988). Effect of sciatic nerve stimulation on pial arterioles in rats. *American Journal of Physiology, 254*, H133–H139.

Nichols, W., O'Rourke, M., & Vlachopoulos, C. (Eds.). (2011). *McDonald's blood flow in arteries: Theoretical, experimental and clinical principles* (6th ed.). London, England: Taylor & Francis Group.

Nichols, W. M., O' Rourke, M. F., & Vlachopoulos, C. (2011). *McDonald's blood flow in arteries*. Boca Raton, FL: CRC Press.

Niedermeyer, E. (2006). Alzheimer disease: Caused by primary deficiency of the cerebral blood flow. *Clinical EEG and Neuroscience, 37*(3), 175–177.

Nilsson, E. D., Elmstahl, S., Minthon, L., Nilsson, P. M., Pihlsgard, M., Tufvesson, E., & Nagga, K. (2014). Nonlinear association between pulse wave velocity and cognitive function: A population-based study. *Journa Hypertension, 32*(11), 2152–2157; discussion 2157. doi:10.1097/hjh.0000000000000329

Niwa, K., Kazama, K., Younkin, L., Younkin, S. G., Carlson, G. A., & Iadecola, C. (2002). Cerebrovascular autoregulation is profoundly impaired in mice overexpressing amyloid precursor protein. *American Journal of Physiology-Heart and Circulatory Physiology, 283*, H315–H323.

O'Rourke, M. F., & Safar, M. E. (2005). Relationship between aortic stiffening and microvascular disease in brain and kidney. *Hypertension, 46*(1), 200–204. doi:10.1161/01.HYP.0000168052.00426.65

O'Rourke, M. F., Safar, M. E., & Dzau, V. (2010). The Cardiovascular Continuum extended: Aging effects on the aorta and microvasculature. *Vascular Medicine, 15*(6), 461–468.

Pase, M. P., Herbert, A., Grima, N. A., Pipingas, A., & O'Rourke, M. F. (2012). Arterial stiffness as a cause of cognitive decline and dementia: A systematic review and meta-analysis. *Internal Medicine Journal, 42*(7), 808–815. doi:10.1111/j.1445-5994.2011.02645.x

Pase, M. P., Stough, C., Grima, N. A., Harris, E., Macpherson, H., Scholey, A. B., & Pipingas, A. (2013). Blood pressure and cognitive function. *Psychological Science, 24*(11), 2173–218. doi:10.1177_0956797613488602

Paulson, O. B., Strandgaard, S., & Edvinsson, L. (1990). Cerebral autoregulation. *Cerebrovascular and Brain Metabolism Reviews, 2,* 161–192.

Poels, M. M., van Oijen, M., Mattace-Raso, F. U., Hofman, A., Koudstaal, P. J., Witteman, J. C. M., & Breteler, M. M. (2007). Arterial stiffness, cognitive decline, and risk of dementia. *Stroke, 38*(3), 888–892. doi:10.1161/01.STR.0000257998.33768.87

Poels, M. M., Vernooij, M. W., Ikram, M. A., Hofman, A., Krestin, G. P., van der Lugt, A., & Breteler, M. M. (2010). Prevalence and risk factors of cerebral microbleeds. *Stroke, 41*(10 Suppl), S103–S106. doi:10.1161/STROKEAHA.110.595181

Qiu, C., Winblad, B., & Fratiglioni, L. (2005). The age-dependent relation of blood pressure to cognitive function and dementia. *Lancet Neurology, 4*(8), 487–499.

Qiu, C., Winblad, B., Viitanen, M., & Fratiglioni, L. (2003). Pulse pressure and risk of Alzheimer disease in persons aged 75 years and older: a community-based, longitudinal study. *Stroke, 34*(3), 594–599. doi:10.1161/01.str.0000060127.96986.f4

Rabkin, S. W., & Jarvie, G. (2011). Comparison of vascular stiffness in vascular dementia, Alzheimer dementia and cognitive impairment. *Blood Pressure, 20*(5), 274–283. doi:10.3109/08037051.2011.566246

Reed, B. R., Eberling, J. L., Mungas, D., Weiner, M., Kramer, J. H., & Jagust, W. J. (2004). Effects of white matter lesions and lacunes on cortical function. *Archives of Neurology, 61*(10), 1545–1550.

Rivera-Rivera, L. A., Turski, P., Johnson, K. M., Hoffman, C., Berman, S. E., Kilgas, P., . . . Wieben, O. (2016). 4D flow MRI for intracranial hemodynamics assessment in Alzheimer's disease. *Journal of Cerebral Blood Flow & Metabolism, 36*(10), 1718–1730.

Robbins, M. A., Elias, M. F., Elias, P. K., & Budge, M. M. (2005). Blood pressure and cognitive function in an African-American: The Maine–Syracuse Study. *Psychosomatic Medicine, 67*(5), 707–714.

Rodrigue, K. M., Rieck, J. R., Kennedy, K. M., Devous, M. D., Sr., Diaz-Arrastia, R., & Park, D. C. (2013). Risk factors for beta-amyloid deposition in healthy aging: Vascular and genetic effects. *JAMA Neurology, 70*(5), 600–606. doi:10.1001/jamaneurol.2013.1342

Roher, A. E., Garami, A., Tyas, S. L., Maarouf, C. L., Kokjohn, T. A., Belohlavek, M., . . . Emmerling, M. R. (2011). Transcranial Doppler ultrasound blood flow velocity and pulsatility index as systemic indicators for Alzheimer's disease. *Alzheimer's & Dementia, 7*(4), 445–455.

Ruitenberg, A., den Heijer, T., Bakker, S. L., van Swieten, J. C., Koudstaal, P. J., Hofman, A., & Breteler, M. M. (2005). Cerebral hypoperfusion and clinical onset of dementia: The Rotterdam Study. *Annals of Neurology, 57*(6), 789–794. doi:10.1002/ana.20493

Sabayan, B., Oleksik, A. M., Maier, A. B., van Buchem, M. A., Poortvliet, R. K., de Ruijter, W., . . . Westendorp, R. G. (2012). High blood pressure and resilience to physical and cognitive decline in the oldest old: the Leiden 85-plus Study. *Journal of the American Geriatrics Society*, *60*(11), 2014–2019. doi:10.1111/j.1532-5415.2012.04203.x

Schmidt, R., Schmidt, H., & Fazekas, F. (2000). Vascular risk factors in dementia. *Journal of Neurology*, *247*(2), 81–87.

Schreiber, S. J., Doepp, F., Spruth, E., Kopp, U. A., & Valdueza, J. M. (2005). Ultrasonographic measurement of cerebral blood flow, cerebral circulation time and cerebral blood volume in vascular and Alzheimer's dementia. *Journal of Neurology*, *252*(10), 1171–1177. doi:10.1007/s00415-005-0826-8

Scuteri, A., Tesauro, M., Guglini, L., Lauro, D., Fini, M., & Di Daniele, N. (2013). Aortic stiffness and hypotension episodes are associated with impaired cognitive function in older subjects with subjective complaints of memory loss. *International Journal of Cardiology*, *169*(5), 371–377. doi:10.1016/j.ijcard.2013.09.009

Selkoe, D. J., & Hardy, J. (2016). The amyloid hypothesis of Alzheimer's disease at 25 years. *EMBO Molecular Medicine*, *8*(6), 595–608. doi:10.15252/emmm.201606210

Shim, Y., Yoon, B., Shim, D. S., Kim, W., An, J., & Yang, D. (2015). Cognitive correlates of cerebral vasoreactivity on transcranial doppler in older adults. *Journal of Stroke and Cerebrovascular Diseases*, *24*(6), 1262–1269.

Skoog, I. (2003). Highs and lows of blood pressure: a cause of Alzheimer's disease? *Neurology*, *2*(6), 334.

Smith, E. E., Vijayappa, M., Lima, F., Delgado, P., Wendell, L., Rosand, J., & Greenberg, S. M. (2008). Impaired visual evoked flow velocity response in cerebral amyloid angiopathy. *Neurology*, *71*, 1424–1430.

Snyder, H. M., Corriveau, R. A., Craft, S., Faber, J. E., Greenberg, S. M., Knopman, D., . . . Carrillo, M. C. (2015). Vascular contributions to cognitive impairment and dementia including Alzheimer's disease. *Alzheimer's & Dementia*, *11*(6), 710–717. doi:10.1016/j.jalz.2014.10.008

Stroobant, N., & Vingerhoets, G. (2000). Transcranial doppler ultrasonography monitoring of cerebral hemodynamics during performance of cognitive tasks: A review. *Neuropsychology Review*, *10*(4), 213–231.

Sutton-Tyrrell, K., Najjar, S. S., Boudreau, R. M., Venkitachalam, L., Kupelian, V., Simonsick, E. M., . . . Newman, A. (2005). Elevated aortic pulse wave velocity, a marker of arterial stiffness, predicts cardiovascular events in well-functioning older adults. *Circulation*, *111*(25), 3384–3390. doi:10.1161/circulationaha.104.483628

Tai, L. M., Thomas, R., Marottoli, F. M., Koster, K. P., Kanekiyo, T., Morris, A. W., & Bu, G. (2016). The role of APOE in cerebrovascular dysfunction. *Acta Neuropathologica*, *131*(5), 709–723.

Tarumi, T., & Zhang, R. (2014). Cerebral hemodynamics of the aging brain: risk of Alzheimer disease and benefit of aerobic exercise. *Frontiers in Physiology*, *5*, 6. doi:10.3389/fphys.2014.00006

Toledo, J. B., Arnold, S. E., Raible, K., Brettschneider, J., Xie, S. X., Grossman, M., . . . Trojanowski, J. Q. (2013a). Contribution of cerebrovascular disease in autopsy confirmed neurodegenerative disease cases in the National Alzheimer's Coordinating Centre. *Brain*, *136*(Pt 9), 2697–2706. doi:10.1093/brain/awt188

Toledo, J. B., Arnold, S. E., Raible, K., Brettschneider, J., Xie, S. X., Grossman, M., . . . Trojanowski, J. Q. (2013b). Contribution of cerebrovascular disease in autopsy confirmed neurodegenerative disease cases in the National Alzheimer's Coordinating Centre. *Brain*, *136*(Pt 9), 2697–2706.

Tsao, C. W., Seshadri, S., Beiser, A. S., Westwood, A. J., Decarli, C., Au, R., . . . Mitchell, G. F. (2013). Relations of arterial stiffness and endothelial function to brain aging in the community. *Neurology*, *81*(11), 984–991. doi:10.1212/WNL.0b013e3182a43e1c

Tzourio, C., Laurent, S., & Debette, S. (2014). Is hypertension associated with an accelerated aging of the brain? *Hypertension*, *63*(5), 894–903. doi:10.1161/HYPERTENSIONAHA.113.00147

van Beek, A. H., Claassen, J. A., Rikkert, M. G., & Jansen, R. W. (2008). Cerebral autoregulation: an overview of current concepts and methodology with special focus on the elderly. *Journal of Cerebral Blood Flow & Metabolism*, *28*, 1071–1085.

van Beek, A. H., Sijbesma, J. C., Jansen, R. W., Olde Rikkert, M. G., & Claassen, J. A. (2010). Cortical oxygen supply during postural hypotension is further decreased in alzheimer's disease, but unrelated to cholinesterase-inhibitor use. *Journal of Alzheimer's Disease*, *21*(2), 519–526.

van Beek, A. H., Sijbesma, J. C., Jansen, R. W., Olde Rikkert, M. G., & Claassen, J. A. (2012). Oscillations in cerebral blood flow and cortical oxygenation in Alzheimer's disease. *Neurobiol Aging*, *33*(2), 428.e421–431.

van Bruchem-Visser, R. L., Mattace-Raso, F. U., & van der Cammen, T. J. (2009). High systolic and pulse pressure levels are associated with better cognitive performance in patients with probable Alzheimer's disease: A cross-sectional observational study in a geriatric outpatient population. *Dementia and Geriatric Cognitive Disorders*, *28*(4), 320–324. doi:10.1159/000249146

van Sloten, T. T., Protogerou, A. D., Henry, R. M., Schram, M. T., Launer, L. J., & Stehouwer, C. D. (2015). Association between arterial stiffness, cerebral small vessel disease and cognitive impairment: A systematic review and meta-analysis. *Neuroscience & Biobehavioral Reviews*, *53*, 121–130. doi:10.1016/j.neubiorev.2015.03.011

Verhaaren, B. F.d, Vernooij, M. W., de Boer, R., Hofman, A., Niessen, W. J., van der Lugt, A., & Ikram, M. A. (2013). High blood pressure and cerebral white matter lesion progression in the general population: novelty and significance. *Hypertension*, *61*(6), 1354–1359. doi:10.1161/HYPERTENSIONAHA.111.00430

Villeneuve, S., Reed, B. R., Madison, C. M., Wirth, M., Marchant, N. L., Kriger, S., . . . Jagust, W. J. (2014). Vascular risk and Abeta interact to reduce cortical thickness in AD vulnerable brain regions. *Neurology*, *83*(1), 40–47. doi:10.1212/WNL.0000000000000550

Waldstein, S. R., Rice, S. C., Thayer, J. F., Najjar, S. S., Scuteri, A., & Zonderman, A. B. (2008). Pulse pressure and pulse wave velocity are related to cognitive decline in the Baltimore Longitudinal Study of Aging. *Hypertension*, *51*(1), 99–104. doi:10.1161/HYPERTENSIONAHA.107.093674

Wang, Z. (2014). Characterizing early Alzheimer's disease and disease progression using hippocampal volume and arterial spin labeling perfusion MRI. *Journal of Alzheimer's Disease*, *42*, S495–S502.

Wang, Z., Yang, D., Zhang, X., Li, T., Li, J., Tang, Y., & Le, W. (2011). Hypoxia-induced down-regulation of neprilysin by histone modification in mouse primary cortical and hippocampal neurons. *PLoS One*, *6*(4), e19229.

Warnert, E. A., Murphy, K., Hall, J. E., & Wise, R. G. (2015). Noninvasive assessment of arterial compliance of human cerebral arteries with short inversion time arterial spin labeling. *Journal of Cerebral Blood Flow & Metabolism*, *35*(3), 461–468. doi:10.1038/jcbfm.2014.219

Watson, N. L., Sutton-Tyrrell, K., Rosano, C., Boudreau, R. M., Hardy, S. E., Simonsick, E. M., . . . Newman, A. B. (2011). Arterial stiffness and cognitive decline in well-functioning older adults. *Journal of Gerontology: Series A, 66A*(12), 1336–1342. doi:10.1093/gerona/glr119

Weller, R. O., Boche, D., & Nicoll, J. A. (2009). Microvasculature changes and cerebral amyloid angiopathy in Alzheimer's disease and their potential impact on therapy. *Acta Neuropathologica, 118*, 87–102.

Weller, R. O., Subash, M., Preston, S. D., Mazanti, I., & Carare, R. O. (2008). Perivascular drainage of amyloid-ß peptides from the brain and its failure in cerebral amyloid angiopathy and Alzheimer's disease. *Brain Pathology, 18*, 253–266.

Wintermark, M., Sesay, M., Barbier, E., Borbély, K., Dillon, W. P., Eastwood, J. D., . . . Yonas, H. (2005). Comparative overview of brain perfusion imaging techniques. *Stroke, 36*(9), e83–e99. doi:10.1161/01.STR.0000177884.72657.8b

Wu, Z., Guo, H., Chow, N., Sallstrom, J., Bell, R. D., Deane, R., . . . Zlokovic, B. V. (2005). Role of the MEOX2 homeobox gene in neurovascular dysfunction in Alzheimer disease. *Nature Medicine, 11*(9), 959–965.

Yan, L., Liu, C. Y., Smith, R. X., Jog, M., Langham, M., Krasileva, K., . . . Wang, D. J. J. (2016). Assessing intracranial vascular compliance using dynamic arterial spin labeling. *NeuroImage, 124*, 433–441. doi:10.1016/j.neuroimage.2015.09.008

Yasar, S., Ko, J. Y., Nothelle, S., Mielke, M. M., & Carlson, M. C. (2011). Evaluation of the effect of systolic blood pressure and pulse pressure on cognitive function: the Women's Health and Aging Study II. *PloS one, 6*(12), e27976.

Yew, B., & Nation, D. A. (2017). Cerebrovascular resistance and cerebral amyloidosis: Effects on cognitive decline, cortical atrophy, and progression to dementia. *Brain, 140*, 1987–2001.

Yoshiura, T., Hiwatashi, A., Yamashita, K., Ohyagi, Y., Monji, A., Takayama, Y., . . . Honda, H. (2009). Simultaneous measurement of arterial transit time, arterial blood volume, and cerebral blood flow using arterial spin labeling in patients with Alzheimer disease. *American Journal of Neuroradiology, 30*, 1388–1393.

Zazulia, A. R., Videen, T. O., Morris, J. C., & Powers, W. J. (2010). Autoregulation of cerebral blood flow to changes in arterial pressure in mild Alzheimer's disease. *Journal of Cerebral Blood Flow and Metabolism, 30*(11), 1883–1889. doi:10.1038/jcbfm.2010.135

Zeki Al Hazzouri, A., Newman, A. B., Simonsick, E., Sink, K. M., Sutton Tyrrell, K., Watson, N., . . . Yaffe, K. (2013). Pulse wave velocity and cognitive decline in elders: The Health, Aging, and Body Composition study. *Stroke, 44*(2), 388–393. doi:10.1161/strokeaha.112.673533

Zhong, W., Cruickshanks, K. J., Schubert, C. R., Carlsson, C. M., Chappell, R. J., Klein, B. E., . . . Acher, C. W. (2014). Pulse wave velocity and cognitive function in older adults. *Alzheimer Disease and Associated Disorders, 28*(1), 44–49. doi:10.1097/WAD.0b013e3182949f06

Zieman, S. J., Melenovsky, V., & Kass, D. A. (2005). Mechanisms, pathophysiology, and therapy of arterial stiffness. *Arteriosclerosis, Thrombosis, and Vascular Biology, 25*(5), 932–943. doi:10.1161/01.ATV.0000160548.78317.29

Zlokovic, B. V. (2011). Neurovascular pathways to neurodegeneration in Alzheimer's disease and other disorders. *Nature Reviews Neuroscience, 12*(12), 723–738. doi:10.1038/nrn3114

13

Hemodynamics in Alzheimer's Disease and Vascular Cognitive Impairment and Dementia

Francis Cambronero and Angela L. Jefferson

1. Introduction

Hemodynamic impairment is one the earliest detectable abnormalities in Alzheimer's disease (AD; Iturria-Medina, Sotero, Toussaint, Mateos-Perez, & Evans, 2016; Sweeney, Sagare, & Zlokovic, 2015; Wierenga, Hays, & Zlatar, 2014) with well-documented cerebral blood flow (CBF) changes occurring in prodromal AD (i.e., mild cognitive impairment [MCI]; Beishon, Haunton, Panerai, & Robinson, 2017; Dai et al., 2009) as well as in cognitively normal older adults at genetic risk for AD (Thambisetty, Beason-Held, An, Kraut, & Resnick, 2010). Chronic cerebral hypoperfusion develops decades before cognitive decline and precedes the earliest detectable in vivo changes in amyloid-β (Aβ) accumulation, hypometabolism, and brain atrophy (Iturria-Medina et al., 2016). These early vascular insufficiencies, including CBF dysfunction and blood–brain barrier (BBB) breakdown, trigger the development of cerebrovascular pathology that drives cognitive impairment and may accelerate AD pathology. In fact, cerebrovascular disease (CVD) is the most common pathology to co-occur with AD (Schneider, Arvanitakis, Bang, & Bennett, 2007), leading to possible additive and synergistic effects of both pathologies on cognitive impairment (Attems & Jellinger, 2014; Kester et al., 2014; Zlokovic, 2011).

The clinical impact of hemodynamic impairment and CVD have been well characterized in vascular cognitive impairment and dementia (VCID). Among aging adults free of clinical dementia, CVD is frequently reported (Lindgren et al., 1994), particularly mild forms of cerebral small vessel disease (SVD), such as microinfarcts detected at autopsy (Esiri, Wilcock, & Morris, 1997) or diffuse white matter damage on magnetic resonance imaging (MRI; Fazekas et al., 1988; K. W. Kim, MacFall, & Payne, 2008; Lindemer, Greve, Fischl, Augustinack, & Salat, 2017). Plus, it is the second most common cause of dementia after AD (Attems & Jellinger, 2014). Emerging evidence suggests there is considerable

Francis Cambronero and Angela L. Jefferson, *Hemodynamics in Alzheimer's Disease and Vascular Cognitive Impairment and Dementia* In: *Vascular Disease, Alzheimer's Disease, and Mild Cognitive Impairment.* Edited by: David J. Libon, Melissa Lamar, Rodney A. Swenson, Kenneth M. Heilman, Oxford University Press (2020).
DOI: 10.1093/oso/9780190634230.003.0014

overlap between VCID and AD and that mixed pathologies account for most clinical dementia syndromes (Schneider et al., 2007). Vascular lesions influence the presence of dementia in AD, both by lowering the threshold at which existing pathology will clinically present as overt dementia (Snowdon et al., 1997) and potentially mediating or amplifying the severity of amyloid effects. Given the growing recognition of the link between cerebrovascular dysfunction and AD, it is important to understand how observed hemodynamic impairments contribute to worse vascular and neuronal health.

This chapter reviews the fundamentals of the cerebrovasculature, the tightly controlled mechanisms underlying CBF regulation, the early hemodynamic differences that emerge in AD and VCID, and how these changes are connected to dysfunction and damage of key neurovascular cells. The chapter also discusses how Aβ pathology in AD contributes to these pathways of damage in the cerebrovasculature and its surrounding tissue. Finally, the relevance of systemic contributions to cerebral vascular dysfunction and hemodynamic impairment, including vascular risk factors and cardiac function, is reviewed.

2. An Introduction to the Cerebrovasculature

Blood flow control is especially critical to neuronal health and is tightly controlled by specific mechanisms at rest and under stress. The brain is one of the most metabolically demanding organs in the human body, consuming 20% of total oxygen and 25% of total glucose. It is incredibly sensitive to metabolic deficits, with hypoxia causing unconsciousness within seconds and irreversible neuronal damage within minutes (Haddad & Jiang, 1993; Prior, 1985; Sohmer, 1987). Tightly controlled systemic and CBF regulation mechanisms are thus required to ensure rapid and continuous delivery of vital substrates across a variety of conditions.

The body must respond to physical activity, external temperature, and other pertinent factors by adjusting blood flow delivery to stressed tissue for proper function. In basic fluid dynamics, flow results when a pressure difference is exerted over a given resistance. In humans, the heart's left ventricular pump creates a large pressure difference every cardiac cycle that is exerted over vascular resistance segments to generate blood flow, analogous to an electrical circuit. The primary determinant of this vascular resistance to flow is vessel diameter, wherein smaller diameters increase resistance and reduce blood flow. However, predictive models of hemodynamics are further complicated by real-life vessel properties, including vessel wall compliance that dampens fluctuations in pressure and diverse vessel architecture that contributes to irregularities in flow patterns. Vessel tortuosity, nonsmooth vascular walls, irregular arterial geometry, and branching patterns all contribute to variabilities in vascular resistance (and thus blood flow) throughout the vasculature.

Influential works like Duvernoy, Delon, and Vannson (1981) have described the complexity of the vascular system of the human brain in detail, and it is important to underscore that vascular architecture varies more than neuronal circuitry. Primary feeding arteries in the neck join near the base of the skull to form the circle of Willis, a structure that supports collateral circulation. There is considerable variation in circle of Willis anatomy across humans, with only 21% of individuals possessing a completely patent structure on postmortem examination (Riggs & Rupp, 1963) and 36% to 42% on in vivo magnetic resonance angiography (Hartkamp, van Der Grond, van Everdingen, Hillen, & Mali, 1999; Krabbe-Hartkamp et al., 1998). The major arteries of the circle of Willis give rise to progressively smaller pial arteries, which run along the surface of the brain in the pia-arachnoid space until they penetrate the brain parenchyma as intracerebral arterioles and begin associating with astrocytes and neurons.

Pial arteries are structurally distinct from the microcirculation in several important ways. First, pial arteries are supported by collateral networks and innervated by perivascular nerves critical for regulation of cerebrovascular tone. In contrast, downstream arterioles are typically long and unbranched, making their flow territories more susceptible to damage from occlusion. Both pial arteries and intracerebral arterioles are surrounded by smooth muscle cell layers that further ensure greater basal tone. As parenchymal arterioles successively branch into capillaries, the smooth muscle cell layer gradually disappears and vascular tone is supplemented by pericyte contractile cells that wrap around capillaries (Hall et al., 2014). At this level of the BBB, vital substrates may be extracted from the blood and toxic metabolites may be cleared (e.g., carbon dioxide) via the selective diffusion barrier at tight junctions between endothelial cells. Blood flow to these capillary beds is primarily driven by smooth muscle cells, which locally control arteriole diameter and help amplify the pressure wave over the entire arterial tree. Thus, the complex and intricate structure of the human cerebrovasculature ensures adequate blood flow delivery to tissue by regulating vascular resistance through a variety of structural and cellular properties.

3. Mechanisms of Hemodynamic Regulation

The cerebral circulatory system is controlled by distinct homeostatic mechanisms that ensure stable blood flow delivery in the face of fluctuating central perfusion pressures (i.e., cerebral autoregulation; Lassen, 1974) and further adapt blood flow to meet the metabolic demands of activated neurons (i.e., functional hyperemia; Buxton & Frank, 1997). Arterioles regulate CBF via adjacent smooth muscle cells, which induce local contractions in response to a variety of stimuli. Depending on how the smooth muscle membrane is polarized, it will either relax (hyperpolarization) or contract (depolarization) to control arteriole diameter and thus resistance to flow. This smooth muscle cell activity is regulated by vascular pressure changes, which form the basis of the myogenic response, and neurovascular coupling mechanisms that coordinate complex signaling cascades from a variety of neurovascular cells. For example, neurons (Drake & Iadecola, 2007), endothelial cells (Busse & Fleming, 2003; Hillman, 2014), and astrocytes (Howarth, 2014; Murphy, Rich, Orgren, Moore, & Faraci, 1994) produce vasoactive substances known to regulate smooth muscle cells. Ultimately, vascular smooth muscle integrates a myriad of vasoactive and vasoconstrictive signals to regulate CBF, including signals propagated through passive diffusion, ligand-gated ion channels, and voltage-gated ion channels.

Cerebrovascular autoregulation mechanisms work at rest and throughout postural changes to protect delicate brain vasculature from changes in blood pressure. Autoregulation ensures that the microvasculature receives a stable level of CBF regardless of cerebral perfusion pressure fluctuations by narrowing arterioles in high-pressure states and dilating arterioles in low-pressure states (Zlokovic, 2011). Although incompletely understood, cerebral autoregulation relies on the ability of blood vessels to dilate in response to a vasoactive stimulus, known as cerebrovascular reactivity (CVR). Autoregulation is traditionally thought to occur in response to cerebral perfusion pressure changes that stimulate stretching of the vascular smooth muscle, including transmural blood pressure forces and linear shear stress (i.e., increased blood-flow velocity). The resultant changes in arteriolar wall tension trigger signaling pathways in smooth muscle cells (Ye, Nesmith, & Parker, 2014) and the endothelium (Baeyens, Bandyopadhyay, Coon, Yun, & Schwartz, 2016; Harder, 1987; Rubanyi, Freay, Kauser, Johns, & Harder, 1990) that work to modulate contractility and restore wall tension. Notably however, the CVR mechanisms that underlie autoregulation are not exclusively linked to changes in cerebral perfusion pressure. Thus, traditional definitions of cerebral autoregulation have expanded in recent years to include influences from other physiological variables that can alter myogenic tone, including arterial gas levels (Meng & Gelb, 2015). In contrast to cerebral autoregulation, functional hyperemia is stimulated exclusively by vasoactive metabolites produced during neural activity. The neurovascular coupling mechanism involves well-characterized signaling pathways (e.g., classical nitric oxide signal transduction; Denninger & Marletta, 1999) with additional contributions from astrocytic end-feet, interneurons (Cauli et al., 2004), and retrograde endothelium signaling (Andresen, Shafi, & Bryan, 2006; B. R. Chen, Bouchard, McCaslin, Burgess, & Hillman, 2011; B. R. Chen, Kozberg, Bouchard, Shaik, & Hillman, 2014) that work to regulate myogenic tone. Neurovascular coupling determines the hemodynamic response function, which is the physiological foundation for functional MRI. The initiators of neurovascular coupling are thought to be located at the capillary bed (Collins, McCullough, & Ellsworth, 1998; Harraz, Longden, & Dabertrand, 2018), and pericytes have recently been implicated as a candidate initiator of the functional MRI signal (Hall et al., 2014).

In addition to autoregulatory and metabolic mechanisms of CBF regulation, chemoregulation mechanisms are critical for clearing carbon dioxide waste in the blood stream arising from respiration or situations of physiological stress. This mechanism is the basis of the hypercapnic response often used in neuroimaging paradigms to assess the quality of CVR. In this paradigm, a hypercapnic stimulus elevates the partial pressure of carbon dioxide in the bloodstream and stimulates CVR, defined as the ability of the cerebrovasculature to increase CBF in response. Hypercapnia-induced CVR is a reliable marker of cerebrovascular reserve capacity (Tajima et al., 2014). CVR mechanisms regulate CBF during hypercapnia via myogenic partial pressure-sensing mechanisms mediated by pH changes in the extracellular fluid and the formation of nitric oxide (Glodzik, Randall, Rusinek, & de Leon, 2013; Lavi, Egbarya, Lavi, & Jacob, 2003). The myogenic behavior of resistance arteries is therefore defined not only by its sustained state of constriction (i.e., myogenic tone) but also by its responsiveness (i.e., myogenic reactivity).

Although there is still conflicting evidence surrounding the underlying mechanisms and overlap between cerebral autoregulation, functional hyperemia, and chemoregulation, these CBF regulation pathways are thought to be the most predominant and fast-acting. Despite well-documented sympathetic innervation of intracerebral arteries, the role of neurogenic regulation remains controversial, with some evidence suggesting it is beneficial in conditions of severe ischemia (ter Laan, van Dijk, Elting, Staal, & Absalom, 2013). With advancing age, these predominant resting and dynamic CBF control mechanisms may be increasingly less effective, particularly if myogenic health or coupling mechanisms are affected. Emerging evidence suggests that the quality of hemodynamics and perfusion appear to be compromised in both typical aging as well as disease, including AD and CVD, such as VCID (Bar et al., 2007; den Abeelen, Lagro, van Beek, & Claassen, 2014). Such compromise ultimately places the brain at risk for oligemia, ischemic damage, and a cascade of pathological changes associated with vascular and neuronal injury.

4. Patterns of Hemodynamic Impairment in Aging and Dementia

Although brain structure, activity, and cognitive abilities all undergo patterned changes with normal aging, some of the earliest patterned changes to emerge are in blood flow. Chronic hypoperfusion is promoted by aging and comorbidities, including hypertension, obesity, and diabetes (Daulatzai, 2017). Early CBF studies using radioligand-based neuroimaging techniques demonstrated global and regional reductions in the aging brain, particularly in limbic or association cortices (Martin, Friston, Colebatch, & Frackowiak, 1991). However, more recent studies have relied on arterial spin labeling MRI for the reproducible quantification of CBF given that this noninvasive, nonionizing neuroimaging technique typically provides better spatial resolution and is more suitable for studies in healthy individuals or studies with repetitive follow-ups (Fan, Jahanian, Holdsworth, & Zaharchuk, 2016). These MRI studies have revealed more complex, bidirectional regional CBF patterns in aging. Although global CBF is still reduced independent of tissue atrophy, particularly in spatial patterns overlapping with the default-mode network (J. J. Chen, Rosas, & Salat, 2011), there are also increases in regional CBF in older adults (Preibisch et al., 2011). Recent evidence indicating that higher flow territory asymmetry (defined as how much an individual's CBF pattern deviates from the symmetrical group pattern) relates to lower memory performance in cognitively normal older adults suggests flow territory asymmetry may serve as a marker of worse cognitive aging, perhaps due to earlier age-related pathology (M. J. Donahue et al., 2014).

Unlike structural tissue measures, drivers of age-related changes in CBF remain harder to isolate and are largely unclear. Nevertheless, there are clear patterns of hypo- and hyperperfusion across the brain. Decreased regional CBF in older adults is likely intimately linked to subtle neuronal dysfunction due to age-related neurodegenerative factors (e.g., changes in neuronal number, size, activity, or synaptic density) as well as neurometabolic dysfunction (Mosconi et al., 2008), neurovascular uncoupling (Park, Anrather, Girouard, Zhou, & Iadecola, 2007; Sorond, Hurwitz, Salat, Greve, & Fisher, 2013), and perturbed cerebral autoregulation (Sorond, Khavari, Serrador, & Lipsitz, 2005). On the other hand, increased regional CBF may indicate neuronal compensation (Beason-Held, Kraut, & Resnick, 2008; Cabeza, Anderson, Locantore, & McIntosh, 2002) or overactivation reflective of more aggressive disease such as hyperactivity (Haberman, Branch, & Gallagher, 2017; Putcha et al., 2011) or hypervascularization (Liebeskind et al., 2011) that emerges due to age-related pathology. It is very likely that a lifetime burden of systemic vascular risk factors contributes to vascular dysfunction and compromised blood delivery, particularly when cerebral autoregulation mechanisms begin to fail in conditions like hypertension, during which higher perfusion pressures are needed to maintain the same level of CBF (Jennings et al., 2005; Strandgaard, Olesen, Skinhoj, & Lassen, 1973). Subtle changes in cerebral autoregulation may make the brain more susceptible to central hemodynamics.

There is consistent evidence of hemodynamic changes in VCID and AD, and both diseases appear to have pronounced CBF disturbances beyond typical aging with neuropathological overlap (Schneider et al., 2007). Although previous Doppler-based CBF studies indicated that the severity of disturbances in cerebral hemodynamics may be higher in VCID compared to AD (Sabayan et al., 2012). Both VCID and AD demonstrate CBF reductions relative to cognitively normal older adults, but it has been harder to distinguish CBF patterns in VCID and AD based on more recent arterial spin labeling MRI studies (Schuff et al., 2009). Interestingly, both groups also have elevated pulsatility indices (Stefani et al., 2009) compared to cognitively normal controls, but patients with VCID demonstrate relatively higher pulsatility indices compared to AD (Stefani et al., 2009). Blood flow pulsatility can be damaging to the microcirculation, contributing to vascular remodeling, increasing resistance, and failing cerebrovascular reserve over time. Accordingly, significant reductions in CVR have been found in VCID compared to cognitive controls (Bar et al., 2007; Smith & Beaudin, 2018). However, similar to arterial spin labeling MRI CBF studies, there are minimal detectable differences in CVR between VCID and AD (Bar et al., 2007; Vicenzini et al., 2007), perhaps because of the neuropathological co-occurrence of these two diseases.

In AD, CBF patterns distinct from normal aging emerge early on, before tissue atrophy, and most noticeably as global hypoperfusion, which eventually correlates with cognitive impairment (Leeuwis et al., 2017). Compared to cognitive controls, there is unique hypoperfusion of medial parietal (i.e., posterior cingulate cortex and precuneus) and lateral temporo-parietal regions in AD (Hu et al., 2010; Mattsson et al., 2014; Yoshiura et al., 2009). AD and MCI tend to reflect similar changes in perfusion, and hypoperfusion in parietal areas further predicts clinical conversion from MCI to AD (Hirao et al., 2005). Interestingly, medial temporal regions display more complex CBF patterns, including distinct patterns of regional hyperperfusion in the hippocampus (Alsop, Casement, de Bazelaire, Fong, & Press, 2008) that suggest compensatory or pathological elevation of neural activity (Desai, Schneider, Li, Carvey, & Hendey, 2009). In support of a compensatory perfusion theory in AD, higher flow territory asymmetry is correlated with better memory performance in MCI but not cognitively normal older adults (Donahue et al., 2014). In cognitively normal older adults, however, higher regional CBF is associated with worse cognition only among Aβ-positive individuals compared to Aβ-negative individuals, suggesting more CBF may be needed to support normal, but declining, memory systems (Bangen et al., 2017).

These observations indicate that higher regional CBF may be needed to maintain cognitive abilities in nondemented individuals closer to developing MCI and that flow asymmetry may later develop as a protective mechanism in early AD to recruit additional resources for tissue operating at maximal cerebrovascular reserve capacity.

Emerging MRI studies of CVR in AD support the notion that cerebrovascular reserve capacity may also be impaired in the earliest disease stages. As a measure of how well vessels respond to excessive carbon dioxide in the bloodstream, CVR reflects myogenic function (i.e., smooth muscle cell contractility) more so than neurovascular coupling, which is dependent on neuroactive substrate release from the tissue. In addition to hypoperfusion, CVR seems to be among the earliest neuroimaging markers of AD on MRI (Glodzik et al., 2013). Significant CVR reductions have been found in MCI and AD, with localizations that may be distinct from CBF reductions (Yezhuvath et al., 2012). Although MRI-based CVR mapping in AD remains limited (Chen, 2018), documented CVR impairments appear to be spatially similar to amyloid neuroimaging findings, suggesting MRI-based CVR may be more sensitive to AD pathology (Yezhuvath et al., 2012). Impairments in CVR mechanisms may contribute to neurovascular uncoupling seen in AD (Lourenco, Ledo, Barbosa, & Laranjinha, 2017; Park et al., 2005, 2008; Tarantini, Tran, Gordon, Ungvari, & Csiszar, 2017), creating an inability of the cerebrovasculature to dilate independent of any dysfunctional signaling between neurons and blood vessels. The effectiveness of any CBF regulatory mechanism relies heavily on the integrity of its cellular components and tightly coupled molecular signaling pathways. Alterations in CBF in both VCID and AD likely reflect microvascular dysfunction that may be driven by declines in capillary health, endothelial dysfunction, and other neurovascular unit cell problems. Eventual patterns of hypoperfusion will drive damage to the immediate vascular tissue and surrounding parenchyma.

5. Hemodynamic Contributions to Vascular Injury and Neurodegeneration

Once hemodynamic impairments develop, they contribute to worse brain health primarily through ischemic and hemorrhagic injury. Subtle CBF reductions may result in oligemia, which promotes suboptimal neuronal activity due to deprivation of vital ions and nutrients as well as the gradual development of hypoxia-triggered oxidative-nitrosative stress and neuroinflammation. However, larger CBF reductions lead to ischemia, resulting in more severe and rapid damage as well as pathological protein homeostasis. Hypoxic conditions in AD may further drive the overexpression of contractile proteins, resulting in arterial hypercontractility and CBF dysregulation (Chow et al., 2007). In addition to ischemia, hemorrhagic damage can also arise secondary to the disruption of the cellular architecture and development of neurotoxic microbleeds (Keep, Hua, & Xi, 2012). The ultimate activation of apoptotic and necrotic cascade pathways drive neuronal damage and clinically detectable cerebrovascular lesions in the parenchyma, seen on MRI as cerebral SVD. These cerebrovascular lesions contribute directly to worse neuronal function, neurodegeneration, and subsequent cognitive impairment. Original definitions of vascular dementia focused on diffuse arteriosclerotic changes (Hershey, Modic, Jaffe, & Greenough, 1986; Loeb, 1995), including large vessel disease. However, a more recent reconceptualization of VCID expands to all forms of cerebrovascular changes that affect cognition, including cerebral SVD, offering a more sophisticated perspective on cerebrovascular underpinnings of cognitive impairment and dementia (Hachinski, Lassen, & Marshall, 1974).

From a neuropathological perspective, cerebral SVD encompasses a variety of degenerative changes affecting small arterioles and microvessels of the brain, primarily driven by arteriolosclerosis, cerebral amyloid angiopathy, microaneurysms, and microvascular degeneration markers, such as fibrinoid necrosis and lipohyalinosis (i.e., arteriolar wall disorganization characterized by thickening and narrowing of small vessels). These pathologies are mostly observed in subcortical brain areas (e.g., basal ganglia and white matter) and lead to lacunar infarcts, hemorrhages, and axonal loss. Although prevalent in white matter, SVD is closely associated with regional grey matter changes, including cortical thinning and volumetric decline, suggesting damage may occur along fiber bundles and white matter disconnection may be significant to disease pathogenesis (Lambert et al., 2015). Importantly, recent evidence indicates the detection of even a few microinfarcts at autopsy implies the presence of hundreds globally, a substantial enough burden of whole-brain SVD capable of driving neurologic dysfunction (Westover, Bianchi, Yang, Schneider, & Greenberg, 2013).

Clinically, the term "cerebral SVD" is also used to describe larger parenchymal damage easily detected on MRI. Conventional MRI markers of SVD include white matter abnormalities, cerebral microbleeds, and lacunar infarcts, which have been shown to exist in up to 85% of aging adults (Lindgren et al., 1994) and associate with cognitive impairment and dementia. White matter abnormalities appear as hyperintensities on T2 fluid-attenuated inversion recovery MRI. While presumably of vascular origin, such as ischemia, microhemorrhages, and damage to small blood vessel walls, they can be of varying pathogenesis, including gliosis, breaches in the cerebrospinal fluid (CSF) and brain barrier, or myelin sheath loss and deformation. Cerebral microbleeds result from impaired small vessel integrity, mainly attributed to either hypertensive vasculopathy or cerebral amyloid angiopathy (Yates et al., 2014). Lacunar infarcts are small (<15 mm in diameter), caused by ischemia, and located in the territory of deep penetrating arteries. While not a common MRI marker of SVD, perivascular spaces are visible fluid-filled spaces adjacent to cerebral vessels thought to reflect tissue damage due to impairments in perivascular drainage, particularly driven by hypertension and abnormal arterial pulsatility in the basal ganglia (Yakushiji et al., 2014). Traditionally, perivascular spaces have been considered benign with limited clinical significance. However, recent work by our group suggests perivascular spaces not only correlate strongly with information processing speed and executive function, but they also appear to have more robust associations with cognition than other SVD markers (Passiak et al., 2019).

In addition to ischemic and hemorrhagic damage, hemodynamic insufficiencies also promote damage to the BBB and neurovascular unit. As previously described, the BBB is critical for both providing the neuron with blood-derived nutrients and minerals and protecting the neuron from toxic blood components that can cause diffuse oxidative damage and outright cell death (e.g., exposure to red blood cells). BBB permeability increases in advanced aging and has become an intense focus of recent AD research (Halliday et al., 2016; Montagne et al., 2015; Montagne, Zhao, & Zlokovic, 2017). The neurotoxic consequences of BBB breakdown include endothelial metabolic dysfunction, pericyte dysfunction, and hypoperfusion/hypoxia. Taken together, current evidence suggests hypoperfusion, SVD, and BBB breakdown are closely related in cognitive impairment and dementia. Going forward, both typical and abnormal brain aging studies seeking to understand drivers of disease will benefit from examining how early vascular changes fit into the larger pathological cascade.

6. Interactions of AD Pathology With Vascular Dysfunction

Cerebrovascular pathology has overlapping and even possibly synergistic effects with amyloid and tau pathologies, the pathological hallmarks of AD (Zlokovic, 2011). In autopsy series, cerebrovascular pathology reflects the second most common pathology after AD (Schneider et al., 2007) and the most common pathology to co-occur with AD (Montine et al., 2014; Petrovitch et al., 2005). Furthermore, vascular dysfunction is common in AD. Both patients with prodromal AD (Montagne et al., 2015) and transgenic AD mouse models (Paul, Strickland, & Melchor, 2007; Zipser et al., 2007) have accelerated BBB breakdown, along with focal microcirculatory changes, such as string vessels, alterations in capillary density, rises in endothelial pinocytosis, decreases in mitochondrial content, accumulation of basement membrane proteins (Lepelletier, Mann, Robinson, Pinteaux, & Boutin, 2017), and loss of tight junctions

(Zlokovic, 2011). These prominent AD-related vascular changes have intimate interactions with Aβ and tau pathology, as described in the following discussion.

Amassing evidence suggest cerebrovascular compromise may contribute to impairments in amyloid transport across various clearance pathways. Aβ is eliminated from extracellular spaces primarily via exchange across the BBB (Zlokovic, 2008). However, a smaller percentage of Aβ clearance is also supported by interstitial fluid (ISF) bulk flow pathways, including traditional perivascular clearance (i.e., ISF drainage through basement membranes of smooth muscle cells in the capillary and arterial walls; Bakker et al., 2016; Hawkes et al., 2012; Weller, Subash, Preston, Mazanti, & Carare, 2008) and glymphatic perivascular clearance (i.e., CSF influx into the periarterial space and CSF–ISF exchange in the parenchyma; Iliff et al., 2012; Tarasoff-Conway et al., 2015). Small vessel injury likely affects Aβ accumulation across varied perivascular (Weller, 1998; Weller, Massey, Kuo, & Roher, 2000) and BBB (Shibata et al., 2000) clearance pathways. Molecular evidence in AD further indicates impairments in Aβ receptor expression along the BBB, including increased receptors for advanced glycation end products involved in Aβ influx into the brain and decreased lipoprotein receptor-related proteins involved in Aβ efflux into the circulation (J. E. Donahue et al., 2006). In addition to clearance impairments, hypoperfusion in AD creates a metabolically deregulated environment (e.g., glucose hypometabolism) and stimulates both entry and aggregation of peripheral Aβ into the vasculature as well as production and deposition of Aβ in the parenchyma (ElAli, Theriault, Prefontaine, & Rivest, 2013; Salvadores, Searcy, Holland, & Horsburgh, 2017). Furthermore, although Aβ is known to be produced from neuronal membranes, local Aβ release from degenerating smooth muscle cells highlights potentially overlapping roles of cerebrovascular cells in Aβ production (Wisniewski & Wegiel, 1994). Chronic hypoperfusion purportedly promotes Aβ pathology across tissues through aberrant amyloid precursor protein processing (e.g., increases in β-secretase/γ-secretase amyloidogenic activity; Cai, Liu, Xiao, Wang, & Tian, 2017). Evidence supporting Aβ-vascular interactions suggests pathological changes in CBF may occur along shared pathways with Aβ pathology. For example, higher global Aβ loads are associated with reduced CBF (Mattsson et al., 2014). Notably, Aβ can impair vessel function as parenchymal plaques, more toxic soluble oligomers (Sakono & Zako, 2010), and widespread vascular deposits (i.e., cerebral amyloid angiopathy), the latter of which occurs in 82% to 98% of AD cases (Attems, 2005). On a cellular level, Aβ pathology promotes oxidative stress and inflammation, which cause endothelial and pericyte damage, basement membrane thickening, and degeneration of smooth muscle cells, a common feature of AD. This Aβ-induced cerebrovascular disruption is thought to promote BBB permeability, inducing angiogenesis as a regenerative response. However, alternative hypotheses suggest Aβ may directly stimulate pathological angiogenesis in AD independent of vascular damage, thereby implicating hypervascularization as the cause of BBB disruption and a potential therapeutic target (Biron, Dickstein, Gopaul, & Jefferies, 2011). Regardless of the underlying mechanism, Aβ-associated loss of vascular integrity compromises the structural and functional integrity of cell types involved in hemodynamic regulation, driving BBB transport impairments, endothelial dysfunction, and CBF dysregulation throughout the arterial tree.

In addition to Aβ pathology, hyperphosphorylated tau oligomers have been shown to accumulate in the microvasculature of AD patients (Castillo-Carranza et al., 2017) and induce blood vessel abnormalities (e.g., spiraling morphologies, lower vessel density) as well as CBF obstructions (Bennett et al., 2018). Although cerebrovascular effects of hyperphosphorylated tau may be a consequence of increased soluble Aβ around cortical arteries (Williams, Chalmers, Wilcock, & Love, 2005), hyperphosphorylated tau may also have Aβ-independent associations with CVD. Recent evidence indicates that neurofibrillary tau pathology mediates cognitive decline independent of Aβ pathology (H. J. Kim et al., 2018). Furthermore, chronic cerebral hypoperfusion enhances tau hyperphosphorylation (L. Qiu et al., 2016), including through hypertension-induced vascular dysfunction (Raz et al., 2019), suggesting that hyperphosphorylated tau production may also be implicated in early CBF dysregulation events. Tau pathology is suggested to induce cerebral arterial remodeling prior to AD-related microvascular cerebral amyloid angiopathy (Merlini, Wanner, & Nitsch, 2016), and tau alone is known to initiate breakdown of the BBB (Blair et al., 2015). Although it is not well-established whether tau pathology predominantly contributes to or is driven by the development of Aβ pathology, it undoubtedly serves a pivotal role as the final common pathway for cognitive impairment due to both vascular and AD pathologies (H. J. Kim et al., 2018).

The previously described vascular structural abnormalities in AD brains likely increase vascular resistance and contribute to hypercontractility and hypoperfusion. Indeed, recent studies show increased pulsatility and resistance indices in AD (Rivera-Rivera et al., 2016). Moreover, functional deficits in neurovascular unit signaling may contribute to neurovascular uncoupling, which is well-documented in AD (Lourenco et al., 2017; Park et al., 2005, 2008; Tarantini et al., 2017). Age- and AD-related alterations in cerebrovascular structure and functional reactivity may reduce the efficacy of cerebral autoregulation (Bar et al., 2007; den Abeelen et al., 2014), especially when vascular risk factors are present (Bar et al., 2007; Jennings et al., 2005; Y. S. Kim et al., 2008; Schroeter, Cutini, Wahl, Scheid, & Yves von Cramon, 2007; Strandgaard et al., 1973). In this manner, the brain may be more vulnerable to damage over time, particularly from exposure to subtle age-related alterations in cardiovascular hemodynamics.

7. Cardiac Contributions to Cerebral Hemodynamics

As the central blood pump of the human body, the heart plays an essential role in hemodynamic regulation and determines critical characteristics of initial blood flow, including volume, pressure, and pulsatility. The brain consumes 15% of cardiac output, a measure of forward stroke volume, despite only accounting for 2% of total body weight. Like dementia, cardiovascular dysfunction becomes increasingly common with advancing age, with 28% of older adults experiencing some form of prevalent cardiovascular disease (e.g., coronary heart disease, angina, heart attack, heart failure, or peripheral artery disease; Blackwell & Villarroel, 2018). Furthermore, as many as 97% of older adults also have at least one key cardiovascular risk factor, including high blood pressure, diabetes, high cholesterol, or smoking, all of which are associated with a higher burden of subclinical cardiovascular dysfunction (Benjamin et al., 2018). Thus, alterations in heart health can have implications for brain health, particularly in older adults with more vulnerable vascular systems.

Severe cardiac dysfunction in the form of clinical heart failure is a known risk factor for cognitive impairment (Hammond et al., 2018; Hoth, Poppas, Moser, Paul, & Cohen, 2008; Sauve, Lewis, Blankenbiller, Rickabaugh, & Pressler, 2009) and incident clinical dementia (Adelborg et al., 2017; C. Qiu et al., 2006), likely through microvascular dysfunction and reduced CBF (Cermakova et al., 2015; Jefferson & Benjamin, 2009). However, evidence from our group (Jefferson et al., 2010, 2015; Jefferson, Poppas, Paul, & Cohen, 2007) and others (Okonkwo, Cohen, Gunstad, & Poppas, 2011; Sabayan et al., 2015) suggests even subclinical reductions in cardiac output are associated with worse cognitive outcomes. Lower cardiac output is associated with worse executive function in aging cardiac patients (Jefferson, Poppas, et al., 2007), worse information processing speed and executive function in middle-age and older community dwelling adults (Jefferson et al., 2010; Sabayan et al., 2015), and a higher risk of incident clinical dementia and AD in community-dwelling aging adults (Jefferson et al., 2015). We have recently shown that cardiac strain, an early MRI marker of changes in contractility of the myocardial fibers, relates to episodic memory and language performance (Kresge et al., 2018). Nearly all of these findings persist when excluding participants with heart failure, prevalent cardiovascular disease, or arrhythmias (Jefferson et al., 2010, 2015; Kresge et al., 2018), suggesting subclinical changes in cardiac function with advancing age correspond to worse cognition and cannot be explained by shared vascular risk factors or disease.

Cardiac hemodynamics may relate to worse cognition through disturbances of cerebral hemodynamics and subsequent neurodegeneration. Indeed, our research has shown that lower cardiac output is associated with smaller cerebral gray matter volume (Jefferson et al., 2010), greater subcortical white matter damage (Jefferson, Tate, et al., 2007), and CBF reductions as recently reported for the first time in humans (Jefferson et al., 2017). While these latter findings were anatomically global, the most robust effects were regionally specific to the temporal lobes. The temporal lobes may be particularly vulnerable to systemic hypoperfusion given they are especially sensitive to hypoxia (Liebeskind, 2003) and the earliest neuroanatomical location of BBB degeneration in aging and MCI (Montagne et al., 2015). Theoretical models linking more severe cardiac dysfunction to AD support reduced systemic perfusion as a primary driver of reduced CBF (as we have recently observed in a subclinical setting; Jefferson et al., 2017) but further implicate maladaptive neurohormonal changes, inflammation, and microvascular dysfunction as secondary contributors to impaired CBF (Cermakova et al., 2015). These more mild, prolonged damage pathways are likely larger drivers of cerebrovascular and neuronal dysfunction in subclinical cardiac dysfunction rather than outright ischemia and neuronal failure. Subtle but chronic reductions in cardiac output likely results in oligemia with a gradual metabolic energy crisis for neurons, leading to inflammation, oxidative stress, and dysfunction of enzymes and protein synthesis. It is important to note that although cerebral autoregulation mechanisms generally serve to maintain a constant CBF level, the accumulation of vascular risk factors and vascular damage with older age may compromise the integrity of these mechanisms (Strandgaard et al., 1973). Thus, in the setting of advanced aging with a lifetime of vascular burden exposure, subtle changes in systemic blood flow and pressure may exert a larger adverse impact on brain health, including the development or progression of SVD, AD pathology, and neurodegeneration.

While a direct pathway between cardiovascular changes and brain health is plausible, alternatively, cardiovascular dysfunction may relate to worse brain health as a consequence of emerging neuropathology (i.e., a brain to heart pathway). Several reports indicate that evolving pathology and neurodegeneration in the AD brain may drive disruptions of autonomic control circuits responsible for heart rate and blood pressure control. Indeed, autonomic dysfunction has been repeatedly described in AD patients (Allan et al., 2007; Beach, Huck, Zhu, & Bozoki, 2017; Elmstahl et al., 1992; Femminella et al., 2014; Idiaquez & Roman, 2011; Meel-van den Abeelen, Lagro, Gommer, Reulen, & Claassen, 2013; Vitiello et al., 1993), including impaired cardiovagal parasympathetic function (Issac et al., 2017; Wang et al., 1994) and vasomotor sympathetic dysfunction (Algotsson, Viitanen, Winblad, & Solders, 1995). Although Braak and Braak (1995) staging criteria do not include evaluation of the brainstem, a central regulator of autonomic function, its early involvement in AD suggests emerging relevance (Simic et al., 2009). AD pathophysiology may cause a disruption of essential brainstem circuitry responsible for cardiovascular control, upstream autonomic control centers responsible for integrating peripheral signals and regulating the brainstem (e.g., hypothalamus and insula; Braak & Braak, 1995; Chu, Tranel, Damasio, & Van Hoesen, 1997), and cortical modulators of these autonomic circuits (Idiaquez, Sandoval, & Seguel, 2002). Moreover, cholinergic signaling pathways associated with cerebral and peripheral nerve dysfunction may be particularly vulnerable in AD (Femminella et al., 2014; van Beek & Claassen, 2011). Ultimately, varied abnormalities in brain structures and networks subserving autonomic regulation may impair cardiovascular function in AD, accounting for previously reported connections between cardiovascular function and abnormal brain changes (Jefferson et al., 2010, 2015, 2017; Jefferson, Poppas, et al., 2007; Jefferson, Tate, et al., 2007; Kresge et al., 2018).

It is also possible that the link between cardiovascular and brain dysfunction is an epiphenomenon. In support of this hypothesis, pleiotropy between AD and cardiovascular risk-associated genes has been increasingly established. For example, variants in the presenilin-1 gene, the same gene associated with early-onset AD, have been reported in idiopathic dilated cardiomyopathy (Gianni et al., 2010). These variants appear to reduce protein expression of the presenilin 1 protein, likely compromising its direct roles in calcium signaling (Green et al., 2008; Sarasija & Norman, 2018) and excitation–contraction coupling (Gianni et al., 2010) rather than amyloid processing. More recent genetic studies have indicated that the polygenetic component of AD is also enriched for cardiovascular risk factors, particularly lipid-associated factors potentially linked to BBB damage and pathological cholesterol metabolism in the brain (Broce et al., 2018; Xue-Shan et al., 2016). In addition to a common genetic profile affecting the heart and brain, studies of cardiovascular protein abnormalities in AD have further demonstrated a common molecular profile. In AD patients, biochemically similar Aβ deposits have been shown to co-exist in the heart and brain, and myocardial Aβ deposits appear to contribute to early diastolic dysfunction, as defined by impaired left ventricular relaxation (Troncone et al., 2016). While cardiovascular amyloid is likely common in advanced age (Cornwell, Murdoch, Kyle, Westermark, & Pitkanen, 1983; Gonzalez-Lopez et al., 2015; Mohammed et al., 2014), cardiovascular $A\beta_{40}$ and $A\beta_{42}$ expression is particularly increased in AD (Troncone et al., 2016). The possibility that Aβ aggregates may directly drive cardiomyocyte defects is strengthened by findings that myocardial Aβ oligomers promote changes in calcium homeostasis that likely mediate cardiomyocyte toxicity and contractile dysfunction in idiopathic dilated cardiomyopathy (Gianni et al., 2010). Future genetic, biochemical, and molecular studies will likely continue to shed light on the shared mechanisms underlying declines in heart and brain health, as well as whether these declines occur independently or through a shared pathway.

8. Conclusions

The clinical diagnosis of dementia is increasingly recognized to be driven by pathophysiological processes decades in the making (Sperling et al., 2011). Early hemodynamic changes likely contribute to and reflect frequently co-occurring cerebrovascular pathology in AD. Although vascular impairments are known to contribute independently and through Aβ interactions to neuronal dysfunction, further research is needed to disentangle additive, mediating, or synergistic effects. Regardless, emerging basic science studies and recent clinical trial results support the notion that preventing and treating vascular disease will reduce incident MCI and dementia, both by reducing the clinical significance of existing AD pathology and decelerating the deposition of emerging AD and vascular pathology. To gain a more comprehensive understanding of VCID and AD pathogenesis, emerging measures of hemodynamic compromise (e.g., onset and time course of CBF response; Duffin et al., 2015), regional distribution patterns, and other key players in cerebral metabolism (e.g., glucose utilization, oxidative metabolism) should be incorporated into a larger framework for understanding vascular dysfunction across the clinical spectrum of dementia.

References

Adelborg, K., Horvath-Puho, E., Ording, A., Pedersen, L., Toft Sorensen, H., & Henderson, V. W. (2017). Heart failure and risk of dementia: A Danish nationwide population-based cohort study. *European Journal of Heart Failure, 19*(2), 253–260. doi:10.1002/ejhf.631

Algotsson, A., Viitanen, M., Winblad, B., & Solders, G. (1995). Autonomic dysfunction in Alzheimer's disease. *Acta neurologica Scandinavica, 91*(1), 14–18.

Allan, L. M., Ballard, C. G., Allen, J., Murray, A., Davidson, A. W., McKeith, I. G., & Kenny, R. A. (2007). Autonomic dysfunction in dementia. *Journal of Neurology, Neurosurgery, and Psychiatry, 78*(7), 671–677. doi:10.1136/jnnp.2006.102343

Alsop, D. C., Casement, M., de Bazelaire, C., Fong, T., & Press, D. Z. (2008). Hippocampal hyperperfusion in Alzheimer's disease. *NeuroImage, 42*(4), 1267–1274. doi:10.1016/j.neuroimage.2008.06.006

Andresen, J., Shafi, N. I., & Bryan, R. M., Jr. (2006). Endothelial influences on cerebrovascular tone. *Journal of Applied Physiology, 100*(1), 318–327.

Attems, J. (2005). Sporadic cerebral amyloid angiopathy: Pathology, clinical implications, and possible pathomechanisms. *Acta neuropathologica, 110*(4), 345–359. doi:10.1007/s00401-005-1074-9

Attems, J., & Jellinger, K. A. (2014). The overlap between vascular disease and Alzheimer's disease--lessons from pathology. *BMC Medicine, 12*, 206. doi:10.1186/s12916-014-0206-2

Baeyens, N., Bandyopadhyay, C., Coon, B. G., Yun, S., & Schwartz, M. A. (2016). Endothelial fluid shear stress sensing in vascular health and disease. *Journal of Clinical Investigation, 126*(3), 821–828. doi:10.1172/jci83083

Bakker, E. N., Bacskai, B. J., Arbel-Ornath, M., Aldea, R., Bedussi, B., Morris, A. W., . . . Carare, R. O. (2016). Lymphatic clearance of the brain: Perivascular, paravascular and significance for neurodegenerative diseases. *Cellular and Molecular Neurobiology, 36*(2), 181–194. doi:10.1007/s10571-015-0273-8

Bangen, K. J., Clark, A. L., Edmonds, E. C., Evangelista, N. D., Werhane, M. L., Thomas, K. R., . . . Delano-Wood, L. (2017). Cerebral blood flow and amyloid-beta interact to affect memory performance in cognitively normal older adults. *Frontiers in Aging Neuroscience, 9*, 181. doi:10.3389/fnagi.2017.00181

Bar, K. J., Boettger, M. K., Seidler, N., Mentzel, H. J., Terborg, C., & Sauer, H. (2007). Influence of galantamine on vasomotor reactivity in Alzheimer's disease and vascular dementia due to cerebral microangiopathy. *Stroke, 38*(12), 3186–3192. doi:10.1161/strokeaha.107.492033

Beach, P. A., Huck, J. T., Zhu, D. C., & Bozoki, A. C. (2017). Altered behavioral and autonomic pain responses in Alzheimer's disease are associated with dysfunctional affective, self-reflective and salience network resting-state connectivity. *Frontiers in Aging Neuroscience, 9*, 297. doi:10.3389/fnagi.2017.00297

Beason-Held, L. L., Kraut, M. A., & Resnick, S. M. (2008). I. Longitudinal changes in aging brain function. *Neurobiology of Aging, 29*(4), 483–496. doi:10.1016/j.neurobiolaging.2006.10.031

Beishon, L., Haunton, V. J., Panerai, R. B., & Robinson, T. G. (2017). Cerebral hemodynamics in mild cognitive impairment: A systematic review. *Journal of Alzheimer's Disease, 59*(1), 369–385. doi:10.3233/jad-170181

Benjamin, E. J., Virani, S. S., Callaway, C. W., Chamberlain, A. M., Chang, A. R., Cheng, S., . . . Muntner, P. (2018). Heart disease and stroke statistics-2018 update: A report from the American Heart Association. *Circulation, 137*(12), e67–e492. doi:10.1161/cir.0000000000000558

Bennett, R. E., Robbins, A. B., Hu, M., Cao, X., Betensky, R. A., Clark, T., . . . Hyman, B. T. (2018). Tau induces blood vessel abnormalities and angiogenesis-related gene expression in P301L transgenic mice and human Alzheimer's disease. *Proceedings of the National Academy of Sciences of the United States of America, 115*(6), E1289–e1298. doi:10.1073/pnas.1710329115

Biron, K. E., Dickstein, D. L., Gopaul, R., & Jefferies, W. A. (2011). Amyloid triggers extensive cerebral angiogenesis causing blood brain barrier permeability and hypervascularity in Alzheimer's disease. *PloS One, 6*(8), e23789. doi:10.1371/journal.pone.0023789

Blackwell, D. L., & Villarroel, M. A. (2018). Tables of summary health statistics for U.S. adults: 2017 National Health Interview Survey. *National Center for Health Statistics*. Retrieved from http://www.cdc.gov/nchs/nhis/SHS/tables.htm

Blair, L. J., Frauen, H. D., Zhang, B., Nordhues, B. A., Bijan, S., Lin, Y. C., . . . Dickey, C. A. (2015). Tau depletion prevents progressive blood–brain barrier damage in a mouse model of tauopathy. *Acta Neuropathologica Communications, 3*, 8. doi:10.1186/s40478-015-0186-2

Braak, H., & Braak, E. (1995). Staging of Alzheimer's disease-related neurofibrillary changes. *Neurobiology of Aging, 16*(3), 271–278; discussion 278–284.

Broce, I. J., Tan, C. H., Fan, C. C., Jansen, I., Savage, J. E., Witoelar, A., . . . Desikan, R. S. (2018). Dissecting the genetic relationship between cardiovascular risk factors and Alzheimer's disease. *Acta Neuropathologica, 137*(2), 209–226. doi:10.1007/s00401-018-1928-6

Busse, R., & Fleming, I. (2003). Regulation of endothelium-derived vasoactive autacoid production by hemodynamic forces. *Trends in Pharmacological Science, 24*(1), 24–29.

Buxton, R. B., & Frank, L. R. (1997). A model for the coupling between cerebral blood flow and oxygen metabolism during neural stimulation. *Journal of Cerebral Blood Flow & Metabolism, 17*(1), 64–72. doi:10.1097/00004647-199701000-00009

Cabeza, R., Anderson, N. D., Locantore, J. K., & McIntosh, A. R. (2002). Aging gracefully: Compensatory brain activity in high-performing older adults. *NeuroImage, 17*(3), 1394–1402.

Cai, Z., Liu, Z., Xiao, M., Wang, C., & Tian, F. (2017). Chronic Cerebral Hypoperfusion Promotes Amyloid-Beta Pathogenesis via Activating beta/gamma-Secretases. *Neurochemical Research, 42*(12), 3446–3455. doi:10.1007/s11064-017-2391-9

Castillo-Carranza, D. L., Nilson, A. N., Van Skike, C. E., Jahrling, J. B., Patel, K., Garach, P., . . . Kayed, R. (2017). Cerebral microvascular accumulation of tau oligomers in Alzheimer's disease and related tauopathies. *Aging and Disease, 8*(3), 257–266. doi:10.14336/ad.2017.0112

Cauli, B., Tong, X. K., Rancillac, A., Serluca, N., Lambolez, B., Rossier, J., & Hamel, E. (2004). Cortical GABA interneurons in neurovascular coupling: Relays for subcortical vasoactive pathways. *Journal of Neuroscience, 24*(41), 8940–8949. doi:10.1523/jneurosci.3065-04.2004

Cermakova, P., Eriksdotter, M., Lund, L., Winblad, B., Religa, P., & Religa, D. (2015). Heart failure and Alzheimer's disease. *Journal of Internal Medicine, 277*(4), 406–425.

Chen, B. R., Bouchard, M. B., McCaslin, A. F., Burgess, S. A., & Hillman, E. M. (2011). High-speed vascular dynamics of the hemodynamic response. *NeuroImage, 54*(2), 1021–1030. doi:10.1016/j.neuroimage.2010.09.036

Chen, B. R., Kozberg, M. G., Bouchard, M. B., Shaik, M. A., & Hillman, E. M. (2014). A critical role for the vascular endothelium in functional neurovascular coupling in the brain. *Journal of the American Heart Association, 3*(3), e000787. doi:10.1161/jaha.114.000787

Chen, J. J. (2018). Cerebrovascular-Reactivity Mapping Using MRI: Considerations for Alzheimer's Disease. *Frontiers in Aging Neuroscience, 10*, 170. doi:10.3389/fnagi.2018.00170

Chen, J. J., Rosas, H. D., & Salat, D. H. (2011). Age-associated reductions in cerebral blood flow are independent from regional atrophy. *NeuroImage, 55*(2), 468–478. doi:10.1016/j.neuroimage.2010.12.032

Chow, N., Bell, R. D., Deane, R., Streb, J. W., Chen, J., Brooks, A., . . . Zlokovic, B. V. (2007). Serum response factor and myocardin mediate arterial hypercontractility and cerebral blood flow dysregulation in Alzheimer's phenotype. *Proceedings of the National Academy of Sciences of the United States of America, 104*(3), 823–828. doi:10.1073/pnas.0608251104

Chu, C. C., Tranel, D., Damasio, A. R., & Van Hoesen, G. W. (1997). The autonomic-related cortex: Pathology in Alzheimer's disease. *Cerebral Cortex, 7*(1), 86–95.

Collins, D. M., McCullough, W. T., & Ellsworth, M. L. (1998). Conducted vascular responses: Communication across the capillary bed. *Microvascular Research, 56*(1), 43–53. doi:10.1006/mvre.1998.2076

Cornwell, G. G., 3rd, Murdoch, W. L., Kyle, R. A., Westermark, P., & Pitkanen, P. (1983). Frequency and distribution of senile cardiovascular amyloid. A clinicopathologic correlation. *American Journal of Medicine*, *75*(4), 618–623.

Dai, W., Lopez, O. L., Carmichael, O. T., Becker, J. T., Kuller, L. H., & Gach, H. M. (2009). Mild cognitive impairment and Alzheimer disease: Patterns of altered cerebral blood flow at MR imaging. *Radiology*, *250*(3), 856–866. doi:10.1148/radiol.2503080751

Daulatzai, M. A. (2017). Cerebral hypoperfusion and glucose hypometabolism: Key pathophysiological modulators promote neurodegeneration, cognitive impairment, and Alzheimer's disease. *Journal of Neuroscience Research*, *95*(4), 943–972. doi:10.1002/jnr.23777

den Abeelen, A. S., Lagro, J., van Beek, A. H., & Claassen, J. A. (2014). Impaired cerebral autoregulation and vasomotor reactivity in sporadic Alzheimer's disease. *Current Alzheimer Research*, *11*(1), 11–17.

Denninger, J. W., & Marletta, M. A. (1999). Guanylate cyclase and the .NO/cGMP signaling pathway. *Biochimica et Biophysica Acta*, *1411*(2–3), 334–350.

Desai, B. S., Schneider, J. A., Li, J. L., Carvey, P. M., & Hendey, B. (2009). Evidence of angiogenic vessels in Alzheimer's disease. *Journal of Neural Transmission*, *116*(5), 587–597. doi:10.1007/s00702-009-0226-9

Donahue, J. E., Flaherty, S. L., Johanson, C. E., Duncan, J. A., 3rd, Silverberg, G. D., Miller, M. C., . . . Stopa, E. G. (2006). RAGE, LRP-1, and amyloid-beta protein in Alzheimer's disease. *Acta Neuropathologica*, *112*(4), 405–415. doi:10.1007/s00401-006-0115-3

Donahue, M. J., Hussey, E., Rane, S., Wilson, T., van Osch, M., Hartkamp, N., . . . Ally, B. A. (2014). Vessel-encoded arterial spin labeling (VE-ASL) reveals elevated flow territory asymmetry in older adults with substandard verbal memory performance. *Journal of Magnetic Resonance Imaging*, *39*(2), 377–386. doi:10.1002/jmri.24150

Drake, C. T., & Iadecola, C. (2007). The role of neuronal signaling in controlling cerebral blood flow. *Brain and Language*, *102*(2), 141–152. doi:10.1016/j.bandl.2006.08.002

Duffin, J., Sobczyk, O., Crawley, A. P., Poublanc, J., Mikulis, D. J., & Fisher, J. A. (2015). The dynamics of cerebrovascular reactivity shown with transfer function analysis. *NeuroImage*, *114*, 207–216. doi:10.1016/j.neuroimage.2015.04.029

Duvernoy, H. M., Delon, S., & Vannson, J. L. (1981). Cortical blood vessels of the human brain. *Brain Research Bulletin*, *7*(5), 519–579.

ElAli, A., Theriault, P., Prefontaine, P., & Rivest, S. (2013). Mild chronic cerebral hypoperfusion induces neurovascular dysfunction, triggering peripheral beta-amyloid brain entry and aggregation. *Acta Neuropathologica Communications*, *1*, 75. doi:10.1186/2051-5960-1-75

Elmstahl, S., Petersson, M., Lilja, B., Samuelsson, S. M., Rosen, I., & Bjuno, L. (1992). Autonomic cardiovascular responses to tilting in patients with Alzheimer's disease and in healthy elderly women. *Age and Ageing*, *21*(4), 301–307.

Esiri, M. M., Wilcock, G. K., & Morris, J. H. (1997). Neuropathological assessment of the lesions of significance in vascular dementia. *Journal of Neurology, Neurosurgery, and Psychiatry*, *63*(6), 749–753.

Fan, A. P., Jahanian, H., Holdsworth, S. J., & Zaharchuk, G. (2016). Comparison of cerebral blood flow measurement with [15O]-water positron emission tomography and arterial spin labeling magnetic resonance imaging: A systematic review. *Journal of Cerebral Blood Flow & Metabolism*, *36*(5), 842–861. doi:10.1177/0271678x16636393

Fazekas, F., Niederkorn, K., Schmidt, R., Offenbacher, H., Horner, S., Bertha, G., & Lechner, H. (1988). White matter signal abnormalities in normal individuals: Correlation with carotid ultrasonography, cerebral blood flow measurements, and cerebrovascular risk factors. *Stroke, 19*(10), 1285–1288.

Femminella, G. D., Rengo, G., Komici, K., Iacotucci, P., Petraglia, L., Pagano, G., . . . Ferrara, N. (2014). Autonomic dysfunction in Alzheimer's disease: Tools for assessment and review of the literature. *Journal of Alzheimer's disease, 42*(2), 369–377. doi:10.3233/jad-140513

Gianni, D., Li, A., Tesco, G., McKay, K. M., Moore, J., Raygor, K., . . . del Monte, F. (2010). Protein aggregates and novel presenilin gene variants in idiopathic dilated cardiomyopathy. *Circulation, 121*(10), 1216–1226. doi:10.1161/circulationaha.109.879510

Glodzik, L., Randall, C., Rusinek, H., & de Leon, M. J. (2013). Cerebrovascular reactivity to carbon dioxide in Alzheimer's disease. *Journal of Alzheimer's Disease, 35*(3), 427–440. doi:10.3233/jad-122011

Gonzalez-Lopez, E., Gallego-Delgado, M., Guzzo-Merello, G., de Haro-Del Moral, F. J., Cobo-Marcos, M., Robles, C., . . . Garcia-Pavia, P. (2015). Wild-type transthyretin amyloidosis as a cause of heart failure with preserved ejection fraction. *European Heart Journal, 36*(38), 2585–2594. doi:10.1093/eurheartj/ehv338

Green, K. N., Demuro, A., Akbari, Y., Hitt, B. D., Smith, I. F., Parker, I., & LaFerla, F. M. (2008). SERCA pump activity is physiologically regulated by presenilin and regulates amyloid beta production. *Journal of Cell Biology, 181*(7), 1107–1116. doi:10.1083/jcb.200706171

Haberman, R. P., Branch, A., & Gallagher, M. (2017). Targeting neural hyperactivity as a treatment to stem progression of late-onset Alzheimer's disease. *Neurotherapeutics, 14*(3), 662–676. doi:10.1007/s13311-017-0541-z

Hachinski, V. C., Lassen, N. A., & Marshall, J. (1974). Multi-infarct dementia: A cause of mental deterioration in the elderly. *Lancet, 2*(7874), 207–210.

Haddad, G. G., & Jiang, C. (1993). O2 deprivation in the central nervous system: On mechanisms of neuronal response, differential sensitivity and injury. *Prog Neurobiol, 40*(3), 277–318.

Hall, C. N., Reynell, C., Gesslein, B., Hamilton, N. B., Mishra, A., Sutherland, B. A., . . . Attwell, D. (2014). Capillary pericytes regulate cerebral blood flow in health and disease. *Nature, 508*(7494), 55–60. doi:10.1038/nature13165

Halliday, M. R., Rege, S. V., Ma, Q., Zhao, Z., Miller, C. A., Winkler, E. A., & Zlokovic, B. V. (2016). Accelerated pericyte degeneration and blood-brain barrier breakdown in apolipoprotein E4 carriers with Alzheimer's disease. *Journal of Cerebral Blood Flow & Metabolism, 36*(1), 216–227. doi:10.1038/jcbfm.2015.44

Hammond, C. A., Blades, N. J., Chaudhry, S. I., Dodson, J. A., Longstreth, W. T., Jr., Heckbert, S. R., . . . Thacker, E. L. (2018). Long-term cognitive decline after newly diagnosed heart failure: Longitudinal analysis in the CHS (Cardiovascular Health Study). *Circulation: Heart Failure, 11*(3), e004476. doi:10.1161/circheartfailure.117.004476

Harder, D. R. (1987). Pressure-induced myogenic activation of cat cerebral arteries is dependent on intact endothelium. *Circulation Research, 60*(1), 102–107.

Harraz, O. F., Longden, T. A., & Dabertrand, F. (2018). Endothelial GqPCR activity controls capillary electrical signaling and brain blood flow through PIP2 depletion. *Proceedings of the National Academy of Sciences of the United States of America, 115*(15), E3569–e3577. doi:10.1073/pnas.1800201115

Hartkamp, M. J., van Der Grond, J., van Everdingen, K. J., Hillen, B., & Mali, W. P. (1999). Circle of Willis collateral flow investigated by magnetic resonance angiography. *Stroke, 30*(12), 2671–2678.

Hawkes, C. A., Sullivan, P. M., Hands, S., Weller, R. O., Nicoll, J. A., & Carare, R. O. (2012). Disruption of arterial perivascular drainage of amyloid-beta from the brains of mice expressing the human APOE epsilon4 allele. *PloS One*, *7*(7), e41636. doi:10.1371/journal.pone.0041636

Hershey, L. A., Modic, M. T., Jaffe, D. F., & Greenough, P. G. (1986). Natural history of the vascular dementias: A prospective study of seven cases. *Canadian Journal of Neurological Sciences*, *13*(4 Suppl), 559–565.

Hillman, E. M. (2014). Coupling mechanism and significance of the BOLD signal: A status report. *Annual Review of Neuroscience*, *37*, 161–181. doi:10.1146/annurev-neuro-071013-014111

Hirao, K., Ohnishi, T., Hirata, Y., Yamashita, F., Mori, T., Moriguchi, Y., . . . Asada, T. (2005). The prediction of rapid conversion to Alzheimer's disease in mild cognitive impairment using regional cerebral blood flow SPECT. *NeuroImage*, *28*(4), 1014–1021. doi:10.1016/j.neuroimage.2005.06.066

Hoth, K. F., Poppas, A., Moser, D. J., Paul, R. H., & Cohen, R. A. (2008). Cardiac dysfunction and cognition in older adults with heart failure. *Cognitive and Behavioral Neurology*, *21*(2), 65–72.

Howarth, C. (2014). The contribution of astrocytes to the regulation of cerebral blood flow. *Frontiers in Neuroscience*, *8*, 103. doi:10.3389/fnins.2014.00103

Hu, W. T., Wang, Z., Lee, V. M., Trojanowski, J. Q., Detre, J. A., & Grossman, M. (2010). Distinct cerebral perfusion patterns in FTLD and AD. *Neurology*, *75*(10), 881–888. doi:10.1212/WNL.0b013e3181f11e35

Idiaquez, J., & Roman, G. C. (2011). Autonomic dysfunction in neurodegenerative dementias. *Journal of the Neurological Sciences*, *305*(1–2), 22–27. doi:10.1016/j.jns.2011.02.033

Idiaquez, J., Sandoval, E., & Seguel, A. (2002). Association between neuropsychiatric and autonomic dysfunction in Alzheimer's disease. *Clinical Autonomic Research*, *12*(1), 43–46.

Iliff, J. J., Wang, M., Liao, Y., Plogg, B. A., Peng, W., Gundersen, G. A., . . . Nedergaard, M. (2012). A paravascular pathway facilitates CSF flow through the brain parenchyma and the clearance of interstitial solutes, including amyloid beta. *Science Translational Medicine*, *4*(147), 147ra111. doi:10.1126/scitranslmed.3003748

Issac, T. G., Chandra, S. R., Gupta, N., Rukmani, M. R., Deepika, S., & Sathyaprabha, T. N. (2017). Autonomic dysfunction: A comparative study of patients with Alzheimer's and frontotemporal dementia - A pilot study. *Journal of Neurosciences in Rural Practice*, *8*(1), 84–88. doi:10.4103/0976-3147.193545

Iturria-Medina, Y., Sotero, R. C., Toussaint, P. J., Mateos-Perez, J. M., & Evans, A. C. (2016). Early role of vascular dysregulation on late-onset Alzheimer's disease based on multifactorial data-driven analysis. *Nature Communications*, *7*, 11934. doi:10.1038/ncomms11934

Jefferson, A. L., Beiser, A. S., Himali, J. J., Seshadri, S., O'Donnell, C. J., Manning, W. J., . . . Benjamin, E. J. (2015). Low cardiac index is associated with incident dementia and Alzheimer disease: The Framingham Heart Study. *Circulation*, *131*(15), 1333–13339. doi:10.1161/CIRCULATIONAHA.114.012438

Jefferson, A. L., & Benjamin, E. J. (2009). Cardiovascular disease, cognitive decline, and dementia. In L. O. Wahlund, T. Erkinjuntti, & S. Gauthier (Eds.), *Vascular cognitive impairment in clinical practice* (pp. 166–177). Cambridge, England: Cambridge University Press.

Jefferson, A. L., Himali, J. J., Beiser, A. S., Au, R., Massaro, J. M., Seshadri, S., . . . Manning, W. J. (2010). Cardiac index is associated with brain aging: The Framingham Heart Study. *Circulation, 122*(7), 690–697. doi:10.1161/CIRCULATIONAHA.109.905091

Jefferson, A. L., Liu, D., Gupta, D. K., Pechman, K. R., Watchmaker, J. M., Gordon, E. A., . . . Donahue, M. J. (2017). Lower cardiac index levels relate to lower cerebral blood flow in older adults. *Neurology, 89*(23), 2327–2334. doi:10.1212/wnl.0000000000004707

Jefferson, A. L., Poppas, A., Paul, R. H., & Cohen, R. A. (2007). Systemic hypoperfusion is associated with executive dysfunction in geriatric cardiac patients. *Neurobiology of Aging, 28*(3), 477–483. doi:10.1016/j.neurobiolaging.2006.01.001

Jefferson, A. L., Tate, D. F., Poppas, A., Brickman, A. M., Paul, R. H., Gunstad, J., & Cohen, R. A. (2007). Lower cardiac output is associated with greater white matter hyperintensities in older adults with cardiovascular disease. *Journal of the American Geriatrics Society, 55*(7), 1044–1048. doi:10.1111/j.1532-5415.2007.01226.x

Jennings, J. R., Muldoon, M. F., Ryan, C., Price, J. C., Greer, P., Sutton-Tyrrell, K., . . . Meltzer, C. C. (2005). Reduced cerebral blood flow response and compensation among patients with untreated hypertension. *Neurology, 64*(8), 1358–1365. doi:10.1212/01.WNL.0000158283.28251.3C

Keep, R. F., Hua, Y., & Xi, G. (2012). Intracerebral haemorrhage: Mechanisms of injury and therapeutic targets. *Lancet Neurology, 11*(8), 720–731. doi:10.1016/s1474-4422(12)70104-7

Kester, M. I., Goos, J. D., Teunissen, C. E., Benedictus, M. R., Bouwman, F. H., Wattjes, M. P., . . . van der Flier, W. M. (2014). Associations between cerebral small-vessel disease and Alzheimer disease pathology as measured by cerebrospinal fluid biomarkers. *JAMA Neurology, 71*(7), 855–862. doi:10.1001/jamaneurol.2014.754

Kim, H. J., Park, S., Cho, H., Jang, Y. K., San Lee, J., Jang, H., . . . Seo, S. W. (2018). Assessment of extent and role of tau in subcortical vascular cognitive impairment using 18F-AV1451 positron emission tomography imaging. *JAMA Neurology, 75*(8), 999-1007. doi:10.1001/jamaneurol.2018.0975

Kim, K. W., MacFall, J. R., & Payne, M. E. (2008). Classification of white matter lesions on magnetic resonance imaging in elderly persons. *Biological Psychiatry, 64*(4), 273–280. doi:10.1016/j.biopsych.2008.03.024

Kim, Y. S., Immink, R. V., Stok, W. J., Karemaker, J. M., Secher, N. H., & van Lieshout, J. J. (2008). Dynamic cerebral autoregulatory capacity is affected early in Type 2 diabetes. *Clinical Science, 115*(8), 255–262. doi:10.1042/cs20070458

Krabbe-Hartkamp, M. J., van der Grond, J., de Leeuw, F. E., de Groot, J. C., Algra, A., Hillen, B., . . . Mali, W. P. (1998). Circle of Willis: Morphologic variation on three-dimensional time-of-flight MR angiograms. *Radiology, 207*(1), 103–111. doi:10.1148/radiology.207.1.9530305

Kresge, H. A., Khan, O. A., Wegener, M. A., Liu, D., Terry, J. G., Nair, S., . . . Jefferson, A. L. (2018). Subclinical compromise in cardiac strain relates to lower cognitive performances in older adults. *Journal of the American Heart Association, 7*(4), e007562. doi:10.1161/JAHA.117.007562

Lambert, C., Sam Narean, J., Benjamin, P., Zeestraten, E., Barrick, T. R., & Markus, H. S. (2015). Characterising the grey matter correlates of leukoaraiosis in cerebral small vessel disease. *NeuroImage: Clinical, 9*, 194–205. doi:10.1016/j.nicl.2015.07.002

Lassen, N. A. (1974). Control of cerebral circulation in health and disease. *Circulation Research, 34*(6), 749–760.

Lavi, S., Egbarya, R., Lavi, R., & Jacob, G. (2003). Role of nitric oxide in the regulation of cerebral blood flow in humans: Chemoregulation versus mechanoregulation. *Circulation, 107*(14), 1901–1905. doi:10.1161/01.cir.0000057973.99140.5a

Leeuwis, A. E., Benedictus, M. R., Kuijer, J. P. A., Binnewijzend, M. A. A., Hooghiemstra, A. M., Verfaillie, S. C. J., . . . van der Flier, W. M. (2017). Lower cerebral blood flow is associated with impairment in multiple cognitive domains in Alzheimer's disease. *Alzheimer's & Dementia, 13*(5), 531–540. doi:10.1016/j.jalz.2016.08.013

Lepelletier, F. X., Mann, D. M., Robinson, A. C., Pinteaux, E., & Boutin, H. (2017). Early changes in extracellular matrix in Alzheimer's disease. *Neuropathology and Applied Neurobiology, 43*(2), 167–182. doi:10.1111/nan.12295

Liebeskind, D. S. (2003). Collateral circulation. *Stroke, 34*(9), 2279–2284. doi:10.1161/01.str.0000086465.41263.06

Liebeskind, D. S., Cotsonis, G. A., Saver, J. L., Lynn, M. J., Turan, T. N., Cloft, H. J., & Chimowitz, M. I. (2011). Collaterals dramatically alter stroke risk in intracranial atherosclerosis. *Annals of Neurology, 69*(6), 963–974. doi:10.1002/ana.22354

Lindemer, E. R., Greve, D. N., Fischl, B. R., Augustinack, J. C., & Salat, D. H. (2017). Regional staging of white matter signal abnormalities in aging and Alzheimer's disease. *NeuroImage: Clinical, 14*, 156–165. doi:10.1016/j.nicl.2017.01.022

Lindgren, A., Roijer, A., Rudling, O., Norrving, B., Larsson, E. M., Eskilsson, J., . . . Johansson, B. B. (1994). Cerebral lesions on magnetic resonance imaging, heart disease, and vascular risk factors in subjects without stroke: A population-based study. *Stroke, 25*(5), 929–934.

Loeb, C. (1995). The history of vascular dementia. *Journal of the History of the Neurosciences, 4*(2), 121–126. doi:10.1080/09647049509525631

Lourenco, C. F., Ledo, A., Barbosa, R. M., & Laranjinha, J. (2017). Neurovascular uncoupling in the triple transgenic model of Alzheimer's disease: Impaired cerebral blood flow response to neuronal-derived nitric oxide signaling. *Experimental Neurology, 291*, 36–43. doi:10.1016/j.expneurol.2017.01.013

Martin, A. J., Friston, K. J., Colebatch, J. G., & Frackowiak, R. S. (1991). Decreases in regional cerebral blood flow with normal aging. *Journal of Cerebral Blood Flow and Metabolism, 11*(4), 684–689. doi:10.1038/jcbfm.1991.121

Mattsson, N., Tosun, D., Insel, P. S., Simonson, A., Jack, C. R., Jr., Beckett, L. A., . . . Weiner, M. W. (2014). Association of brain amyloid-beta with cerebral perfusion and structure in Alzheimer's disease and mild cognitive impairment. *Brain, 137*(Pt 5), 1550–1561. doi:10.1093/brain/awu043

Meel-van den Abeelen, A. S., Lagro, J., Gommer, E. D., Reulen, J. P., & Claassen, J. A. (2013). Baroreflex function is reduced in Alzheimer's disease: A candidate biomarker? *Neurobiology of Aging, 34*(4), 1170–1176. doi:10.1016/j.neurobiolaging.2012.10.010

Meng, L., & Gelb, A. W. (2015). Regulation of cerebral autoregulation by carbon dioxide. *Anesthesiology, 122*(1), 196–205. doi:10.1097/aln.0000000000000506

Merlini, M., Wanner, D., & Nitsch, R. M. (2016). Tau pathology-dependent remodelling of cerebral arteries precedes Alzheimer's disease-related microvascular cerebral amyloid angiopathy. *Acta Neuropathologica, 131*(5), 737–752. doi:10.1007/s00401-016-1560-2

Mohammed, S. F., Mirzoyev, S. A., Edwards, W. D., Dogan, A., Grogan, D. R., Dunlay, S. M., . . . Redfield, M. M. (2014). Left ventricular amyloid deposition in patients with heart failure and preserved ejection fraction. *JACC: Heart Failure, 2*(2), 113–122. doi:10.1016/j.jchf.2013.11.004

Montagne, A., Barnes, S. R., Sweeney, M. D., Halliday, M. R., Sagare, A. P., Zhao, Z., . . . Zlokovic, B. V. (2015). Blood-brain barrier breakdown in the aging human hippocampus. *Neuron, 85*(2), 296–302. doi:10.1016/j.neuron.2014.12.032

Montagne, A., Zhao, Z., & Zlokovic, B. V. (2017). Alzheimer's disease: A matter of blood-brain barrier dysfunction? *Journal of Experimental Medicine, 214*(11), 3151–3169. doi:10.1084/jem.20171406

Montine, T. J., Koroshetz, W. J., Babcock, D., Dickson, D. W., Galpern, W. R., Glymour, M. M., . . . Corriveau, R. A. (2014). Recommendations of the Alzheimer's disease-related dementias conference. *Neurology, 83*(9), 851–860. doi:10.1212/wnl.0000000000000733

Mosconi, L., De Santi, S., Li, J., Tsui, W. H., Li, Y., Boppana, M., . . . de Leon, M. J. (2008). Hippocampal hypometabolism predicts cognitive decline from normal aging. *Neurobiology of Aging, 29*(5), 676–692. doi:10.1016/j.neurobiolaging.2006.12.008

Murphy, S., Rich, G., Orgren, K. I., Moore, S. A., & Faraci, F. M. (1994). Astrocyte-derived lipoxygenase product evokes endothelium-dependent relaxation of the basilar artery. *Journal of Neuroscience Research, 38*(3), 314–318. doi:10.1002/jnr.490380309

Okonkwo, O. C., Cohen, R. A., Gunstad, J., & Poppas, A. (2011). Cardiac output, blood pressure variability, and cognitive decline in geriatric cardiac patients. *Journal of Cardiopulmonary Rehabilitation and Prevention, 31*(5), 290–297. doi:10.1097/HCR.0b013e318220a817

Park, L., Anrather, J., Girouard, H., Zhou, P., & Iadecola, C. (2007). Nox2-derived reactive oxygen species mediate neurovascular dysregulation in the aging mouse brain. *Journal of Cerebral Blood Flow & Metabolism, 27*(12), 1908–1918. doi:10.1038/sj.jcbfm.9600491

Park, L., Anrather, J., Zhou, P., Frys, K., Pitstick, R., Younkin, S., . . . Iadecola, C. (2005). NADPH-oxidase-derived reactive oxygen species mediate the cerebrovascular dysfunction induced by the amyloid beta peptide. *Journal of Neuroscience, 25*(7), 1769–1777. doi:10.1523/jneurosci.5207-04.2005

Park, L., Zhou, P., Pitstick, R., Capone, C., Anrather, J., Norris, E. H., . . . Iadecola, C. (2008). Nox2-derived radicals contribute to neurovascular and behavioral dysfunction in mice overexpressing the amyloid precursor protein. *Proceedings of the National Academy of Sciences of the United States of America, 105*(4), 1347–1352.

Passiak, B. S., Liu, D., Kresge, H. A., Cambronero, F. E., Pechman, K. R., Osborn, K. E., . . . Jefferson, A. L. (2019). Perivascular spaces contribute to cognition beyond other small vessel disease markers. *Neurology, 92*(12), e1309–e1321.

Paul, J., Strickland, S., & Melchor, J. P. (2007). Fibrin deposition accelerates neurovascular damage and neuroinflammation in mouse models of Alzheimer's disease. *Journal of Experimental Medicine, 204*(8), 1999–2008. doi:10.1084/jem.20070304

Petrovitch, H., Ross, G. W., Steinhorn, S. C., Abbott, R. D., Markesbery, W., Davis, D., . . . White, L. R. (2005). AD lesions and infarcts in demented and non-demented Japanese-American men. *Annals of Neurology, 57*(1), 98–103. doi:10.1002/ana.20318

Preibisch, C., Sorg, C., Forschler, A., Grimmer, T., Sax, I., Wohlschlager, A. M., . . . Alexopoulos, P. (2011). Age-related cerebral perfusion changes in the parietal and temporal lobes measured by pulsed arterial spin labeling. *Journal of Magnetic Resonance Imaging, 34*(6), 1295–1302. doi:10.1002/jmri.22788

Prior, P. F. (1985). EEG monitoring and evoked potentials in brain ischaemia. *British Journal of Anaesthesia, 57*(1), 63–81.

Putcha, D., Brickhouse, M., O'Keefe, K., Sullivan, C., Rentz, D., Marshall, G., . . . Sperling, R. (2011). Hippocampal hyperactivation associated with cortical thinning in Alzheimer's disease signature regions in non-demented elderly adults. *Journal of Neuroscience, 31*(48), 17680–17688. doi:10.1523/jneurosci.4740-11.2011

Qiu, C., Winblad, B., Marengoni, A., Klarin, I., Fastbom, J., & Fratiglioni, L. (2006). Heart failure and risk of dementia and Alzheimer disease: A population-based cohort study. *Archives of Internal Medicine, 166*(9), 1003–1008. doi:10.1001/archinte.166.9.1003

Qiu, L., Ng, G., Tan, E. K., Liao, P., Kandiah, N., & Zeng, L. (2016). Chronic cerebral hypoperfusion enhances tau hyperphosphorylation and reduces autophagy in Alzheimer's disease mice. *Scientific Reports, 6*, 23964. doi:10.1038/srep23964

Raz, L., Bhaskar, K., Weaver, J., Marini, S., Zhang, Q., Thompson, J. F., . . . Rosenberg, G. A. (2019). Hypoxia promotes tau hyperphosphorylation with associated neuropathology in vascular dysfunction. *Neurobiology of Disease, 126*, 124–136. doi:10.1016/j.nbd.2018.07.009

Riggs, H. E., & Rupp, C. (1963). Variation in form of circle of Willis. The relation of the variations to collateral circulation: Anatomic analysis. *Archives of Neurology, 8*, 8–14.

Rivera-Rivera, L. A., Turski, P., Johnson, K. M., Hoffman, C., Berman, S. E., Kilgas, P., . . . Wieben, O. (2016). 4D flow MRI for intracranial hemodynamics assessment in Alzheimer's disease. *Journal of Cerebral Blood Flow and Metabolism, 36*(10), 1718–1730. doi:10.1177/0271678x15617171

Rubanyi, G. M., Freay, A. D., Kauser, K., Johns, A., & Harder, D. R. (1990). Mechanoreception by the endothelium: Mediators and mechanisms of pressure- and flow-induced vascular responses. *Blood Vessels, 27*(2–5), 246–257.

Sabayan, B., Jansen, S., Oleksik, A. M., van Osch, M. J., van Buchem, M. A., van Vliet, P., . . . Westendorp, R. G. (2012). Cerebrovascular hemodynamics in Alzheimer's disease and vascular dementia: A meta-analysis of transcranial Doppler studies. *Ageing Research Reviews, 11*(2), 271–277. doi:10.1016/j.arr.2011.12.009

Sabayan, B., van Buchem, M. A., Sigurdsson, S., Zhang, Q., Harris, T. B., Gudnason, V., . . . Launer, L. J. (2015). Cardiac hemodynamics are linked with structural and functional features of brain aging: The age, gene/environment susceptibility (AGES)–Reykjavik Study. *Journal of the American Heart Association, 4*(1), e001294. doi:10.1161/jaha.114.001294

Sakono, M., & Zako, T. (2010). Amyloid oligomers: Formation and toxicity of Abeta oligomers. *FEBS Journal, 277*(6), 1348–1358. doi:10.1111/j.1742-4658.2010.07568.x

Salvadores, N., Searcy, J. L., Holland, P. R., & Horsburgh, K. (2017). Chronic cerebral hypoperfusion alters amyloid-beta peptide pools leading to cerebral amyloid angiopathy, microinfarcts and haemorrhages in Tg-SwDI mice. *Clinical Science, 131*(16), 2109–2123. doi:10.1042/cs20170962

Sarasija, S., & Norman, K. R. (2018). Role of presenilin in mitochondrial oxidative stress and neurodegeneration in caenorhabditis elegans. *Antioxidants, 7*(9). doi:10.3390/antiox7090111

Sauve, M. J., Lewis, W. R., Blankenbiller, M., Rickabaugh, B., & Pressler, S. J. (2009). Cognitive impairments in chronic heart failure: A case controlled study. *Journal of Cardiac Failure, 15*(1), 1–10. doi:10.1016/j.cardfail.2008.08.007

Schneider, J. A., Arvanitakis, Z., Bang, W., & Bennett, D. A. (2007). Mixed brain pathologies account for most dementia cases in community-dwelling older persons. *Neurology, 69*(24), 2197–2204. doi:10.1212/01.wnl.0000271090.28148.24

Schroeter, M. L., Cutini, S., Wahl, M. M., Scheid, R., & Yves von Cramon, D. (2007). Neurovascular coupling is impaired in cerebral microangiopathy--An event-related Stroop study. *NeuroImage, 34*(1), 26–34.

Schuff, N., Matsumoto, S., Kmiecik, J., Studholme, C., Du, A., Ezekiel, F., . . . Weiner, M. W. (2009). Cerebral blood flow in ischemic vascular dementia and Alzheimer's disease, measured by arterial spin-labeling magnetic resonance imaging. *Alzheimer's & Dementia*, *5*(6), 454–462. doi:10.1016/j.jalz.2009.04.1233

Shibata, M., Yamada, S., Kumar, S. R., Calero, M., Bading, J., Frangione, B., . . . Zlokovic, B. V. (2000). Clearance of Alzheimer's amyloid-ss(1-40) peptide from brain by LDL receptor-related protein-1 at the blood-brain barrier. *Journal of Clinical Investigation*, *106*(12), 1489–1499. doi:10.1172/JCI10498

Simic, G., Stanic, G., Mladinov, M., Jovanov-Milosevic, N., Kostovic, I., & Hof, P. R. (2009). Does Alzheimer's disease begin in the brainstem? *Neuropathology and Applied Neurobiology*, *35*(6), 532–554. doi:10.1111/j.1365-2990.2009.01038.x

Smith, E. E., & Beaudin, A. E. (2018). New insights into cerebral small vessel disease and vascular cognitive impairment from MRI. *Current Opinions in Neurology*, *31*(1), 36–43. doi:10.1097/wco.0000000000000513

Snowdon, D. A., Greiner, L. H., Mortimer, J. A., Riley, K. P., Greiner, P. A., & Markesbery, W. R. (1997). Brain infarction and the clinical expression of Alzheimer disease. The Nun Study. *JAMA*, *277*(10), 813–817.

Sohmer, H. (1987). Auditory evoked potentials during deviations from homeostasis: Theoretical and clinical implications. *Electroencephalography and Clinical Neurophysiology: Supplement*, *39*, 267–275.

Sorond, F. A., Hurwitz, S., Salat, D. H., Greve, D. N., & Fisher, N. D. (2013). Neurovascular coupling, cerebral white matter integrity, and response to cocoa in older people. *Neurology*, *81*(10), 904–909. doi:10.1212/WNL.0b013e3182a351aa

Sorond, F. A., Khavari, R., Serrador, J. M., & Lipsitz, L. A. (2005). Regional cerebral autoregulation during orthostatic stress: Age-related differences. *Journals of Gerontology. Series A, Biological Sciences and Medical Sciences*, *60*(11), 1484–1487.

Sperling, R. A., Aisen, P. S., Beckett, L. A., Bennett, D. A., Craft, S., Fagan, A. M., . . . Phelps, C. H. (2011). Toward defining the preclinical stages of Alzheimer's disease: Recommendations from the National Institute on Aging–Alzheimer's Association workgroups on diagnostic guidelines for Alzheimer's disease. *Alzheimer's & Dementia*, *7*(3), 280–292. doi:10.1016/j.jalz.2011.03.003

Stefani, A., Sancesario, G., Pierantozzi, M., Leone, G., Galati, S., Hainsworth, A. H., & Diomedi, M. (2009). CSF biomarkers, impairment of cerebral hemodynamics and degree of cognitive decline in Alzheimer's and mixed dementia. *Journal of the Neurological Sciences*, *283*(1–2), 109–115. doi:10.1016/j.jns.2009.02.343

Strandgaard, S., Olesen, J., Skinhoj, E., & Lassen, N. A. (1973). Autoregulation of brain circulation in severe arterial hypertension. *British Medical Jouranl*, *1*(5852), 507–510.

Sweeney, M. D., Sagare, A. P., & Zlokovic, B. V. (2015). Cerebrospinal fluid biomarkers of neurovascular dysfunction in mild dementia and Alzheimer's disease. *Journal of Cerebral Blood Flow & Metabolism*, *35*(7), 1055–1068. doi:10.1038/jcbfm.2015.76

Tajima, Y., Takuwa, H., Kokuryo, D., Kawaguchi, H., Seki, C., Masamoto, K., . . . Ito, H. (2014). Changes in cortical microvasculature during misery perfusion measured by two-photon laser scanning microscopy. *Journal of Cerebral Blood Flow and Metabolism*, *34*(8), 1363–1372. doi:10.1038/jcbfm.2014.91

Tarantini, S., Tran, C. H. T., Gordon, G. R., Ungvari, Z., & Csiszar, A. (2017). Impaired neurovascular coupling in aging and Alzheimer's disease: Contribution of astrocyte dysfunction and endothelial impairment to cognitive decline. *Experimental Gerontology*, *94*, 52–58. doi:10.1016/j.exger.2016.11.004

Tarasoff-Conway, J. M., Carare, R. O., Osorio, R. S., Glodzik, L., Butler, T., Fieremans, E., . . . de Leon, M. J. (2015). Clearance systems in the brain-implications for Alzheimer disease. *Nature Reviews Neurology, 11*(8), 457–470. doi:10.1038/nrneurol.2015.119

ter Laan, M., van Dijk, J. M., Elting, J. W., Staal, M. J., & Absalom, A. R. (2013). Sympathetic regulation of cerebral blood flow in humans: A review. *British Journal of Anaesthesia, 111*(3), 361–367. doi:10.1093/bja/aet122

Thambisetty, M., Beason-Held, L., An, Y., Kraut, M. A., & Resnick, S. M. (2010). APOE epsilon4 genotype and longitudinal changes in cerebral blood flow in normal aging. *Archives of Neurology, 67*(1), 93–98. doi:10.1001/archneurol.2009.913

Troncone, L., Luciani, M., Coggins, M., Wilker, E. H., Ho, C. Y., Codispoti, K. E., . . . Del Monte, F. (2016). Abeta amyloid pathology affects the hearts of patients with Alzheimer's disease: Mind the heart. *Journal of the American College of Cardiology, 68*(22), 2395–2407. doi:10.1016/j.jacc.2016.08.073

van Beek, A. H., & Claassen, J. A. (2011). The cerebrovascular role of the cholinergic neural system in Alzheimer's disease. *Behavioural Brain Research, 221*(2), 537–542. doi:10.1016/j.bbr.2009.12.047

Vicenzini, E., Ricciardi, M. C., Altieri, M., Puccinelli, F., Bonaffini, N., Di Piero, V., & Lenzi, G. L. (2007). Cerebrovascular reactivity in degenerative and vascular dementia: A transcranial Doppler study. *European Neurology, 58*(2), 84–89. doi:10.1159/000103642

Vitiello, B., Veith, R. C., Molchan, S. E., Martinez, R. A., Lawlor, B. A., Radcliffe, J., . . . Sunderland, T. (1993). Autonomic dysfunction in patients with dementia of the Alzheimer type. *Biological Psychiatry, 34*(7), 428–433.

Wang, S. J., Liao, K. K., Fuh, J. L., Lin, K. N., Wu, Z. A., Liu, C. Y., & Liu, H. C. (1994). Cardiovascular autonomic functions in Alzheimer's disease. *Age & Ageing, 23*(5), 400–404.

Weller, R. O. (1998). Pathology of cerebrospinal fluid and interstitial fluid of the CNS: Significance for Alzheimer disease, prion disorders and multiple sclerosis. *Journal of Neuropathology and Experimental Neurology, 57*(10), 885–894.

Weller, R. O., Massey, A., Kuo, Y. M., & Roher, A. E. (2000). Cerebral amyloid angiopathy: Accumulation of A beta in interstitial fluid drainage pathways in Alzheimer's disease. *Annals of the New York Academy of Sciences, 903*, 110–117.

Weller, R. O., Subash, M., Preston, S. D., Mazanti, I., & Carare, R. O. (2008). Perivascular drainage of amyloid-beta peptides from the brain and its failure in cerebral amyloid angiopathy and Alzheimer's disease. *Brain Pathology, 18*(2), 253–266. doi:10.1111/j.1750-3639.2008.00133.x

Westover, M. B., Bianchi, M. T., Yang, C., Schneider, J. A., & Greenberg, S. M. (2013). Estimating cerebral microinfarct burden from autopsy samples. *Neurology, 80*(15), 1365–1369. doi:10.1212/WNL.0b013e31828c2f52

Wierenga, C. E., Hays, C. C., & Zlatar, Z. Z. (2014). Cerebral blood flow measured by arterial spin labeling MRI as a preclinical marker of Alzheimer's disease. *Journal of Alzheimer's Disease, 42*(Suppl 4), S411–419. doi:10.3233/jad-141467

Williams, S., Chalmers, K., Wilcock, G. K., & Love, S. (2005). Relationship of neurofibrillary pathology to cerebral amyloid angiopathy in Alzheimer's disease. *Neuropathology and Applied Neurobiology, 31*(4), 414–421. doi:10.1111/j.1365-2990.2005.00663.x

Wisniewski, H. M., & Wegiel, J. (1994). Beta-amyloid formation by myocytes of leptomeningeal vessels. *Acta Neuropathologica, 87*(3), 233–241.

Xue-Shan, Z., Juan, P., Qi, W., Zhong, R., Li-Hong, P., Zhi-Han, T., . . . Lu-Shan, L. (2016). Imbalanced cholesterol metabolism in Alzheimer's disease. *Clinica Chimica Acta, 456*, 107–114. doi:10.1016/j.cca.2016.02.024

Yakushiji, Y., Charidimou, A., Hara, M., Noguchi, T., Nishihara, M., Eriguchi, M., . . . Hara, H. (2014). Topography and associations of perivascular spaces in healthy adults: The Kashima scan study. *Neurology, 83*(23), 2116–2123. doi:10.1212/wnl.0000000000001054

Yates, P. A., Villemagne, V. L., Ellis, K. A., Desmond, P. M., Masters, C. L., & Rowe, C. C. (2014). Cerebral microbleeds: A review of clinical, genetic, and neuroimaging associations. *Frontiers in Neurology, 4*, 205. doi:10.3389/fneur.2013.00205

Ye, G. J., Nesmith, A. P., & Parker, K. K. (2014). The role of mechanotransduction on vascular smooth muscle myocytes' [corrected] cytoskeleton and contractile function. *Anatomical Record, 297*(9), 1758–1769. doi:10.1002/ar.22983

Yezhuvath, U. S., Uh, J., Cheng, Y., Martin-Cook, K., Weiner, M., Diaz-Arrastia, R., . . . Lu, H. (2012). Forebrain-dominant deficit in cerebrovascular reactivity in Alzheimer's disease. *Neurobiology of Aging, 33*(1), 75–82. doi:10.1016/j.neurobiolaging.2010.02.005

Yoshiura, T., Hiwatashi, A., Noguchi, T., Yamashita, K., Ohyagi, Y., Monji, A., . . . Honda, H. (2009). Arterial spin labelling at 3-T MR imaging for detection of individuals with Alzheimer's disease. *European Radiology, 19*(12), 2819–2825. doi:10.1007/s00330-009-1511-6

Zipser, B. D., Johanson, C. E., Gonzalez, L., Berzin, T. M., Tavares, R., Hulette, C. M., . . . Stopa, E. G. (2007). Microvascular injury and blood–brain barrier leakage in Alzheimer's disease. *Neurobiology of Aging, 28*(7), 977–986. doi:10.1016/j.neurobiolaging.2006.05.016

Zlokovic, B. V. (2008). The blood-brain barrier in health and chronic neurodegenerative disorders. *Neuron, 57*(2), 178–201. doi:10.1016/j.neuron.2008.01.003

Zlokovic, B. V. (2011). Neurovascular pathways to neurodegeneration in Alzheimer's disease and other disorders. *Nature Reviews Neuroscience, 12*(12), 723–738. doi:10.1038/nrn3114

PART 4

NEUROPATHOLOGICAL AND NEUROPHYSIOLOGICAL MECHANISMS

14
Neuropathology of Alzheimer's Disease and Vascular Dementia

Alifiya Kapasi and Julia A. Schneider

1. Neuropathological Basis of Dementia

The main characteristics for the pathologic diagnosis of Alzheimer's disease (AD) and vascular dementia (VaD) have remained largely unchanged for decades. In AD, molecular specific markers of pathology has advanced diagnosis, whereas in VaD our knowledge regarding the heterogeneity of vessel disease and vascular tissue injury has expanded, with imaging playing an increasingly large role, although not incorporated into the pathologic diagnosis. In addition, both disorders tend lie on a continuum ranging from mild to severe. AD and vascular pathology often co-exist within the same brain, a phenomenon known by various names including mixed pathologies. There are well-established neuropathological criteria for a diagnosis of AD used to confirm a clinical diagnosis. The neuropathological guidelines for confirming a clinical diagnosis of vascular or mixed dementia are more complex given that there are no well-established criteria to determine what extent of underlying cerebrovascular pathology is sufficient to cause or add to cognitive impairment. Both AD and vascular pathology are diagnosed using qualitative, semiquantitative, and topographical staging. AD neuropathology is defined by the extracellular accumulation of pathological Aβ-plaques, with specifically neuritic plaques, and deposition of hyperphosphorylated tau neurofibrillary tangles (NFTs) in cortical neurons. Although these pathological changes represent the critical elements in the pathogenesis of AD and are present in persons with diagnosed clinically with AD, these pathological changes are also observed in persons without any cognitive impairment, a phenomenon often described as resilience. There have been several standardized approaches for the pathological diagnosis of AD with recent criteria proposed by the National Institute on Aging–Alzheimer's Association (NIA-AA; Montine et al., 2014). This recent guideline provided a turning point for the conceptualization of AD pathology as a diagnostic entity separate from an associated clinical syndrome. The NIA-AA guideline provides a framework for tissue sampling and diagnostic analysis to determine the level of

Alifiya Kapasi and Julia A. Schneider, *Neuropathology of Alzheimer's Disease and Vascular Dementia* In: *Vascular Disease, Alzheimer's Disease, and Mild Cognitive Impairment.* Edited by: David J. Libon, Melissa Lamar, Rodney A. Swenson, Kenneth M. Heilman, Oxford University Press (2020).
DOI: 10.1093/oso/9780190634230.003.0015

AD neuropathological changes. These guidelines include an ABC score by incorporating histological assessment for Thal amyloid phase (Thal, Rub, Orantes, & Braak, 2002), Braak neurofibrillary tangle staging (Braak & Braak, 1995), and the Consortium to Establish a Registry for Alzheimer's Disease (CERAD) neuritic plaque semiquantitative scoring (Mirra et al., 1991). The combined measures can be interpreted as not, low, intermediate, and high levels of AD neuropathologic changes. Intermediate or high levels of Alzheimer's disease neuropathic changes (ADNC) are considered sufficient for a pathologic diagnosis of AD in the presence or absence of cognitive impairment. However, new to these criteria are additional detailed approaches for assessing co-existing pathologies including Lewy body disease, microvascular pathology, hippocampal sclerosis (HS), and TDP-43 staging.

The importance of vascular disease in the development of dementia has been widely recognized for decades; however, the importance of co-existing vascular disease in patients whom may otherwise qualify for a diagnosis of AD has been accumulating in recent years. Moreover, it is now recognized that cardiovascular risk factors and presence of cerebrovascular pathology increase the risk and severity of cognitive impairment associated with AD in both human- and animal-based studies (Corrada, Sonnen, Kim, & Kawas, 2016; Hainsworth et al., 2017; Pfeifer, White, Ross, Petrovitch, & Launer, 2002; Schneider, Boyle, Arvanitakis, Bienias, & Bennett, 2007; Schneider & Bennett, 2010; Wijesinghe et al., 2016). Whereas neuropathological examinations in multiple longitudinal cohorts have provided evidence that both neurodegenerative and vascular pathologies (mixed pathologies) are often present person's otherwise diagnosed with an Alzheimer's clinical syndrome, understanding the full spectrum of vascular cognitive impairment (VCI) and the vascular association with AD pathology remains unclear for multiple reasons including but not limited to (a) the heterogeneous nature of cerebrovascular lesions, (b) variations in vascular lesion size, location, and number, and (c) multiple pathogenic mechanisms including changes in cerebral blood flow, neuroinflammation, and disruption of axonal tracts. Unfortunately, there is currently no reliable and harmonized diagnostic protocol to assess vascular pathology burden in postmortem brain tissue.

Despite these caveats, there is compelling evidence that vascular disease plays an important role in most insidious onset, age-related dementias. Epidemiologic studies report that better control of vascular risk factors results in a downward trend for both the incidence of stroke and prevalence of dementia (Fillit, Nash, Rundek, & Zuckerman, 2008) providing evidence for the importance of a vascular component in dementia. These studies underscore the importance of cerebrovascular disease (CVD) as a contributing factor in the development of dementia encouraging health care workers to manage and treat risk factors to prevent cognitive impairment and dementia (Corriveau et al., 2017).

2. Neuropathology of Alzheimer's Disease

The pattern of distribution of NFTs across brain regions is predictable and has been proposed by Braak and Braak (1995) to occur in six stages (I–VI). Deposition begins in the transentorhinal regions (Stage I), extending into entorhinal cortex and hippocampus (Stages II and III), abundant involvement of limbic regions and spreading to neocortical regions (Stages IV and V), with final involvement of primary motor, sensory, and visual cortices (Stage VI; Braak & Braak, 1995). Thal et al. (2002) proposed that the distribution of amyloid plaques occurs in five phases. Amyloid plaques primarily accumulate in the isocortex ex (Phase 1), progressing to the allocortical regions (Phase 2), to subcortical nuclei (Phase 3), to brainstem structures (Phase 4), and lastly to cerebellum and pons (Phase 5; Thal, Rub, Orantes, & Braak, 2002).

Neuropathological criteria to diagnose AD have undergone several revisions in the last few decades. The first criteria proposed was based on the highest density of amyloid plaques including both neuritic and diffuse plaques in any cortical field (Khachaturian, 1985). The density of plaques needed for a diagnosis of AD was based on age and diagnosis. A few years later, CERAD revised this to only to include neuritic plaques. A semiquantitative score was suggested to evaluate the highest density of neuritic plaques in any neocortical region (frontal, temporal, or parietal cortices; Mirra et al., 1991). CERAD score was incorporated with clinical information (age and diagnosis) to give a level of certainty that dementia is explained by AD pathological changes: not, possible, probable, and definite. In 1997, the National Institute of Aging and the Reagan Institute (NIA-Reagan) consensus recommended combining CERAD and NFT Braak staging. Depending on the combinations of semiquantitative score of CERAD and Braak, staging the diagnostic categories falls into either high likelihood, intermediate likelihood, or low likelihood. For example, high likelihood indicates that the dementia could be explained by AD if the CERAD score was definite (frequent neuritic plaques) and Braak staging was either V/VI (NFTs in isocortical regions; Hyman & Trojanowski, 1997). This version of the criteria recently underwent revisions (i.e., the ABC/ NIA-AA criteria scoring for amyloid; Thal stage), Braak NFT staging, and CERAD neuritic plaque scores. This scoring system provides a severity of level of AD neuropathological changes without consideration of age or clinical diagnosis. Thus, for the first time, with this scoring system the neuropathology of AD was separated from the clinical diagnosis of Alzheimer's dementia

(Montine et al., 2014). Another change in this version is that the presence of amyloid is required to denote any AD neuropathological changes, whereas NFT alone is not adequate to diagnose AD neuropathological changes. Given the importance of mixed pathologies, this version also requires the neuropathologist to include other co-existing pathology in the diagnosis. In general, intermediate or high ADNC is necessary to confirm the existence of an AD dementia syndrome. A recent study to determine compatibility of NIA-AA evaluation showed high agreement between ten AD centers (Montine et al., 2016). However, there is considerable variability regarding how CERAD, Braak, and Thal scores can predict neuropsychological test performance, with Thal scores being less associated with cognition than CERAD or Braak (Serrano-Pozo et al., 2016).

3. Common Vessel Pathologies With Aging and Dementia

Degenerative processes together with vascular changes can result in multiple cerebrovascular lesions, most frequently but not limited to infarcts, hemorrhages, and alterations of subcortical white matter. In this section, we describe neuropathological basis of large vessel atherosclerosis, small vessel disease (SVD), including arteriolosclerosis and cerebral amyloid angiopathy (CAA), and venous collagenosis all of which are commonly observed in older persons (Figure 14.1). Other vascular disorders including aneurysms and arteriovenous malformations that also give rise to tissue injury; however, these lesions occur less frequently in older persons.

3.1. Large Vessel Atherosclerosis

In the brain, atherosclerosis typically affects the large- and medium-sized arteries, most commonly the carotid, middle cerebral and basilar arteries, as well as the circle of Willis. Smaller penetrating arteries are also affected but are considered under the rubric of SVD (see following discussion). Formation of an atherosclerotic plaque is a result of proliferation and accumulation of cholesterol-laden macrophages within the vessel wall, occurring very slowly over decades of years. This process can lead to calcification and development of a mature atherosclerotic plaque causing further fibrotic/necrotic changes that injured the vessel wall. Consequently, these changes lead to endothelial damage, predisposing the vessel to thrombosis with partial or complete occlusion. Alternatively, small emboli can break loose from an atherosclerotic plaque formation within intra- and extracranial arteries, leading to embolic infarctions of the brain. Both types of lesions can create global or local hypoxic-ischemic events in the brain and can lead to a variety of brain lesions (Thal, Grinberg, & Attems, 2012).

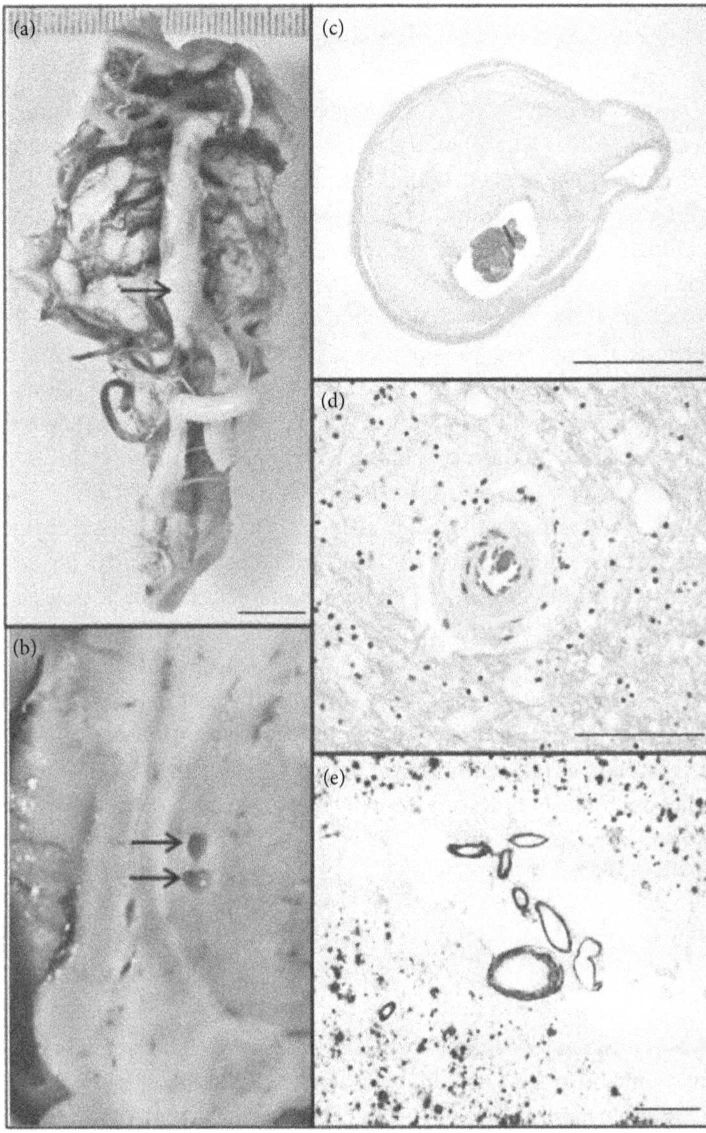

Figure 14.1. Vessel disease in the aging brain. Presence of atherosclerotic plaque, which appears yellow in the basilar artery, can transform arteries into stiffened and nontransparent tubes (A, arrow). Eccentric atheroma plaque impinges onto the lumen causing it to narrow. Other common histologic features of an atheroma often include fibromuscular intima hyperplasia with an intact endothelium and the presence of cholesterol clefts (C). Macroscopic finding of enlarged perivascular spaces (B, arrows). Small vessel disease including arteriolosclerosis of the smaller penetrating arteries (D) and cerebral amyloid angiopathy in the meningeal and parenchymal vessels (E).

Notes: Scale bars: 10mm (images A, B); 1mm (image C); 50µm (image D); and 100µm (image E).

3.2. Small Vessel Disease

SVDs (termed *nonamyloid SVD* or *sporadic nonamyloid microangiopathy*) have also been described (Charidimou et al., 2017). This represents a spectrum of vessel disorders that cause necrotic/degenerative changes within small perforating arteries vessels enter the brain parenchyma from leptomeningeal vessels. SVD is often associated with hypertension, diabetes, and other age-related vascular risk factors. Pathological SVD subtypes include small vessel atherosclerosis, arteriolosclerosis, lipohyalinosis, and hypertensive arteriopathy. Pathogenesis of small vessel atherosclerosis is similar to large vessel atherosclerosis but involves smaller vessels, sized from 200 to 800 μm, and results in the formation of microatheromas (McAleese et al., 2016). Vascular changes underlying arteriolosclerosis, the most common form of SVD, include concentric hyaline thickening of small arteries and arterioles, sized 40 to 150 μm in diameter, and are often associated with accumulation of plasma proteins. Lipohyalinosis, originally use to denote alterations in the arterioles or capillaries (vessels with a diameter of 40–300 μm) in the brain, are characterized by increased vessel wall thickening and a resultant reduction in luminal diameter. The term "lipohyalinosis" is often used synonymously with arteriolosclerosis (Kapasi & Schneider, 2016). Finally, *hypertensive arteriopathy* (a term also used synonymously with arteriolosclerosis) results from collagenous thickening leading to loss of smooth muscle cells within the vessel wall. Together, SVD-induced vascular changes can lead to loss of elasticity and an inability to dilate or constrict in response to systemic blood pressure, leading to fluctuations in blood flow and changes in perfusion.

3.3. Cerebral Amyloid Angiopathy

CAA (also considered as part of the SVD spectrum) is characterized by the deposition of amyloid in the basement membrane or in the smooth muscle cell layer of arteries and arterioles. Involvement typically occurs in the leptomeningeal and cortical vessels with a topographical distribution favoring the posterior lobar regions (Charidimou et al., 2017). CAA can be subtyped as capillary CAA when there is amyloid deposits in capillaries (Attems, Jellinger, Thal, & Van Nostrand, 2011). CAA has a distinct role in the spectrum of AD and SVD. While there is significant overlapping between AD pathology and CAA, not every patient with CAA has a pathologic diagnosis of AD, and, conversely, not all persons with a pathologic diagnosis of AD exhibit CAA (Keage et al., 2009). While nearly half of older persons with a pathologic diagnosis of AD have moderate to severe CAA, by contrast only 20% of persons without a pathologic diagnosis of AD have CAA

(Yu, Boyle, Nag et al., 2015). Amyloid in both neuritic plaques and CAA is a consequence of abnormal cleavage of amyloid precursor protein generating a pathogenic amyloid-β (Aβ) protein. However, unlike amyloid in neuritic plaques, which is predominantly composed of Aβ42 variant, amyloid in CAA is composed of mainly the Aβ40 variant, a more soluble isoform (Love et al., 2014). The effects of vascular Aβ deposition can lead to vascular degeneration, in particular degeneration of pericytes (Verbeek, de Waal, Schipper, & Van Nostrand, 1997), endothelial cell damage (Thomas, Thomas, McLendon, Sutton, & Mullan, 1996), and smooth muscle degeneration (Haglund, Kalaria, Slade, & Englund, 2006). These changes can lead to decreased vascular compliance and elasticity. In addition, CAA can contribute to both hemorrhagic and ischemic lesions in the brain including intracerebral lobar hemorrhages, microbleeds (Renard et al., 2018), white matter hyperintensities (WMH; Charidimou et al., 2016), microinfarcts (van den Brink et al., 2018), and cortical superficial siderosis, with hemosiderin deposits in the superficial cortical layers or the subarachnoid space (Charidimou et al., 2015). CAA is an extremely common finding in the elderly population and has been correlated with atrophy patterns (Kim et al., 2018), age-related cognitive impairment (Banerjee et al., 2018), and cognitive decline independent of AD and other degenerative pathologies (Boyle et al., 2015).

3.4. Venous Collagenosis

Venous collagenosis is characterized by collagen proliferation within the wall of veins and venules, most commonly in the periventricular regions. It is proposed that dysfunction of arteries and arterioles may result in activation of downstream oxidative stress leading to collagen proliferation in venules and veins (Pettersen, Keith, Gao, Spence, & Black, 2017). There is emerging evidence to suggest that with aging venous collagenosis has a role in the pathological changes involving white matter; however, more studies are warranted to further understand the role of venous collagenosis in CVD (Hartmann, Hyacinth, Liao, & Shih, 2017; Keith et al., 2017) and its potential role in VCI.

3.5. Genetics and Cerebral Vessel Disease

Hereditary SVD encompasses a small group of monogenic disorders that have overlapping clinical presentations, often characterized by stroke, VaD, motor and cognitive dysfunction, migraine with visual aura, and mood disturbances. Disorders identified in this group are cerebral autosomal dominant arteriopathy with subcortical infarcts and leukoencephalopathy (CADASIL), cerebral autosomal recessive arteriopathy with subcortical infarcts and leukoencephalopathy (CARASIL), collagen type IV mutations, cereboretinal vasculopathy, Fabry disorder, and hereditary cerebral hemorrhage with amyloidosis (Sondergaard, Nielsen, Hansen, & Christensen, 2017). Imaging and laboratory tests play a crucial role in diagnosing monogenic disorders; however, molecular genetic testing from tissue biopsies is considered the gold standard.

CADASIL is the most common form of hereditary SVD and caused by an autosomal dominant mutation in the NOTCH3 gene. Neuroimaging studies of CADASIL patients show white matter hyperintensity lesions distributed in both subcortical and periventricular white matter regions; lacunar infarcts involving the basal ganglia, thalamus, and pons; and cerebral microbleeds in various brain regions (Puy et al., 2017; Stojanov et al., 2015). There are a limited number of studies investigating neuropathological changes in CADASIL. Microvascular changes include apoptosis of smooth muscle cells, dilation of Virchow–Robin spaces (Gray et al., 2007), a granular osmiophilic material deposition within the media and adventitia causing thickening of the vessel wall and axonal abnormalities in the frontal white matter (Craggs et al., 2014). Furthermore, abnormalities in frontal white matter axons disrupt cortico–subcortical networks, which may result in executive dysfunction and motor deficits are commonly observed in CADASIL patients (Gray et al., 2007).

When compared to the sporadic forms of CAA, hereditary forms of CAA presents in families with autosomal dominant mutations. These are rare disorders that are characterized by earlier age of onset with a more severe clinical course. Hereditary cerebral hemorrhage with amyloidosis is associated with the Dutch, Finnish, and Icelandic forms of familial CAA and often involves an early fatal onset of cerebral hemorrhage/hemorrhagic stroke. Those surviving the initial hemorrhagic episode may go on to develop dementia (Biffi & Greenberg, 2011). Sporadic CAA is extremely common affecting elderly individuals with and without clinical dementia, and in those with and without AD. AD pathology and sporadic CAA have a strong overlap and share many common risk factors, but both remain independent risk factors for dementia (Boyle et al., 2015). The apolipoprotein E (APOE) gene is well-known risk factor for late onset of AD. APOE isoforms differentially interact and regulate clearance of Aβ, and likely to be involved in amyloidosis in both the brain vasculature and parenchyma (Holtzman, 2001). As a result, compared to E3, APOE4 increases the risk for AD dementia, while APOE2 is protective. Interestingly, the association of APOE with CAA is discordant with that of AD. Whereas APOE4 is associated with higher risk of CAA, APOE2 is also an independent risk factors associated with increased sporadic CAA and lobar hemorrhages (Nelson et al., 2013; Yu, Boyle, Nag et al., 2015).

4. Neuropathology of Cerebrovascular Tissue Injury in Aging

4.1. Brain Infarcts

Brain infarcts are caused by insufficient blood flow, resulting in parenchyma necrosis. Macroscopic changes in the brain after a stroke or infarct correspond to the sequence of microscopic changes. Macroscopic changes in an acute infarct occurring 12 to 36 hours prior to death includes discoloration and slight softening of the brain tissue. An infarct in subacute stages, which occurs within the interval of 2 days to several weeks, is typically associated with cytotoxic edema, resulting in blurring between the demarcation of the white and gray matter. Lastly, the changes associated with a chronic infarct, which can occur after an interval of a few months, revealing liquefactive necrosis and cavitation. Microscopic changes in an acute infarct include pyknosis of neurons result in loss of Nissl substance in neurons and the appearance of a "red" (eosinophilic) neuron. Often there is pallor and vacuolation of the neuropil in acute infarcts. In subacute stages, reactive astrocytes are present, and there may be a sparse infiltration of neutrophils and formation of foamy-macrophages, (hemosiderin-laden macrophages with a hemorrhagic infarct). In chronic stages, there are an abundant number of reactive astrocytes and microglia, surrounding the infarct region and foamy-macrophages or hemosiderin-laden macrophages within the central area of necrosis. An infarct typically comprises of a central ischemic core and an ischemic penumbra zone (surrounding the ischemic brain tissue). In comparison to the central core, which has necrotic tissue and is irreversibly damaged, there are many active pathogenic mechanisms evolving in the penumbra, making this surrounding tissue potentially salvageable with appropriate treatments (Liu, Levine, & Winn, 2010).

There are many different types of brain infarcts that can occur in the aging brain, which can differ in size, location, underlying pathophysiological mechanisms, and their clinical effects. First, large brain infarcts (larger than 15 mm^3) are often a result of thrombotic events or thromboembolic occlusion of larger blood vessels. Large hemorrhagic infarcts are associated with a variety of mechanisms, most commonly from a cardiac embolism, with reperfusion in the ischemic infarcted area. Second, rupture of fragile CAA- or SVD-affected vessels (Kalaria, 2016) can occur causing a hemorrhage. However, for these events infarct size and location are not typically definitive indicators of the mechanism of injury. Watershed (or border zone) infarcts are lesions which occur at the distal ends between two or more arterial territories. For example, an anterior watershed infarct may occur at the distal ends of the anterior and middle cerebral arterial territories. Depending on anatomical location, these infarcts can be classified into external (cortical) or internal (subcortical) watershed infarcts. In the event of hemodynamic compromise in the brain (usually in patients with internal carotid stenosis), watershed regions have lower perfusion, creating a hypoxic environment and making them more susceptible to hypoxic-ischemic lesions (Kapasi et al., 2018; Mangla, Kolar, Almast, & Ekholm, 2011).

Lacunar infarcts are small irregular lesions ranging from 1 to 15 mm in size most commonly located in the subcortical nuclei (putamen, caudate, globus pallidus, and thalamus), internal capsule, pons, and perhaps less commonly in the subcortical white matter and cerebellum (Figure 14.2).

Significant vascular and/or occlusive changes in smaller penetrating arteries or arterioles, which branch off from the large arteries in the brain, can lead to decreased perfusion and result in the development of a lacunar infarct. Age, smoking, hypertension, and diabetes are all well-known risk factors for SVD and for lacunar infarcts (Caplan, 2015). In addition to arterial strokes or infarctions, venous infarcts are caused by an obstruction to the venous system (e.g., cerebral

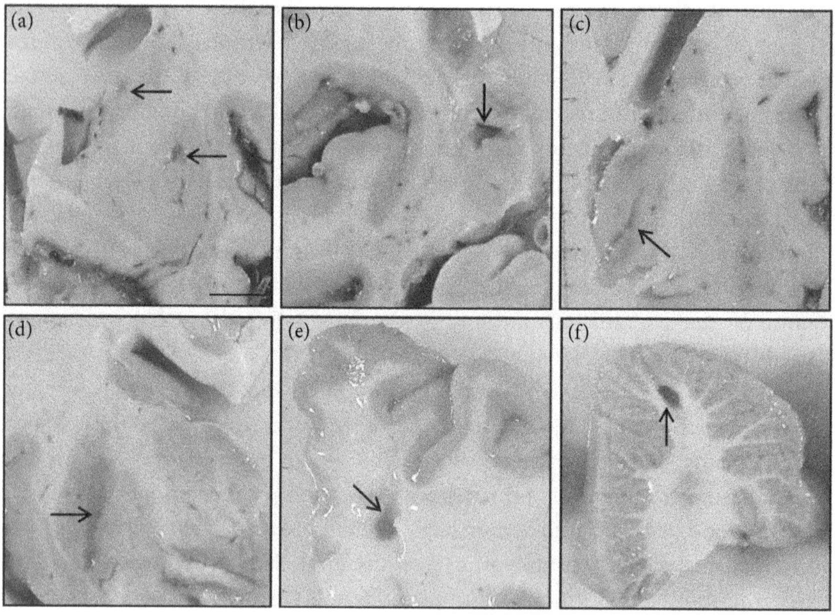

Figure 14.2. Macroscopic appearance of lacunar infarcts. Top panel shows lacunar infarcts involving the caudate and putamen (A), mid-thalamus (B), and anterior thalamus (C) in formalin-fixed tissue. Bottom panel shows lacunar infarcts involving putamen (D), subcortical frontal white matter (E), and cerebellar white matter (F) in fresh brain tissue.

Note: Scale bar 10mm for all images.

venous thrombosis). However, these types of infarcts are related to specific risk factors such as hypercoagulable states and are relatively uncommon (Kowoll et al., 2016).

Finally, microinfarcts are microscopic lesions that are not visible to the naked eye and vary in size between 100 μm to only a few of millimeters. While newer imaging modalities have improved the ability to detect these microscopic lesions, imaging techniques generally detect lesions >1 mm in size and therefore only capturing the tip of the iceberg, leaving the smallest of lesions (from 100 μm in size) only detectable by neuropathological examination. Similar to macroscopic infarcts, microinfarcts can be categorized into acute, subacute, and chronic ages based on their histological appearance. Acute microinfarcts often have a focal area of neuronal injury, while chronic microinfarcts lesions are associated with cavitation, gliosis, and presence of macrophages (van Veluw, Shih et al., 2017). On a routine neuropathological examination, microinfarct counts can range from one to very few lesions. However mathematical studies show that finding one microinfarct implies there is a vascular burden of over 500 microinfarcts, and finding two implies there are over 1,000 microinfarcts throughout the whole brain (Westover, Bianchi, Yang, Schneider, & Greenberg, 2013), reinforcing the idea we are only detecting the tip of the iceberg, and microscopic vascular lesions are perhaps major contributors to cognitive impairments.

4.2. Cerebral Hemorrhages and Microbleeds

There are many different underlying causes a blood vessel to rupture resulting in extravasation of blood into the brain parenchyma resulting in cerebral hemorrhages. Generally, hypertensive vasculopathy or SVD (commonly associated with hypertension) and CAA are primarily the most common vessel pathologies accompanying hemorrhages and microbleeds in the elderly. Other nontraumatic causes of hemorrhages can include aneurysms and arteriovenous malformations; however, these are relatively less common in the older population. Large hemorrhages can cause displacement of the brain tissue and cerebral edema resulting in increased intracranial pressure leading to brain herniation. CAA is considered the major cause of lobar intracerebral hemorrhage, most commonly occurring in parietal-occipital locations. Hypertensive vasculopathy or SVD is also associated with hemorrhages and/or microbleeds often located in the basal ganglia, thalamus, cerebellum, and brainstem (Fazekas et al., 1999; Greenberg, Vernooij et al., 2009; Figure 14.3).

Microbleeds are small lesions that are usually less than 10 mm in diameter and are typically defined radiographically. Histologically, microbleeds present with extravasated or lysed erythrocytes. The presence of hemosiderin-laden

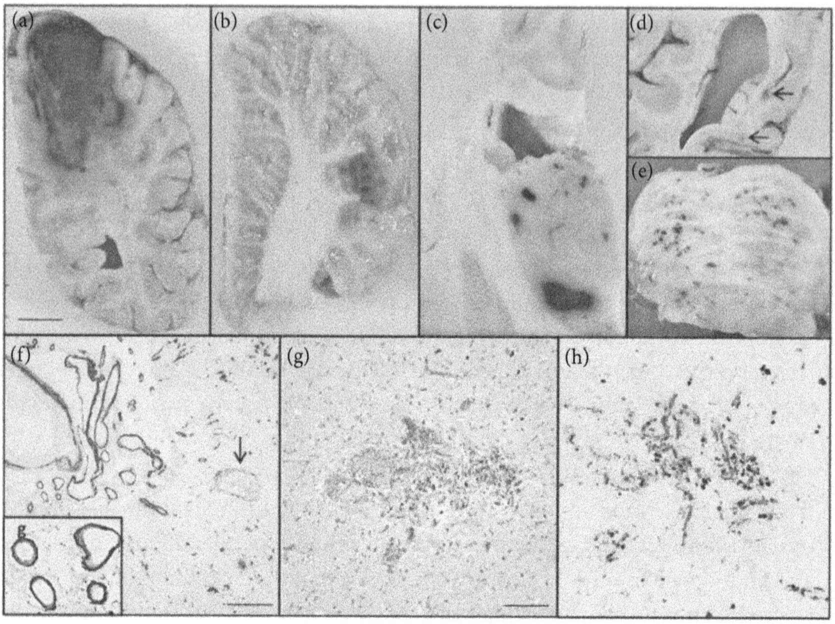

Figure 14.3. Pathology of hemorrhages and microbleeds. Macroscopic images: An acute (recent) intracerebral lobar hemorrhage in the superior parietal lobule extending into the parietal white matter (A). Macroscopic acute hemorrhages, which could be detected as microbleeds with neuroimaging, in the cerebellar lateral cortex (B), thalamus (C), and pons (E). Of note, petechial hemorrhage in the pons (E) may be association with disseminated intravascular coagulation. Two chronic (old) microbleeds present in occipital temporal cortex (arrows; D). Microscopic images: Immunohistochemistry for amyloid in the inferior parietal lobule shows amyloid angiopathy, involving leptomeningeal and parenchymal vessels, with a chronic microhemorrhage in the cortex (arrow; F). Circumferential amyloid deposition in leptomeningeal vessels (G). Histology of a chronic (old) microbleed with a routine hematoxylin and eosin stain shows disruption of vessel wall with accumulation of hemosiderin-laden macrophages (brown deposits; H). Perls iron stain of a chronic (old) microbleed (I).

Notes: Scale bar 10mm (images A–E); 250μm (images F and G); and 100μm (images H and I).

macrophages or iron, with varying degrees of astrocytosis and tissue damage, may indicate a chronic stage (van Veluw, Biessels, Klijn, & Rozemuller, 2016; van Veluw et al., 2017). The primary pathological mechanism of microbleeds is leakage of blood (or extravasated erythrocyte hemoglobin) from nearby damaged vessels. Additional mechanism for microbleeds revolve iron released by oligodendrocytes (Janaway et al., 2014), the presence of hemorrhagic microinfarcts (Tanskanen et al., 2012), or phagocytosis of a microemboli in the perivascular space (Grutzendler et al., 2014).

Cortical/lobar microbleeds identified on imaging are most indicative of CAA, while deep microbleeds observed in white matter are more associated with arteriolosclerosis (Greenberg et al., 2009; Hommet et al., 2011; van Es et al., 2011). In a magnetic resonance imaging (MRI) study, microbleeds were preferentially localized with increased concentration of Aβ detected by 11C-Pittsburgh Compound B positron emission tomography (PiB PET) imaging, suggesting this tool may be useful in predicting incident hemorrhages (Gurol et al., 2012). However, PiB-PET cannot reliably detect Aβ in parenchymal vessels (Kovari et al., 2015). There is strong evidence to suggest cortical microbleeds are strongly associated with CAA; however, studies are raising the possibility that other mechanisms may also be involved in the pathophysiology of these microbleeds. For example, a neuropathological study in a large autopsy series showed no direct evidence between CAA and the presence of cortical microbleeds, raising the possibility of involvement of nonamyloid SVD or other pathogenic mechanisms in the pathophysiology of cortical microbleeds (Kovari et al., 2015). Another study also showed low levels of Aβ in the microenvironment of cortical microbleeds (van Veluw et al., 2017). Microbleeds visualized on imaging have variable pathological correlates, most often including focal accumulation of hemosiderin deposits, but also (less likely) small lacunes with hemosiderin or microaneurysms (Gouw et al., 2011; Schrag et al., 2010). Together, these findings demonstrate the need for MRI–histopathology validation studies to bridge the gap between imaging and neuropathology.

Both hemorrhages and microbleeds can be accompanied by other age-related vascular pathologies, including white matter changes and microinfarcts (De Reuck et al., 2016; Lauer et al., 2016). An interesting area of ongoing investigation is how small microbleeds can be related to their larger counterparts; that is, is there a snowball effect where rupture of one vessel leads to a rupture on surrounding vessels? It has also been suggested that the hemorrhagic process may occur after an ischemic process; however, direct evidence for this is lacking (Greenberg, Vernooij et al., 2009).

4.3. White Matter Lesions

White matter lesions are synonymous with leukoaraiosis as seen on computed tomography images, and MRI high signal T2-weighted WMH are heterogeneous in etiology and clinical manifestations and therefore are diagnostically challenging. They are typically observed as a clinical surrogate for cerebral SVD and have been associated with increased likelihood of cognitive impairment and dementia including AD (Benedictus et al., 2013; Boyle et al., 2016; Joutel & Chabriat, 2017). However, WMH are not specific to AD and can also been seen in cognitively healthy persons and in other neurological diseases including migraines, multiple sclerosis, other autoimmune and inflammatory diseases, and leukodystophies (Hamedani et al., 2013; Zhong, Utriainen, Wang, Kang, & Haacke, 2014). Pathological features are consistent with white matter pallor, demyelination and axonal loss, tissue rarefaction, gliosis, and macrophage activation, with sparing of subcortical U-fibers. Patients with CVD or those with vascular risk factors often present with an increase of white mater lesions (Kalaria et al., 2004). Pathological heterogeneity in community-based older persons can occur depending on the type of white matter lesions, for example, in punctate versus confluent lesions (Schmidt et al., 2003, 2011). There may also be differences depending on anatomical location of the white matter involved, for example, periventricular white matter versus subcortical (Murray et al., 2012) and watershed versus non-watershed regions (Mangla et al., 2011). Minor pathological changes limited to the capping or the rim of periventricular regions are hypothesized to be associated with disturbed CSF transports and edema. More progressive/advanced lesions are thought to have a vascular etiology (DeCarli, Fletcher, Ramey, Harvey, & Jagust, 2005). Finally, accumulating evidence suggests that white matter lesions are attributed to SVD-related ischemia/hypoxic injury. However, in the context of cortical degenerative pathology, Wallerian degeneration (axonal injury) may be also be involved (McAleese et al., 2017). Whereas the common views of the pathophysiology accounting for white matter lesions include chronic hypoperfusion, blood–brain barrier (BBB) dysfunction, and changes in cerebral blood flow (Joutel & Chabriat, 2017), there is some speculation AD pathology may be related to WMH through vascular and/or nonvascular processes (Lee et al., 2016).

5. Vascular Dementia

VaD is a dementia syndrome caused solely by vascular injuries to brain tissue typically from ischemic and/or hemorrhagic etiologies. Because some clinicians believe that dementia syndromes require memory impairment, and some patients with cognitive impairment from vascular disease do not necessarily present with an amnestic disorder, the term "vascular cognitive impairment" has been introduced (Bowler, 2004, 2005; Bowler & Hachinski, 1995). VCI can include mild cognitive impairment, often revolving around the presence of a dysexecutive syndrome and is sometimes used interchangeably with VaD. More recently, because of mixed pathologies as well as vascular contributions to AD and other degenerative pathologies, the term "vascular contributions to cognitive impairment" has also been considered. In epidemiology literature, the term "vascular dementia" is frequently used, but these studies often do not separate between those with pure VaD, VCI, and mixed pathologies (i.e. those where vascular pathology contributes to dementia; van der Flier et al., 2018).

Over the years, many criteria to operationally define VaD have been proposed. All current criteria for VCI are based on two factors: (a) the presentation of cognitive impairment and (b) either a clinical history of stroke or presence of vascular disease by imaging (Gorelick et al., 2011). VaD often presents as a heterogeneous syndrome and can co-exist with other cerebral and systemic disorders, all of which can lead to cognitive dysfunction. Epidemiology studies show that the prevalence of clinical VaD among adults older than 68 years accounts for 14.5% of dementia cases (Goodman et al., 2017). Pathologically confirmed diagnosis of "pure" VaD is relatively uncommon in older persons with dementia (with most having vascular mixed with other pathologies), and often cerebrovascular pathologies, like infarcts and WMH, can go unrecognized clinically. Therefore, the contribution of vascular disease burden to cognitive impairment and dementia is often underestimated in these epidemiology studies. Data from two large autopsy series in the United States, the Religious Orders Study and the Rush Memory and Aging Project, showed approximately only 16% of persons had isolated vascular pathology irrespective of clinical diagnosis (Kapasi, DeCarli, & Schneider, 2017). Isolated vascular pathology frequency further decreases to <10% in persons with a clinical diagnosis of dementia (Schneider, 2007). In comparison to isolated vascular pathologies, there is a higher burden of "mixed" vascular pathologies, including AD and/or other degenerative pathologies mixed with vascular pathologies among participants with and without dementia (Kapasi et al., 2017). Other Western population-based studies have also shown similar proportion rates of "pure" VaD (Thal et al., 2012). However, in Asian and Japanese population studies, there is a higher prevalence of VaD (Ikeda et al., 2001).

One study identified pathological changes in persons clinically diagnosed with VaD. Cystic infarcts were present in 25% of participants, but the most common finding was the presence of lacunar infarcts and microinfarcts in over 50% of persons. This study did not include watershed or border zone infarcts, which could also be present (Kalaria, Akinyemi, & Ihara, 2016; Vinters et al., 2000). Furthermore, remote hippocampal injury was also present in 55% of persons diagnosed with VaD (Vinters et al., 2000). Vascular brain lesions underlying VaD can occur either as multi-infarct dementia, strategic infarct dementia, or subcortical ischemic VaD. Multi-infarct dementia is characterized by multiple large and small infarcts, lacunar infarcts, and microinfarcts in the cortical and subcortical brain regions. The etiology can be multiple, and infarcts can be a result of atherosclerosis in large brain arteries, embolic events, and SVD. Strategic infarct dementia involves strategically localized infarcts in particular brain regions, for example bilateral lesions in the thalamus or hippocampus. A predominant feature of VCI is disruption of fronto-cortical networks, resulting in dysfunction of executive functions (Kalaria & Erkinjuntti, 2006; Thal et al., 2012). Subcortical ischemic VaD, also known as Binswanger's disease, is characterized by the presence of multiple lacunar infarcts with diffuse white matter demyelination and sparing the subcortical U-fibers.

6. Poststroke Dementia

Development of dementia after a stroke depends on the presence of several factors: (a) the location and volume of the stroke), (b) if there was pre-existing cognitive impairment, (c) incidence of co-occurring cerebral pathologies, and (d) the degree of neuronal damage or dysfunction. The etiology can be complex often including both small and large vessel disease, and other neurodegenerative pathologies. Often patients with poststroke cognitive impairment or dementia present with a history of multiple stroke events. However, a strategic infarct or hemorrhage in critical locations could also result in VCI. There is a temporal relationship between the onset of stroke and cognitive impairment. By definition, poststroke dementia is defined by cognitive impairment or dementia occurring within 3 months or after a stable period of a year after stroke injury (Kalaria et al., 2016). Like VaD, and VCI, the underlying biology of poststroke dementia includes pure vascular disorders as well as mixed pathologies. Pathological changes in patients with clinical variants of VCI including poststroke subcortical ischemia and mixed AD and VaD subtypes. These pathological changes are positive for decrease in cell volume of the prefrontal cortex associated with impaired executive functions (Foster et al., 2014). In poststroke cohorts, presence of executive impairment together with depression predicts poorer long-term survival than just depression itself (Melkas et al., 2010).

7. Age-Related Neuropathology Associated, Cognitive Impairment, and Dementia

As previously noted, vascular disease often co-exists with AD and other non-AD neurodegenerative diseases. Therefore, it is often difficult to assign the consequence of cognitive dysfunction to vascular disease, AD pathology, and/or other non-AD neurodegenerative pathologies (Figure 14.4).

Some of these difficulties may partly be due to the complexity and heterogeneity of vascular diseases; for example, infarcts vary by size, number, and location (Schneider et al., 2003; Sonnen et al., 2007) that occur in persons with and without degenerative dementia (Jellinger & Attems, 2012). These

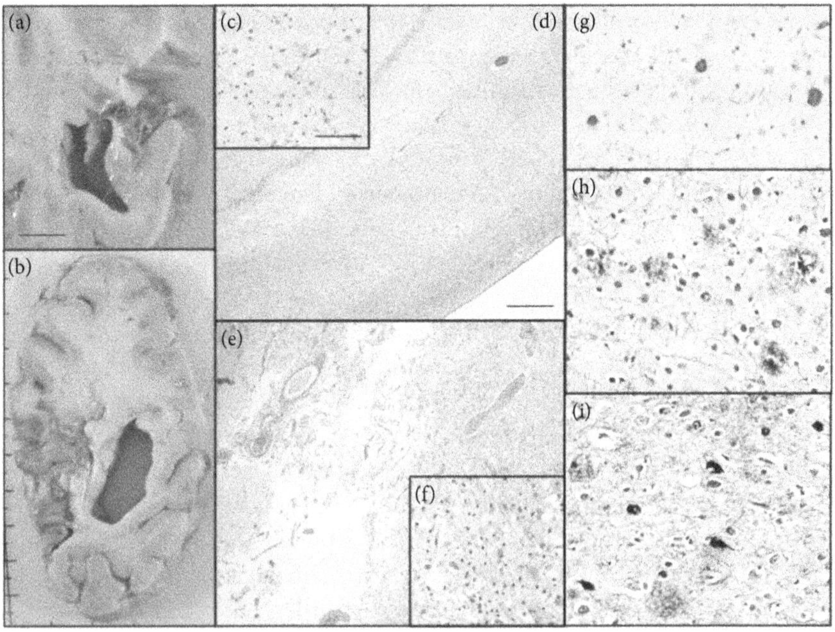

Figure 14.4. Mixed Alzheimer's disease (AD), vascular and non-AD degenerative pathologies, in a 68-year-old man with a history of motor and cognitive impairment. Neuropathological findings show multiple pathologies coexisting in the brain meeting the criteria for several pathological diagnoses. Macroscopic examination of the left hemisphere showed atrophy of the hippocampus (A) and a large chronic infarct involving the parietal and temporal lobes (B). Hematoxylin and eosin stain shows severe neuronal loss and gliosis in the CA1 region of the hippocampus (C and D). Microscopy of chronic infarct shows cavitation in the central ischemic core and reactive astrocytes and accumulation of foamy macrophages in the surrounding ischemic penumbra (E and F). Alpha-synuclein immunohistochemistry shows presence of Lewy bodies and Lewy-positive neurites in the Amygdala (G). Bielschowsky silver stain indicates presence of AD pathology, neuritic plaques (H) and neurofibrillary tangles (I). Neuropathological changes were consistent with a pathological diagnosis of high likelihood of Alzheimer's disease, dementia with Lewy body disease (Amygdala-predominant), hippocampal sclerosis involving the CA1 region, and the presence of a chronic macroscopic infarct.

Notes: Scale bars 10mm (images A and B); 250μm (images D and E); and 100μm (images C, F, and G–I).

neuropathological alterations can fail to be recognized as they are often not associated with clinical stroke (Longstreth, 1998). Use of clinical data proximate to death and quantitative neuropathological data in community-based studies from persons with and without dementia can overcome some obstacles. These data have provided new insights into the contribution of vascular disease and vascular pathology to cognitive impairment and dementia. The types of neurodegenerative pathologies identified in community-based pathological studies include AD, Lewy body, HS, and TAR DNA binding protein 43 (TDP-43), and a wide variety of vascular pathologies include macro- and microinfarcts, and vessel pathologies including atherosclerosis, arteriolosclerosis, and CAA.

A large number of community-based studies indicate older persons with and without dementia present with mixed pathologies (Brayne et al., 2009; Brenowitz et al., 2016; James, Bennett, Boyle, Leurgans, & Schneider, 2012; Schneider, Arvanitakis, Bang, & Bennett, 2007; Schneider, Aggarwal, Barnes, Boyle, & Bennett, 2009). Specifically, persons with AD might not only have a confirmed pathological changes diagnostic of AD but also present with evidence of vascular disease and other non-AD neurodegenerative pathologies. Pathological studies of patients with dementia from the Religious Orders Study and Rush Memory and Aging project showed that 85% of persons with a clinical diagnosis of probable AD did, indeed, have a confirmed pathologic diagnosis of AD. However, isolated AD pathology was rare (3%). Nearly 90% of people with a clinical diagnosis of probable AD had one or more type of vascular pathologies. Over 45% presenting with AD, vascular, and other degenerative (Kapasi et al., 2017). Other studies have also reported high frequency of cerebrovascular pathologies in older persons (Neuropathology Group; Medical Research Council Cognitive Function and Aging Study, 2001).

8. Clinical Pathological Correlates of Mixed AD and Vascular Pathologies

8.1. Infarction

Several studies suggest concomitant CVD including brain infarction in persons meeting neuropathological criteria for AD increases the risk and severity for clinical dementia. Some researchers have suggested a synergistic relationship between AD and vascular alterations such that concomitant vascular lesions can be seen along with fewer Alzheimer's plaques and neurofibrillary tangles needed to reach threshold for clinical dementia (Esiri, Nagy, Smith, Barnetson, & Smith, 1999; Petrovitch et al., 2000; Snowdon et al., 1997). Other researchers have suggested an additive effect between AD and vascular pathology in lowering cognitive functioning (Schneider et al., 2007). Indeed, brain infarcts have been shown to lower function in specific cognitive domains including episodic memory, the hallmark of clinical AD, even after accounting for AD pathology (Schneider, Wilson, Bienias, Evans, & Bennett, 2004; Schneider et al., 2007).

In some studies microinfarct frequency is more common than macroscopic infarcts (Sonnen et al., 2007; White et al., 2002). Increasingly, studies suggest cortical microinfarcts are important independent contributors to cognitive dysfunction and dementia (Arvanitakis, Leurgans, Barnes, Bennett, & Schneider, 2011; Corrada et al., 2016; Kovari et al., 2004) with multiple cortical infarct associated with significant cognitive impairment (Arvanitakis et al., 2011; Sonnen et al., 2007). Furthermore, sophisticated statistical approaches when microinfarcts are present on a neuropathological evaluation often suggests the presence of thousands of additional microscopic lesions in the brain (Westover et al., 2013). These unrecognized lesions may disrupt structural networks, further contributing to cognitive dysfunction. The odds of having cortical microinfarcts are increased with the presence of CAA, while the odds of having subcortical microinfarcts are increased with arteriolar- and atherosclerosis (Arvanitakis et al., 2017). Toledo et al. (2013) found that concurrent CVD is a common neuropathological finding in persons with dementia; is more common in AD than in other neurodegenerative disorders, especially in younger subjects; and lowers the threshold for dementia due to AD and synucleinopathies, In keeping with this, persons having advanced Lewy body pathology show less CVD (Ghebremedhin et al., 2010). However, age-at-death of persons with advanced Lewy body pathology may be much younger. This may explain the lower burden of vascular pathology. Lower incidence of CVD has also been found in patients with frontotemporal lobe dementia (FTLD), with 17% for FTLD–TDP-43 and 5% for FTLD–tau (Toledo et al., 2013). Again, these individuals are often younger, and this may at least partially explain the lower amount of CVDs.

8.2. Atherosclerosis

Atherosclerosis commonly occurs in cerebral arteries and circle of Willis in the brain in older persons. Data from participants of the Rotterdam study, a population-based cohort, suggests atherosclerosis increases the risk of dementia independent of AD pathology (Dolan et al., 2010; van Oijen et al., 2007). Pathologic data showed that the relation of intracranial atherosclerosis with global cognitive dysfunction was independent of gross and microscopic infarcts as well as SVD (Arvanitakis, Capuano, Leurgans, Bennett, & Schneider, 2016). There are conflicting studies on the relationship between atherosclerosis and AD pathology. Some studies report a relationship between atherosclerosis in cerebral arteries and circle of Willis with AD pathology (Beach et al., 2007; Honig, Kukull, & Mayeux, 2005) while others showing conflicting data (Dolan et al., 2010). Indeed, new neuroimaging techniques measuring cerebral blood flow in circle of Willis will be important in understanding the role of atherosclerosis with AD pathology and cognitive impairment.

8.3. Small Vessel Disease

SVD markers represent a potential link between aging, stroke, cognitive dysfunction, and dementia, yet they have not emerged as candidates for clinical trials, perhaps due to their uncertain pathological mechanism and undefined MRI markers. However, there is significant effort to develop SVD biomarkers to understand their contribution to cognitive impairment. The most common alterations as related to SVD and, perhaps the earliest vascular changes, are arteriolosclerosis and CAA (Deramecourt et al., 2012). Sporadic CAA has been shown to be associated with cognitive impairment (Pfeifer et al., 2002) and increased odds of clinical AD dementia (Boyle et al., 2015). Indeed, CAA may occur independently of AD and is commonly associated with other pathologies including lobar hemorrhages, microbleeds, and microinfarcts in older persons, all of which have been implicated in cognitive dysfunction (Lauer et al., 2016; Summers et al., 2017). Similar to microinfarcts, the number and location of microbleeds need to be considered in determining the specific impact microbleeds have on cognition. A higher number of microbleeds (≥4 bleeds) is associated with cognitive decline (Akoudad et al., 2016) and in particular lobar/cortical microbleeds (more likely to be related to CAA) are found to predict poorer cognitive performance than deep microbleeds (more likely to be related to hypertension; Poels et al., 2012). It seems likely that microbleeds partly mediate the relationship between CAA and cognition, but other factors are likely. Lastly, arteriolosclerosis has also been shown to be independently associated with lowered global cognition, poorer performance specifically in episodic memory and perceptual speed, and increased odds of developing dementia (Arvanitakis et al., 2016; Ighodaro et al., 2017).

9. Impact of Mixed Pathologies on Cognitive Impairment and Clinical Phenotype

There is significant heterogeneity with mixed pathologies, and the extent to which these additional pathologies impact cognition. In cross-sectional studies,

AD pathology had the strongest effect on episodic memory with infarcts showing their strongest effect on tests assessing information processing speed. However, it is important to note that there is tremendous overlap in the effects of infarcts and AD pathology on cognitive domains (Schneider & Bennett, 2010). Previous studies have suggested neurodegenerative pathologies may account for a larger percentage of cognitive decline and have been weighted in order of the impact on neurocognitive impairment, starting neurofibrillary tangles, Lewy bodies, amyloid plaques, and macroscopic infarcts (Boyle et al., 2013).

Recent research has shown that multiple types of vascular pathology accounted for over 30% of the association between age and dementia (Power et al., 2018). In persons with AD vascular pathology was present in over 25% of cases (Boyle et al., 2018). Interestingly, AD pathology accounted for 22% to 100% of cognitive loss, whereas macroscopic infarct and other vascular pathologies had a less potent effect, ranging from 10% to 30% (Boyle et al., 2018). The timing of cognitive decline may also vary by pathology. While infarct pathology has been associated with early cognitive decline, Lewy body pathology has been implicated in later stages (Yu, Boyle, Leurgans et al., 2015). Moreover, the presence of single versus a combination of pathologies also has an effect on the clinical progression to dementia. Faster progression to clinical dementia was identified in persons with mixed AD/Lewy body disease pathology compared to persons with mixed AD/Vascular Brain Injury (VBI) or AD alone (Brenowitz et al., 2016).

Taken together, AD pathology including neuritic plaques and neurofibrillary tangles; along with macroinfarcts, microinfarcts, and Lewy body pathologies accounted for 40% of the variance of cognitive decline (Boyle et al., 2013). HS is pathologically defined as severe neuronal loss and gliosis in the CA1 and/or subiculum subfields of the hippocampus. HS may accompany neurodegenerative and vascular disorders including AD, FTLD, VaD, dementia with Lewy body disease, and tauopathies. Indeed, HS pathology has also been described in non-neurodegenerative disorders including temporal lobe epilepsy and multiple sclerosis (Hatanpaa et al., 2014). In comparison to younger individuals with HS, older persons with HS have a significantly increase probability of cognitive dysfunction (Nelson et al., 2011). In persons with dementia, HS is particularly common in those who are very old (over 90 years; Nag et al., 2015). There are two main views regarding the etiology of HS: hypoxic-ischemic injury or neurodegeneration. A hypoxic-ischemic origin is supported by the fact CA1 neurons have an increased number of glutamate receptors and therefore would be more susceptible to excitotoxic cell death in a hypoxic environment (Amador-Ortiz, Ahmed, Zehr, & Dickson, 2007). Further supporting the notion of a ischemic etiology, there have been reports of patients with HS showing ischemic damage (Volpe BT, 1985), and increased prevalence of cardiac and CVD (Crystal et al., 2000; Kril, Patel, Harding, & Halliday, 2002; Wegiel et al., 2002). However, there are conflicting data regarding the association of HS with CVD or vascular risk factors, with some autopsy studies showing a lack of association (Leverenz et al., 2002; Nelson et al., 2011). In contrast, the hypothesis of a neurodegenerative cause is supported by the fact HS is commonly accompanied by other types of pathology including AD pathology and TDP-43 proteinopathy. Furthermore, recent clinical pathological studies have shown older persons with HS mixed with TDP-43 proteinopathy or AD pathology show poorer performance in multiple cognitive domains (Josephs et al., 2008; Nag et al., 2015). Given that the hippocampus is vulnerable to both ischemic and neurodegenerative diseases and HS is observed in multiple disorders, it is quite likely that HS in aging is etiologically heterogeneous. The presence of co-existing TDP-43 may suggest a degenerative etiology, and the absence of such in an older person is more likely to be vascular in etiology (Amador-Ortiz, Ahmed, Zehr, & Dickson, 2007). Interestingly, HS with TDP-43 pathology may also have links to vascular pathogenesis (Nelson et al., 2016).

10. Mechanisms Contributing to Vascular Disease

10.1. Inflammation

In the aging brain the neuroinflammatory processes include endothelial activation, recruitment of perivascular macrophages, activation of microglia, and induction of inflammatory-related proteins. On a molecular and cellular level, it is clear that an inflammatory response accompanies AD pathology as well as other non-AD neurodegenerative diseases. Neuropathological studies show the presence of inflammatory-related markers and activated microglia around fibrillary amyloid plaques in both animal and human studies (Eikelenboom et al., 2010). Indeed, age-related changes in microglia may also play a role in the pathogenesis of AD (Wong, 2013). The cerebral white matter consists of various glial cell types including astrocytes, oligodendrocytes, and microglia. There is emerging literature to suggest inflammation may be a feature of WMH, suggesting that inflammation is associated with SVD (Giwa et al., 2012; Satizabal, Zhu, Mazoyer, Dufouil, & Tzourio, 2012). There is an increase in activated microglia in white matter lesions in both subcortical and periventricular regions, but the pathological nature of microglia differs. While activated microglia (ramified) in the periventricular region are likely due to immune response, activated microglia (amoeboid) in subcortical regions have a role in removing myelin breakdown debris (Simpson et al., 2007).

10.2. Dysfunction of Blood–Brain Barrier

The neurovascular unit comprises a specialized network of cells including pericytes, endothelial cells, astrocytes, and neurons, all of which play an important role in maintaining the BBB and regulate cerebral blood flow. Neuropathological assessment of BBB dysfunction can be difficult to assess and, therefore, in clinical-pathological studies the relationship between BBB dysfunction with the various forms of dementia remains less clear; however, there is some evidence to suggest BBB dysfunction increases in the aging brain. Indeed, a large number of studies using animal models provide compelling evidence to suggest these factors play a role in pathophysiological mechanisms contributing to cognitive impairment.

Several neuropathological studies show older persons have some degree of BBB permeability, evidenced by extravasation of plasma proteins such as fibrinogen, albumin, and immunoglobulins (Bridges et al., 2014; Hainsworth et al., 2017; Tomimoto et al., 1996), which may be partly due to accumulation of Aβ surrounding and within cerebral vessels, and associated neuroinflammation in the microenvironment (Takeda, Sato, & Morishita, 2014). Additionally, contrast MRI studies (Wardlaw et al., 2009; Zhang et al., 2017) have demonstrated the presence of extravagated plasma proteins due to BBB leakage. Some suggest BBB dysfunction is an early process in aging and in AD (Montagne et al., 2015). In addition, evidence suggests BBB dysfunction in defined areas of white matter lesions increase the risk of developing clinical dementia. This increased risk may be due to the toxic brain environment, as consequence of extravasated plasma proteins (Hainsworth et al., 2017). Findings regarding the association of BBB dysfunction with SVD remain unclear with some studies suggesting there is an association (Tomimoto et al., 1996; Utter et al., 2008) and others showing conflicting data (Bridges et al., 2014). Nonetheless, several studies consistently suggest that BBB dysfunction is common in the elderly and relevant to the cognitive changes associated with aging and dementia.

10.3. Neuropathological Correlates of Vascular Risk Factors

A number of vascular risk factors have been identified that induce neuropathological changes in brain structure and are associated with an increased risk of cognitive impairment and dementia. Diabetes mellitus is common condition. Several neuropathological studies have revealed that diabetes is associated with increased number of brain microinfarcts and lacunar infarcts, but not AD pathology (Arvanitakis et al., 2006; Peila, Rodriguez, Launer, & Honolulu–Asia Aging Study, 2002; Sonnen et al., 2009). Brain imaging studies also show a relation between diabetes with lacunar infarcts and white matter changes (Longstreth et al., 1998; Schmidt et al., 2004). While diabetes affects both amnestic and other cognitive functions, the association between diabetes and nonamnestic cognitive dysfunctions is greater in magnitude (Luchsinger et al., 2007). This dysfunction is often related to disruption of fronto-parietal connectivity via white matter injury as a result of cerebrovascular lesions (Knopman & Roberts, 2010).

In the elderly, high blood pressure is extremely common and has also been shown to be associated with cerebrovascular pathology (Brickman et al., 2010) as well as cognitive impairment, in particular when onset occurs in midlife. Recent studies show that in addition to the presence or absence of high blood pressure the trajectory and change in blood pressure over time is important as related to cognitive decline (Arvanitakis et al., 2018; J. Graff-Radford et al., 2018). Elevated blood pressure in late life is related to an increased number of cerebral infarcts as well as neurofibrillary tangles (Arvanitakis et al., 2018). Other studies have also reported an association between midlife hypertension with AD neuropathologic changes in late life (Hoffman et al., 2009; Petrovitch et al., 2000). Furthermore, studies have shown persons treated with antihypertensive medication had less AD pathology than those who had untreated hypertension (Hoffman et al., 2009). Imaging studies have also shown that midlife vascular risk factors are associated with late-life amyloid deposition (Gottesman et al., 2017), accelerated volume and progression of WMH, and an increase in temporal horn volume (an imaging surrogate for hippocampal atrophy; Debette et al., 2011).

11. Neuropathological Assessment in Specialized Populations/Cohorts

11.1. Community-Based and Clinic-Based Cohorts

Traditional clinical pathological studies of aging and dementia using clinic-based cohorts have been important in understanding clinical pathological relationships. However, these findings must be carefully considered as they may not be representative of older persons living in the community. Selection bias is important to consider as persons referred from a hospital or specialty clinics may not be representative of the community. Previous studies have shown important differences in sociodemographic variables (Kokmen, Ozsarfati, Beard, O'Brien, & Rocca, 1996), clinical features (Massoud et al., 1999), and genetic factors between clinic-based and community-based cohorts. Compared to community-based studies there is an overrepresentation of the younger population in clinic-based studies. Thus, incorrect conclusions might be drawn and may have important ramifications if generalized to older persons with dementia (Schoenmaker & Van Gool, 2004). Most persons who are referred to specialized clinics already have a certain degree of suspected or documented cognitive impairment and/or have been clinically diagnosed as having dementia. Risk factors identified in these people who have been referred may be different than those people who live in a community and who have not yet developed dementia. Therefore, in these studies, it is important to include persons who are representative of the community and who are without known dementia or cognitive impairment (Barnes & Bennett, 2014).

There are also likely to be neuropathological differences between those referred to specialty clinic and people who are representative of the community (Massoud et al., 1999; Schneider et al., 2009). Compared to clinic patients, people with AD who live in the community had less AD pathology in their brains resulting in a pathological diagnosis of intermediate likelihood of AD (Schneider et al., 2009). There are, perhaps, multiple factors that could explain this difference. In the community, persons with dementia may have less severe cognitive impairment (Bennett et al., 2006). In addition, the average age of community-based participants is older than clinic participants resulting in a higher incidence of mixed pathologies with concomitant less AD pathology. Finally, clinic patients referred on the basis of severe behavioral abnormalities may have more severe cognitive impairments and, perhaps, higher burden of AD pathology. Greater Lewy body pathology and atypical pathologies are also observed in clinic-based patients compared to community-based participants (Schneider et al., 2009). This may be expected as Lewy body pathologies are associated with behavioral and sleep disorders (Ferman et al., 2014). These disturbance are likely to result in families and patients seeking out medical attention from tertiary-care specialty centers. Mixed and cerebrovascular pathologies were more common in the community than the clinic (Massoud et al., 1999; Schneider et al., 2009). Together, these findings emphasize caution needs to be taken when inferring results from clinic studies to the community.

11.2. Minority Aging Populations

The racial and ethnic population of people living in the United States is changing with an increase in diversity. There is increasing evidence that prevalence of dementia is higher in non-White populations (Corriveau et al., 2017). Studies using neuropathological data in non-White populations show that there are racial differences in brain pathology with an increase in mixed pathology suggesting that "pure" AD is less likely in these non-White populations. In particular, mixed AD and Lewy body pathology is quite common, a finding that perhaps resulted from selection bias. Mixed AD pathology, along with infarcts and Lewy bodies, is also very common (Barnes et al., 2015). Although infarcts were not more common in African Americans than Whites in this study, the African American patients did show more severe small and large vessel disease. A study using data from the National Alzheimer's Coordinating Center (NACC), which harmonizes data from 30 different Alzheimer's disease centers across the United States, showed that African Americans had increased AD-related, vascular, and Lewy body pathologies than Whites (N. R. Graff-Radford, Besser, Crook, Kukull, & Dickson, 2016). Another study using NACC data showed Latinos have increased vascular and neuritic plaque pathology compared to non-Latino Whites and these pathological changes were associated with lower Mini-Mental State Examination scores (Mehta et al., 2008). However, use of NACC data may not be generalizable since participants in these Alzheimer's disease centers are not always derived from population based cohorts. In addition with various different centers participating, procedures for data acquisition are highly variable (N. R. Graff-Radford et al., 2016). Vascular pathology associated with AD-related changes are also common in the South Asian population (Wijesinghe et al., 2016). Special populations such as the oldest old, the fastest-growing segment of our population, also show a rise in mixed AD and vascular pathology profiles (James et al., 2012).

Overall, the role of vascular pathology and mixed pathologies is a growing public health issue, where vascular pathologies occur frequently in combination and can account for about 30% of dementia cases (Power, Boyle 2018). To better understand the clinical–pathological relationships associated with dementia, more research is need to investigate neuropathological data from minority populations. To reach this goal, there is a need to improve liaison and educational outreach programs to effectively translate and communicate research efforts in minority aging populations. Effective strategies need to be multidimensional and need to address the communities concerns and expectations.

12. A Perspective of Neuropathology Assessment in Studies of Aging and Dementia

Dementia is a clinical syndrome caused by multiple disorders and often associated with overlapping cognitive and functional symptoms, as well as variable clinical presentations making a clinical diagnosis challenging (Montine et al., 2014). A neuropathological examination remains the primary method by which a definitive diagnosis can be made. There are, however, limitations.

Neuropathological findings are the cumulative burden of injury during life and is a cross-sectional observation. Moreover, there is a need for in vivo measures of vascular and neurodegenerative pathologies. Recent research suggests that clinical pathological studies have advanced our understanding of disease etiology and the impact of mixed pathologies as related to cognition decline. Nonetheless, advanced technology is important to optimize information that is available from neuropathological assessments including the development of methods for objective quantification of neuropathological alterations (Nelson et al., 2016; Walker et al., 2015). Sophisticated statistical modelling approaches allow investigation of trajectories of longitudinal cognitive data in relation to pathology in the context of epidemiological studies (Boyle et al., 2017; Capuano et al., 2016). Novel approaches using MRI techniques are also being used to help identify pathological changes associated with aging and cognitive decline (McAleese et al., 2016).

Widely used consensus criteria for both AD and Lewy body disease have been used for many years (Braak & Braak, 1995; Braak et al., 2003; Hyman et al., 2012; McKeith, 2006; Mirra et al., 1991). By contrast, there are currently no accepted validated neuropathological criteria to assess VaD, VCI, or vascular pathology, a consequence likely due to the complexity and heterogeneity of vascular pathologies. Different AD and aging research centers have different methodologies in evaluating CVD and vascular pathologies. For example, some research studies define microscopic infarcts as lesions not visible to the naked eye (Dolan et al., 2010; Schneider et al., 2007), while others rely on the size of the lesion, for example, lesions smaller than 1 mm in diameter (Ince et al., 2016). In addition to these differences, there are may be differences in the brain sampling strategy, markers/stains used for histological evaluation, and techniques used to detect vascular pathology (neuropathology vs. imaging). Although different approaches have advanced our knowledge and understanding of the pathologies contributing to the clinical picture of AD and dementia, more objective criteria and quantitative measures are needed.

For a standardized approach for reproducible and comparable data between different centers, the NIA-AA recommends a macroscopic examination of the brain to evaluate large vessel disease, macroscopic infarcts, and hemorrhages of a minimum of six brain regions including four cortical (middle frontal gyrus, middle/superior temporal gyrus, inferior parietal, and calcarine cortices) and two subcortical regions (basal ganglia and thalamus). The NIA-AA guidelines also call for the examination of the white matter serves by the anterior, middle, and posterior cerebral arteries and watershed brain regions. In addition, these guidelines also provides guidance when evaluating co-existing pathologies including AD, Lewy body disease, HS, and TDP-43 staging (Hyman et al., 2012).

13. Summary and Future Directions

The contribution of vascular disease to cognitive decline and progression of VaD, Alzheimer's dementia, and mixed dementias is complicated and diverse. It is clear that AD and vascular pathologies rarely occur in isolation and more commonly co-exist in the same brain of older persons. Because of the high incidence of mixed pathologies, it is important to investigate risk factors and pathogenic mechanisms which underlie these multiple pathologies, for example the role of APOE isoforms and neuroinflammation. Future collaborative efforts are needed to understand the pathogenic diversity of vascular pathology. Use of animal model systems that recapitulate key features of the disease process are also needed as well as the development of tools for cell-specific genotyping and phenotyping (Montine et al., 2012). There is an increasing need to validate and standardize an approach to evaluate vascular pathology in post-mortem brain tissue. However, the use of ex vivo imaging techniques has continued to complement postmortem neuropathologic evaluations (Gorelick et al., 2011). Further, the use of biochemical assessments are a promising means to evaluate ischemic injury.

While there have been advances in imaging biomarkers to identify hemorrhages and large infarcts in vivo, specific structural biomarkers are necessary to identify other pathologies including microvascular disease, with microinfarcts, TDP-43, and HS, to further understand and aid diagnosis of mixed dementia. More studies are needed to better understand relationship between vascular tissue pathology and cognitive outcomes. It is possible that there are yet unrecognized pathologies that may play important roles in cognitive decline. We have incomplete understanding how mid- and late-life vascular risk factors are associated with dementia and how treatment of these risk factors can impact cognitive outcomes. Finally, we understand very little in regard to neurobiological basis of other risk factors for dementia including depression, education, stress, and other psychological factors. Since adequate tissue perfusion is necessary for normal brain functioning and is associated with optimal neuronal activity and cerebral blood flow (Burrage, Marshall, Santanam, & Chantler, 2018), the prevention and treatment of dementia will depend on further studies that help us understand the relationships between these risk factors and alterations of the cerebrovasculature.

References

Akoudad, S., Wolters, F. J., Viswanathan, A., de Bruijn, R. F., van der Lugt, A., Hofman, A., ... Vernooij, M. W. (2016). Association of cerebral microbleeds with cognitive decline and dementia. *JAMA Neurology*, *73*(8), 934–943. doi:10.1001/jamaneurol.2016.1017

Amador-Ortiz, C., Ahmed, Z., Zehr, C., & Dickson, D. W. (2007). Hippocampal sclerosis dementia differs from hippocampal sclerosis in frontal lobe degeneration. *Acta Neuropathologica*, *113*(3), 245–252. doi:10.1007/s00401-006-0183-4

Arvanitakis, Z., Capuano, A. W., Lamar, M., Shah, R. C., Barnes, L. L., Bennett, D. A., & Schneider, J. A. (2018). Late-life blood pressure association with cerebrovascular and Alzheimer disease pathology. *Neurology*, *91*(6), e517–e525. doi:10.1212/WNL.0000000000005951 [doi]

Arvanitakis, Z., Capuano, A. W., Leurgans, S. E., Bennett, D. A., & Schneider, J. A. (2016). Relation of cerebral vessel disease to Alzheimer's disease dementia and cognitive function in elderly people: A cross-sectional study. *Lancet Neurology*, *15*(9), 934–943. doi:10.1016/S1474-4422(16)30029-1

Arvanitakis, Z., Capuano, A. W., Leurgans, S. E., Buchman, A. S., Bennett, D. A., & Schneider, J. A. (2017). The relationship of cerebral vessel pathology to brain microinfarcts. *Brain Pathology (Zurich, Switzerland)*, *27*(1), 77–85. doi:10.1111/bpa.12365

Arvanitakis, Z., Leurgans, S. E., Barnes, L. L., Bennett, D. A., & Schneider, J. A. (2011). Microinfarct pathology, dementia, and cognitive systems. *Stroke*, *42*(3), 722–727. doi:10.1161/STROKEAHA.110.595082

Arvanitakis, Z., Schneider, J. A., Wilson, R. S., Li, Y., Arnold, S. E., Wang, Z., & Bennett, D. A. (2006). Diabetes is related to cerebral infarction but not to AD pathology in older persons. *Neurology*, *67*(11), 1960–1965. doi:67/11/1960

Attems, J., Jellinger, K., Thal, D. R., & Van Nostrand, W. (2011). Review: Sporadic cerebral amyloid angiopathy. *Neuropathology and Applied Neurobiology*, *37*(1), 75–93. doi:10.1111/j.1365-2990.2010.01137.x

Banerjee, G., Wilson, D., Ambler, G., Osei-Bonsu Appiah, K., Shakeshaft, C., Lunawat, S., . . . Werring, D. J.; CROMIS-2 Collaborators. (2018). Cognitive impairment before intracerebral hemorrhage is associated with cerebral amyloid angiopathy. *Stroke*, *49*(1), 40–45. doi:10.1161/STROKEAHA.117.019409

Barnes, L. L., & Bennett, D. A. (2014). Alzheimer's disease in African Americans: Risk factors and challenges for the future. *Health Affairs (Project Hope)*, *33*(4), 580–586. doi:10.1377/hlthaff.2013.135

Barnes, L. L., Leurgans, S., Aggarwal, N. T., Shah, R. C., Arvanitakis, Z., James, B. D., . . . Schneider, J. A. (2015). Mixed pathology is more likely in black than white decedents with Alzheimer dementia. *Neurology*, *85*(6), 528–534. doi:10.1212/WNL.0000000000001834

Beach, T. G., Wilson, J. R., Sue, L. I., Newell, A., Poston, M., Cisneros, R., . . . Roher, A. E. (2007). Circle of Willis atherosclerosis: Association with Alzheimer's disease, neuritic plaques and neurofibrillary tangles. *Acta Neuropathologica*, *113*(1), 13–21. doi:10.1007/s00401-006-0136-y

Benedictus, M. R., Goos, J. D., Binnewijzend, M. A., Muller, M., Barkhof, F., Scheltens, P., . . . van der Flier, W. M. (2013). Specific risk factors for microbleeds and white matter hyperintensities in Alzheimer's disease. *Neurobiology of Aging*, *34*(11), 2488–2494. doi:10.1016/j.neurobiolaging.2013.04.023

Bennett, D. A., Schneider, J. A., Aggarwal, N. T., Arvanitakis, Z., Shah, R. C., Kelly, J. F., . . . Wilson, R. S. (2006). Decision rules guiding the clinical diagnosis of Alzheimer's disease in two community-based cohort studies compared to standard practice in a clinic-based cohort study. *Neuroepidemiology*, *27*(3), 169–176. doi:96129

Biffi, A., & Greenberg, S. M. (2011). Cerebral amyloid angiopathy: A systematic review. *Journal of Clinical Neurology (Seoul, Korea)*, *7*(1), 1–9. doi:10.3988/jcn.2011.7.1.1

Bowler, J. V. (2004). Vascular cognitive impairment. *Stroke, 35*(2), 386–388.

Bowler, J. V. (2005). Vascular cognitive impairment. *Journal of Neurology, Neurosurgery & Psychiatry, 76*(suppl 5), v35–v44.

Bowler, J. V., & Hachinski, V. (1995). Vascular cognitive impairment: A new approach to vascular dementia. *Bailliere's Clinical Neurology, 4*(2), 357–376.

Boyle, P. A., Wilson, R. S., Yu, L., Barr, A. M., Honer, W. G., Schneider, J. A., & Bennett, D. A. (2013). Much of late life cognitive decline is not due to common neurodegenerative pathologies. *Annals of Neurology, 74*(3), 478–489. doi:10.1002/ana.23964

Boyle, P. A., Yang, J., Yu, L., Leurgans, S. E., Capuano, A. W., Schneider, J. A., . . . Bennett, D. A. (2017). Varied effects of age-related neuropathologies on the trajectory of late life cognitive decline. *Brain, 140*(3), 804–812. doi:aww341 [pii]

Boyle, P. A., Yu, L., Fleischman, D. A., Leurgans, S., Yang, J., Wilson, R. S., . . . Bennett, D. A. (2016). White matter hyperintensities, incident mild cognitive impairment, and cognitive decline in old age. *Annals of Clinical and Translational Neurology, 3*(10), 791–800. doi:10.1002/acn3.343

Boyle, P. A., Yu, L., Leurgans, S. E., Wilson, R. S., Brookmeyer, R., Schneider, J. A., & Bennett, D. A. (2018). Attributable risk of Alzheimer's dementia due to age-related neuropathologies. *Annals of Neurology, 85*(1), 114–124. doi:10.1002/ana.25380

Boyle, P. A., Yu, L., Nag, S., Leurgans, S., Wilson, R. S., Bennett, D. A., & Schneider, J. A. (2015). Cerebral amyloid angiopathy and cognitive outcomes in community-based older persons. *Neurology, 85*(22), 1930–1936. doi:10.1212/WNL.0000000000002175

Boyle, P. A., Yu, L., Wilson, R. S., Leurgans, S. E., Schneider, J. A., & Bennett, D. A. (2018). Person-specific contribution of neuropathologies to cognitive loss in old age. *Annals of Neurology, 83*(1), 74–83. doi:10.1002/ana.25123 [doi]

Braak, H., & Braak, E. (1995). Staging of Alzheimer's disease-related neurofibrillary changes. *Neurobiology of Aging, 16*(3), 271–8; discussion 278–84. doi:0197458095000216 [pii]

Braak, H., Del Tredici, K., Rub, U., de Vos, R. A., Jansen Steur, E. N., & Braak, E. (2003). Staging of brain pathology related to sporadic Parkinson's disease. *Neurobiology of Aging, 24*(2), 197–211. doi:S0197458002000659

Brayne, C., Richardson, K., Matthews, F. E., Fleming, J., Hunter, S., Xuereb, J. H., . . . Dening, T.; Cambridge City Over-75s Cohort Cc75c Study Neuropathology Collaboration. (2009). Neuropathological correlates of dementia in over-80-year-old brain donors from the population-based Cambridge City Over-75s Cohort (CC75C) study. *Journal of Alzheimer's Disease, 18*(3), 645–658. doi:10.3233/JAD-2009-1182

Brenowitz, W. D., Hubbard, R. A., Keene, C. D., Hawes, S. E., Longstreth, W. T., Jr., Woltjer, R. L., & Kukull, W. A. (2016). Mixed neuropathologies and estimated rates of clinical progression in a large autopsy sample. *Alzheimer's & Dementia, 13*(6), 654–662. doi:S1552-5260(16)33057-6

Brickman, A. M., Reitz, C., Luchsinger, J. A., Manly, J. J., Schupf, N., Muraskin, J., . . . Mayeux, R. (2010). Long-term blood pressure fluctuation and cerebrovascular disease in an elderly cohort. *Archives of Neurology, 67*(5), 564–569. doi:10.1001/archneurol.2010.70

Bridges, L. R., Andoh, J., Lawrence, A. J., Khoong, C. H. L., Poon, W., Esiri, M. M., . . . Hainsworth, A. H. (2014). Blood–brain barrier dysfunction and cerebral small vessel disease (arteriolosclerosis) in brains of older people. *Journal of Neuropathology and Experimental Neurology*, *73*(11), 1026–1033. doi:10.1097/NEN.0000000000000124

Burrage, E., Marshall, K. L., Santanam, N., & Chantler, P. D. (2018). Cerebrovascular dysfunction with stress and depression. *Brain Circulation*, *4*(2), 43–53. doi:10.4103/bc.bc_6_18

Caplan, L. R. (2015). Lacunar infarction and small vessel disease: Pathology and pathophysiology. *Journal of Stroke*, *17*(1), 2–6. doi:10.5853/jos.2015.17.1.2

Capuano, A. W., Wilson, R. S., Leurgans, S. E., Dawson, J. D., Bennett, D. A., & Hedeker, D. (2016). Sigmoidal mixed models for longitudinal data. *Statistical Methods in Medical Research*, *27*(3), 863–875. doi:0962280216645632

Charidimou, A., Boulouis, G., Gurol, M. E., Ayata, C., Bacskai, B. J., Frosch, M. P., . . . Greenberg, S. M. (2017). Emerging concepts in sporadic cerebral amyloid angiopathy. *Brain*, *140*(7), 1829–1850. doi:10.1093/brain/awx047

Charidimou, A., Boulouis, G., Haley, K., Auriel, E., van Etten, E. S., Fotiadis, P., . . . Gurol, M. E. (2016). White matter hyperintensity patterns in cerebral amyloid angiopathy and hypertensive arteriopathy. *Neurology*, *86*(6), 505–511. doi:10.1212/WNL.0000000000002362

Charidimou, A., Linn, J., Vernooij, M. W., Opherk, C., Akoudad, S., Baron, J. C., . . . Werring, D. J. (2015). Cortical superficial siderosis: Detection and clinical significance in cerebral amyloid angiopathy and related conditions. *Brain*, *138*(Pt 8), 2126–2139. doi:10.1093/brain/awv162

Corrada, M. M., Sonnen, J. A., Kim, R. C., & Kawas, C. H. (2016). Microinfarcts are common and strongly related to dementia in the oldest-old: The 90+ study. *Alzheimer's & Dementia*, *12*(8), 900–908. doi:10.1016/j.jalz.2016.04.006

Corriveau, R. A., Koroshetz, W. J., Gladman, J. T., Jeon, S., Babcock, D., Bennett, D. A., . . . Holtzman, D. M. (2017). Alzheimer's disease-related dementias summit 2016: National research priorities. *Neurology*, *89*(23), 2381–2391. doi:10.1212/WNL.0000000000004717

Craggs, L. J., Yamamoto, Y., Ihara, M., Fenwick, R., Burke, M., Oakley, A. E., . . . Kalaria, R. N. (2014). White matter pathology and disconnection in the frontal lobe in cerebral autosomal dominant arteriopathy with subcortical infarcts and leukoencephalopathy (CADASIL). *Neuropathology and Applied Neurobiology*, *40*(5), 591–602. doi:10.1111/nan.12073

Crystal, H. A., Dickson, D., Davies, P., Masur, D., Grober, E., & Lipton, R. B. (2000). The relative frequency of "dementia of unknown etiology" increases with age and is nearly 50% in nonagenarians. *Archives of Neurology*, *57*(5), 713–719. doi:noc90020

De Reuck, J., Deramecourt, V., Cordonnier, C., Pasquier, F., Leys, D., Maurage, C. A., & Bordet, R. (2016). The incidence of post-mortem neurodegenerative and cerebrovascular pathology in mixed dementia. *Journal of the Neurological Sciences*, *366*, 164–166. doi:10.1016/j.jns.2016.05.021

Debette, S., Seshadri, S., Beiser, A., Au, R., Himali, J. J., Palumbo, C., . . . DeCarli, C. (2011). Midlife vascular risk factor exposure accelerates structural brain aging and cognitive decline. *Neurology*, *77*(5), 461–468. doi:10.1212/WNL.0b013e318227b227

DeCarli, C., Fletcher, E., Ramey, V., Harvey, D., & Jagust, W. J. (2005). Anatomical mapping of white matter hyperintensities (WMH): Exploring the relationships between periventricular WMH, deep WMH, and total WMH burden. *Stroke*, *36*(1), 50–55. doi:01.STR.0000150668.58689.f2

Deramecourt, V., Slade, J. Y., Oakley, A. E., Perry, R. H., Ince, P. G., Maurage, C. A., & Kalaria, R. N. (2012). Staging and natural history of cerebrovascular pathology in dementia. *Neurology, 78*(14), 1043–1050. doi:10.1212/WNL.0b013e31824e8e7f

Dolan, H., Crain, B., Troncoso, J., Resnick, S. M., Zonderman, A. B., & Obrien, R. J. (2010). Atherosclerosis, dementia, and Alzheimer disease in the Baltimore longitudinal study of aging cohort. *Annals of Neurology, 68*(2), 231–240. doi:10.1002/ana.22055 [doi]

Eikelenboom, P., van Exel, E., Hoozemans, J. J., Veerhuis, R., Rozemuller, A. J., & van Gool, W. A. (2010). Neuroinflammation: An early event in both the history and pathogenesis of Alzheimer's disease. *Neuro-Degenerative Diseases, 7*(1–3), 38–41. doi:10.1159/000283480

Esiri, M. M., Nagy, Z., Smith, M. Z., Barnetson, L., & Smith, A. D. (1999). Cerebrovascular disease and threshold for dementia in the early stages of Alzheimer's disease. *Lancet (London, England), 354*(9182), 919–920. doi:S0140-6736(99)02355-7

Fazekas, F., Kleinert, R., Roob, G., Kleinert, G., Kapeller, P., Schmidt, R., & Hartung, H. P. (1999). Histopathologic analysis of foci of signal loss on gradient-echo T2*-weighted MR images in patients with spontaneous intracerebral hemorrhage: Evidence of microangiopathy-related microbleeds. *American Journal of Neuroradiology, 20*(4), 637–642.

Ferman, T. J., Smith, G. E., Dickson, D. W., Graff-Radford, N. R., Lin, S. C., Wszolek, Z., . . . Boeve, B. F. (2014). Abnormal daytime sleepiness in dementia with Lewy bodies compared to Alzheimer's disease using the multiple sleep latency test. *Alzheimer's Research & Therapy, 6*(9), 76-014-0076-z. doi:10.1186/s13195-014-0076-z

Fillit, H., Nash, D. T., Rundek, T., & Zuckerman, A. (2008). Cardiovascular risk factors and dementia. *American Journal of Geriatric Pharmacotherapy, 6*(2), 100–118. doi:10.1016/j.amjopharm.2008.06.004

Foster, V., Oakley, A. E., Slade, J. Y., Hall, R., Polvikoski, T. M., Burke, M., . . . Kalaria, R. N. (2014). Pyramidal neurons of the prefrontal cortex in post-stroke, vascular and other ageing-related dementias. *Brain, 137*(Pt 9), 2509–2521. doi:10.1093/brain/awu172

Ghebremedhin, E., Rosenberger, A., Rub, U., Vuksic, M., Berhe, T., Bickeboller, H., . . . Deller, T. (2010). Inverse relationship between cerebrovascular lesions and severity of Lewy body pathology in patients with Lewy body diseases. *Journal of Neuropathology and Experimental Neurology, 69*(5), 442–448. doi:10.1097/NEN.0b013e3181d88e63

Giwa, M. O., Williams, J., Elderfield, K., Jiwa, N. S., Bridges, L. R., Kalaria, R. N., . . . Hainsworth, A. H. (2012). Neuropathologic evidence of endothelial changes in cerebral small vessel disease. *Neurology, 78*(3), 167–174. doi:10.1212/WNL.0b013e3182407968

Goodman, R. A., Lochner, K. A., Thambisetty, M., Wingo, T. S., Posner, S. F., & Ling, S. M. (2017). Prevalence of dementia subtypes in United States Medicare fee-for-service beneficiaries, 2011–2013. *Alzheimer's & Dementia, 13*(1), 28–37. doi:S1552-5260(16)30052-8

Gorelick, P. B., Scuteri, A., Black, S. E., Decarli, C., Greenberg, S. M., Iadecola, C., . . . Seshadri, S.; American Heart Association Stroke Council, Council on Epidemiology and Prevention, Council on Cardiovascular Nursing, Council on Cardiovascular Radiology and Intervention, and Council on Cardiovascular Surgery and Anesthesia. (2011). Vascular contributions to cognitive impairment and dementia: A statement for healthcare professionals from the American Heart Association/American Stroke Association. *Stroke; a Journal of Cerebral Circulation, 42*(9), 2672–2713. doi:10.1161/STR.0b013e3182299496

Gottesman, R. F., Schneider, A. L., Zhou, Y., Coresh, J., Green, E., Gupta, N., . . . Mosley, T. H. (2017). Association between midlife vascular risk factors and estimated brain amyloid deposition. *JAMA*, *317*(14), 1443–1450. doi:10.1001/jama.2017.3090

Gouw, A. A., Seewann, A., van der Flier, W. M., Barkhof, F., Rozemuller, A. M., Scheltens, P., & Geurts, J. J. (2011). Heterogeneity of small vessel disease: A systematic review of MRI and histopathology correlations. *Journal of Neurology, Neurosurgery, and Psychiatry*, *82*(2), 126–135. doi:10.1136/jnnp.2009.204685

Graff-Radford, J., Raman, M. R., Rabinstein, A. A., Przybelski, S. A., Lesnick, T. G., Boeve, B. F., . . . Kantarci, K. (2018). Association between microinfarcts and blood pressure trajectories. *JAMA Neurology*, *75*(2), 212–218. doi:10.1001/jamaneurol.2017.3392

Graff-Radford, N. R., Besser, L. M., Crook, J. E., Kukull, W. A., & Dickson, D. W. (2016). Neuropathologic differences by race from the National Alzheimer's Coordinating Center. *Alzheimer's & Dementia*, *12*(6), 669–677. doi:10.1016/j.jalz.2016.03.004

Gray, F., Polivka, M., Viswanathan, A., Baudrimont, M., Bousser, M. G., & Chabriat, H. (2007). Apoptosis in cerebral autosomal-dominant arteriopathy with subcortical infarcts and leukoencephalopathy. *Journal of Neuropathology and Experimental Neurology*, *66*(7), 597–607. doi:10.1097/nen.0b013e318093e574

Greenberg, S. M., Nandigam, R. N., Delgado, P., Betensky, R. A., Rosand, J., Viswanathan, A., . . . Smith, E. E. (2009). Microbleeds versus macrobleeds: Evidence for distinct entities. *Stroke*, *40*(7), 2382–2386. doi:10.1161/STROKEAHA.109.548974

Greenberg, S. M., Vernooij, M. W., Cordonnier, C., Viswanathan, A., Al-Shahi Salman, R., Warach, S., . . . Breteler, M. M.; Microbleed Study Group. (2009). Cerebral microbleeds: A guide to detection and interpretation. *Lancet Neurology*, *8*(2), 165–174. doi:10.1016/S1474-4422(09)70013-4

Grutzendler, J., Murikinati, S., Hiner, B., Ji, L., Lam, C. K., Yoo, T., . . . Rodriguez, G. (2014). Angiophagy prevents early embolus washout but recanalizes microvessels through embolus extravasation. *Science Translational Medicine*, *6*(226), 226ra31. doi:10.1126/scitranslmed.3006585

Gurol, M. E., Dierksen, G., Betensky, R., Gidicsin, C., Halpin, A., Becker, A., . . . Greenberg, S. M. (2012). Predicting sites of new hemorrhage with amyloid imaging in cerebral amyloid angiopathy. *Neurology*, *79*(4), 320–326. doi:10.1212/WNL.0b013e31826043a9

Haglund, M., Kalaria, R., Slade, J. Y., & Englund, E. (2006). Differential deposition of amyloid beta peptides in cerebral amyloid angiopathy associated with Alzheimer's disease and vascular dementia. *Acta Neuropathologica*, *111*(5), 430–435. doi:10.1007/s00401-006-0054-z

Hainsworth, A. H., Minett, T., Andoh, J., Forster, G., Bhide, I., Barrick, T. R., . . . Bridges, L. R. (2017). Neuropathology of white matter lesions, blood–brain barrier dysfunction, and dementia. *Stroke*, *48*(10), 2799–2804. doi:10.1161/STROKEAHA.117.018101

Hamedani, A. G., Rose, K. M., Peterlin, B. L., Mosley, T. H., Coker, L. H., Jack, C. R., . . . Gottesman, R. F. (2013). Migraine and white matter hyperintensities: The ARIC MRI study. *Neurology*, *81*(15), 1308–1313. doi:10.1212/WNL.0b013e3182a8235b

Hartmann, D. A., Hyacinth, H. I., Liao, F. F., & Shih, A. Y. (2017). Does pathology of small venules contribute to cerebral microinfarcts and dementia? *Journal of Neurochemistry*, doi:10.1111/jnc.14228

Hatanpaa, K. J., Raisanen, J. M., Herndon, E., Burns, D. K., Foong, C., Habib, A. A., & White, C. L., III. (2014). Hippocampal sclerosis in dementia, epilepsy, and ischemic injury: Differential vulnerability of hippocampal subfields. *Journal of Neuropathology and Experimental Neurology*, *73*(2), 136–142. doi:10.1097/OPX.0000000000000170

Hilal, S., Sikking, E., Shaik, M. A., Chan, Q. L., van Veluw, S. J., Vrooman, H., . . . Ikram, M. K. (2016). Cortical cerebral microinfarcts on 3T MRI: A novel marker of cerebrovascular disease. *Neurology, 87*(15), 1583–1590. doi:WNL.0000000000003110

Hoffman, L. B., Schmeidler, J., Lesser, G. T., Beeri, M. S., Purohit, D. P., Grossman, H. T., & Haroutunian, V. (2009). Less Alzheimer disease neuropathology in medicated hypertensive than nonhypertensive persons. *Neurology, 72*(20), 1720–1726. doi:10.1212/01.wnl.0000345881.82856.d5

Holtzman, D. M. (2001). Role of apoe/Abeta interactions in the pathogenesis of Alzheimer's disease and cerebral amyloid angiopathy. *Journal of Molecular Neuroscienc, 17*(2), 147–155. doi:JMN:17:2:147

Hommet, C., Mondon, K., Constans, T., Beaufils, E., Desmidt, T., Camus, V., & Cottier, J. P. (2011). Review of cerebral microangiopathy and Alzheimer's disease: Relation between white matter hyperintensities and microbleeds. *Dementia and Geriatric Cognitive Disorders, 32*(6), 367–378. doi:10.1159/000335568

Honig, L. S., Kukull, W., & Mayeux, R. (2005). Atherosclerosis and AD: Analysis of data from the US national Alzheimer's coordinating center. *Neurology, 64*(3), 494–500. doi:64/3/494

Hyman, B. T., Phelps, C. H., Beach, T. G., Bigio, E. H., Cairns, N. J., Carrillo, M. C., . . . Montine, T. J. (2012). National Institute on Aging–Alzheimer's Association guidelines for the neuropathologic assessment of Alzheimer's disease. *Alzheimer's & Dementia, 8*(1), 1–13. doi:10.1016/j.jalz.2011.10.007

Hyman, B. T., & Trojanowski, J. Q. (1997). Consensus recommendations for the postmortem diagnosis of alzheimer disease from the national institute on aging and the Reagan Institute working group on diagnostic criteria for the neuropathological assessment of Alzheimer disease. *Journal of Neuropathology and Experimental Neurology, 56*(10), 1095–1097.

Ighodaro, E. T., Abner, E. L., Fardo, D. W., Lin, A. L., Katsumata, Y., Schmitt, F. A., . . . Nelson, P. T. (2017). Risk factors and global cognitive status related to brain arteriolosclerosis in elderly individuals. *Journal of Cerebral Blood Flow and Metabolism, 37*(1), 201–216. doi:0271678X15621574

Ikeda, M., Hokoishi, K., Maki, N., Nebu, A., Tachibana, N., Komori, K., . . . Tanabe, H. (2001). Increased prevalence of vascular dementia in japan: A community-based epidemiological study. *Neurology, 57*(5), 839–844.

Ince, P. G., Minett, T., Forster, G., Brayne, C., & Wharton, S. B.; Medical Research Council Cognitive Function and Ageing Neuropathology Study. (2016). Microinfarcts in an Older population-representative brain donor cohort (MRC CFAS): Prevalence, relation to dementia and mobility, and implications for the evaluation of cerebral small vessel disease. *Neuropathology and Applied Neurobiology, 43*(5), 409–41. doi:10.1111/nan.12363 [doi]

James, B. D., Bennett, D. A., Boyle, P. A., Leurgans, S., & Schneider, J. A. (2012). Dementia from Alzheimer disease and mixed pathologies in the oldest old. *JAMA, 307*(17), 1798–1800. doi:10.1001/jama.2012.3556

Janaway, B. M., Simpson, J. E., Hoggard, N., Highley, J. R., Forster, G., Drew, D., . . . Ince, P. C.; MRC Cognitive Function and Ageing Neuropathology Study. (2014). Brain haemosiderin in older people: Pathological evidence for an ischaemic origin of magnetic resonance imaging (MRI) microbleeds. *Neuropathology and Applied Neurobiology, 40*(3), 258–269. doi:10.1111/nan.12062

Jellinger, K. A., & Attems, J. (2012). Neuropathology and general autopsy findings in nondemented aged subjects. *Clinical Neuropathology, 31*(2), 87–98. doi:9524

Josephs, K. A., Whitwell, J. L., Knopman, D. S., Hu, W. T., Stroh, D. A., Baker, M., . . . Dickson, D. W. (2008). Abnormal TDP-43 immunoreactivity in AD modifies clinicopathologic and radiologic phenotype. *Neurology, 70*(19 Pt 2), 1850–1857. doi:10.1212/01.wnl.0000304041.09418.b1

Joutel, A., & Chabriat, H. (2017). Pathogenesis of white matter changes in cerebral small vessel diseases: Beyond vessel-intrinsic mechanisms. *Clinical Science (London, England : 1979), 131*(8), 635–651. doi:10.1042/CS20160380

Kalaria, R. N. (2016). Neuropathological diagnosis of vascular cognitive impairment and vascular dementia with implications for Alzheimer's disease. *Acta Neuropathologica, 131*(5), 659–685. doi:10.1007/s00401-016-1571-z

Kalaria, R. N., Akinyemi, R., & Ihara, M. (2016). Stroke injury, cognitive impairment and vascular dementia. *Biochimica Et Biophysica Acta, 1862*(5), 915–925. doi:S0925-4439(16)30002-3

Kalaria, R. N., & Erkinjuntti, T. (2006). Small vessel disease and subcortical vascular dementia. *Journal of Clinical Neurology (Seoul, Korea), 2*(1), 1–11. doi:10.3988/jcn.2006.2.1.1

Kalaria, R. N., Kenny, R. A., Ballard, C. G., Perry, R., Ince, P., & Polvikoski, T. (2004). Towards defining the neuropathological substrates of vascular dementia. *Journal of the Neurological Sciences, 226*(1–2), 75–80. doi:S0022-510X(04)00298-9

Kapasi, A., DeCarli, C., & Schneider, J. A. (2017). Impact of multiple pathologies on the threshold for clinically overt dementia. *Acta Neuropathologica, 134*(2), 171–186. doi:10.1007/s00401-017-1717-7

Kapasi, A., Leurgans, S. E., James, B. D., Boyle, P. A., Arvanitakis, Z., Nag, S., . . . Schneider, J. A. (2018). Watershed microinfarct pathology and cognition in older persons. *Neurobiology of Aging, 70*, 10–17. doi:S0197-4580(18)30195-7

Kapasi, A., & Schneider, J. A. (2016). Vascular contributions to cognitive impairment, clinical Alzheimer's disease, and dementia in older persons. *Biochimica et Biophysica Acta*, doi:S0925-4439(15)00387-7

Keage, H. A., Carare, R. O., Friedland, R. P., Ince, P. G., Love, S., Nicoll, J. A., . . . Brayne, C. (2009). Population studies of sporadic cerebral amyloid angiopathy and dementia: A systematic review. *BMC Neurology, 9*, 3–2377-9–3. doi:10.1186/1471-2377-9-3

Keith, J., Gao, F. Q., Noor, R., Kiss, A., Balasubramaniam, G., Au, K., . . . Black, S. E. (2017). Collagenosis of the deep medullary veins: An underrecognized pathologic correlate of white matter hyperintensities and periventricular infarction? *Journal of Neuropathology and Experimental Neurology, 76*(4), 299–312. doi:10.1093/jnen/nlx009

Khachaturian, Z. S. (1985). Diagnosis of Alzheimer's disease. *Archives of Neurology, 42*(11), 1097–1105.

Kim, J., Na, H. K., Shin, J. H., Kim, H. J., Seo, S. W., Seong, J. K., & Na, D. L. (2018). Atrophy patterns in cerebral amyloid angiopathy with and without cortical superficial siderosis. *Neurology, 90*(20), e1751–e1758. doi:10.1212/WNL.0000000000005524

Knopman, D. S., & Roberts, R. (2010). Vascular risk factors: Imaging and neuropathologic correlates. *Journal of Alzheimer's Disease, 20*(3), 699–709. doi:10.3233/JAD-2010-091555

Kokmen, E., Ozsarfati, Y., Beard, C. M., O'Brien, P. C., & Rocca, W. A. (1996). Impact of referral bias on clinical and epidemiological studies of Alzheimer's disease. *Journal of Clinical Epidemiology, 49*(1), 79–83. doi:0895435695000313

Kovari, E., Charidimou, A., Herrmann, F. R., Giannakopoulos, P., Bouras, C., & Gold, G. (2015). No neuropathological evidence for a direct topographical relation between microbleeds and cerebral amyloid angiopathy. *Acta Neuropathologica Communications, 3*, 49-015-0228-9. doi:10.1186/s40478-015-0228-9

Kovari, E., Gold, G., Herrmann, F. R., Canuto, A., Hof, P. R., Michel, J. P., . . . Giannakopoulos, P. (2004). Cortical microinfarcts and demyelination significantly affect cognition in brain aging. *Stroke, 35*(2), 410–414. doi:10.1161/01.STR.0000110791.51378.4E

Kowoll, C. M., Kaminski, J., Weiss, V., Bosel, J., Dietrich, W., Juttler, E., . . . Dohmen, C. (2016). Severe cerebral venous and sinus thrombosis: Clinical course, imaging correlates, and prognosis. *Neurocritical Care, 25*(3), 392–399. doi:10.1007/s12028-016-0256-8

Kril, J. J., Patel, S., Harding, A. J., & Halliday, G. M. (2002). Patients with vascular dementia due to microvascular pathology have significant hippocampal neuronal loss. *Journal of Neurology, Neurosurgery, and Psychiatry, 72*(6), 747–751.

Lauer, A., van Veluw, S. J., William, C. M., Charidimou, A., Roongpiboonsopit, D., Vashkevich, A., . . . Viswanathan, A. (2016). Microbleeds on MRI are associated with microinfarcts on autopsy in cerebral amyloid angiopathy. *Neurology, 87*(14), 1488–1492. doi:WNL.0000000000003184

Lee, S., Viqar, F., Zimmerman, M. E., Narkhede, A., Tosto, G., Benzinger, T. L., . . . Brickman, A. M.; Dominantly Inherited Alzheimer Network. (2016). White matter hyperintensities are a core feature of Alzheimer's disease: Evidence from the Dominantly Inherited Alzheimer Network. *Annals of Neurology, 79*(6), 929–939. doi:10.1002/ana.24647

Leverenz, J. B., Agustin, C. M., Tsuang, D., Peskind, E. R., Edland, S. D., Nochlin, D., . . . Larson, E. B. (2002). Clinical and neuropathological characteristics of hippocampal sclerosis: A community-based study. *Archives of Neurology, 59*(7), 1099–1106. doi:noc10247

Liu, S., Levine, S. R., & Winn, H. R. (2010). Targeting ischemic penumbra: Part I. From pathophysiology to therapeutic strategy. *Journal of Experimental Stroke & Translational Medicine, 3*(1), 47–55.

Longstreth, W. T., Jr. (1998). Brain abnormalities in the elderly: Frequency and predictors in the united states (the cardiovascular health study). cardiovascular health study collaborative research group. *Journal of Neural Transmission Supplementum, 53*, 9–16.

Longstreth, W. T., Jr, Bernick, C., Manolio, T. A., Bryan, N., Jungreis, C. A., & Price, T. R. (1998). Lacunar infarcts defined by magnetic resonance imaging of 3660 elderly people: The cardiovascular health study. *Archives of Neurology, 55*(9), 1217–1225.

Love, S., Chalmers, K., Ince, P., Esiri, M., Attems, J., Jellinger, K., . . . Kehoe, P. G. (2014). Development, appraisal, validation and implementation of a consensus protocol for the assessment of cerebral amyloid angiopathy in post-mortem brain tissue. *American Journal of Neurodegenerative Disease, 3*(1), 19–32.

Luchsinger, J. A., Reitz, C., Patel, B., Tang, M. X., Manly, J. J., & Mayeux, R. (2007). Relation of diabetes to mild cognitive impairment. *Archives of Neurology, 64*(4), 570–575. doi:64/4/570

Mangla, R., Kolar, B., Almast, J., & Ekholm, S. E. (2011). Border zone infarcts: Pathophysiologic and imaging characteristics. *Radiographics, 31*(5), 1201–1214. doi:10.1148/rg.315105014

Massoud, F., Devi, G., Stern, Y., Lawton, A., Goldman, J. E., Liu, Y., . . . Mayeux, R. (1999). A clinicopathological comparison of community-based and clinic-based cohorts of patients with dementia. *Archives of Neurology, 56*(11), 1368–1373.

McAleese, K. E., Alafuzoff, I., Charidimou, A., De Reuck, J., Grinberg, L. T., Hainsworth, A. H., . . . Attems, J. (2016). Post-mortem assessment in vascular dementia: Advances and aspirations. *BMC Medicine*, *14*(1), 129–016-0676–5. doi:10.1186/s12916-016-0676-5

McAleese, K. E., Walker, L., Graham, S., Moya, E. L. J., Johnson, M., Erskine, D., . . . Attems, J. (2017). Parietal white matter lesions in Alzheimer's disease are associated with cortical neurodegenerative pathology, but not with small vessel disease. *Acta Neuropathologica*, doi:10.1007/s00401-017-1738-2

McKeith, I. G. (2006). Consensus guidelines for the clinical and pathologic diagnosis of dementia with Lewy bodies (DLB): Report of the Consortium on DLB International Workshop. *Journal of Alzheimer's Disease*, *9*(3 Suppl), 417–423.

Mehta, K. M., Yaffe, K., Perez-Stable, E. J., Stewart, A., Barnes, D., Kurland, B. F., & Miller, B. L. (2008). Race/ethnic differences in AD survival in US Alzheimer's disease centers. *Neurology*, *70*(14), 1163–1170. doi:01.wnl.0000285287.99923.3c

Melkas, S., Vataja, R., Oksala, N. K., Jokinen, H., Pohjasvaara, T., Oksala, A., . . . Erkinjuntti, T. (2010). Depression-executive dysfunction syndrome relates to poor poststroke survival. *The American Journal of Geriatric Psychiatry*, *18*(11), 1007–1016. doi:10.1097/JGP.0b013e3181d695d7

Mirra, S. S., Heyman, A., McKeel, D., Sumi, S. M., Crain, B. J., Brownlee, L. M., . . . Berg, L. (1991). The consortium to establish a registry for Alzheimer's disease (CERAD): Part II. Standardization of the neuropathologic assessment of Alzheimer's disease. *Neurology*, *41*(4), 479–486.

Montagne, A., Barnes, S. R., Sweeney, M. D., Halliday, M. R., Sagare, A. P., Zhao, Z., . . . Zlokovic, B. V. (2015). Blood–brain barrier breakdown in the aging human hippocampus. *Neuron*, *85*(2), 296–302. doi:10.1016/j.neuron.2014.12.032

Montine, T. J., Koroshetz, W. J., Babcock, D., Dickson, D. W., Galpern, W. R., Glymour, M. M., . . . Corriveau, R. A.; ADRD 2013 Conference Organizing Committee. (2014). Recommendations of the Alzheimer's disease-related dementias conference. *Neurology*, *83*(9), 851–860. doi:10.1212/WNL.0000000000000733

Montine, T. J., Monsell, S. E., Beach, T. G., Bigio, E. H., Bu, Y., Cairns, N. J., . . . Hyman, B. T. (2016). Multisite assessment of NIA-AA guidelines for the neuropathologic evaluation of Alzheimer's disease. *Alzheimer's & Dementia*, *12*(2), 164–169. doi:S1552-5260(15)02669-2

Montine, T. J., Phelps, C. H., Beach, T. G., Bigio, E. H., Cairns, N. J., Dickson, D. W., . . . Hyman, B. T. (2012). National Institute on Aging–Alzheimer's Association guidelines for the neuropathologic assessment of Alzheimer's disease: A practical approach. *Acta Neuropathologica*, *123*(1), 1–11. doi:10.1007/s00401-011-0910-3

Murray, M. E., Vemuri, P., Preboske, G. M., Murphy, M. C., Schweitzer, K. J., Parisi, J. E., . . . Dickson, D. W. (2012). A quantitative postmortem MRI design sensitive to white matter hyperintensity differences and their relationship with underlying pathology. *Journal of Neuropathology and Experimental Neurology*, *71*(12), 1113–1122. doi:10.1097/NEN.0b013e318277387e

Nag, S., Yu, L., Capuano, A. W., Wilson, R. S., Leurgans, S. E., Bennett, D. A., & Schneider, J. A. (2015). Hippocampal sclerosis and TDP-43 pathology in aging and Alzheimer disease. *Annals of Neurology*, *77*(6), 942–952. doi:10.1002/ana.24388

Nelson, P. T., Pious, N. M., Jicha, G. A., Wilcock, D. M., Fardo, D. W., Estus, S., & Rebeck, G. W. (2013). APOE-epsilon2 and APOE-epsilon4 correlate with increased amyloid accumulation in cerebral vasculature. *Journal of Neuropathology and Experimental Neurology*, *72*(7), 708–715. doi:10.1097/NEN.0b013e31829a25b9

Nelson, P. T., Schmitt, F. A., Lin, Y., Abner, E. L., Jicha, G. A., Patel, E., . . . Kryscio, R. J. (2011). Hippocampal sclerosis in advanced age: Clinical and pathological features. *Brain : A Journal of Neurology*, *134*(Pt 5), 1506–1518. doi:10.1093/brain/awr053

Nelson, P. T., Trojanowski, J. Q., Abner, E. L., Al-Janabi, O. M., Jicha, G. A., Schmitt, F. A., . . . Ighodaro, E. T. (2016). "New old pathologies": AD, PART, and cerebral age-related TDP-43 with sclerosis (CARTS). *Journal of Neuropathology and Experimental Neurology*, *75*(6), 482–498. doi:10.1093/jnen/nlw033

Neuropathology Group, Medical Research Council Cognitive Function and Aging Study. (2001). Pathological correlates of late-onset dementia in a multicentre, community-based population in England and Wales: Neuropathology group of the medical research council cognitive function and ageing study (MRC CFAS). *Lancet*, *357*(9251), 169–175. doi:S0140673600035893

Peila, R., Rodriguez, B. L., & Launer, L. J.; Honolulu–Asia Aging Study. (2002). Type 2 diabetes, APOE gene, and the risk for dementia and related pathologies: The Honolulu–Asia aging study. *Diabetes*, *51*(4), 1256–1262.

Petrovitch, H., White, L. R., Izmirilian, G., Ross, G. W., Havlik, R. J., Markesbery, W., . . . Launer, L. J. (2000). Midlife blood pressure and neuritic plaques, neurofibrillary tangles, and brain weight at death: The HAAS: Honolulu–Asia Aging Study. *Neurobiology of Aging*, *21*(1), 57–62. doi:S0197458000001068

Pettersen, J. A., Keith, J., Gao, F., Spence, J. D., & Black, S. E. (2017). CADASIL accelerated by acute hypotension: Arterial and venous contribution to leukoaraiosis. *Neurology*, *88*(11), 1077–1080. doi:10.1212/WNL.0000000000003717

Pfeifer, L. A., White, L. R., Ross, G. W., Petrovitch, H., & Launer, L. J. (2002). Cerebral amyloid angiopathy and cognitive function: The HAAS autopsy study. *Neurology*, *58*(11), 1629–1634.

Poels, M. M., Ikram, M. A., van der Lugt, A., Hofman, A., Niessen, W. J., Krestin, G. P., . . . Vernooij, M. W. (2012). Cerebral microbleeds are associated with worse cognitive function: The Rotterdam Scan Study. *Neurology*, *78*(5), 326–333. doi:10.1212/WNL.0b013e3182452928

Power, M. C., Mormino, E., Soldan, A., James, B. D., Yu, L., Armstrong, N. M., . . . Schneider, J. (2018). Combined neuropathological pathways account for age-related risk of dementia. *Annals of Neurology*, *84*(1), 10–22. doi:10.1002/ana.25246

Puy, L., De Guio, F., Godin, O., Duering, M., Dichgans, M., Chabriat, H., & Jouvent, E. (2017). Cerebral microbleeds and the risk of incident ischemic stroke in CADASIL (cerebral autosomal dominant arteriopathy with subcortical infarcts and leukoencephalopathy). *Stroke*, *48*(10), 2699–2703. doi:10.1161/STROKEAHA.117.017839

Renard, D., Tatu, L., Collombier, L., Wacongne, A., Ayrignac, X., Charif, M., . . . Thouvenot, E. (2018). Cerebral amyloid angiopathy and cerebral amyloid angiopathy-related inflammation: Comparison of hemorrhagic and DWI MRI features. *Journal of Alzheimer's Disease*, *64*(4), 1113–1121. doi:10.3233/JAD-180269

Satizabal, C. L., Zhu, Y. C., Mazoyer, B., Dufouil, C., & Tzourio, C. (2012). Circulating IL-6 and CRP are associated with MRI findings in the elderly: The 3C-dijon study. *Neurology*, *78*(10), 720–727. doi:10.1212/WNL.0b013e318248e50f

Schmidt, R., Enzinger, C., Ropele, S., Schmidt, H., Fazekas, F., & Austrian Stroke Prevention Study. (2003). Progression of cerebral white matter lesions: 6-year results of the Austrian Stroke Prevention Study. *Lancet*, *361*(9374), 2046–2048. doi:S0140673603136161

Schmidt, R., Launer, L. J., Nilsson, L. G., Pajak, A., Sans, S., Berger, K., . . . Hofman, A.; CASCADE Consortium. (2004). Magnetic resonance imaging of the brain in diabetes: The cardiovascular determinants of dementia (CASCADE) study. *Diabetes*, *53*(3), 687–692.

Schmidt, R., Schmidt, H., Haybaeck, J., Loitfelder, M., Weis, S., Cavalieri, M., . . . Jellinger, K. (2011). Heterogeneity in age-related white matter changes. *Acta Neuropathologica*, *122*(2), 171–185. doi:10.1007/s00401-011-0851-x

Schneider, J. A., Aggarwal, N. T., Barnes, L., Boyle, P., & Bennett, D. A. (2009). The neuropathology of older persons with and without dementia from community versus clinic cohorts. *Journal of Alzheimer's Disease*, *18*(3), 691–701. doi:10.3233/JAD-2009-1227

Schneider, J. A., Arvanitakis, Z., Bang, W., & Bennett, D. A. (2007). Mixed brain pathologies account for most dementia cases in community-dwelling older persons. *Neurology*, *69*(24), 2197–2204. doi:01.wnl.0000271090.28148.24

Schneider, J. A., & Bennett, D. A. (2010). Where vascular meets neurodegenerative disease. *Stroke; a Journal of Cerebral Circulation*, *41*(10 Suppl), S144–S146. doi:10.1161/STROKEAHA.110.598326

Schneider, J. A., Boyle, P. A., Arvanitakis, Z., Bienias, J. L., & Bennett, D. A. (2007). Subcortical infarcts, Alzheimer's disease pathology, and memory function in older persons. *Annals of Neurology*, *62*(1), 59–66. doi:10.1002/ana.21142

Schneider, J. A., Wilson, R. S., Bienias, J. L., Evans, D. A., & Bennett, D. A. (2004). Cerebral infarctions and the likelihood of dementia from Alzheimer disease pathology. *Neurology*, *62*(7), 1148–1155.

Schneider, J. A., Wilson, R. S., Cochran, E. J., Bienias, J. L., Arnold, S. E., Evans, D. A., & Bennett, D. A. (2003). Relation of cerebral infarctions to dementia and cognitive function in older persons. *Neurology*, *60*(7), 1082–1088.

Schoenmaker, N., & Van Gool, W. A. (2004). The age gap between patients in clinical studies and in the general population: A pitfall for dementia research. *Lancet Neurology*, *3*(10), 627–630. doi:10.1016/S1474-4422(04)00884-1

Schrag, M., McAuley, G., Pomakian, J., Jiffry, A., Tung, S., Mueller, C., . . . Kirsch, W. M. (2010). Correlation of hypointensities in susceptibility-weighted images to tissue histology in dementia patients with cerebral amyloid angiopathy: A postmortem MRI study. *Acta Neuropathologica*, *119*(3), 291–302. doi:10.1007/s00401-009-0615-z

Serrano-Pozo, A., Qian, J., Muzikansky, A., Monsell, S. E., Montine, T. J., Frosch, M. P., . . . Hyman, B. T. (2016). Thal amyloid stages do not significantly impact the correlation between neuropathological change and cognition in the Alzheimer disease continuum. *Journal of Neuropathology and Experimental Neurology*, *75*(6), 516–526. doi:10.1093/jnen/nlw026

Simpson, J. E., Ince, P. G., Higham, C. E., Gelsthorpe, C. H., Fernando, M. S., Matthews, F., . . . Wharton, S. B.; MRC Cognitive Function and Ageing Neuropathology Study Group. (2007). Microglial activation in white matter lesions and nonlesional white matter of ageing brains. *Neuropathology and Applied Neurobiology*, *33*(6), 670–683. doi:NAN890

Snowdon, D. A., Greiner, L. H., Mortimer, J. A., Riley, K. P., Greiner, P. A., & Markesbery, W. R. (1997). Brain infarction and the clinical expression of Alzheimer disease. The Nun Study. *JAMA*, *277*(10), 813–817.

Sondergaard, C. B., Nielsen, J. E., Hansen, C. K., & Christensen, H. (2017). Hereditary cerebral small vessel disease and stroke. *Clinical Neurology and Neurosurgery*, *155*, 45–57. doi:S0303-8467(17)30050-1

Sonnen, J. A., Larson, E. B., Brickell, K., Crane, P. K., Woltjer, R., Montine, T. J., & Craft, S. (2009). Different patterns of cerebral injury in dementia with or without diabetes. *Archives of Neurology*, *66*(3), 315–322. doi:10.1001/archneurol.2008.579

Sonnen, J. A., Larson, E. B., Crane, P. K., Haneuse, S., Li, G., Schellenberg, G. D., . . . Montine, T. J. (2007). Pathological correlates of dementia in a longitudinal, population-based sample of aging. *Annals of Neurology*, *62*(4), 406–413. doi:10.1002/ana.21208

Stojanov, D., Vojinovic, S., Aracki-Trenkic, A., Tasic, A., Benedeto-Stojanov, D., Ljubisavljevic, S., & Vujnovic, S. (2015). Imaging characteristics of cerebral autosomal dominant arteriopathy with subcortical infarcts and leucoencephalopathy (CADASIL). *Bosnian Journal of Basic Medical Sciences/Udruzenje Basicnih Mediciniskih Znanosti*, *15*(1), 1–8. doi:10.17305/bjbms.2015.247

Summers, P. M., Hartmann, D. A., Hui, E. S., Nie, X., Deardorff, R. L., McKinnon, E. T., . . . Shih, A. Y. (2017). Functional deficits induced by cortical microinfarcts. *Journal of Cerebral Blood Flow and Metabolism*, *37*(11), 3599–3614. doi:10.1177/0271678X16685573

Takeda, S., Sato, N., & Morishita, R. (2014). Systemic inflammation, blood–brain barrier vulnerability and cognitive/non-cognitive symptoms in Alzheimer disease: Relevance to pathogenesis and therapy. *Frontiers in Aging Neuroscience*, *6*, 171. doi:10.3389/fnagi.2014.00171

Tanskanen, M., Makela, M., Myllykangas, L., Rastas, S., Sulkava, R., & Paetau, A. (2012). Intracerebral hemorrhage in the oldest old: A population-based study (Vantaa 85+). *Frontiers in Neurology*, *3*, 103. doi:10.3389/fneur.2012.00103

Thal, D. R., Grinberg, L. T., & Attems, J. (2012). Vascular dementia: Different forms of vessel disorders contribute to the development of dementia in the elderly brain. *Experimental Gerontology*, *47*(11), 816–824. doi:10.1016/j.exger.2012.05.023

Thal, D. R., Rub, U., Orantes, M., & Braak, H. (2002). Phases of A beta-deposition in the human brain and its relevance for the development of AD. *Neurology*, *58*(12), 1791–1800.

Thomas, T., Thomas, G., McLendon, C., Sutton, T., & Mullan, M. (1996). Beta-amyloid-mediated vasoactivity and vascular endothelial damage. *Nature*, *380*(6570), 168–171. doi:10.1038/380168a0

Toledo, J. B., Arnold, S. E., Raible, K., Brettschneider, J., Xie, S. X., Grossman, M., . . . Trojanowski, J. Q. (2013). Contribution of cerebrovascular disease in autopsy confirmed neurodegenerative disease cases in the National Alzheimer's Coordinating Centre. *Brain*, *136*(Pt 9), 2697–2706. doi:10.1093/brain/awt188

Tomimoto, H., Akiguchi, I., Suenaga, T., Nishimura, M., Wakita, H., Nakamura, S., & Kimura, J. (1996). Alterations of the blood–brain barrier and glial cells in white-matter lesions in cerebrovascular and Alzheimer's disease patients. *Stroke*, *27*(11), 2069–2074.

Utter, S., Tamboli, I. Y., Walter, J., Upadhaya, A. R., Birkenmeier, G., Pietrzik, C. U., . . . Thal, D. R. (2008). Cerebral small vessel disease-induced apolipoprotein E leakage is associated with Alzheimer disease and the accumulation of amyloid beta-protein in perivascular astrocytes. *Journal of Neuropathology and Experimental Neurology*, *67*(9), 842–856. doi:10.1097/NEN.0b013e3181836a71

van den Brink, H., Zwiers, A., Switzer, A. R., Charlton, A., McCreary, C. R., Goodyear, B. G., . . . Smith, E. E. (2018). Cortical microinfarcts on 3T magnetic resonance imaging in cerebral amyloid angiopathy. *Stroke*, *49*(8), 1899–1905. doi:10.1161/STROKEAHA.118.020810 van der Flier, W. M., Skoog, I., Schneider, J. A., Pantoni, L., Mok, V., Chen, C. L. H., & Scheltens, P. (2018). Vascular cognitive impairment. *Nature Reviews Disease Primers*, *4*, 18003. doi:10.1038/nrdp.2018.3

van Es, A. C., van der Grond, J., de Craen, A. J., Westendorp, R. G., Bollen, E. L., Blauw, G. J., . . . van Buchem, M. A.; PROSPER Study Group. (2011). Cerebral microbleeds and cognitive functioning in the PROSPER study. *Neurology*, *77*(15), 1446–1452. doi:10.1212/WNL.0b013e318232ab1d

van Oijen, M., de Jong, F. J., Witteman, J. C., Hofman, A., Koudstaal, P. J., & Breteler, M. M. (2007). Atherosclerosis and risk for dementia. *Annals of Neurology*, *61*(5), 403–410. doi:10.1002/ana.21073

van Veluw, S. J., Biessels, G. J., Klijn, C. J., & Rozemuller, A. J. (2016). Heterogeneous histopathology of cortical microbleeds in cerebral amyloid angiopathy. *Neurology*, *86*(9), 867–871. doi:10.1212/WNL.0000000000002419

van Veluw, S. J., Kuijf, H. J., Charidimou, A., Viswanathan, A., Biessels, G. J., Rozemuller, A. J., . . . Greenberg, S. M. (2017). Reduced vascular amyloid burden at microhemorrhage sites in cerebral amyloid angiopathy. *Acta Neuropathologica*, *133*(3), 409–415. doi:10.1007/s00401-016-1635-0

van Veluw, S. J., Shih, A. Y., Smith, E. E., Chen, C., Schneider, J. A., Wardlaw, J. M., . . . Biessels, G. J. (2017). Detection, risk factors, and functional consequences of cerebral microinfarcts. *The Lancet.Neurology*, *16*(9), 730–740. doi:S1474-4422(17)30196-5

Verbeek, M. M., de Waal, R. M., Schipper, J. J., & Van Nostrand, W. E. (1997). Rapid degeneration of cultured human brain pericytes by amyloid beta protein. *Journal of Neurochemistry*, *68*(3), 1135–1141.

Vinters, H. V., Ellis, W. G., Zarow, C., Zaias, B. W., Jagust, W. J., Mack, W. J., & Chui, H. C. (2000). Neuropathologic substrates of ischemic vascular dementia. *Journal of Neuropathology and Experimental Neurology*, *59*(11), 931–945.

Volpe, B. T., & Petito, C. K. (1985). Dementia with bilateral medial temporal lobe ischemia. *Neurology, 35*(12), 1793–1793.

Walker, L., McAleese, K. E., Thomas, A. J., Johnson, M., Martin-Ruiz, C., Parker, C., . . . Attems, J. (2015). Neuropathologically mixed Alzheimer's and Lewy body disease: Burden of pathological protein aggregates differs between clinical phenotypes. *Acta Neuropathologica*, *129*(5), 729–748. doi:10.1007/s00401-015-1406-3

Wardlaw, J. M., Doubal, F., Armitage, P., Chappell, F., Carpenter, T., Munoz Maniega, S., . . . Dhillon, B. (2009). Lacunar stroke is associated with diffuse blood–brain barrier dysfunction. *Annals of Neurology*, *65*(2), 194–202. doi:10.1002/ana.21549

Wegiel, J., Kuchna, I., Wisniewski, T., de Leon, M. J., Reisberg, B., Pirttila, T., . . . Lehtimaki, T. (2002). Vascular fibrosis and calcification in the hippocampus in aging, Alzheimer disease, and down syndrome. *Acta Neuropathologica*, *103*(4), 333–343. doi:10.1007/s00401-001-0471-y

Westover, M. B., Bianchi, M. T., Yang, C., Schneider, J. A., & Greenberg, S. M. (2013). Estimating cerebral microinfarct burden from autopsy samples. *Neurology*, *80*(15), 1365–1369. doi:10.1212/WNL.0b013e31828c2f52

White, L., Petrovitch, H., Hardman, J., Nelson, J., Davis, D. G., Ross, G. W., . . . Markesbery, W. R. (2002). Cerebrovascular pathology and dementia in autopsied Honolulu–Asia Aging Study participants. *Annals of the New York Academy of Sciences*, *977*, 9–23.

Wijesinghe, P., Shankar, S. K., Yasha, T. C., Gorrie, C., Amaratunga, D., Hulathduwa, S., . . . De Silva, K. R. (2016). Vascular contributions in Alzheimer's disease-related neuropathological changes: First autopsy evidence from a South Asian aging population. *Journal of Alzheimer's Disease, 54*(4), 1607–1618. doi:JAD160425

Wong, W. T. (2013). Microglial aging in the healthy CNS: Phenotypes, drivers, and rejuvenation. *Frontiers in Cellular Neuroscience, 7*, 22. doi:10.3389/fncel.2013.00022

Yu, L., Boyle, P. A., Leurgans, S., Schneider, J. A., Kryscio, R. J., Wilson, R. S., & Bennett, D. A. (2015). Effect of common neuropathologies on progression of late life cognitive impairment. *Neurobiology of Aging, 36*(7), 2225–2231. doi:10.1016/j.neurobiolaging.2015.04.006

Yu, L., Boyle, P. A., Nag, S., Leurgans, S., Buchman, A. S., Wilson, R. S., . . . Schneider, J. A. (2015). APOE and cerebral amyloid angiopathy in community-dwelling older persons. *Neurobiology of Aging, 36*(11), 2946–2953. doi:S0197-4580(15)00419-4

Zhang, C. E., Wong, S. M., van de Haar, H. J., Staals, J., Jansen, J. F., Jeukens, C. R., . . . Backes, W. H. (2017). Blood–brain barrier leakage is more widespread in patients with cerebral small vessel disease. *Neurology, 88*(5), 426–432. doi:10.1212/WNL.0000000000003556

Zhong, Y., Utriainen, D., Wang, Y., Kang, Y., & Haacke, E. M. (2014). Automated white matter hyperintensity detection in multiple sclerosis using 3D T2 FLAIR. *International Journal of Biomedical Imaging, 2014*, 239123. doi:10.1155/2014/239123

15

Potential of Blood- and CSF-Based Biomarkers for Alzheimer's Disease Diagnostics

Eric L. Goldwaser and Robert G. Nagele

AD and the Need for Biomarkers for Early-Stage Detection and Monitoring

1. Introduction

Alzheimer's disease (AD), a progressive and devastating neurodegenerative disorder afflicting the elderly, is hallmarked by dramatic cognitive and memory impairment caused by a loss of neurons and their synapses and brain atrophy in selected brain regions (Bertoni-Freddari et al., 2003; D'Andrea, 2001; Hamos, DeGennaro, & Drachman, 1989; Selkoe, 2002). Well-known pathological features include the deposition of amyloid-beta (Aβ) peptides (especially the 42-amino acid peptide [$A\beta_{42}$]), primarily in pyramidal neurons, amyloid plaques, and in the walls of brain blood vessels, and the appearance of neurofibrillary tangles (NFTs) containing hyperphosphorylated tau protein, reactive gliosis, and widespread inflammation (Clifford et al., 2007; D'Andrea, 2001; Dickson, 1997; Gouras, Almeida, & Takahashi, 2005; Gouras et al., 2000; R. G. Nagele, D'Andrea, Anderson, & Wang, 2002; Schwab & McGeer, 2008). The underlying mechanisms and factors contributing to the development of these features remain elusive and controversial. Available treatments for AD, at best, only slow the course of some symptoms and provide no relief from pathological progression. Current methods of diagnosing AD remain exceptionally difficult, especially at early stages, and usually involve a combination of a detailed history obtained from the patient and family and the results of neuropsychological, laboratory, and brain imaging studies. The current diagnosis of AD according to the fifth edition of the *Diagnostic and Statistical Manual of Mental Disorders* (American Psychiatric Association, 2013) does not incorporate the

Eric L. Goldwaser and Robert G. Nagele, *Potential of Blood- and CSF-Based Biomarkers for Alzheimer's Disease Diagnostics* In: *Vascular Disease, Alzheimer's Disease, and Mild Cognitive Impairment.* Edited by: David J. Libon, Melissa Lamar, Rodney A. Swenson, Kenneth M. Heilman, Oxford University Press (2020).
DOI: 10.1093/oso/9780190634230.003.0016

use of biomarkers, despite the push from organizations like the Alzheimer's Association (2015) to do so (Alzheimer's Association, 2015; Ronald and Nancy Reagan Research Institute of the Alzheimer's Association and the National Institute on Aging Working Group, 1998; Ganguli et al., 2011; Hendrix et al., 2015; Sachdev et al., 2014; Van Assche, Persoons, & Vandenbulcke, 2014). Some advancements in diagnosing AD have been made in the area of neuroimaging, such as magnetic resonance imaging (MRI) and positron emission tomography (PET), using tracers such as florbetapir (^{18}F), Pittsburgh compound B (PiB), and fluorodeoxyglucose (FDG; Weiner et al., 2016). However, their utility for early-stage AD detection is still being explored. Also, the high cost of imaging procedures, lack of standardized cross-institution protocols, and inconsistencies in interpretation of results prohibits their utility as initial disease screeners, and they may not be readily available to individuals in economically disadvantaged areas or remote geographical locations.

The high prevalence of AD is alarming with one in nine people at age 65 and older diagnosed, over 5.1 million Americans currently affected, and over 13 million expected to have the disease by 2050 (Alzheimer's Association, 2015). The annual economic and social burdens of AD are already staggering with an estimated $200 billion expended for care and $44 billion attributed to out-of-pocket spending. In response to these anticipated future clinical and financial burdens, the National Institutes of Health has significantly increased funding for AD research in recent years with the hope and goal of curtailing the impact of this disease before this devastating forecast becomes a reality (Alzheimer's Association, 2015). Particularly worrisome is the fact that research efforts aimed at developing therapeutics for AD have been met with a more than 99% failure rate in clinical trials over the past two decades (Cavanaugh, 2014; Cummings, Morstorf, & Zhong, 2014). Immunologic therapies employing various iterations of antiamyloid antibodies aimed at reducing brain amyloid levels and promoting amyloid clearance from the brain have yielded disappointing results in the form of little or no clinical improvement from a number of clinical trials (Dodel et al., 2011; Fuller et al., 2015; Needham & Zandi, 2014; Niewoehner et al., 2014; Panza et al., 2012; Salloway et al., 2009; Vandenberghe et al., 2016). However, one avenue of hope has arisen from retrospective analyses of some clinical trials that have suggested that patients at earlier stages of AD (e.g., at the prodromal or mild cognitive impairment [MCI] stage), did show some delay in progression from MCI to full-blown dementia as well as some signs of cognitive improvement. Although further testing is certainly required to validate these beneficial effects, this finding clearly emphasizes the need to focus AD-related therapeutic efforts on earlier disease stages. There is general agreement that treatment of AD at an early point in disease pathogenesis (i.e., before extensive brain devastation has occurred) offers the best chance of slowing AD pathological progression or perhaps stopping it altogether (Aggarwal, Shah, & Bennett, 2015; Cummings et al., 2014; Siemers et al., 2016).

It is now known that AD has a very long preclinical stage, as pathological changes are thought to be initiated 15 to 20 years before emergence of clinical signs and symptoms (Gandy & DeKosky, 2013). Roughly 10% to 15% of these predementia MCI patients convert to full-blown AD each year (Alzheimer's Association, 2015; Ronald and Nancy Reagan Research Institute of the Alzheimer's Association and the National Institute on Aging Working Group, 1998; Hendrix et al., 2015; Reitz & Mayeux, 2014; Sosa-Ortiz, Acosta-Castillo, & Prince, 2012). Although the preclinical status eliminates our ability to make use of symptoms to detect and diagnose AD, it also provides a new window of opportunity for discovering new disease biomarkers and developing early disease detection and diagnostic approaches that rely instead on the presence of ongoing early-stage AD pathology. At present, the hope is that drugs used to treat early-stage AD, perhaps some already available or in the pipeline, will soon be shown to have beneficial effects on these early stages and that these new preclinical and prodromal AD biomarkers will also have clinical utility for tracking the efficacy of potential disease-modifying therapies. In view of this, we turn our attention in this chapter to the rapidly evolving field of biomarker discovery for the detection and diagnosis of AD, using blood and cerebrospinal fluid (CSF) as body fluid sources.

2. Biomarkers: Goals and Obstacles

The discovery, development, and optimization of biomarkers for detection and diagnosis of AD are still in the early stages, but an enormous amount of work carried out thus far is very encouraging and highly suggestive that these efforts will ultimately be successful. Desired features and goals for useful biomarker efforts include a utility for early detection and disease progression monitoring while under treatment, minimally invasive, sensitive and specific, reliable, reproducible, simple to perform, and affordable (Ronald and Nancy Reagan Research Institute of the Alzheimer's Association and the National Institute on Aging Working Group, 1998; H. Hampel et al., 2010; Hendrix et al., 2015).

In recent years, much effort has been devoted to identifying soluble components in the blood and CSF that can serve as useful and reliable biomarkers to detect and diagnose AD. A serious limitation to widespread use of CSF, in general, has been the means by which it is obtained (i.e., via a lumbar spinal puncture), as this is considered invasive, requires a higher level of skill from the practitioner, and is accompanied by some risk. Also, the handling of CSF samples is much less standardized than it is for blood, and compositional differences are often noted when comparing the first milliliter taken to the next (Fourier et al., 2015; Lucey et al., 2015; Reiber, 1994, 2001). By contrast, obtaining blood by venipuncture is much easier, less invasive, and carries minimal risk, and blood tends to be more uniform in composition in the volumes typically drawn. A major obstacle that has arisen from both blood-based and CSF-based biomarker studies has been the lack of reproducibility among tests carried out at multiple laboratory testing sites. For this reason, O'Bryant and colleagues (O'Bryant et al., 2014, 2016, 2017; O'Bryant, Xiao, Barber, Huebinger et al., 2011; O'Bryant, Xiao, Barber, Reisch et al., 2011) have recently called for the standardization of sample procurement, preanalytical processing, and the means by which the various assays are analyzed and interpreted among different testing sites to facilitate cross-validation, which should make a significant contribution to advancing this important field.

3. CSF-Based Biomarkers

CSF, which fills the brain ventricles and spinal canal, is produced at a rate of 500 to 700 mL per day, largely by the choroid plexus located within the brain ventricles. It is in direct contact with the interstitial fluid that bathes neurons and their processes and synapses as well as glial cells. As a result, the complex byproducts of pathological events (or debris) that occur within the brain, including that from dead or dying neurons and glia, readily enter the CSF and thus can be detected in the small samples of CSF removed by spinal puncture. In CSF, the most established biomarkers are assayed using enzyme-linked immunosorbent assay (ELISA)-based systems and include $A\beta_{42}$, total tau, and phosphorylated tau (p-tau; e.g., phosphorylated at threonine residue 181) and their relative ratios. Measured values of these biomarkers are now thought to reflect the amyloid plaque and NFT burden in the brain.

3.1. $A\beta_{42}$

Low CSF $A\beta_{42}$ levels in individuals with MCI are now considered to be strongly indicative of the presence of early ongoing AD pathology, particularly plaque deposition, as well as predictive of the likelihood of rapid disease progression from the prodromal phase to full-blown AD. During early-stage clinical AD, there is an inverse relationship between CSF $A\beta_{42}$ levels and the level of amyloid deposition in the brain, with CSF levels consistently dropping to roughly 50% of that seen in corresponding normal controls (Andreasen & Blennow, 2002; Andreasen et al., 1999, 2001; Blennow et al., 2015; Buchhave et al., 2012; Forlenza et al., 2015; Hansson et al., 2006; Jack et al., 2016; Lewczuk, Mroczko,

Fagan, & Kornhuber, 2015; Mattsson et al., 2014; Mehta et al., 2000; Parnetti, Lanari, Silvestrelli, Saggese, & Reboldi, 2006; Shams et al., 2016; Sunderland et al., 2003; Toledo et al., 2014; Trushina, Dutta, Persson, Mielke, & Petersen, 2013; Wurtman, 2015; Zetterberg, Blennow, & Hanse, 2010). One possible explanation for this seemingly counterintuitive finding is chronic intraneuronal deposition and accumulation of soluble $A\beta_{42}$ in vulnerable neurons (e.g., pyramidal neurons) that is widespread in early disease stages, leading to progressive synaptic loss and eventual cell death prior to plaque formation (Choi et al., 2012; D'Andrea, 2001; Gouras et al., 2005; Ikonomovic et al., 2008; R. G. Nagele et al., 2002, 2011; Wurtman, 2015). In this case, the neurons are serving as a "sink" for soluble $A\beta_{42}$, thus removing it from the interstitial fluid and resulting in lower levels of $A\beta_{42}$ in the communicating CSF compartment. Moreover, in this context, it is noteworthy to point out that progressive Aβ deposition occurs within living neurons, as has been shown in humans and AD mouse models, thus rendering intraneuronal $A\beta_{42}$ undetectable by imaging agents such as PiB and florbetapir by PET until it is released from these cells (Clifford et al., 2007). This provides a plausible explanation for why a significant percentage of patients exhibiting symptoms at early stages of AD appear to lack a demonstrable Aβ burden when using PET neuroimaging. At present, low CSF $A\beta_{42}$ levels have now been accepted by most leaders in the field to best reflect ongoing early-stage AD pathology, with a reported sensitivity of over 96% before changes in tau levels are noted (Buchhave et al., 2012; Shaw et al., 2011).

3.2. Tau

Tau is a member of the class of proteins known as "microtubule associated proteins." Its function is to promote microtubule assembly and stabilization, and thus it is found in all nucleated cells (Aggarwal et al., 2015; Andreasen et al., 2001; Castellani & Perry, 2014; Harald Hampel et al., 2010; Jack et al., 2016; Kontsekova, Zilka, Kovacech, Skrabana, & Novak, 2014; Panza et al., 2012). Although it is normally in a phosphorylated state, tau may become hyperphosphorylated by kinases (e.g., glycogen synthase kinase 3) and other enzymes, leaving it unable to perform its wide gamut of structural functions (de Barry, Liégeois, & Janoshazi, 2010; Isla, Vazquez-Cuevas, & Pena-Ortega, 2016; Mouton-Liger et al., 2012). Structural imbalances that ensue as a result of tau hyperphosphorylation generate large aggregates of spiraling fibrils that disrupt cellular transport and architecture and cause irreparable neuronal damage. These so-called NFTs eventually fill much of the cell volume and are left as persistent remnants of dead neurons. It is established that NFT formation occurs as a downstream event to Aβ accumulation, and it is suspected that the latter may stimulate a cascade of cellular events that culminate in various kinase activation states that can drive tau phosphorylation. Upon neuronal death and lysis, soluble tau proteins and their fragments that have not been incorporated into NFTs will be mobile within the brain interstitial fluid and can be later detected in the CSF. Thus, higher CSF levels of total tau and p-tau suggest ongoing tau pathology (an increased abundance of NFTs) and AD pathogenesis in general (Andreasen et al., 2001; Forlenza et al., 2015; Hampel et al., 2010; Y. Y. Hu et al., 2002; Kohnken et al., 2000; Vanmechelen et al., 2000). Higher CSF tau levels are considered to be more directly linked to neuronal injury during AD pathogenesis than is $A\beta_{42}$, but this is most likely due to the fact that tau levels are increased at a later point in disease progression when a higher percentage of neurons are dying (Counts, Ikonomovic, Mercado, Vega, & Mufson, 2017; Tiernan et al., 2016).

3.3. Combined $A\beta_{42}$ and Tau

As previously described, CSF levels of $A\beta_{42}$ in patients at the MCI stage are reportedly decreased, while total tau or p-tau are increased compared to cognitively normal individuals and, further, are used to indicate a rapid progression to full-blown disease (Buchhave, Minthon, Zetterberg, Wallin et al., 2012; Hansson et al., 2006; Johnson et al., 2013; Mattsson et al., 2014; Parnetti et al., 2006; Toledo et al., 2014; Toledo, Korff, Shaw, Trojanowski, & Zhang, 2013; Visser et al., 2009; Yang et al., 2013; Zetterberg, Wahlund, & Blennow, 2003). There has been some international consensus regarding the concentrations of CSF biomarkers that are useful for the diagnosis of AD using ELISA-based assays; for example, $A\beta_{42}$ cutoff values of less than 500 pg/mL, p-tau (T181) greater than 60 pg/mL, and total tau ranging between 450 and 600 pg/mL. Control values for $A\beta_{42}$ are roughly 800 pg/mL, total tau between 100 and 400 pg/mL, and p-tau 20 pg/mL (Andreasen et al., 2001; Forlenza et al., 2015; Fourier et al., 2015; Humpel, 2011; Parnetti et al., 2006; Sauvee et al., 2014; Slaets et al., 2014). Combining measurements of CSF p-tau (T181) with $A\beta_{42}$ has been shown to result in improved diagnostic performance, yielding a sensitivity of 86% and specificity of 97% (Maddalena et al., 2003). Additional longitudinal studies have explored the utility of combined CSF $A\beta_{42}$ and total tau and p-tau for predicting conversion of preclinical AD to prodromal MCI and MCI to AD. The combination of high levels of total tau and p-tau and low $A\beta_{42}$ in the CSF was demonstrated in 90% of MCI subjects that transitioned to AD (Riemenschneider et al., 2002). Also, the combination of high total tau with a low $A\beta_{42}$/p-tau ratio detected initial AD with 95% sensitivity and 87% specificity and high CSF total tau/$A\beta_{42}$ and p-tau/$A\beta_{42}$ ratios significantly predicted a faster rate of conversion from MCI to AD (Fagan et al., 2007;

Hansson et al., 2006). Inconsistent results from one testing site to another were initially problematic, but the recent emphasis on standardizing CSF collection and handling methods as well as sample analysis, as is now being implemented at the Alzheimer's Disease Neuroimaging Initiative (ADNI), is clearly a major stride toward minimizing these shortcomings (Verwey et al., 2009). A recent meta-analysis and systematic review by Olsson and colleagues (2016) had similar aims in mind when parlaying various "core" biomarkers for AD across over 200 studies. They were able to normalize the disparities between sites where samples were gathered and of different immunologic assay techniques to yield comparative results, which showed an ability for CSF biomarkers including total tau, p-tau, and $A\beta_{42}$ to reliably distinguish AD and MCI from controls.

3.4. Other CSF Proteins and Inflammation-Associated Proteins

Although $A\beta_{42}$ and the various forms of tau in CSF have shown great promise as useful biomarkers of early-stage and perhaps even preclinical AD, patients at these early stages of disease progression exhibit considerable heterogeneity in the brain locations and amounts of amyloid and tangles, and the presence of co-incident comorbidities tends to collectively dampen the diagnostic accuracy of these useful biomarkers (Counts & Mufson, 2010; Perrin et al., 2011; Roe et al., 2011). To remedy this, some effort has been given to combining measurements of CSF $A\beta_{42}$ and tau with other novel and pathologically relevant proteins that are also detectable in CSF, including brain-derived neurotrophic factor (G. Li et al., 2009), apolipoproteins (Puchades et al., 2003; Zhang et al., 2008), synucleins (Mukaetova-Ladinska et al., 2008; J. B. Toledo, Korff, Shaw, Trojanowski, & Zhang, 2013), ubiquitin (Iqbal et al., 2005; Iqbal & Grundke-Iqbal, 1997), visinin-like protein 1 (VILIP-1), and the neurofilament light chain (NFL) and the postsynaptic protein neurogranin (Kvartsberg et al., 2015; Portelius et al., 2015; Skillback et al., 2014; Skillback, Zetterberg, Blennow, & Mattsson, 2013; Tarawneh et al., 2016; Zetterberg et al., 2016). For example, in longitudinal studies, AD patients who converted to AD from MCI revealed significantly higher neurogranin levels than controls and other MCI subjects who failed to convert to AD, thus reflecting an increase in synaptic degeneration during this interval. Higher levels of neurogranin were also better correlated with CSF tau levels and reduced cognitive performance than $A\beta_{42}$ (Portelius et al., 2015). Similarly, higher NFL levels, reflecting a collapse of neuronal processes, have been linked to more rapid degeneration of the hippocampus, one of the main areas of memory formation affected by AD, and reduced cognitive performance (Kaj Blennow, 2017; Zetterberg et al., 2016).

Given that major features of AD pathogenesis are a loss of synapses and their supportive axons and dendrites, neuron and glial death, and associated inflammation, additional CSF biomarkers linked to these events have been preferentially sought after for use as AD diagnostic indicators. The most promising recent candidates for detection of MCI and AD include protein components of the endosome-lysosome system (Counts et al., 2017; Counts & Mufson, 2010), which is clearly disturbed in neurons and glia (Ginsberg et al., 2010; Nixon, 2013; Tiernan et al., 2016), protein and lipid biomarkers linked to oxidative stress (Di Domenico et al., 2016; Montine et al., 1999; Pratico et al., 2002), and altered microRNA (miRNA) profiles (Denk et al., 2015; Liu, Wang, Li, & Wang, 2014; Sala Frigerio et al., 2013). The hope is that the use of some of these biomarkers will work in unison with the core CSF biomarkers ($A\beta_{42}$, tau, and p-tau) and serve to bolster overall diagnostic accuracy for detecting early-stage AD and its later progression as well as help to distinguish AD-related pathology from that of other dementias and neurodegenerative diseases. If so, then these biomarkers will have valuable utility by serving as a screening tool to identify patients needing early therapeutic intervention as well as for early recruitment into clinical trials. An example of this utility is seen with α-synuclein, a protein highly relevant to Parkinson's disease (PD) pathology, where its use as an adjuvant biomarker to the core CSF biomarkers has been met with some success in detecting AD with concomitant Lewy body pathology (the classic lesions associated with PD; Slaets et al., 2014; J. B. Toledo et al., 2013). Growth factors and inflammatory markers such as cytokines and chemokines in the CSF are being explored to aid in this diagnostic effort, a list that includes nerve growth factor, hepatocyte growth factor, and vascular endothelial growth factor, interleukin-6, interleukin-11, and macrophage migration inhibitor factor (Bacher et al., 2010; Blasko et al., 2006; Fiala & Veerhuis, 2010; Galimberti et al., 2008; Llano et al., 2012; Marksteiner et al., 2008; Popp et al., 2009; Tsuboi, Kakimoto, Akatsu, Daikuhara, & Yamada, 2002; Tsuboi et al., 2003).

3.5. Blood–Brain Barrier Biomarkers

Given the considerable attention devoted to research on the involvement of the cerebrovasculature in AD, the role of the blood–brain barrier (BBB) has been widely studied. Numerous studies have presented evidence that BBB integrity is compromised, especially in focal regions of AD pathology early in disease development and, later on, more globally (Shams et al., 2016). S100B, an established surrogate protein for detecting BBB dysfunction, is used as a nonspecific biomarker supporting a diagnosis of AD. S100B is a calcium channel protein that is an accepted means of assaying for glial and astrocyte activation, generally in response to cellular damage to the neurovascular unit, leading to BBB breakdown. It is detected at significantly higher levels in CSF of patients with AD compared to healthy controls (Peskind, Griffin, Akama, Raskind, & Van Eldik, 2001; Petzold et al., 2003; Sørensen, Nygaard, & Christensen, 2016). Olsson and colleagues (2016) also included albumin quotients in their meta-analysis, which establishes a ratio of CSF to serum albumin concentrations that correlate to the extent of BBB breakdown and can differentiate AD patients from nondemented controls (Olsson et al., 2016). In interpreting these albumin ratios, it is understood that albumin leaks into the CSF through a permeabilized BBB; however, the location of the BBB breach within the brain vasculature cannot be ascertained. In another study, Skillbäck and colleagues (2017) assayed for CSF/serum albumin ratios across a host of neurodegenerative, neurocognitive, and neuropsychiatric conditions, including AD, MCI, PD, vascular dementia, and Lewy body dementia. These authors found a significant increase in albumin ratio, again suggesting BBB breakdown in AD and MCI compared to control subjects. However, it was not possible to clearly differentiate one form of neurocognitive condition from another, perhaps owing to a common feature shared among these conditions (i.e., cerebrovascular dysfunction).

3.6. MicroRNAs

A family of small, noncoding RNA molecules now known to play a key role in regulation of gene expression has been under intense investigation for use as disease-specific biomarkers in recent years. These 22-nucleotide RNA species, called microRNAs (miRNAs), generally mediate gene silencing by repressing translation of messenger RNAs (mRNAs) after they bind to complementary RNA sequences on the target transcript. miRNAs can now be assayed with commercialized kits, and their discovery has given birth to new field of biomarker discovery that spans many diseases. In the context of AD, for example, investigators have detected that the levels of the following miRNA species in the CSF differ in AD patients compared to controls and other forms of dementia: miR27a, miR-29a, miR-29b, miR-125b, let-71-5p, miR-15a-5p, and miR-29c-3p (Müller et al., 2016; Sørensen et al., 2016; Van Giau & An, 2016). Exploration of the pathophysiologic relevance of these miRNAs to AD has led to the finding that miR-15a can regulate the amyloid precursor protein (APP) and beta-secretase-1 (BACE1), the latter an enzyme that cleaves the APP protein into fragments that facilitate $A\beta_{42}$ production (Müller et al., 2016; Sørensen et al., 2016).

3.7. Future Prospects

The list of useful CSF biomarkers used alone and in combination will undoubtedly continue to grow in parallel with additional technical refinements that culminate in increased efficacy, accessibility, ease of use, and more precise and reliable analytic detection methods. The ever-growing landscape of candidate CSF biomarkers is now shifting the emphasis from biomarker discovery research focused on their utility to diagnosis emergent illness. Also, recent attention given to standardization of sample procurement, handling and storage methods as well as to the various biomarker detection and quantification assays will no doubt have a great and positive impact on the success of these efforts.

4. Blood-Based Biomarkers

In recent years, a great deal of research has been aimed at identifying blood-based biomarkers that are useful for the detection and diagnosis of AD and related disorders (Henriksen et al., 2014; Lista, Faltraco, Prvulovic, & Hampel, 2013; O'Bryant, 2016; Snyder et al., 2014). The goals are twofold: to develop screening tools that would work in a primary care setting and efficiently direct patients to seek additional, more costly confirming tests and to develop accurate diagnostic tools (Blasko et al., 2010; Chang et al., 2016; O'Bryant et al., 2016, 2017). Using blood as the source of biomarkers for detection of disease has a number of advantages over the use of CSF for the same purpose. First and foremost, blood samples are much more easily obtained by a relatively noninvasive venipuncture, in sharp contrast to the need for lumbar spinal puncture for CSF (Lista et al., 2013; O'Bryant et al., 2016). The latter requires individuals with special training and cannot be performed without moderate risk. For blood-based biomarkers to be useful for early AD detection and disease monitoring, they must satisfy several important criteria. To start, blood-based biomarkers should reflect pathophysiological processes linked to disease such that measured levels in the blood should change in response to administration of disease-modifying treatments reflecting a reduction in existing pathology. Second, blood-based biomarkers should display high sensitivity and specificity with results reproducible over time and in different laboratory settings. Lastly, the entire process of obtaining, storing, and analyzing blood-based biomarkers should be affordable (Humpel, 2011). Currently, the resources and costs required for widespread use of CSF- and imaging-based biomarkers are prohibitive for making them part of routine clinical practice.

As it now stands, even the most promising blood-based biomarkers have not yet been tested as extensively as the core CSF biomarkers. One inherent problem with blood-based biomarkers is the fact that the blood, much more so than CSF, can vary significantly in composition from one individual to the next and even in the same individual depending on circadian or time of day variations in when the sample is drawn. Other factors contributing to variation in blood composition include the health status of the individual and the presence and mode of progression of diseases that can alter blood composition. In addition, while neuronal and glial debris produced by ongoing brain pathology can deposit potentially useful biomarkers directly within the CSF, these biomarkers must first escape the CSF and enter into the systemic circulation to become detectable as blood-based biomarkers. The rate at which they leave the CSF and travel within the blood can be influenced by many factors, each of which can affect measurable levels to varying degrees. Thus far, the development of blood-based biomarkers has been plagued by a lack of reproducibility. Despite these inherent potential shortcomings, as described in the following sections, work on the discovery and validation of blood-based biomarkers is progressing remarkably quickly and shows great promise for eventual success. Furthermore, it seems that the most likely use for blood-based biomarkers will be a first-stage primary care screening which will serve to justify directing patients to additional, more costly, and invasive diagnostic procedures (i.e., CSF $A\beta_{42}$ and tau quantifications and PET amyloid neuroimaging) with the goal of confirming the presence of AD pathology. As accuracy and reliability improve and are validated, additional applications will include stand-alone diagnostics, determination of risk for developing AD or risk for progression from MCI to AD, monitoring of disease progression, early enrollment of subjects with confirmed disease into clinical trials, and monitoring of disease progression in patients under their physician's care or in clinical trials of new drugs (Gold, Klein, Carr, Kessler, & Sullivan, 2012; O'Bryant et al., 2017).

4.1. $A\beta_{42}$ and Tau

Unfortunately, unlike in CSF, blood levels of the most prevalent Aβ peptides ($A\beta_{42}$ and $A\beta_{40}$) and tau have not proven to be particularly useful for detection and diagnosis of AD. Levels of both Aβ peptides in the blood are often quite variable, ranging from unchanged to higher levels with little reliability and considerable overlap when comparing patients and controls or when attempting to use these parameters as biomarkers of risk for AD (Graff-Radford et al., 2007; Irizarry, 2004; Mayeux et al., 2003; Pomara, Willoughby, Sidtis, & Mehta, 2005). These findings strongly suggest that there is no meaningful relationship between plasma Aβ levels and the amyloid load status of the brain (Fagan et al., 2006; Mehta et al., 2000). One potential contributor to the difficulty in quantifying the absolute amount of circulating soluble Aβ (especially $A\beta_{42}$) is the fact that these peptides can interact with many other proteins present in the blood, such as albumin and a number of cellular membrane proteins. An additional complication comes from the fact that the APP and its metabolites are normally produced throughout the body, most prominently in platelets and skeletal muscle. In fact, a number of sources suggest that these two cell types make a major contribution to the pool of Aβ in the blood (Abdullah et al., 2007; Kuo et al., 2000; O'Bryant et al., 2016; Roher et al., 2009). Given that skeletal muscle represents a significant percentage of total body weight (roughly 25%), it is easy to understand how this tissue can deposit a sizable fraction of the total circulating Aβ peptide pool. With BBB compromise common in brain regions exhibiting AD pathology, it is reasonable to suspect that skeletal muscle and platelets represent major sources of soluble monomeric and oligomeric Aβ peptides that eventually make their way into the brain parenchyma, thus, providing the raw materials for deposition of Aβ peptides in vulnerable neurons and amyloid plaques during disease pathogenesis (R. G. Nagele et al., 2011). Lastly, several studies have shown that the increased lipophilicity of $Aβ_{42}$ over $Aβ_{40}$ (an alternatively processed fragment of APP) makes the former much more difficult to extract from the soluble fraction of blood than $Aβ_{40}$ (Borroni, Agosti, Marcello, Di Luca, & Padovani, 2010; Evin & Li, 2012; Gustaw-Rothenberg et al., 2010; Q Li, Gordon, Cao, Ugen, & Morgan, 2007; Niederst, Reyna, & Goldstein, 2015; Nixon, 2007; O'Bryant et al., 2016; Zetterberg et al., 2010). Historically, this has confounded results from one study to the next and, ultimately, has left plasma Aβ as a yet to be validated tool in the diagnosis of AD (H. Hampel et al., 2010; Henriksen et al., 2014; O'Bryant et al., 2014; O'Bryant, Xiao, Barber, Huebinger et al., 2011; Snyder et al., 2014). However, a recent study by Nakamura et al. (2018) has raised new hope for this approach by showing that Aβ peptides can be detected accurately in plasma using immunoprecipitation coupled to mass spectroscopy and that this assay can be a reliable indicator of brain Aβ burden. This once again opens the door to more feasible and accessible blood-based detection and efficient screening of the population. Attempts to accurately assay the levels of the various forms of tau have also generally been unsuccessful, as no clear correlation has been found between plasma and CSF total tau concentrations, also in stark contrast to that found in the CSF (Olsson et al., 2016; Nakamura et al., 2018; Zetterberg et al., 2013).

4.2. Proteins Associated With Cell Signaling and Inflammation

A number of recent studies have reported promising novel blood-based biomarkers for AD and have raised the hope that this approach will be fruitful. For example, an analysis of the levels of plasma proteins associated with cell signaling and inflammation led to the selection of a panel of 18 proteins that could distinguish patients with AD from controls and accurately predict later AD in subjects with MCI (Ray et al., 2007). O'Bryant, Xiao, Barber, Huebinger et al. (2011) carried out multianalyte profiling in a study of over 500 AD patient and control samples obtained from both the Texas Alzheimer's Research Consortium and the ADNI and identified a panel of 11 proteins that were differentially expressed between AD and control groups. When combined with other biological and demographic parameters, these biomarkers yielded an overall accuracy comparable to that of CSF total tau/Aβ_{42} for these patients (O'Bryant, Xiao, Barber, Huebinger et al., 2011). In another study, a group of 18 proteins (including cortisol, APOE, pancreatic polypeptide and epidermal growth factor receptor) was used successfully to distinguish AD patients from controls with high sensitivity (85%) and specificity (93%; Doecke et al., 2012). W. T. Hu et al. (2012) described 17 proteins and peptides linked to AD-associated MCI, two of which were correlated with CSF levels of Aβ_{42} and total tau. Lastly, an evaluation of 1129 plasma proteins using the SomaScan® platform led to the identification of five proteins in blood samples that could distinguish AD patients from healthy controls with high overall accuracy (sensitivity = 90.0%; specificity = 84.2%) and even higher values in a subsequent validation study (sensitivity = 96.7%; specificity = 80.0%; Zhao et al., 2015). NFL levels in the plasma and CSF have shown good correlation with increased levels in CSF and plasma in both MCI and AD (Bacioglu et al., 2016; Gisslen et al., 2016; Olsson et al., 2016). Also, a large longitudinal study of subjects from the Framingham Study Offspring Cohort monitored plasma APOJ (clusterin) and showed higher levels in both MCI and AD that were linked to PET amyloid levels and changes in hippocampal volume, suggesting that this approach has potential to be useful for determination of risk for conversion of MCI to AD (Gupta et al., 2016; Weinstein et al., 2016).

4.3. Platelet Biomarkers

Platelets express APP and BACE1, contain serotonin-filled vesicles, and recently have been described to also exhibit pathological variations of tau as part of their proteomic repertoire (Bermejo-Bescos et al., 2013; Borroni et al., 2010; Colciaghi et al., 2004; Decourt et al., 2013; Evin & Li, 2012; Roher et al., 2009; Tang, Hynan, Baskin, & Rosenberg, 2006). Platelet activation and coating events are reflected by changes in the number of surface membrane proteins, and certain members of these protein families have been shown to be preferentially increased when assayed in AD patients compared to controls (Decourt et al., 2013; Evin & Li, 2012; Tang et al., 2006). Serotonin metabolism and APP processing are altered in the platelets of AD patients and can also be used to distinguish the blood of MCI patients from controls (Arora, Emery, & Meltzer, 1991; Johnston et al., 2008;

Spigset, Wilhelmsson, Mjorndal, & Eriksson, 2000). Studies on phosphorylated tau in platelets have revealed conflicting results but monitoring certain tau ratios have yielded promising data suggesting that this approach may be able to accurately differentiate AD patients and control subjects (Farias, Perez, Slachevsky, & Maccioni, 2012; Mukaetova-Ladinska et al., 2012; Neumann, Farias, Slachevsky, Perez, & Maccioni, 2011).

4.4. Exosomes and Their Contents

Blood-based proteins, lipids, and miRNAs enclosed within exosomes have all shown promise as blood-based biomarkers for early detection of AD pathology (Bermejo-Bescos et al., 2013; Borroni et al., 2010; Chang et al., 2016; Colas, Shinohara, Dalli, Chiang, & Serhan, 2014; Hall et al., 2013; Henriksen et al., 2014; Mapstone et al., 2014; O'Bryant, Xiao, Barber, Huebinger et al., 2011; O'Bryant, Xiao, Barber, Reisch et al., 2011; Snyder et al., 2014). Exosomes are small (30–100 nm in diameter) cell-derived vesicles found in many of the body's fluids, most notably blood, urine, and CSF (Cheng et al., 2015; Van Giau & An, 2016). They are thought to contribute to the formation of multivesicular bodies and can be released from cells into the surrounding extracellular space. Evidence is accumulating that exosomes are not simply membrane-enclosed packets of cell debris; they may have specialized functions and play a key role in processes such as coagulation, intercellular signaling, and waste management. Their contents have been shown to reflect their cell of origin and include specific proteins, RNAs, miRNAs and double-stranded DNA. Although exosomal protein composition varies with the parent cell and tissue, most exosomes contain a common set of protein molecules as cargo. Because their contents reflect the type and health status of the cell of origin, the contents of exosomes are currently being investigated for their potential utility as biomarkers for health and disease. Exosomes originating from brain cells also find their way into the blood. Plasma lipids as well as proteins and miRNAs enclosed within exosomes and lysosomal derivatives have all shown promise as biomarkers for early detection of AD pathology. For example, levels of total tau, p-tau, and $A\beta_{42}$ in blood exosomes were shown to be significantly higher in patients with AD than in matched controls, with combined levels showing 96% sensitivity. Moreover, analysis of exosomes taken from a group of AD patients at two different time points showed that levels of these biomarkers were elevated in cognitively normal subjects, years before they developed AD (Fiandaca et al., 2015). Recently, the utility of brain-derived exosomes for predicting the progression of MCI to dementia was evaluated (Winston et al., 2016). Alterations in the levels of several biomarkers, including p-tau, $A\beta_{42}$, neurogranin, and repressor element 1-silencing transcription factor were detected in exosomes obtained from AD as well as in MCI subjects who converted to AD within 36 months compared to normal controls and MCI cases that failed to convert. Although much work needs to be done to standardize exosome isolation and processing protocols, it is clear that brain-derived exosomes show great promise as sources of biomarkers linked to pathology that may prove useful for detection and diagnosis of all stages of AD progression.

The identification of miRNAs in exosomes in the blood has led to investigations probing the relationship between their presence and various disease states (Cheng et al., 2015; Van Giau & An, 2016; Winston et al., 2016). Exosomes in CSF and blood of AD patients were found to have certain miRNA species that appear to facilitate identification of specific diseases. Given the novelty of miRNA detection in exosomes and the limited understanding of their pathophysiology, the ability to translate these research findings into clinical practice is far from within grasp. However, there have been some notable successes that enable miRNA species found in blood exosomes to be used to accurately differentiate AD subjects from controls and those with MCI, much like in CSF. miRNAs in blood that differentiated AD from controls include miR-590-5- and miR-142-5p, miR-194-5p, miR342-3p, and a panel of others reported in similar studies (Cheng et al., 2015; Van Giau & An, 2016; Winston et al., 2016).

5. Autoantibodies and the Diagnosis of Mild Cognitive Impairment and Dementia

Autoantibodies are self-reactive antibodies that have been widely implicated as causal agents of autoimmune diseases and have also been shown to be useful for the detection and diagnosis of these diseases. Well-known examples include rheumatoid arthritis, systemic lupus erythematosus, and vasculitis. Individuals afflicted with these diseases are now routinely screened for rheumatoid factor, antinuclear antibodies, and antineutrophil cytoplasmic antibodies, respectively, to confirm these diseases. Until recently, detection of disease-linked autoantibodies was largely serendipitous. However, during the past decade, great advancements in the development of human protein microarray technology have provided a platform on which thousands of potential antigen targets can be immobilized and used as bait to attract their cognate autoantibodies. These arrays can be probed with human serum, plasma, CSF, or saliva to gain a better appreciation of the true scale and diversity of autoantibody expression in the body.

Recently, in a study of sera obtained from 166 individuals, we used human protein microarrays containing nearly 10,000 potential antigen target proteins to demonstrate that thousands of immunoglobulin G autoantibodies are ubiquitously present in human blood, a finding that runs counter to a central tenant of immunology (i.e., the principle of self-tolerance) (E. P. Nagele et al., 2013). We further showed that the detected number, titer, and diversity of autoantibodies represented were clearly influenced by age, gender, and the presence of disease (E. P. Nagele et al., 2013).

While the underlying purpose for the ubiquity of autoantibodies in the blood remains unknown, we have found that similarly complex autoantibody profiles are evolutionarily conserved, at least among mammals, suggesting that they have an important function. We have hypothesized that the main function of these autoantibodies is clearance of blood-borne cell and tissue debris that is universally generated in both healthy and diseased individuals on a daily basis. Assuming this to be true, otherwise healthy subjects have been shown to exhibit baseline levels of thousands of autoantibodies in the blood. However, one would also expect that the presence of disease should result in the production of excessive debris from the affected organ(s), some of which inevitably makes its way into the blood. We believe that this transient increase in disease-associated debris in the blood is met with a concordant increase in the production of specific autoantibodies targeting this debris that act collectively to remove it from the blood. Following this scenario, the appearance of common and specific perturbations in individual autoantibody profiles should directly reflect the status of ongoing pathology, and detection of these changes may reveal the identities of some very early and specific blood-based biomarkers of disease.

As an early test of the utility of autoantibodies as blood-based biomarkers of disease, Reddy and Kodadek (2005) implemented combinatorial library screening using microarrays containing thousands of unnatural synthetic molecules, referred to as peptoids, designed to mimic native autoantigens. They showed disease-associated differences in the peptoid binding patterns of autoantibodies in the blood of AD patients compared to healthy controls. In this study, three candidate peptoids were selected as the top discriminators, which were then used to distinguish AD patient from controls with an overall accuracy ranging from 93% to 96% (sensitivity = 93.7%; specificity = 93.7%–100%). Similarly, Restrepo, Stafford, Magee, and Johnston (2011) created an array-based platform consisting of 10,000 random-sequence peptides composed of 17 residues that was able to detect a single common immunoglobulin G binding pattern in the plasma of six of eight subjects with AD that were distinct from two binding patterns present in nine age-matched controls without dementia and eight cognitively normal subjects.

In initial proof-of-concept studies using human protein microarrays containing nearly 10,000 potential antigen targets, we identified panels of selected autoantibodies that can serve as diagnostic biomarkers of mild/moderate AD and PD with overall accuracies of 96.0% and 97.1%, respectively (DeMarshall et al., 2016; Han, Nagele, DeMarshall, Acharya, & Nagele, 2012; E. Nagele, Han,

Demarshall, Belinka, & Nagele, 2011). Since the practical utility of potential AD or PD biomarkers for disease screening and diagnostics depends on their capacity to detect these diseases at early stages, we then focused our efforts on early detection of both diseases. In a larger study of 357 patients, including 103 early-stage PD patients (with 90% confidence in diagnosis), we showed that a panel of as few as four serum autoantibodies biomarkers was capable of distinguishing early-stage PD patients from age- and gender-matched controls with an overall accuracy of 87.9%, a sensitivity of 94.1% and specificity of 85.5% (DeMarshall et al., 2015). These biomarkers were also capable of "staging" PD (i.e., differentiating early-stage PD from mild/moderate-stage PD) with an overall accuracy of 97.5% and showing that disease staging may be achieved through the use of distinct panels of biomarkers for each stage. Lastly, our early-stage PD biomarker panel was able to distinguish early-stage PD patients from those with other neurological (e.g., early-stage and mild/moderate-stage AD and multiple sclerosis) and no-neurological (e.g., breast cancer) diseases with comparable overall accuracies (DeMarshall et al., 2015).

Most recently, in a proof of concept study of 236 patients, our objective was to determine if autoantibodies can be used as biomarkers to accurately diagnose individuals with MCI caused by early-stages of AD pathology. We obtained sera from 50 MCI subjects from the ADNI. Each MCI patients also exhibited CSF biomarker ($A\beta_{42,}$ total tau, $A\beta_{42}$/tau ratio, and phosphorylated tau) levels consistent with the presence of ongoing early-stage AD pathology and a high likelihood of rapid progression to AD. Results showed that a small panel of as few as 10 autoantibody biomarkers can readily differentiate AD-driven MCI patients from matched controls with an overall accuracy, sensitivity, and specificity of 98% (DeMarshall et al., 2016). The selected panel of AD-associated MCI biomarkers was disease stage-specific in that it was also possible to differentiate MCI patients from individuals at a more advanced (mild/moderate) stage of AD. These biomarkers showed high disease-specificity since they were also capable of distinguishing AD-associated MCI patients from those with mild-moderate AD and other neurological and nonneurological diseases with high overall accuracy, suggesting the potential of this approach for even earlier (preclinical) AD diagnosis as well as for monitoring discrete stages of AD progression.

6. Conclusions and Perspectives

The last decade has witnessed tremendous progress in the identification of biomarkers in the blood and CSF that can be used for early detection and diagnosis of AD as well as monitoring of disease progression through preclinical, prodromal, and full-blown disease stages. Ideal features of diagnostic tests

Origin and Fate of Alzheimer's Disease Biomarkers in Blood and CSF
Sagittal View of an Alzheimer's Brain Showing Neurodegeneration

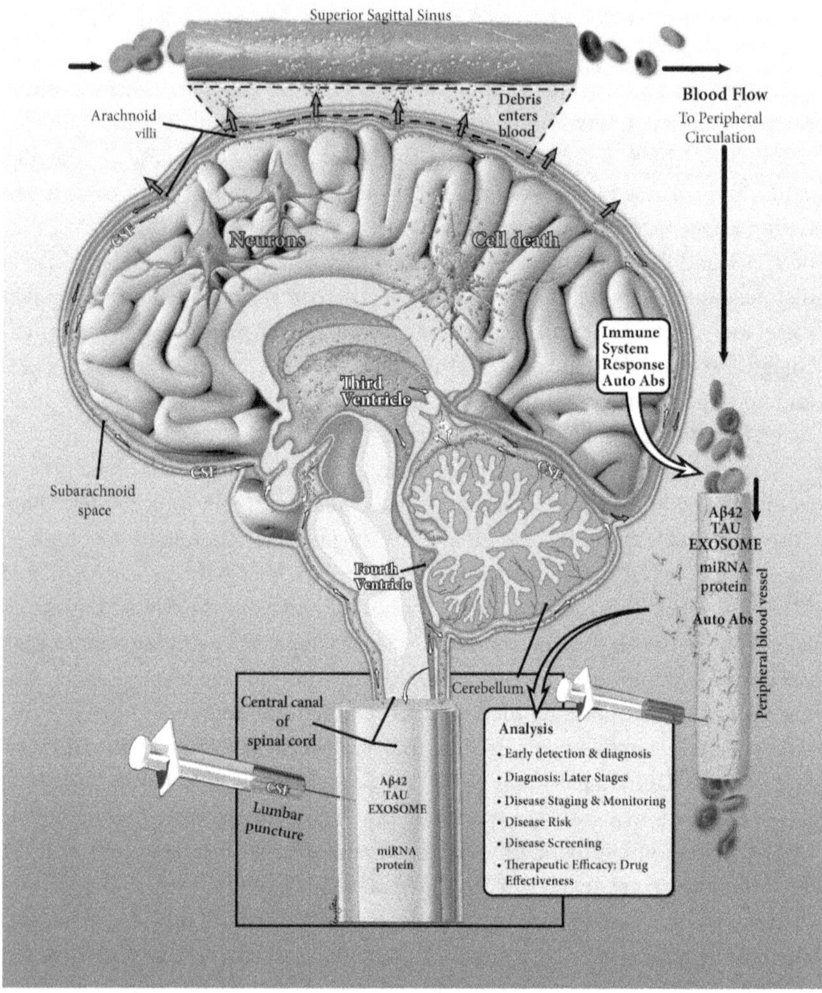

employing these biomarkers include that they should be simple to use, highly accurate and reproducible, minimally invasive, and affordable. With the general agreement that AD pathology is underway for many years prior to the appearance of telltale symptoms, a focus on identifying biomarkers that have a direct link to the pathology opens the door to early (perhaps even preclinical) detection of AD. Early detection and diagnosis enables earlier access to available treatments, thus greatly improving the chances for a favorable outcome if the treatment is administered before the disease has progressed beyond the point where it can be slowed or stopped without adverse loss of functionality. The ability to develop specific biomarker panels for different stages of disease progression should enable patient monitoring while under treatment by their physicians or while participating as subjects in clinical trials. Also, identification of new and useful disease-specific biomarkers may help to identify disease-relevant molecular pathways that have thus far escaped detection and could lead to identification of novel therapeutic targets. Although there is still a great deal of work to be done, the continued discovery and refinement of existing and new blood- and CSF-based biomarkers for AD and the development of highly accurate and reproducible assays for their detection and quantification will undoubtedly have a profound and positive impact on clinical outcomes for future AD patients. Likewise, the application of refinements in these technologies to other diseases may effect a major change in the strategies used for disease diagnostics in general.

References

Abdullah, L., Paris, D., Luis, C., Quadros, A., Parrish, J., Valdes, L., . . . Mullan, M. (2007). The influence of diagnosis, intra- and inter-person variability on serum and plasma Abeta levels. *Neuroscience Letters*, *428*(2–3), 53–58. doi:10.1016/j.neulet.2007.09.058

Aggarwal, N. T., Shah, R. C., & Bennett, D. A. (2015). Alzheimer's disease: Unique markers for diagnosis & new treatment modalities. *Indian Journal of Medical Research*, *142*(4), 369–382. doi:10.4103/0971-5916.169193

American Psychiatric Association. (2013). *Diagnostic and statistical manual of mental disorders* (5th ed.). Washington, DC: Author.

Andreasen, N., & Blennow, K. (2002). Beta-amyloid (Abeta) protein in cerebrospinal fluid as a biomarker for Alzheimer's disease. *Peptides*, *23*(7), 1205–1214.

Andreasen, N., Hesse, C., Davidsson, P., Minthon, L., Wallin, A., Winblad, B., . . . Blennow, K. (1999). Cerebrospinal fluid beta-amyloid(1-42) in Alzheimer disease: Differences between early- and late-onset Alzheimer disease and stability during the course of disease. *Archives of Neurology*, *56*(6), 673–680.

Andreasen, N., Minthon, L., Davidsson, P., Vanmechelen, E., Vanderstichele, H., Winblad, B., & Blennow, K. (2001). Evaluation of CSF-tau and CSF-Abeta42 as diagnostic markers for Alzheimer disease in clinical practice. *Archives of Neurology*, *58*(3), 373–379.

Arora, R. C., Emery, O. B., & Meltzer, H. Y. (1991). Serotonin uptake in the blood platelets of Alzheimer's disease patients. *Neurology*, *41*(8), 1307–1309.

Alzheimer's Association. (2015). 2015 Alzheimer's disease facts and figures. *Alzheimer's & Dementia*, *11*(3), 332–384.

Bacher, M., Deuster, O., Aljabari, B., Egensperger, R., Neff, F., Jessen, F., . . . Dodel, R. (2010). The role of macrophage migration inhibitory factor in Alzheimer's disease. *Molecular Medicine*, *16*(3–4), 116–121. doi:10.2119/molmed.2009.00123

Bacioglu, M., Maia, L. F., Preische, O., Schelle, J., Apel, A., Kaeser, S. A., . . . Jucker, M. (2016). Neurofilament light chain in blood and CSF as marker of disease progression in mouse models and in neurodegenerative diseases. *Neuron*, *91*(1), 56–66. doi:10.1016/j.neuron.2016.05.018

Bermejo-Bescos, P., Martin-Aragon, S., Jimenez-Aliaga, K., Benedi, J., Felici, E., Gil, P., . . . Villar, A. M. (2013). Processing of the platelet amyloid precursor protein in the mild cognitive impairment (MCI). *Neurochemical Research*, *38*(7), 1415–1423. doi:10.1007/s11064-013-1039-7

Bertoni-Freddari, C., Fattoretti, P., Solazzi, M., Giorgetti, B., Di Stefano, G., Casoli, T., & Meier-Ruge, W. (2003). Neuronal death versus synaptic pathology in Alzheimer's disease. *Annals of the New York Academy of Sciences*, *1010*, 635–638.

Blasko, I., Kemmler, G., Jungwirth, S., Wichart, I., Krampla, W., Weissgram, S., . . .Fischer, P. (2010). Plasma amyloid beta-42 independently predicts both late-onset depression and Alzheimer disease. *American Journal of Geriatric Psychiatry*, *18*(11), 973–982. doi:10.1097/JGP.0b013e3181df48be

Blasko, I., Lederer, W., Oberbauer, H., Walch, T., Kemmler, G., Hinterhuber, H., . . . Humpel, C. (2006). Measurement of thirteen biological markers in CSF of patients with Alzheimer's disease and other dementias. *Dementia and Geriatric Cognitive Disorders*, *21*(1), 9–15. doi:10.1159/000089137

Blennow, K. (2017). A review of fluid biomarkers for Alzheimer's disease: Moving from CSF to blood. *Neurology and Therapy*, *6*(Suppl 1), 15–24. doi:10.1007/s40120-017-0073-9

Blennow, K., Dubois, B., Fagan, A. M., Lewczuk, P., de Leon, M. J., & Hampel, H. (2015). Clinical utility of cerebrospinal fluid biomarkers in the diagnosis of early Alzheimer's disease. *Alzheimer's & Dementia*, *11*(1), 58–69. doi:10.1016/j.jalz.2014.02.004

Borroni, B., Agosti, C., Marcello, E., Di Luca, M., & Padovani, A. (2010). Blood cell markers in Alzheimer disease: Amyloid precursor protein form ratio in platelets. *Experimental Gerontology*, *45*(1), 53–56. doi:10.1016/j.exger.2009.08.004

Buchhave, P., Minthon, L., Zetterberg, H., Wallin, A. K., Blennow, K., & Hansson, O. (2012). Cerebrospinal fluid levels of beta-amyloid 1-42, but not of tau, are fully changed already 5 to 10 years before the onset of Alzheimer dementia. *Archives of General Psychiatry*, *69*(1), 98–106. doi:10.1001/archgenpsychiatry.2011.155

Castellani, R. J., & Perry, G. (2014). The complexities of the pathology-pathogenesis relationship in Alzheimer disease. *Biochemical Pharmacology*, *88*(4), 671–676. doi:10.1016/j.bcp.2014.01.009

Cavanaugh, S. E. (2014). Animal models of Alzheimer disease: Historical pitfalls and a path forward. *Altex*, *31*(3), 279–302. doi:10.14573/altex.1310071

Chang, K.-A., Shin, K. Y., Nam, E., Lee, Y.-B., Moon, C., Suh, Y.-H., & Lee, S. H. (2016). Plasma soluble neuregulin-1 as a diagnostic biomarker for Alzheimer's disease. *Neurochemistry International*, *97*, 1–7. doi:http://dx.doi.org/10.1016/j.neuint.2016.04.012

Cheng, L., Doecke, J. D., Sharples, R. A., Villemagne, V. L., Fowler, C. J., Rembach, A., . . . Hill, A. F. (2015). Prognostic serum miRNA biomarkers associated with Alzheimer's disease shows concordance with neuropsychological and neuroimaging assessment. *Molecular Psychiatry*, *20*(10), 1188–1196. doi:10.1038/mp.2014.127

Choi, S. R., Schneider, J. A., Bennett, D. A., Beach, T. G., Bedell, B. J., Zehntner, S. P., . . . Clark, C. M. (2012). Correlation of amyloid PET ligand florbetapir F 18 binding with Abeta aggregation and neuritic plaque deposition in postmortem brain tissue. *Alzheimer Disease and Associated Disorders*, *26*(1), 8–16. doi:10.1097/WAD.0b013e31821300bc

Clifford, P. M., Zarrabi, S., Siu, G., Kinsler, K. J., Kosciuk, M. C., Venkataraman, V., . . . Nagele, R. G. (2007). Abeta peptides can enter the brain through a defective blood-brain barrier and bind selectively to neurons. *Brain Research*, *1142*, 223–236. doi:10.1016/j.brainres.2007.01.070

Colas, R. A., Shinohara, M., Dalli, J., Chiang, N., & Serhan, C. N. (2014). Identification and signature profiles for pro-resolving and inflammatory lipid mediators in human tissue. *American Journal of Physiology–Cell Physiology*, *307*(1), C39–C54. doi:10.1152/ajpcell.00024.2014

Colciaghi, F., Marcello, E., Borroni, B., Zimmermann, M., Caltagirone, C., Cattabeni, F., . . . Di Luca, M. (2004). Platelet APP, ADAM 10 and BACE alterations in the early stages of Alzheimer disease. *Neurology*, *62*(3), 498–501.

Counts, S. E., Ikonomovic, M. D., Mercado, N., Vega, I. E., & Mufson, E. J. (2017). Biomarkers for the Early Detection and Progression of Alzheimer's Disease. *Neurotherapeutics*, *14*(1), 35–53. doi:10.1007/s13311-016-0481-z

Counts, S. E., & Mufson, E. J. (2010). Putative CSF protein biomarker candidates for amnestic mild cognitive impairment. *Translational Neuroscience*, *1*(1), 2–8. doi:10.2478/v10134-010-0004-0

Cummings, J. L., Morstorf, T., & Zhong, K. (2014). Alzheimer's disease drug-development pipeline: Few candidates, frequent failures. *Alzheimer's Research & Therapy*, *6*(4), 37. doi:10.1186/alzrt269

D'Andrea, M. R., Nagele, R. G., Wang, H-Y., Peterson, P. A., Lee, D. H. (2001). Evidence that neurones accumulating amyloid can undergo lysis to form amyloid plaques in Alzheimer's disease. *Histopathology*, *38*, 120–134.

de Barry, J., Liégeois, C. M., & Janoshazi, A. (2010). Protein kinase C as a peripheral biomarker for Alzheimer's disease. *Experimental Gerontology*, *45*(1), 64–69. doi:10.1016/j.exger.2009.10.015

Decourt, B., Walker, A., Gonzales, A., Malek-Ahmadi, M., Liesback, C., Davis, K., . . . Sabbagh, M. (2013). Platelet BACE1 levels as a possible biomarker for Alzheimer's disease. *Molecular Neurodegeneration*, *8*(1), P14. doi:10.1186/1750-1326-8-s1-p14

DeMarshall, C. A., Han, M., Nagele, E. P., Sarkar, A., Acharya, N. K., Godsey, G., . . . Nagele, R. G. (2015). Potential utility of autoantibodies as blood-based biomarkers for early detection and diagnosis of Parkinson's disease. *Immunology Letters*, *168*(1), 80–88. doi:10.1016/j.imlet.2015.09.010

DeMarshall, C. A., Nagele, E. P., Sarkar, A., Acharya, N. K., Godsey, G., Goldwaser, E. L., . . . Nagele, R. G. (2016). Detection of Alzheimer's disease at mild cognitive impairment and disease progression using autoantibodies as blood-based biomarkers. *Alzheimer's & Dementia*, *3*, 51–62. doi:10.1016/j.dadm.2016.03.002

Denk, J., Boelmans, K., Siegismund, C., Lassner, D., Arlt, S., & Jahn, H. (2015). MicroRNA profiling of CSF reveals potential biomarkers to detect Alzheimer`s disease. *PLoS One*, *10*(5), e0126423. doi:10.1371/journal.pone.0126423

Di Domenico, F., Pupo, G., Giraldo, E., Badia, M. C., Monllor, P., Lloret, A., . . . Perluigi, M. (2016). Oxidative signature of cerebrospinal fluid from mild cognitive impairment and Alzheimer disease patients. *Free Radical Biology and Medicine*, *91*, 1–9. doi:10.1016/j.freeradbiomed.2015.12.004

Dickson, D. W. (1997). The pathogenesis of senile plaques. *Journal of Neuropathology & Experimental Neurology*, *56*(4), 321–339.

Dodel, R., Balakrishnan, K., Keyvani, K., Deuster, O., Neff, F., Andrei-Selmer, L. C., . . . Bacher, M. (2011). Naturally occurring autoantibodies against beta-amyloid: investigating their role in transgenic animal and in vitro models of Alzheimer's disease. *Journal of Neuroscience*, *31*(15), 5847–5854. doi:10.1523/jneurosci.4401-10.2011

Doecke, J. D., Laws, S. M., Faux, N. G., Wilson, W., Burnham, S. C., Lam, C. P., . . . Martins, R. N. (2012). Blood-based protein biomarkers for diagnosis of Alzheimer disease. *Archives of Neurology*, *69*(10), 1318–1325. doi:10.1001/archneurol.2012.1282

Evin, G., & Li, Q. X. (2012). Platelets and Alzheimer's disease: Potential of APP as a biomarker. *World Journal of Psychiatry*, *2*(6), 102–113. doi:10.5498/wjp.v2.i6.102

Fagan, A. M., Mintun, M. A., Mach, R. H., Lee, S. Y., Dence, C. S., Shah, A. R., . . . Holtzman, D. M. (2006). Inverse relation between in vivo amyloid imaging load and cerebrospinal fluid Abeta42 in humans. *Annals of Neurology*, *59*(3), 512–519. doi:10.1002/ana.20730

Fagan, A. M., Roe, C. M., Xiong, C., Mintun, M. A., Morris, J. C., & Holtzman, D. M. (2007). Cerebrospinal fluid tau/beta-amyloid(42) ratio as a prediction of cognitive decline in nondemented older adults. *Archives of Neurology*, *64*(3), 343–349. doi:10.1001/archneur.64.3.noc60123

Farias, G., Perez, P., Slachevsky, A., & Maccioni, R. B. (2012). Platelet tau pattern correlates with cognitive status in Alzheimer's disease. *Journal of Alzheimer's Disease*, *31*(1), 65–69. doi:10.3233/jad-2012-120304

Fiala, M., & Veerhuis, R. (2010). Biomarkers of inflammation and amyloid-β phagocytosis in patients at risk of Alzheimer disease. *Experimental Gerontology*, *45*(1), 57–63. doi:http://dx.doi.org/10.1016/j.exger.2009.08.003

Fiandaca, M. S., Kapogiannis, D., Mapstone, M., Boxer, A., Eitan, E., Schwartz, J. B., . . . Goetzl, E. J. (2015). Identification of preclinical Alzheimer's disease by a profile of pathogenic proteins in neurally derived blood exosomes: A case-control study. *Alzheimer's & Dementia*, *11*(6), 600–607.e601. doi:10.1016/j.jalz.2014.06.008

Forlenza, O. V., Radanovic, M., Talib, L. L., Aprahamian, I., Diniz, B. S., Zetterberg, H., & Gattaz, W. F. (2015). Cerebrospinal fluid biomarkers in Alzheimer's disease: Diagnostic accuracy and prediction of dementia. *Alzheimer's & Dementia*, *1*(4), 455–463. doi:http://dx.doi.org/10.1016/j.dadm.2015.09.003

Fourier, A., Portelius, E., Zetterberg, H., Blennow, K., Quadrio, I., & Perret-Liaudet, A. (2015). Pre-analytical and analytical factors influencing Alzheimer's disease cerebrospinal fluid biomarker variability. *Clinica Chimica Acta*, *449*, 9–15. doi:10.1016/j.cca.2015.05.024

Fuller, J. P., Stavenhagen, J. B., Christensen, S., Kartberg, F., Glennie, M. J., & Teeling, J. L. (2015). Comparing the efficacy and neuroinflammatory potential of three anti-abeta antibodies. *Acta Neuropathologica*, *130*(5), 699–711. doi:10.1007/s00401-015-1484-2

Galimberti, D., Venturelli, E., Fenoglio, C., Guidi, I., Villa, C., Bergamaschini, L., . . . Scarpini, E. (2008). Intrathecal levels of IL-6, IL-11 and LIF in Alzheimer's disease and frontotemporal lobar degeneration. *Journal of Neurology*, *255*(4), 539–544. doi:10.1007/s00415-008-0737-6

Gandy, S., & DeKosky, S. T. (2013). Toward the treatment and prevention of Alzheimer's disease: Rational strategies and recent progress. *Annual Review of Medicine*, *64*, 367–383. doi:10.1146/annurev-med-092611-084441

Ganguli, M., Blacker, D., Blazer, D. G., Grant, I., Jeste, D. V., Paulsen, J. S., . . . Sachdev, P. S. (2011). Classification of neurocognitive disorders in DSM-5: A work in progress. *American Journal of Geriatric Psychiatry*, *19*(3), 205–210.

Ginsberg, S. D., Alldred, M. J., Counts, S. E., Cataldo, A. M., Neve, R. L., Jiang, Y., . . . Che, S. (2010). Microarray analysis of hippocampal CA1 neurons implicates early endosomal dysfunction during Alzheimer's disease progression. *Biological Psychiatry, 68*(10), 885–893. doi:10.1016/j.biopsych.2010.05.030

Gisslen, M., Price, R. W., Andreasson, U., Norgren, N., Nilsson, S., Hagberg, L., . . . Zetterberg, H. (2016). Plasma concentration of the neurofilament light protein (NFL) is a biomarker of CNS injury in HIV infection: A cross-sectional study. *EBioMedicine, 3*, 135–140. doi:10.1016/j.ebiom.2015.11.036

Gold, L. S., Klein, G., Carr, L., Kessler, L., & Sullivan, S. D. (2012). The emergence of diagnostic imaging technologies in breast cancer: Discovery, regulatory approval, reimbursement, and adoption in clinical guidelines. *Cancer Imaging, 12*, 13–24. doi:10.1102/1470-7330.2012.0003

Gouras, G. K., Almeida, C. G., & Takahashi, R. H. (2005). Intraneuronal Abeta accumulation and origin of plaques in Alzheimer's disease. *Neurobiology of Aging, 26*(9), 1235–1244. doi:10.1016/j.neurobiolaging.2005.05.022

Gouras, G. K., Tsai, J., Naslund, J., Vincent, B., Edgar, M., Checler, F., . . . Relkin, N. R. (2000). Intraneuronal Abeta42 accumulation in human brain. *American Journal of Pathology, 156*(1), 15–20.

Graff-Radford, N. R., Crook, J. E., Lucas, J., Boeve, B. F., Knopman, D. S., Ivnik, R. J., . . . Younkin, S. G. (2007). Association of low plasma Abeta42/Abeta40 ratios with increased imminent risk for mild cognitive impairment and Alzheimer disease. *Archives of Neurology, 64*(3), 354–362. doi:10.1001/archneur.64.3.354

Gupta, V. B., Doecke, J. D., Hone, E., Pedrini, S., Laws, S. M., Thambisetty, M., . . . Martins, R. N. (2016). Plasma apolipoprotein J as a potential biomarker for Alzheimer's disease: Australian Imaging, Biomarkers and Lifestyle study of aging. *Alzheimer's & Dementia, 3*, 18–26. doi:10.1016/j.dadm.2015.12.001

Gustaw-Rothenberg, K. A., Siedlak, S. L., Bonda, D. J., Lerner, A., Tabaton, M., Perry, G., & Smith, M. A. (2010). Dissociated amyloid-β antibody levels as a serum biomarker for the progression of Alzheimer's disease: A population-based study. *Experimental Gerontology, 45*(1), 47–52. doi:10.1016/j.exger.2009.10.003

Hall, J. R., Wiechmann, A. R., Johnson, L. A., Edwards, M., Barber, R. C., Winter, A. S., . . . O'Bryant, S. E. (2013). Biomarkers of vascular risk, systemic inflammation, and microvascular pathology and neuropsychiatric symptoms in Alzheimer's disease. *Journal of Alzheimer's Disease, 35*(2), 363–371. doi:10.3233/JAD-122359

Hamos, J. E., DeGennaro, L. J., & Drachman, D. A. (1989). Synaptic loss in Alzheimer's disease and other dementias. *Neurology, 39*(3), 355–361.

Hampel, H., Blennow, K., Shaw, L. M., Hoessler, Y. C., Zetterberg, H., & Trojanowski, J. Q. (2010). Total and phosphorylated tau protein as biological markers of Alzheimer's disease. *Experimental Gerontology, 45*(1), 30–40. doi:10.1016/j.exger.2009.10.010

Hampel, H., Frank, R., Broich, K., Teipel, S. J., Katz, R. G., Hardy, J., . . . Blennow, K. (2010). Biomarkers for Alzheimer's disease: Academic, industry and regulatory perspectives. *Nature Reviews Drug Discovery, 9*(7), 560–574. doi:10.1038/nrd3115

Han, M., Nagele, E., DeMarshall, C., Acharya, N., & Nagele, R. (2012). Diagnosis of Parkinson's disease based on disease-specific autoantibody profiles in human sera. *PLoS One, 7*(2), e32383. doi:10.1371/journal.pone.0032383

Hansson, O., Zetterberg, H., Buchhave, P., Londos, E., Blennow, K., & Minthon, L. (2006). Association between CSF biomarkers and incipient Alzheimer's disease in patients with mild cognitive impairment: a follow-up study. *Lancet Neurology*, *5*(3), 228–234. doi:10.1016/s1474-4422(06)70355-6

Hendrix, J. A., Finger, B., Weiner, M. W., Frisoni, G. B., Iwatsubo, T., Rowe, C. C., . . . Carrillo, M. C. (2015). The Worldwide Alzheimer's Disease Neuroimaging Initiative: An update. *Alzheimer's & Dementia*, *11*(7), 850–859. doi:10.1016/j.jalz.2015.05.008

Henriksen, K., O'Bryant, S. E., Hampel, H., Trojanowski, J. Q., Montine, T. J., Jeromin, A., . . . Weiner, M. R.; Blood-Based Biomarker Interest Group. (2014). The future of blood-based biomarkers for Alzheimer's disease. *Alzheimer's & Dementia*, *10*(1), 115–131. doi:10.1016/j.jalz.2013.01.013

Hu, W. T., Holtzman, D. M., Fagan, A. M., Shaw, L. M., Perrin, R., Arnold, S. E., . . . Soares, H. (2012). Plasma multianalyte profiling in mild cognitive impairment and Alzheimer disease. *Neurology*, *79*(9), 897–905. doi:10.1212/WNL.0b013e318266fa70

Hu, Y. Y., He, S. S., Wang, X., Duan, Q. H., Grundke-Iqbal, I., Iqbal, K., & Wang, J. (2002). Levels of nonphosphorylated and phosphorylated tau in cerebrospinal fluid of Alzheimer's disease patients: An ultrasensitive bienzyme-substrate-recycle enzyme-linked immunosorbent assay. *American Journal of Pathology*, *160*(4), 1269–1278. doi:10.1016/s0002-9440(10)62554-0

Humpel, C. (2011). Identifying and validating biomarkers for Alzheimer's disease. *Trends Biotechnology*, *29*(1), 26–32. doi:10.1016/j.tibtech.2010.09.007

Ikonomovic, M. D., Klunk, W. E., Abrahamson, E. E., Mathis, C. A., Price, J. C., Tsopelas, N. D., . . . DeKosky, S. T. (2008). Post-mortem correlates of in vivo PiB-PET amyloid imaging in a typical case of Alzheimer's disease. *Brain*, *131*(Pt 6), 1630–1645. doi:10.1093/brain/awn016

Iqbal, K., Flory, M., Khatoon, S., Soininen, H., Pirttila, T., Lehtovirta, M., . . . Grundke-Iqbal, I. (2005). Subgroups of Alzheimer's disease based on cerebrospinal fluid molecular markers. *Annals of Neurology*, *58*(5), 748–757. doi:10.1002/ana.20639

Iqbal, K., & Grundke-Iqbal, I. (1997). Elevated levels of tau and ubiquitin in brain and cerebrospinal fluid in Alzheimer's disease. *International Psychogeriatrics*, *9*(Suppl 1), 289–296; discussion 317–221.

Irizarry, M. C. (2004). Biomarkers of Alzheimer disease in plasma. *NeuroRx*, *1*(2), 226–234. doi:10.1602/neurorx.1.2.226

Isla, A. G., Vazquez-Cuevas, F. G., & Pena-Ortega, F. (2016). Exercise prevents amyloid-beta-induced hippocampal network disruption by inhibiting GSK3beta activation. *Journal of Alzheimer's Disease*, *52*(1), 333–343. doi:10.3233/jad-150352

Jack, C. R., Jr., Bennett, D. A., Blennow, K., Carrillo, M. C., Feldman, H. H., Frisoni, G. B., . . . Dubois, B. (2016). A/T/N: An unbiased descriptive classification scheme for Alzheimer disease biomarkers. *Neurology*, *87*(5), 539–547. doi:10.1212/wnl.0000000000002923

Johnson, K. A., Sperling, R. A., Gidicsin, C. M., Carmasin, J. S., Maye, J. E., Coleman, R. E., . . . Skovronsky, D. M.; AV45-A11 Study Group. (2013). Florbetapir (F18-AV-45) PET to assess amyloid burden in Alzheimer's disease dementia, mild cognitive impairment, and normal aging. *Alzheimer's & Dementia*, *9*(5 Suppl), S72–83. doi:10.1016/j.jalz.2012.10.007

Johnston, J. A., Liu, W. W., Coulson, D. T., Todd, S., Murphy, S., Brennan, S., . . . Passmore, A. P. (2008). Platelet beta-secretase activity is increased in Alzheimer's disease. *Neurobiology of Aging*, *29*(5), 661–668. doi:10.1016/j.neurobiolaging.2006.11.003

Kohnken, R., Buerger, K., Zinkowski, R., Miller, C., Kerkman, D., DeBernardis, J., . . . Hampel, H. (2000). Detection of tau phosphorylated at threonine 231 in cerebrospinal fluid of Alzheimer's disease patients. *Neuroscience Letters*, *287*(3), 187–190.

Kontsekova, E., Zilka, N., Kovacech, B., Skrabana, R., & Novak, M. (2014). Identification of structural determinants on tau protein essential for its pathological function: Novel therapeutic target for tau immunotherapy in Alzheimer's disease. *Alzheimer's Research & Therapy*, *6*(4), 45. doi:10.1186/alzrt277

Kuo, Y. M., Kokjohn, T. A., Watson, M. D., Woods, A. S., Cotter, R. J., Sue, L. I., . . . Roher, A. E. (2000). Elevated abeta42 in skeletal muscle of Alzheimer disease patients suggests peripheral alterations of AbetaPP metabolism. *American Journal of Pathology*, *156*(3), 797–805.

Kvartsberg, H., Duits, F. H., Ingelsson, M., Andreasen, N., Ohrfelt, A., Andersson, K., . . . Blennow, K. (2015). Cerebrospinal fluid levels of the synaptic protein neurogranin correlates with cognitive decline in prodromal Alzheimer's disease. *Alzheimer's & Dementia*, *11*(10), 1180–1190. doi:10.1016/j.jalz.2014.10.009

Lewczuk, P., Mroczko, B., Fagan, A., & Kornhuber, J. (2015). Biomarkers of Alzheimer's disease and mild cognitive impairment: A current perspective. *Advances in Medical Sciences*, *60*(1), 76–82. doi:10.1016/j.advms.2014.11.002

Li, G., Peskind, E. R., Millard, S. P., Chi, P., Sokal, I., Yu, C. E., . . . Montine, T. J. (2009). Cerebrospinal fluid concentration of brain-derived neurotrophic factor and cognitive function in non-demented subjects. *PLoS One*, *4*(5), e5424. doi:10.1371/journal.pone.0005424

Li, Q., Gordon, M., Cao, C., Ugen, K. E., & Morgan, D. (2007). Improvement of a low pH antigen-antibody dissociation procedure for ELISA measurement of circulating anti-Abeta antibodies. *BMC Neuroscience*, *8*, 22. doi:10.1186/1471-2202-8-22

Lista, S., Faltraco, F., Prvulovic, D., & Hampel, H. (2013). Blood and plasma-based proteomic biomarker research in Alzheimer's disease. *Progress in Neurobiology*, *101-102*, 1–17. doi:10.1016/j.pneurobio.2012.06.007

Liu, C. G., Wang, J. L., Li, L., & Wang, P. C. (2014). MicroRNA-384 regulates both amyloid precursor protein and beta-secretase expression and is a potential biomarker for Alzheimer's disease. *International Journal of Molecular Medicine*, *34*(1), 160–166. doi:10.3892/ijmm.2014.1780

Llano, D. A., Li, J., Waring, J. F., Ellis, T., Devanarayan, V., Witte, D. G., & Lenz, R. A. (2012). Cerebrospinal fluid cytokine dynamics differ between Alzheimer disease patients and elderly controls. *Alzheimer Disease and Associated Disorders*, *26*(4), 322–328. doi:10.1097/WAD.0b013e31823b2728

Lucey, B. P., Gonzales, C., Das, U., Li, J., Siemers, E. R., Slemmon, J. R., . . . Waring, J. F. (2015). An integrated multi-study analysis of intra-subject variability in cerebrospinal fluid amyloid-beta concentrations collected by lumbar puncture and indwelling lumbar catheter. *Alzheimer's Research & Therapy*, *7*(1), 53. doi:10.1186/s13195-015-0136-z

Maddalena, A., Papassotiropoulos, A., Muller-Tillmanns, B., Jung, H. H., Hegi, T., Nitsch, R. M., & Hock, C. (2003). Biochemical diagnosis of Alzheimer disease by measuring the cerebrospinal fluid ratio of phosphorylated tau protein to beta-amyloid peptide42. *Archives of Neurology*, *60*(9), 1202–1206. doi:10.1001/archneur.60.9.1202

Mapstone, M., Cheema, A. K., Fiandaca, M. S., Zhong, X., Mhyre, T. R., MacArthur, L. H., . . . Federoff, H. J. (2014). Plasma phospholipids identify antecedent memory impairment in older adults. *Nature Medicine*, *20*(4), 415–418. doi:10.1038/nm.3466

Marksteiner, J., Pirchl, M., Ullrich, C., Oberbauer, H., Blasko, I., Lederer, W., . . . Humpel, C. (2008). Analysis of cerebrospinal fluid of Alzheimer patients. Biomarkers and toxic properties. *Pharmacology*, *82*(3), 214–220. doi:10.1159/000156487

Mattsson, N., Insel, P. S., Landau, S., Jagust, W., Donohue, M., Shaw, L. M., . . . Weiner, M.; Alzheimer's Disease Neuroimaging Initiative. (2014). Diagnostic accuracy of CSF Ab42 and florbetapir PET for Alzheimer's disease. *Annals of Clinical and Translational Neurology, 1*(8), 534–543. doi:10.1002/acn3.81

Mayeux, R., Honig, L. S., Tang, M. X., Manly, J., Stern, Y., Schupf, N., & Mehta, P. D. (2003). Plasma A[beta]40 and A[beta]42 and Alzheimer's disease: Relation to age, mortality, and risk. *Neurology, 61*(9), 1185–1190.

Mehta, P. D., Pirttila, T., Mehta, S. P., Sersen, E. A., Aisen, P. S., & Wisniewski, H. M. (2000). Plasma and cerebrospinal fluid levels of amyloid beta proteins 1-40 and 1-42 in Alzheimer disease. *Archives of Neurology, 57*(1), 100–105.

Montine, T. J., Beal, M. F., Cudkowicz, M. E., O'Donnell, H., Margolin, R. A., McFarland, L., . . . Morrow, J. D. (1999). Increased CSF F2-isoprostane concentration in probable AD. *Neurology, 52*(3), 562–565.

Mouton-Liger, F., Paquet, C., Dumurgier, J., Lapalus, P., Gray, F., Laplanche, J.-L., & Hugon, J. (2012). Increased cerebrospinal fluid levels of double-stranded RNA-dependant protein kinase in Alzheimer's disease. *Biological Psychiatry, 71*(9), 829–835. doi:10.1016/j.biopsych.2011.11.031

Mukaetova-Ladinska, E. B., Abdel-All, Z., Dodds, S., Andrade, J., Alves da Silva, J., Kalaria, R. N., & O'Brien, J. T. (2012). Platelet immunoglobulin and amyloid precursor protein as potential peripheral biomarkers for Alzheimer's disease: Findings from a pilot study. *Age & Ageing, 41*(3), 408–412. doi:10.1093/ageing/afr171

Mukaetova-Ladinska, E. B., Milne, J., Andras, A., Abdel-All, Z., Cerejeira, J., Greally, E., . . . Milton, I. (2008). Alpha- and gamma-synuclein proteins are present in cerebrospinal fluid and are increased in aged subjects with neurodegenerative and vascular changes. *Dementia and Geriatric Cognitive Disorders, 26*(1), 32–42. doi:10.1159/000141039

Müller, M., Jäkel, L., Bruinsma, I. B., Claassen, J. A., Kuiperij, H. B., & Verbeek, M. M. (2016). MicroRNA-29a is a candidate biomarker for alzheimer's disease in cell-free cerebrospinal fluid. *Molecular Neurobiology, 53*(5), 2894–2899. doi:10.1007/s12035-015-9156-8

Nakamura, A., Kaneko, N., Villemagne, V. L., Kato, T., Doecke, J., Dore, V., . . . Yanagisawa, K. (2018). High performance plasma amyloid-beta biomarkers for Alzheimer's disease. *Nature, 554*(7691), 249–254. doi:10.1038/nature25456

Nagele, E., Han, M., Acharya, N. K., DeMarshall, C., Kosciuk, M. C., & Nagele, R. G. (2013). Natural IgG autoantibodies are abundant and ubiquitous in human sera, and their number is influenced by age, gender, and disease. *PLoS One, 8*(4), e60726. doi:10.1371/journal.pone.0060726

Nagele, E., Han, M., Demarshall, C., Belinka, B., & Nagele, R. (2011). Diagnosis of Alzheimer's disease based on disease-specific autoantibody profiles in human sera. *PLoS One, 6*(8), e23112. doi:10.1371/journal.pone.0023112

Nagele, R. G., Clifford, P. M., Siu, G., Levin, E. C., Acharya, N. K., Han, M., . . . Levitas, A. (2011). Brain-reactive autoantibodies prevalent in human sera increase intraneuronal amyloid-beta(1-42) deposition. *Journal of Alzheimer's Disease, 25*(4), 605–622. doi:10.3233/JAD-2011-110098

Nagele, R. G., D'Andrea, M. R., Anderson, W. J., & Wang, H. Y. (2002). Intracellular accumulation of beta-amyloid(1-42) in neurons is facilitated by the alpha 7 nicotinic acetylcholine receptor in Alzheimer's disease. *Neuroscience, 110*(2), 199–211.

Needham, E., & Zandi, M. S. (2014). Recent advances in the neuroimmunology of cell-surface CNS autoantibody syndromes, Alzheimer's disease, traumatic brain injury and schizophrenia. *Journal of Neurology*, *261*(10), 2037–2042. doi:10.1007/s00415-014-7473-x

Neumann, K., Farias, G., Slachevsky, A., Perez, P., & Maccioni, R. B. (2011). Human platelets tau: A potential peripheral marker for Alzheimer's disease. *Journal of Alzheimer's Disease*, *25*(1), 103–109. doi:10.3233/jad-2011-101641

Niederst, E. D., Reyna, S. M., & Goldstein, L. S. (2015). Axonal amyloid precursor protein and its fragments undergo somatodendritic endocytosis and processing. *Molecular Biology of the Cell*, *26*(2), 205–217. doi:10.1091/mbc.E14-06-1049

Niewoehner, J., Bohrmann, B., Collin, L., Urich, E., Sade, H., Maier, P., . . . Freskgard, P. O. (2014). Increased brain penetration and potency of a therapeutic antibody using a monovalent molecular shuttle. *Neuron*, *81*(1), 49–60. doi:10.1016/j.neuron.2013.10.061

Nixon, R. A. (2007). Autophagy, amyloidogenesis and Alzheimer disease. *Journal of Cell Science*, *120*(Pt 23), 4081–4091. doi:10.1242/jcs.019265

Nixon, R. A. (2013). The role of autophagy in neurodegenerative disease. *Nature Medicine*, *19*(8), 983–997. doi:10.1038/nm.3232

O'Bryant, S. E. (2016). Introduction to special issue on Advances in blood-based biomarkers of Alzheimer's disease. *Alzheimer's & Dementia*, *3*, 110–112. doi:10.1016/j.dadm.2016.06.003

O'Bryant, S. E., Edwards, M., Johnson, L., Hall, J., Villarreal, A. E., Britton, G. B., . . . Graff-Radford, N. R. (2016). A blood screening test for Alzheimer's disease. *Alzheimer's & Dementia*, *3*, 83–90. doi:10.1016/j.dadm.2016.06.004

O'Bryant, S. E., Lista, S., Rissman, R. A., Edwards, M., Zhang, F., Hall, J., . . . Hampel, H. (2016). Comparing biological markers of Alzheimer's disease across blood fraction and platforms: Comparing apples to oranges. *Alzheimer's & Dementia*, *3*, 27–34. doi:10.1016/j.dadm.2015.12.003

O'Bryant, S. E., Mielke, M. M., Rissman, R. A., Lista, S., Vanderstichele, H., Zetterberg, H., . . . Hampel, H. (2017). Blood-based biomarkers in Alzheimer disease: Current state of the science and a novel collaborative paradigm for advancing from discovery to clinic. *Alzheimer's & Dementia*, *13*(1), 45–58. doi:10.1016/j.jalz.2016.09.014

O'Bryant, S. E., Xiao, G., Barber, R., Cullum, C. M., Weiner, M., Hall, J., . . . Diaz-Arrastia, R. (2014). Molecular neuropsychology: Creation of test-specific blood biomarker algorithms. *Dementia and Geriatric Cognitive Disorders*, *37*(1–2), 45–57.

O'Bryant, S. E., Xiao, G., Barber, R., Huebinger, R., Wilhelmsen, K., Edwards, M., . . . Diaz-Arrastia, R.; Texas Alzheimer's Research & Care Consortium; Alzheimer's Disease Neuroimaging Initiative. (2011). A blood-based screening tool for Alzheimer's disease that spans serum and plasma: Findings from TARC and ADNI. *PLoS One*, *6*(12), e28092. doi:10.1371/journal.pone.0028092

O'Bryant, S. E., Xiao, G., Barber, R., Reisch, J., Hall, J., Cullum, C. M., . . . Care, C. (2011). A blood-based algorithm for the detection of Alzheimer's disease. *Dementia and Geriatric Cognitive Disorders*, *32*(1), 55–62. doi:10.1159/000330750

Olsson, B., Lautner, R., Andreasson, U., Ohrfelt, A., Portelius, E., Bjerke, M., . . . Zetterberg, H. (2016). CSF and blood biomarkers for the diagnosis of Alzheimer's disease: A systematic review and meta-analysis. *Lancet Neurology*, *15*(7), 673–684. doi:10.1016/s1474-4422(16)00070-3

Panza, F., Frisardi, V., Solfrizzi, V., Imbimbo, B. P., Logroscino, G., Santamato, A., . . . Pilotto, A. (2012). Immunotherapy for Alzheimer's disease: From anti-beta-amyloid to tau-based immunization strategies. *Immunotherapy*, *4*(2), 213–238. doi:10.2217/imt.11.170

Parnetti, L., Lanari, A., Silvestrelli, G., Saggese, E., & Reboldi, P. (2006). Diagnosing prodromal Alzheimer's disease: Role of CSF biochemical markers. *Mechanisms of Ageing and Development, 127*(2), 129–132. doi:10.1016/j.mad.2005.09.022

Perrin, R. J., Craig-Schapiro, R., Malone, J. P., Shah, A. R., Gilmore, P., Davis, A. E., . . . Fagan, A. M. (2011). Identification and validation of novel cerebrospinal fluid biomarkers for staging early Alzheimer's disease. *PLoS One, 6*(1), e16032. doi:10.1371/journal.pone.0016032

Peskind, E. R., Griffin, W. S., Akama, K. T., Raskind, M. A., & Van Eldik, L. J. (2001). Cerebrospinal fluid S100B is elevated in the earlier stages of Alzheimer's disease. *Neurochemistry International, 39*(5–6), 409–413.

Petzold, A., Jenkins, R., Watt, H. C., Green, A. J., Thompson, E. J., Keir, G., . . . Rossor, M. N. (2003). Cerebrospinal fluid S100B correlates with brain atrophy in Alzheimer's disease. *Neuroscience Letters, 336*(3), 167–170.

Pomara, N., Willoughby, L. M., Sidtis, J. J., & Mehta, P. D. (2005). Selective reductions in plasma Abeta 1-42 in healthy elderly subjects during longitudinal follow-up: A preliminary report. *American Journal of Geriatric Psychiatry, 13*(10), 914–917. doi:10.1176/appi.ajgp.13.10.914

Popp, J., Bacher, M., Kolsch, H., Noelker, C., Deuster, O., Dodel, R., & Jessen, F. (2009). Macrophage migration inhibitory factor in mild cognitive impairment and Alzheimer's disease. *Journal of Psychiatric Research, 43*(8), 749–753. doi:10.1016/j.jpsychires.2008.10.006

Portelius, E., Zetterberg, H., Skillback, T., Tornqvist, U., Andreasson, U., Trojanowski, J. Q., . . . Blennow, K. (2015). Cerebrospinal fluid neurogranin: Relation to cognition and neurodegeneration in Alzheimer's disease. *Brain, 138*(Pt 11), 3373–3385. doi:10.1093/brain/awv267

Pratico, D., Clark, C. M., Liun, F., Rokach, J., Lee, V. Y., & Trojanowski, J. Q. (2002). Increase of brain oxidative stress in mild cognitive impairment: A possible predictor of Alzheimer disease. *Archives of Neurology, 59*(6), 972–976.

Puchades, M., Hansson, S. F., Nilsson, C. L., Andreasen, N., Blennow, K., & Davidsson, P. (2003). Proteomic studies of potential cerebrospinal fluid protein markers for Alzheimer's disease. *Molecular Brain Research, 118*(1–2), 140–146.

Ray, S., Britschgi, M., Herbert, C., Takeda-Uchimura, Y., Boxer, A., Blennow, K., . . . Wyss-Coray, T. (2007). Classification and prediction of clinical Alzheimer's diagnosis based on plasma signaling proteins. *Nature Medicine, 13*(11), 1359–1362. doi:10.1038/nm1653

Reddy, M. M., & Kodadek, T. (2005). Protein "fingerprinting" in complex mixtures with peptoid microarrays. *Proceedings of the National Academy of Sciences of the United States of America, 102*(36), 12672–12677. doi:10.1073/pnas.0501208102

Reiber, H. (1994). Flow rate of cerebrospinal fluid (CSF): A concept common to normal blood-CSF barrier function and to dysfunction in neurological diseases. *Journal of Neurology Sci, 122*(2), 189–203.

Reiber, H. (2001). Dynamics of brain-derived proteins in cerebrospinal fluid. *Clinica Chimica Acta, 310*(2), 173–186.

Reitz, C., & Mayeux, R. (2014). Alzheimer disease: Epidemiology, diagnostic criteria, risk factors and biomarkers. *Biochemical Pharmacology, 88*(4), 640–651. doi:10.1016/j.bcp.2013.12.024

Restrepo, L., Stafford, P., Magee, D. M., & Johnston, S. A. (2011). Application of immunosignatures to the assessment of Alzheimer's disease. *Annals of Neurology, 70*(2), 286–295. doi:10.1002/ana.22405

Riemenschneider, M., Lautenschlager, N., Wagenpfeil, S., Diehl, J., Drzezga, A., & Kurz, A. (2002). Cerebrospinal fluid tau and beta-amyloid 42 proteins identify Alzheimer disease in subjects with mild cognitive impairment. *Archives of Neurology*, *59*(11), 1729–1734.

Roe, C. M., Fagan, A. M., Williams, M. M., Ghoshal, N., Aeschleman, M., Grant, E. A., . . . Morris, J. C. (2011). Improving CSF biomarker accuracy in predicting prevalent and incident Alzheimer disease. *Neurology*, *76*(6), 501–510. doi:10.1212/WNL.0b013e31820af900

Roher, A. E., Esh, C. L., Kokjohn, T. A., Castano, E. M., Van Vickle, G. D., Kalback, W. M., . . . Sabbagh, M. N. (2009). Amyloid beta peptides in human plasma and tissues and their significance for Alzheimer's disease. *Alzheimer's & Dementia*, *5*(1), 18–29. doi:10.1016/j.jalz.2008.10.004

Ronald and Nancy Reagan Research Institute of the Alzheimer's Association and the National Institute on Aging Working Group. (1998). Consensus report of the Working Group on "Molecular and Biochemical Markers of Alzheimer's Disease." *Neurobiology of Aging*, *19*(2), 109–116.

Sachdev, P. S., Blacker, D., Blazer, D. G., Ganguli, M., Jeste, D. V., Paulsen, J. S., & Petersen, R. C. (2014). Classifying neurocognitive disorders: The DSM-5 approach. *Nature Reviews Neurology*, *10*(11), 634–642. doi:10.1038/nrneurol.2014.181

Sala Frigerio, C., Lau, P., Salta, E., Tournoy, J., Bossers, K., Vandenberghe, R., . . . De Strooper, B. (2013). Reduced expression of hsa-miR-27a-3p in CSF of patients with Alzheimer disease. *Neurology*, *81*(24), 2103–2106. doi:10.1212/01.wnl.0000437306.37850.22

Salloway, S., Sperling, R., Gilman, S., Fox, N. C., Blennow, K., Raskind, M., . . . Grundman, M. (2009). A phase 2 multiple ascending dose trial of bapineuzumab in mild to moderate Alzheimer disease. *Neurology*, *73*(24), 2061–2070. doi:10.1212/WNL.0b013e3181c67808

Sauvee, M., DidierLaurent, G., Latarche, C., Escanye, M. C., Olivier, J. L., & Malaplate-Armand, C. (2014). Additional use of Abeta(4)(2)/Abeta(4)(0) ratio with cerebrospinal fluid biomarkers P-tau and Abeta(4)(2) increases the level of evidence of Alzheimer's disease pathophysiological process in routine practice. *Journal of Alzheimer's Disease*, *41*(2), 377–386. doi:10.3233/jad-131838

Schwab, C., & McGeer, P. L. (2008). Inflammatory aspects of Alzheimer disease and other neurodegenerative disorders. *Journal of Alzheimer's Disease*, *13*(4), 359–369.

Selkoe, D. J. (2002). Deciphering the genesis and fate of amyloid beta-protein yields novel therapies for Alzheimer disease. *Journal of Clinical Investigation*, *110*(10), 1375–1381. doi:10.1172/jci16783

Shams, S., Granberg, T., Martola, J., Li, X., Shams, M., Fereshtehnejad, S. M., . . . Wahlund, L. O. (2016). Cerebrospinal fluid profiles with increasing number of cerebral microbleeds in a continuum of cognitive impairment. *Journal of Cerebral Blood Flow & Metabolism*, *36*(3), 621–628. doi:10.1177/0271678X15606141

Shaw, L. M., Vanderstichele, H., Knapik-Czajka, M., Figurski, M., Coart, E., Blennow, K., . . . Trojanowski, J. Q. (2011). Qualification of the analytical and clinical performance of CSF biomarker analyses in ADNI. *Acta Neuropathologica*, *121*(5), 597–609. doi:10.1007/s00401-011-0808-0

Siemers, E. R., Sundell, K. L., Carlson, C., Case, M., Sethuraman, G., Liu-Seifert, H., . . . Demattos, R. (2016). Phase 3 solanezumab trials: Secondary outcomes in mild Alzheimer's disease patients. *Alzheimer's & Dementia*, *12*(2), 110–120. doi:10.1016/j.jalz.2015.06.1893

Skillback, T., Farahmand, B., Bartlett, J. W., Rosen, C., Mattsson, N., Nagga, K., . . . Zetterberg, H. (2014). CSF neurofilament light differs in neurodegenerative diseases and predicts severity and survival. *Neurology, 83*(21), 1945–1953. doi:10.1212/wnl.0000000000001015

Skillback, T., Zetterberg, H., Blennow, K., & Mattsson, N. (2013). Cerebrospinal fluid biomarkers for Alzheimer disease and subcortical axonal damage in 5,542 clinical samples. *Alzheimer's Research & Therapy, 5*(5), 47. doi:10.1186/alzrt212

Skillbäck, T., Delsing, L., Synnergren, J., Mattsson, N., Janelidze, S., Nägga, K., . . . Zetterberg, H. (2017). CSF/serum albumin ratio in dementias: A cross-sectional study on 1861 patients. *Neurobiology of Aging, 59*, 1–9.

Slaets, S., Vanmechelen, E., Le Bastard, N., Decraemer, H., Vandijck, M., Martin, J.-J., . . . Engelborghs, S. (2014). Increased CSF α-synuclein levels in Alzheimer's disease: Correlation with tau levels. *Alzheimer's & Dementia, 10*(5 Suppl), S290–S298. doi:10.1016/j.jalz.2013.10.004

Snyder, H. M., Carrillo, M. C., Grodstein, F., Henriksen, K., Jeromin, A., Lovestone, S., . . . Fillit, H. M. (2014). Developing novel blood-based biomarkers for Alzheimer's disease. *Alzheimer's & Dementia, 10*(1), 109–114. doi:10.1016/j.jalz.2013.10.007

Sørensen, S. S., Nygaard, A.-B., & Christensen, T. (2016). miRNA expression profiles in cerebrospinal fluid and blood of patients with Alzheimer's disease and other types of dementia – an exploratory study. *Translational Neurodegeneration, 5*(1), 6. doi:10.1186/s40035-016-0053-5

Sosa-Ortiz, A. L., Acosta-Castillo, I., & Prince, M. J. (2012). Epidemiology of dementias and Alzheimer's disease. *Archives of Medical Research, 43*(8), 600–608. doi:10.1016/j.arcmed.2012.11.003

Spigset, O., Wilhelmsson, C., Mjorndal, T., & Eriksson, S. (2000). Serotonin 5-HT2A receptor binding in platelets from patients with Alzheimer's disease or vascular dementia. *International Psychogeriatrics, 12*(4), 537–545.

Sunderland, T., Linker, G., Mirza, N., Putnam, K. T., Friedman, D. L., Kimmel, L. H., . . . Cohen, R. M. (2003). Decreased beta-amyloid1-42 and increased tau levels in cerebrospinal fluid of patients with Alzheimer disease. *JAMA, 289*(16), 2094–2103. doi:10.1001/jama.289.16.2094

Tang, K., Hynan, L. S., Baskin, F., & Rosenberg, R. N. (2006). Platelet amyloid precursor protein processing: A bio-marker for Alzheimer's disease. *Journal of Neurological Sciences, 240*(1–2), 53–58. doi:10.1016/j.jns.2005.09.002

Tarawneh, R., D'Angelo, G., Crimmins, D., Herries, E., Griest, T., Fagan, A. M., . . . Holtzman, D. M. (2016). Diagnostic and prognostic utility of the synaptic marker neurogranin in Alzheimer disease. *JAMA Neurology, 73*(5), 561–571. doi:10.1001/jamaneurol.2016.0086

Tiernan, C. T., Ginsberg, S. D., Guillozet-Bongaarts, A. L., Ward, S. M., He, B., Kanaan, N. M., . . . Counts, S. E. (2016). Protein homeostasis gene dysregulation in pretangle-bearing nucleus basalis neurons during the progression of Alzheimer's disease. *Neurobiology of Aging, 42*, 80–90. doi:10.1016/j.neurobiolaging.2016.02.031

Toledo, J. B., Da, X., Weiner, M. W., Wolk, D. A., Xie, S. X., Arnold, S. E., . . . Trojanowski, J. Q. (2014). CSF Apo-E levels associate with cognitive decline and MRI changes. *Acta Neuropathologica, 127*(5), 621–632. doi:10.1007/s00401-013-1236-0

Toledo, J. B., Korff, A., Shaw, L. M., Trojanowski, J. Q., & Zhang, J. (2013). CSF alpha-synuclein improves diagnostic and prognostic performance of CSF tau and Abeta in Alzheimer's disease. *Acta Neuropathologica*, *126*(5), 683–697. doi:10.1007/s00401-013-1148-z

Trushina, E., Dutta, T., Persson, X. M., Mielke, M. M., & Petersen, R. C. (2013). Identification of altered metabolic pathways in plasma and CSF in mild cognitive impairment and Alzheimer's disease using metabolomics. *PLoS One*, *8*(5), e63644. doi:10.1371/journal.pone.0063644

Tsuboi, Y., Kakimoto, K., Akatsu, H., Daikuhara, Y., & Yamada, T. (2002). Hepatocyte growth factor in cerebrospinal fluid in neurologic disease. *Acta Neurologica Scandinavica*, *106*(2), 99–103.

Tsuboi, Y., Kakimoto, K., Nakajima, M., Akatsu, H., Yamamoto, T., Ogawa, K., . . . Yamada, T. (2003). Increased hepatocyte growth factor level in cerebrospinal fluid in Alzheimer's disease. *Acta Neurologica Scandinavica*, *107*(2), 81–86.

Van Assche, L., Persoons, P., & Vandenbulcke, M. (2014). [Neurocognitive disorders in DSM-5: a critical review]. *Tijdschrift voor psychiatrie*, *56*(3), 211–216.

Van Giau, V., & An, S. S. A. (2016). Emergence of exosomal miRNAs as a diagnostic biomarker for Alzheimer's disease. *Journal of Neurological Sciences*, *360*, 141–152. doi:10.1016/j.jns.2015.12.005

Vandenberghe, R., Rinne, J. O., Boada, M., Katayama, S., Scheltens, P., Vellas, B., . . . Black, R. S. (2016). Bapineuzumab for mild to moderate Alzheimer's disease in two global, randomized, phase 3 trials. *Alzheimer's Research & Therapy*, *8*(1), 18. doi:10.1186/s13195-016-0189-7

Vanmechelen, E., Vanderstichele, H., Davidsson, P., Van Kerschaver, E., Van Der Perre, B., Sjogren, M., . . . Blennow, K. (2000). Quantification of tau phosphorylated at threonine 181 in human cerebrospinal fluid: A sandwich ELISA with a synthetic phosphopeptide for standardization. *Neuroscience Letters*, *285*(1), 49–52.

Verwey, N. A., van der Flier, W. M., Blennow, K., Clark, C., Sokolow, S., De Deyn, P. P., . . . Blankenstein, M. A. (2009). A worldwide multicentre comparison of assays for cerebrospinal fluid biomarkers in Alzheimer's disease. *Annals of Clinical Biochemistry*, *46*(Pt 3), 235–240. doi:10.1258/acb.2009.008232

Visser, P. J., Verhey, F., Knol, D. L., Scheltens, P., Wahlund, L.-O., Freund-Levi, Y., . . . Blennow, K. (2009). Prevalence and prognostic value of CSF markers of Alzheimer's disease pathology in patients with subjective cognitive impairment or mild cognitive impairment in the DESCRIPA study: A prospective cohort study. *Lancet Neurology*, *8*(7), 619–627. doi:10.1016/S1474-4422(09)70139-5

Weiner, M. W., Veitch, D. P., Aisen, P. S., Beckett, L. A., Cairns, N. J., Green, R. C., . . . Trojanowski, J. Q. (2016). The Alzheimer's Disease Neuroimaging Initiative 3: Continued innovation for clinical trial improvement. *Alzheimer's & Dementia*, *13*(5), 561–571. doi:10.1016/j.jalz.2016.10.006

Weinstein, G., Beiser, A. S., Preis, S. R., Courchesne, P., Chouraki, V., Levy, D., & Seshadri, S. (2016). Plasma clusterin levels and risk of dementia, Alzheimer's disease, and stroke. *Alzheimer's & Dementia*, *3*, 103–109. doi:10.1016/j.dadm.2016.06.005

Winston, C. N., Goetzl, E. J., Akers, J. C., Carter, B. S., Rockenstein, E. M., Galasko, D., . . . Rissman, R. A. (2016). Prediction of conversion from mild cognitive impairment to dementia with neuronally derived blood exosome protein profile. *Alzheimer's & Dementia*, *3*, 63–72. doi:10.1016/j.dadm.2016.04.001

Wurtman, R. (2015). Biomarkers in the diagnosis and management of Alzheimer's disease. *Metabolism*, *64*(3, Suppl 1), S47–S50. doi:10.1016/j.metabol.2014.10.034

Yang, S. T., Lee, J. D., Chang, T. C., Huang, C. H., Wang, J. J., Hsu, W. C., . . . Li, K. Y. (2013). Discrimination between Alzheimer's disease and mild cognitive impairment using SOM and PSO-SVM. *Computational and Mathematical Methods in Medicine, 2013*, 253670. doi:10.1155/2013/253670

Zetterberg, H., Blennow, K., & Hanse, E. (2010). Amyloid β and APP as biomarkers for Alzheimer's disease. *Experimental Gerontology*, *45*(1), 23–29. doi:10.1016/j.exger.2009.08.002

Zetterberg, H., Skillback, T., Mattsson, N., Trojanowski, J. Q., Portelius, E., Shaw, L. M., . . . Blennow, K. (2016). Association of cerebrospinal fluid neurofilament light concentration with Alzheimer disease progression. *JAMA Neurology*, *73*(1), 60–67. doi:10.1001/jamaneurol.2015.3037

Zetterberg, H., Wahlund, L.-O., & Blennow, K. (2003). Cerebrospinal fluid markers for prediction of Alzheimer's disease. *Neuroscience Letters*, *352*(1), 67–69. doi:10.1016/j.neulet.2003.08.011

Zetterberg, H., Wilson, D., Andreasson, U., Minthon, L., Blennow, K., Randall, J., & Hansson, O. (2013). Plasma tau levels in Alzheimer's disease. *Alzheimer's Research & Therapy*, *5*(2), 9. doi:10.1186/alzrt163

Zhang, J., Sokal, I., Peskind, E. R., Quinn, J. F., Jankovic, J., Kenney, C., . . . Montine, T. J. (2008). CSF multianalyte profile distinguishes Alzheimer and Parkinson diseases. *American Journal of Clinical Pathology*, *129*(4), 526–529. doi:10.1309/w01y0b808emeh12l

Zhao, X., Lejnine, S., Spond, J., Zhang, C., Ramaraj, T. C., Holder, D. J., . . . Laterza, O. F. (2015). A candidate plasma protein classifier to identify Alzheimer's disease. *Journal of Alzheimer's Disease*, *43*(2), 549–563. doi:10.3233/jad-141149

16

Unraveling the Role of Mitochondria in Alzheimer's Disease

Toward Assembling the Puzzle

Sónia C. Correia, Paula I. Moreira, and George Perry

1. Introduction

Since the first clinical case reported more than 100 years ago by Alois Alzheimer, it has been a long and winding road toward the development of effective disease-modifying and symptomatic therapeutics, in part, because the exact etiology underlying Alzheimer's disease (AD) remains puzzling. Currently recognized as the most prevalent age-related neurodegenerative disease, AD comprises approximately 60% to 70% of all dementia cases and affects more than 30 million people worldwide (Mielke, Vemuri, & Rocca, 2014; Querfurth & LaFerla 2010). Perhaps most alarming, AD has emerged as one of the major global epidemics of the 21st century being projected that AD prevalence will triple by 2050 (Prince et al., 2013). Within this scenario, there is an urgent need to unveil and join the initial pathological "pieces" involved in the AD puzzle o develop novel strategies aimed to prevent and/or tackle this devastating neurodegenerative disease in a timely manner.

Existing in both familial and sporadic forms, the clinical symptoms of AD can sometime revolve around impairment in episodic memory As the illness progresses, other cognitive deficits emerge culminating in the premature loss of mental and physical capacities (Correia, Santos, Cardoso et al., 2012; Querfurth & LaFerla 2010). The pathological signature is defined by the presence of two distinctive brain lesions—extracellular deposition of amyloid-β (Aβ) peptide in senile plaques and intracellular accumulation of neurofibrillary tangles containing hyperphosphorylated tau protein—accompanied by synaptic and neuronal loss, the early pathology occurring selectively in the entorhinal cortex and hippocampus (Braak & Braak, 1995; Price, Davis, Morris, & White, 1991). Importantly, the cognitive and behavioral symptoms constitute only the "tip of the iceberg" of AD pathology since the disruption of brain structure and

Sónia C. Correia, Paula I. Moreira, and George Perry, *Unraveling the Role of Mitochondria in Alzheimer's Disease* In: *Vascular Disease, Alzheimer's Disease, and Mild Cognitive Impairment.* Edited by: David J. Libon, Melissa Lamar, Rodney A. Swenson, Kenneth M. Heilman, Oxford University Press (2020).
DOI: 10.1093/oso/9780190634230.003.0017

function and consequent neuronal loss precede the clinical signs of the disease by 20 to 30 years (Braak & Braak, 1995).

Over the time, considerable progress in basic and clinical research has been made to identify the molecular entities that are the roots of the cognitive decline in AD. The detection of Aβ in the senile plaques in combination with genetic studies in familial cases of AD identifying mutations in the Aβ precursor protein (AβPP) and presenilin-1 and -2 genes resulted in the formulation of the amyloid cascade hypothesis (Hardy & Higgins, 1992; Prince et al., 2013). According to this prevailing hypothesis, the abnormal deposition of Aβ is the primary root cause of the degenerative events that occurs in the AD brain (Hardy & Higgins, 1992; Prince et al., 2013). However, following successive failures of Aβ-targeted therapeutics in clinical trials and the gap of this hypothesis to explain the sporadic form of this neurodegenerative disease, the search for alternative AD triggers and drivers brought mitochondrial abnormalities into the mainstream scientific limelight (Drachman, 2014; Karran & De Strooper, 2016; Swerdlow et al., 2017). Indeed, it is now widely recognized that faulty brain glucose metabolism and disrupted mitochondrial function and morphology are consistent antecedents in AD pathology (Atlante, de Bari, Bobba, & Amadoro, 2017; Cardoso, Carvalho, Correia, Seiça, & Moreira, 2016; Correia, Santos, Carvalho et al., 2012). In this sense, in 2004 Swerdlow and Khan (Swerdlow & Khan, 2004; Swerdlow, Burns, & Khan, 2014) proposed the *mitochondrial cascade hypothesis*, which states that age-related mitochondrial alterations, influenced by both hereditary and environmental factors, are the primary events underlying the emergence of AD neuropathology and symptoms.

Given the physiological relevance of mitochondria in the maintenance of neuronal homeostasis, the present chapter is aimed to summarize the current views on how mitochondrial abnormalities integrate the AD puzzle and their close association with the occurrence of AD, including, Aβ deposition, and tau hyperphosphorylation. The incontestable value of mitochondrial medicine will be also summarized in this chapter as a promising approach to re-establish mitochondrial "health" and counteract the AD-related pathological phenotype.

2. Mitochondrial Role in Neuronal Populations: What Is Behind the "Power Stations"?

To comprehend the intricate involvement of mitochondria in the context of AD pathology, it is important, first, to address why these fascinating organelles are so vital for neuronal physiology and integrity. Characterized by a complex morphology, long lifespan, reduced glycolytic capacity, and energetic requirements that fluctuate in time and space, neurons critically rely on a functional, properly organized, and dynamic mitochondrial network have been recognized (Barnhart, 2016; Harris, Jolivet, & Attwell, 2012; Kann & Kovacs, 2007; Z. H. Sheng & Cai, 2012; ZH Sheng, 2014). To maintain a healthy mitochondrial pool and fulfill neuronal energetic demands, mitochondrial network is continuously reshaped and renewed through the befitting interplay among mitochondrial biogenesis, fusion–fission, transport, and degradation by autophagy (mitophagy; Seo et al., 2010). Mitochondrial biogenesis and mitophagy represent two opposing but coordinated processes that determine mitochondrial quantity and quality (Palikaras, Lionaki, & Tavernarakis, 2015). Briefly, mitochondrial biogenesis is a dynamic process where mitochondria are generated de novo through the growth and division of pre-existing organelles in the soma. Thereafter, "new" and functional mitochondria are transported along the microtubule tracks in the anterograde direction to distant and metabolically demanding structures such as synapses, where these organelles function as "power stations" providing ATP and meticulously regulate Ca^{2+} homeostasis and thus sustaining synaptic transmission, plasticity, and vesicle recycling (Barnhart, 2016; Correia et al., 2016). Of note, the generation of reactive oxygen species (ROS) is a by-product of oxidative metabolism in the course of ATP production (Finkel & Holbrook, 2000). Being considered a double-edged sword for neurons, ROS at low to moderate levels act as signaling molecules playing a vital role in normal neuronal functioning, while supraphysiological ROS levels may directly "attack" mitochondrial components triggering mitochondrial and, subsequently, neuronal oxidative damage (Angelova & Abramov, 2018; Kim, Kim, Rhie, & Yoon, 2015). Once irreversible damaged, mitochondria are transported in the retrograde direction toward the soma to fuse with locally resident lysosomes and degraded by mitophagy (Correia et al., 2016; Lin & Sheng, 2015; Z. H. Sheng, 2014; Z. H. Sheng & Cai, 2012). In this sense and having in mind the postmitotic nature and limited regenerative capacity of neurons, mitophagy constitutes an important mitochondrial quality control mechanism that allows the removal of "old" mitochondria and restrict the deleterious accumulation of oxidative damage (Cummins & Götz, 2017; Misgeld & Schwarz, 2017; Rodolfo, Campello, & Cecconi, 2017). Notably, mitochondrial bioenergetics and dynamics are also influenced by fusion and fission events. Mitochondrial fusion may act as a self-repair mechanism that allows the exchange of contents between healthy and damaged mitochondria, rescuing the functional properties of these organelles. On the flipside, mitochondrial fission facilitates the bidirectional transport of mitochondria and is also an essential prerequisite for mitophagy initiation (Z. H. Sheng & Cai, 2012; Westermann, 2010).

Taking into account the previous discussion, it is irrefutable that the strict regulation of mitochondrial morphology, function, positioning, and turnover represents an immutable control node for the maintenance of a healthy mitochondrial pool in neurons. Therefore, even subtle disturbances in mitochondrial homeostasis are expected to have functional consequences to neuronal functioning and integrity and were proposed to participate in the neurodegenerative processes that occur in AD pathology.

3. Mitochondrial Bioenergetics and Oxidative Stress in Alzheimer's Disease

As previously outlined, AD is characterized by a long latent period before the discernible clinical onset of the disease where the signs of faulty brain glucose metabolism and reduced mitochondrial bioenergetic capacity and redox status are noticeable (Wang et al., 2014). As a matter of fact, positron-emission tomography (PET) imaging revealed that a reduction in brain glucose transport and utilization in the hippocampal and entorhinal cortical regions precede the clinical diagnosis of AD by decades (Friedland et al., 1989; Jagust et al., 1991) and predict the cognitive decline in normal aging (Calsolaro & Edison, 2016) or the progression of subjects from mild cognitive impairment (MCI) to AD with high accuracy (Chetelat et al., 2003). Importantly, this reduction in brain glucose metabolism was found to be accompanied by a decrease in both glucose transporter-1 and -3 levels, which leads to an aggravation of the AD-related pathological phenotype (Shah, Desilva, & Abbruscato, 2012). In terms of metabolism, two essential glucose metabolic pathways within mitochondria have been extensively described to be distressed in AD, the Krebs cycle, and oxidative phosphorylation. In support of a mitocentric chronological sequence of events in AD, compelling evidence demonstrates that this altered mitochondrial metabolism precedes the occurrence of both Aβ and tau pathologies (Chou et al., 2011; Correia et al., 2013; Nunomura et al., 2001; Resende et al., 2008; Yao et al., 2009). Noteworthy, an impairment in the activity of three key enzymes of the Krebs cycle—pyruvate, isocitrate, and α-ketoglutarate dehydrogenases—was shown to be correlated with the clinical state of AD, pinpointing for a causal relation between the progressive deterioration of mitochondrial functioning with the severity of the disease (Bubber, Haroutunian, Fisch, Blass, & Gibson, 2005; Mastrogiacomo, Bergeron, & Kish, 1993). However, the most well-documented and characterized defect in mitochondrial metabolism in AD is the reduction in cytochrome *c* oxidase (COX) activity. First described in the platelets of AD subjects, impaired COX activity was subsequently confirmed in lymphocytes and postmortem brain tissue from AD subjects (Bosetti et al., 2002; Kish et al., 1992; Parker, Filley, & Parks, 1990; Valla et al., 2006). To explain the origin of

COX loss of activity in AD, a role as been attributed to oxidative modifications (Tretter & Adam-Vizi 2000). Indeed, mitochondrial proteins and, in particular, COX are oxidatively modified during the pathological course of AD as evidenced by elevated levels of protein carbonyl and nitration of tyrosine residues (Sultana & Butterfield, 2013). In turn, impaired COX activity also potentiates the generation of mitochondrial-derived ROS, corroborating the idea that mitochondrial bioenergetic deficits mitochondrial bioenergetics and oxidative stress are coupled in a vicious circle (Mutisya, Bowling, & Beal, 1994).

In a step further, one of the most captivating dilemma in the AD field is whether mitochondrial dysfunction could represent a downstream effect of Aβ and tau pathologies. Acting as a driving force underlying the familial forms of AD, Aβ was shown to directly target mitochondria, perturbing the normal functioning of these organelles. Indeed, clinical and experimental studies revealed Aβ monomers and oligomers progressively accumulate within mitochondria (Caspersen et al., 2005; Devi, Prabhu, Galati, Avadhani, & Anandatheerthavarada, 2006; Manczak et al., 2006). But how these amyloidogenic species reach mitochondria? An elegant study from Hansson and collaborators (2008) reported that Aβ is primarily imported into mitochondria via the translocase of the outer membrane (TOM) import machinery and then transported through the inner mitochondrial membrane by the translocase of the inner membrane (TIM). Once inside mitochondria, Aβ has the ability to binds to heme groups, which constitute critical redox centers of COX, and interact with the mitochondrial protein Aβ-binding alcohol dehydrogenase, leading to hampered COX activity, mitochondrial ROS overproduction, and ATP depletion (Atamna & Frey, 2004; Atamna, 2006). Additionally, Devi and collaborators (2006) also found that Aβ disturbs COX activity by blocking TOM40 and TIM23 from importing COX subunits into the mitochondria. Concerning tau pathology, it was found that the interaction of hyperphosphorylated tau with the voltage-dependent anion channel 1 (VDAC1) protein disrupts the balance of the opening and closure of mitochondrial pores, triggering mitochondrial dysfunction (Manczak & Reddy, 2012b). Proteomic and functional studies found that the expression and activity of mitochondrial complex I and COX are deregulated in the triple transgenic mouse model of AD (3×Tg-AD), the deregulation of complex I being remarkably tau-dependent and the deregulation of COX being Aβ-dependent (Rhein et al., 2009). In this way, disturbances in mitochondrial metabolism seem to result from a convergence of Aβ and tau on mitochondria, which act in a synergistic manner to accelerate the defects on mitochondrial respiratory chain, exacerbate oxidative stress, and consequently to promote neuronal demise (Rhein et al., 2009).

4. Mitochondrial Dynamics in Alzheimer's Disease

Scientific advances performed during the last decades in the AD field revealed that mitochondrial pathobiology is not only restricted to mitochondrial bioenergetic deficits and oxidative stress but also comprises perturbations in mitochondrial dynamics. This is not surprising taking into account that mitochondrial metabolism is tightly connected to mitochondrial dynamics, the membrane-bound complexes of the electron transport chain and ROS metabolism being influenced by mitochondrial network connectivity (Princz, Kounakis, & Tavernarakis, 2018). Using cutting-edge cell biology and microscopy techniques, scientific breakthroughs showed that AD neurons exhibit mitochondrial ultrastructural alterations, mislocalization, and reduced mass, possibly suggesting that the catastrophic combination of defective mitochondrial biogenesis, fusion–fission, transport, and turnover is another key piece of the AD puzzle (Cardoso et al., 2016; Correia, Santos, Cardoso et al., 2012; Gao et al., 2017). So, the next subsections are mainly devoted to revisit the role of defective mitochondrial dynamics on AD and how it could be influenced by Aβ and tau pathologies.

4.1. Mitochondrial Fusion–Fission in Alzheimer's Disease

Far from being solitary and statistic structures as portrayed in textbooks, mitochondria are in reality dynamic organelles that experience consecutive cycles of fusion and fission to rapidly adjust mitochondrial network morphology to moment-to-moment fluctuations in metabolic requirements (Bertholet et al., 2016; Chen & Chan, 2009; Misgeld & Schwarz, 2017). Thus, the overall morphological appearance of mitochondrial network is dictated by the action of two opposing processes—mitochondrial fusion and fission. The molecular machinery that governs mitochondrial fusion is composed by mitofusins (Mfn-1 and Mfn-2) and optic atrophy protein-1 (OPA-1). Succinctly, mitofusins promote the fusion of the outer membranes of two separated mitochondria, whereas OPA-1 participates in the lengthening and tethering of the inner mitochondrial membranes, which is crucial for the maintenance and remodeling of cristae structure (Burté, Carelli, Chinnery, & Yu-Wai-Man, 2015; Ni, Williams, & Ding, 2015). In this sense, mitochondrial fusion ensures the communication between mitochondria, the redistribution of the mitochondrial DNA (mtDNA) pool, and the maintenance/restoration of mitochondrial membrane potential. On the flipside, the core components of mitochondrial fission machinery are the dynamin-like protein 1 (DRP-1) and its outer mitochondrial membrane recruiters mitochondrial fission protein 1 (Fis1), mitochondrial fission factor (Mff), and mitochondrial dynamics proteins 49 and 51 kDa (MiD49 and MiD51, respectively; Burté et al., 2015; Ni et al., 2015). As previously mentioned, in face of a dysfunctional mitochondrial network (e.g., loss of mitochondrial membrane potential and ROS overproduction), mitochondrial fission allows the spatial isolation and priming of damaged mitochondria for removal by mitophagy (Z. H. Sheng & Cai, 2012; Westermann, 2010).

At this point and taking in consideration that mitochondrial network can be reconfigured according to the metabolic state of neurons, several questions arise: Is mitochondrial morphology altered in AD? Are mitochondrial fusion and fission events occurring in a balanced manner in this neurodegenerative disease? Are mitochondrial fusion and fission acting properly to maintain a healthy mitochondrial pool in AD? Using postmortem brain tissue from AD subjects, Hirai and collaborators (2001) provided the first clue that mitochondrial morphology suffers drastic alterations during the pathological course of the disease as denoted by smaller mitochondrial size and higher percentage of mitochondria with broken internal membrane cristae. Importantly, a subsequent morphometric study revealed that these ultrastructural mitochondrial alterations are particularly conspicuous in neurons exhibiting loss of dendritic spines and abbreviation of the dendritic arborization, establishing an early pathological link between mitochondrial abnormalities and synaptic dysfunction in AD (Baloyannis, 2006). Consistently, it was reported that AD cybrids also posses a marked alteration in mitochondrial netowork evidenced by the presence of fragmented, misshaped, and bleb-like mitochondria, which corroborates the idea this neurodegenerative disease is associated with a shift in mitochondrial fusion–fission balance toward fission (Gan et al., 2014). Surprisingly, an outstanding study performed in postmortem brain tissue from AD patients using three-dimensional electron microscopy (3D EM) reconstruction to visualize mitochondrial morphology also revealed the occurrence of a mitochondrial fission arrest phenotype that results in elongated interconnected organelles, denominated by "mitochondria-on-a-string" (MOAS; L. Zhang et al., 2016). Representing a transition state, MOAS phenotype was proposed to delay mitochondrial fission during AD progression as a compensatory adaption of mitochondria to cope with bioenergetic stress and to sustain neuronal survival (L. Zhang et al., 2016).

But, what are the molecular basis underlying altered mitochondrial morphology in AD? An exhaustive study from Wang and collaborators (2009) reported reduced levels of the mitochondrial fusion proteins OPA-1, Mnf-1, and Mnf-2 in postmortem hippocampal tissue from AD subjects. In the same line, it was found that AβPP overexpression in M17 neuroblastoma cells also promotes a significant decrease in OPA-1 protein levels (Wang et al., 2008). Additionally, the fragmentation of mitochondrial network in AD cybrids was shown to result from the combination of increased translocation of the mitochondrial fission DRP-1 to mitochondria and reduced Mnf-2 protein levels (Gan et al., 2014).

In a step further, increased levels of DRP-1 S-nitrosylation were observed in the AD brain (Cho et al., 2009). By modulating the GTPase activity of DRP-1, this posttranslation modification favors the occurrence of mitochondrial fission and hampers mitochondrial bioenergetics, contributing to synaptic damage and neuronal demise (Cho et al., 2009). Noteworthy, altered DRP-1 protein levels and activity has been attributed to the interaction of this mitochondrial shaping protein with Aβ and hyperphosphorylated tau, leading to excessive mitochondrial fragmentation and disruption of inter-mitochondrial connectivity (Manczak, Calkins, & Reddy, 2011; Manczak & Reddy, 2012a). Additionally, Pérez, Vergara-Pulgar, Jara, Cabezas-Opazo, and Quintanilla (2018) revealed recently that the presence of tau pathology, specially truncated form of tau, promotes mitochondrial fragmentation and sensitize mitochondria to Aβ-driven neurotoxicity by hampering mitochondrial fusion-fission cycles through the downregulation of OPA-1. In this sense, tau and Aβ seem to act in a synergistic way to modulate mitochondrial morphology in AD pathology.

4.2. Mitochondrial Turnover in Alzheimer's Disease

Considering that excessive mitochondrial fission acts as an "eat me" signal that tags dysfunctional mitochondria for removal by autophagy, the next questions that emerge are, Is mitophagy an efficient "cleaning-service" in AD? Are defective mitochondria being properly replenished in AD to maintain the mitochondrial pool in terms of quantity and quality? Previous studies reported a reduction in mitochondrial content in susceptible hippocampal neurons from AD subjects, providing an indication of a faulty mitochondrial turnover in this neurodegenerative disease (Baloyannis, 2006; Hirai et al., 2001). However, in face of this evidence, it is important to clarify if reduced mitochondrial content result from excessive mitophagy, impaired mitochondrial biogenesis, or both.

As previously mentioned, mitophagy, a type of cargo-specific autophagy, is an essential component of quality control and maintenance of a healthy mitochondrial population. Mechanistically, irreparable damaged mitochondrial are first primed for elimination through the accumulation of PTEN-induced putative kinase 1 (PINK1) that serves as a bioenergetic sensor that recruits the E3 ubiquitin ligase Parkin from the cytosol to the damaged mitochondria. In turn, Parkin ubiquitinates a myriad of substrates that resides in the outer mitochondrial membrane, which will function as a molecular code required for the recruitment of the machinery that drives the mitophagic process (Kane et al., 2014; McWilliams & Muqit, 2017; Wild & Dikic, 2010; Yamano, Matsuda, & Tanaka, 2016). The first sign that defective mitophagy may represent a crucial piece of the AD puzzle arises from a study reporting that the AD brain is characterized by the overcrowding of autophagosomes containing improperly digested autophagic substrates (e.g., mitochondria) in swollen neurites, being later proposed that compromised autophagy in AD resulted from the combination of defects in the transport of autophagosomes and lysosomal dysfunction (Correia, Resende, Moreira, & Pereira, 2015; Nixon et al., 2005; Nixon, 2007). Consistently, two elegant studies from Moreira, Siedlak et al. (2007a, 2007b) performed postmortem brain tissue from AD patients revealed that this neurodegenerative disease is characterized by an increased rate in mitochondrial degradation by autophagy as evidenced by the massive accumulation of mitochondrial components (i.e., COX and lipoic acid) within autophagosomes. But some questions still persist. Are some of the steps of the mitophagic process affected by AD pathology? Is mitophagy doing well its job? In 2014, Shaerzadeh, Motamedi, Minai-Tehrani, and Khodagholi (2014) proposed that during the early phases of AD disease the overinduction of mitophagy constitute a compensatory strategy of the neuronal populations to circumvent and deal with the preeminent energetic crisis. Indeed, these authors found that mitophagy markers reach a maximum level and then return to basal levels as apoptotic markers start to increase, in the hippocampus of Aβ-injected rats (Shaerzadeh et al., 2014). In the same line, under AD-linked pathophysiological conditions, enhanced mitophagy was attributed to increased translocation of cytosolic Parkin to depolarized mitochondria in the somatodendritic regions coupled with augmented retrograde transport of axonal mitochondria (Ye, Sun, Starovoytov, & Cai, 2015). However, as disease progresses the aberrant accumulation of undesirable and irreparable damaged mitochondria in AD-affected neurons result from the failure in the recruitment of the autophagic machinery to mitochondria (Ye et al., 2015). In a step further, two recent and challenging studies differentiated the mechanisms behind mitophagy failure in both sporadic and familial forms of AD (Martin-Maestro, Gargini, Perry, Avila, & García-Escudero, 2016; Martin-Maestro et al., 2017). Interestingly, the authors found that mitophagy failure in sporadic AD is related with a defective labeling of mitochondria to be degraded by mitophagy, whereas in familial AD mitochondria are correctly tagged for recycling, but a deficiency in the degradation step of the mitophagic process occurs (Martin-Maestro et al., 2016, 2017).

Closely associated to mitophagy is mitochondrial biogenesis, a process governed by the transcription factor peroxisome proliferator-activated receptor gamma (PPARγ) co-activator (PGC-1α) and that allows the replacement of mitochondrial pool. In 2009, Qin and collaborators (2009) reported for the first time a reduction in PGC-1α levels in postmortem brain tissue from AD patients, which indicates that mitochondrial biogenesis and the consequent refurbishment of mitochondrial pool is compromised in AD pathology. In the same line, a subsequent study reported a significant shift in the expression pattern of proteins involved in mitochondrial biogenesis in AD (B. Sheng et al., 2012). Using post-mortem hippocampal tissue from AD subjects and a cell line overexpressing AβPP, these authors observed a drastic reduction not only in PGC-1α levels but also in nuclear respiratory factors, mtDNA-to-nuclear DNA ratio and mitochondrial content (B. Sheng et al., 2012). Notably, the overexpression of PGC-1α in this in vitro model of AD boosted both mitochondrial biogenesis and mitochondrial function (B. Sheng et al., 2012), suggesting a role for compromised mitochondrial biogenesis in AD-related mitoenergetic failure.

4.3. Mitochondrial Transport in Alzheimer's Disease

In face of a unique and complex architecture composed by subcellular compartments with distinct metabolic requirements and a limited regenerative capacity, neurons critically rely on the vigorous transport of mitochondria to properly distribute these organelles in a nonuniform fashion according to the temporal and spatial energy demands and to eliminate the irreversible damaged mitochondria (Misgeld & Schwarz, 2017). Succinctly, microtubules serve as the main "rails" for the long-range transport of mitochondria. The motility pattern of mitochondria is characterized by bidirectional movements with frequent pauses, changes in direction, or persistent docking. Importantly, the precise regulation of mitochondrial trafficking and correct positioning of mitochondria within neurons is ensured by their coupling with motor and adaptor proteins and anchoring machinery. Mitochondrial movement is steered by two classes of motors proteins, kinesin and dynein, which use ATP hydrolysis to power the shuttling of these organelles in the anterograde and retrograde direction, respectively. Additionally, the adaptor complex Miro-Milton was shown to favor the anterograde movement of mitochondria by facilitating the tethering of these organelles to kinesin motors. Concerning the anchoring machinery, syntaphilin functions as a "static anchor" that immobilizes mitochondria, leading to the arrestment of mitochondria at specific locations with high energy demands (Lin & Sheng, 2015; Z. H. Sheng, 2014; Z. H. Sheng & Cai, 2012).

In the context of AD pathology, the observation that the early stages of the disease are characterized by defective transport of mitochondria leading to a massive accumulation of these organelles within large swellings along dystrophic and degenerating neuritis represented a one of the most groundbreaking finding in the field (Stokin et al., 2005). Afterward, several studies tried to dissect the basis underlying this mitochondrial "traffic jam" in AD by identifying the potential molecular "roadblocks" (Correia et al., 2016). Being a microtubule-associated protein that possesses as main function the assembly and stabilization of the microtubular network (Morris, Maeda, Vossel, & Mucke, 2011), tau is the most obvious molecular obstacle involved in defective mitochondrial transport in AD. A flurry of experimental studies revealed that tau overexpression and hyperphosphorylation hampers mitochondrial trafficking, leading to an inappropriate mitochondrial distribution and positioning that further potentiates axonal and synaptic pathology (Ebneth et al., 1998; Kopeikina et al., 2011; Rodriguez-Martin et al., 2013; Shahpasand et al., 2012). Using an animal model of the disease, Kopeikina and collaborators (2011) found that the distribution of mitochondria in neurites containing tau aggregates was disrupted in an age-dependent manner. In parallel, these data were corroborated in postmortem human brain tissue of AD patients being observed an association of tau accumulation with mitochondrial translocation deficits (Kopeikina et al., 2011). Notably, the observed mitochondrial mislocalization caused by tau overexpression is caused by the binding of tau to microtubules tracks, which slows down the anterograde transport (Ebneth et al., 1998). Abnormal phosphorylation of tau at AT8 sites (Ser199, Ser202, and Thr205) was also shown to obstruct mitochondrial movement in axons (Shahpasand et al., 2012). Of note, abnormal phosphorylation of tau at AT8 sites resulted in an expansion of the space between microtubules, suggesting that AT8 phosphorylation affects mitochondrial transport by controlling the intermicrotubule spacing (Shahpasand et al., 2012).

Besides tau, Aβ has also been pinpointed as a molecular obstacle to the normal mitochondrial trafficking in AD. Taking advantage of time-lapse microscopy, Wang, Perry, Smith, and Zhu (2010) reported that the oligomeric form of Aβ disturbs the axonal transport of mitochondria in cultured hippocampal neurons. In the same line, it was found that oligomeric Aβ reduces mitochondrial motility (the percentage of motile mitochondria over total mitochondria) in both anterograde and retrograde directions (Du et al., 2010). However, oligomeric Aβ induces a more severe effect on anterograde movement of mitochondria than on their retrograde movement (Calkins & Reddy, 2011; Calkins, Manczak, Mao, Shirendeb, & Reddy, 2011; Du et al., 2010). Likewise, studies performed in *Drosophila melanogaster* exhibiting Aβ pathology revealed that Aβ slows down the bidirectional transport of axonal mitochondria and, consequently, promotes mitochondrial mislocalization as denoted by reduced the number of mitochondria in axons and dendrites, mitochondrial accumulation in the soma, and the concomitant depletion of these organelles in presynaptic terminals (Iijima-Ando et al., 2009; Zhao et al., 2010). Interestingly, tau and Aβ were also found to act in synergistic and overlapping ways to hampers mitochondrial transport in AD. For instance, Quintanilla, Dolan, Jin, and Johnson (2012) found that the presence of truncated tau protein and Aβ decreases the anterograde transport of mitochondria resulting in an increase in the stationary mitochondrial population at the soma. Conversely, it was observed that the genetic ablation of tau protein prevents the inhibition of mitochondrial transport promoted by oligomeric Aβ, suggesting that Aβ affects mitochondrial trafficking in a tau-dependent manner (Vossel et al., 2010). Finally, and considering that ATP is the "fuel" used by the protein motors to shuttle mitochondria between the neuronal compartments, the mitochondrial bioenergetics deficits previously described also represent major obstacles for the normal mitochondrial movement in AD (Correia et al., 2016).

5. Are Mitochondria Feasible Therapeutic Targets to Postpone AD Symptomatology and Neuropathology?

To demystify the initial trigger(s) and develop new and effective strategies aimed to modify and/or reverse the pathological course of the disease represent the "holy grail" for AD therapy. Incited by the limited clinical benefits of current therapies and the successive failure of Aβ-directed therapies in late-stage clinical trials (Feldman et al., 2014; Karran, Mercken, & De Strooper, 2011), the scientific community has been attracted to mitochondria as potential therapeutic targets to counteract AD-related symptomatic and neuropathological. From a therapeutic perspective, this section is devoted to highlight more recent and promising advances in mitochondrial medicine applied in the context of AD pathology.

Antioxidants have emerged as the first form of mitochondrial medicine able to prevent and/or postpone AD pathology. Based on the premise that oxidative stress occurs early during the course of this neurodegenerative disease, the hypothesis was formulated that compounds able to scavenge free radicals and boost oxidative stress defense mechanisms may present therapeutic benefits in AD (Wojsiat, Zoltowska, Laskowska-Kaszub, & Wojda, 2018). In this sense, several natural antioxidants, such as vitamin E and C, α-lipoic acid, co-enzyme Q_{10} (CoQ_{10}) and melatonin have been employed in preclinical studies, as these compounds have consistently demonstrated that they are able to reduce oxidative stress, improve mitochondrial bioenergetics, avert Aβ pathology, and restore cognitive performance (Dumont et al., 2011; Li, Zou, Cao, & Yang, 2005; Matsubara et al., 2003; Moreira et al., 2005; Moreira, Harris et al., 2007; Rudnitskaya et al., 2015; Stefanova et al., 2015; Sung et al., 2004; Swerdlow 2009; Yang, Yang, Li, Wang, & Yang, 2008; Yang, Dai, Li, & Yang, 2010). However, despite these positive outcomes, none of these natural antioxidants showed efficacy in clinical trial. Why does this happens? First and foremost, the most important caveat resides in the conception of the experimental design of the clinical trials. In fact, most clinical trials enrolled subjects with moderate to severe AD (Persson, Popescu, & Cedazo-Minguez, 2014), these stages being associated with the abrupt loss of neuronal populations in selected brain regions and thus representing phases of the disease where a "point of no return" was already installed. Additionally, it is important to be conscious that mitochondrial-derived ROS are important signaling molecules and their neutralization could compromise some ROS-triggered survival pathways in neurons. Finally, another important aspect is related with ability of these natural antioxidants to cross the blood–brain barrier and reach mitochondria to neutralize free radical overproduction (Persson et al., 2014).

To circumvent this last caveat, during the last decades mitochondrial-targeted molecules have been developed with the purpose of enhancing the delivery and accumulation of antioxidants into mitochondria, the MitoQ and Szeto-Schiller (SS) peptides being the most promising to tackle AD pathology. For instance, McManus and collaborators (2011) demonstrated that MitoQ is effective in averting cognitive decline and delaying the early neuropathological phenotype (oxidative stress, Aβ deposition, astrogliosis, caspase activation, and loss of synaptic integrity) in the 3×Tg-AD mouse model. SS-31, the most effective and potent SS peptide, was also shown to restore mitochondrial trafficking and synaptic viability and decrease the number of damaged mitochondria in primary neurons from Tg2756 mice treated with $A\beta_{25\text{-}35}$ (Reddy et al., 2012). So far, there are no clinical data regarding the beneficial effects of these mitochondria-targeted antioxidants in AD pathology.

More recently, scientific advances in mitochondrial medicine also cast light in the potential of mitochondrial quality control mechanisms and dynamics as promising therapeutic targets to counteract AD. Within this scenario, the mitochondrial fission inhibitor mdivi-1 emerged a new candidate in AD therapy. Using AD cybrids, this inhibitor of DRP-1 GTPase activity was found to eradicate both structural and functional mitochondrial defects (Gan et al., 2014). Particularly, this study revealed that the pharmacological blockage of excessive mitochondrial fragmentation with mdivi-1 improves mitochondrial length and density, restores COX activity and ATP levels, and suppresses ROS overproduction (Gan et al., 2014). Similarly, another in vitro study reported that mdivi-1 is able to protect against Aβ-associated mitochondrial fragmentation and synaptic damage. (Reddy, Manczak, & Yin, 2017). More recently, an exciting study represented a new step in the direction for a better therapeutic approach in AD by combining the mitochondrial-targeted antioxidant SS-31 and the mdivi-1, as these compounds have demonstrated that they exert synergistic protective effects in Aβ-induced in vitro models of the disease (Reddy, Manczak, Yin, & Reddy, 2018). Alternatively, the modulation of mitochondrial biogenesis also seems to be a plausible strategy to "fight" AD. Briefly, W. Zhang and collaborators (2015) found that neural stem cell transplantation leads to an upregulation of mitochondrial biogenesis, thus generating a more functional and "stronger" mitochondrial pool able to rescue mitochondrial dysfunction and cognitive deficits in a transgenic mouse model of AD. Compelling preclinical studies also demonstrated that the induction of mitochondrial biogenesis with resveratrol via sirtuin 1 exerts protective effects against AD-related pathological phenotype. In vitro data revealed that resveratrol abrogates Aβ-induced reduced mitochondrial mass and abnormal expression of mitochondrial structural genes and preserves mitochondrial function (Manczak et al., 2010). Moreover, resveratrol was also shown to attenuate cognitive deficits, tau pathology, and oxidative stress in a rat model of sporadic AD induced by the intracerebroventricular administration of streptozotocin (Du et al., 2014; Sharma & Gupta, 2002). Importantly, a phase II clinical trial on mild to moderate AD subjects revealed that resveratrol is safe, is well-tolerated, and alters some AD biomarker trajectories (Turner et al., 2015).

Lastly, besides pharmacological approaches, mitochondrial medicine also includes lifestyle interventions. Day by day, the old saying "We are what we eat" reflects the importance of dietary nutrition interventions in age-related neurodegenerative disease, including AD. The Mediterranean diet and caloric restriction have been shown to have a positive impact in the course of AD pathology by modulating mitochondrial healthy homeostasis (Morris, Maeda, Vossel, & Mucke, 2015; Van Cauwenberghe et al., 2016). Specifically, caloric restriction, which is known to activate a PGC-1α-dependent metabolic reprogramming and improve mitochondrial bioenergetic efficiency, was found to ameliorate behavioral performance and attenuate both Aβ and tau pathologies in transgenic mouse models of the disease (Brownlow et al., 2014; J. Wang et al., 2005; Wu et al., 2008). Finally, epidemiological evidence repeatedly documents the positive effects of physical exercise in reducing cognitive decline in AD subjects (Archer 2011; Venturelli, Scarsini, & Schena, 2011; Winchester et al., 2013). There is no clear-cut relation between the positive effects of physical exercise in AD and mitochondria. However, based on studies demonstrating that physical exercise stimulates mitochondrial biogenesis, improves mitochondrial bioenergetics, and positively regulates mitochondrial fusion–fission and mitophagy in the brain cortex (Marques-Aleixo et al., 2015; Steiner et al., 2011), it is tempting to speculate that these fascinating organelles are playing a role.

Overall, in face of these promising effects of pharmacological and nonpharmacological strategies to re-establish mitochondrial homeostasis, it is very clear that more in-depth preclinical studies are needed to define new molecular routes and time points in mitochondrial medicine before the translation to human medicine.

6. Final Remarks

Over the last decades, considerable progress has been made to ascertain the initial pieces involved the AD puzzle. Despite the current open questions, it is incontestable that mitochondrial pathobiology is an early contributing factor for the neurodegenerative processes that occur during the pathological course of AD. Particularly, AD-related mitochondrial pathobiology is manifested by mitochondrial bioenergetics deficits, ultrastructural abnormalities, and mislocalization and faulty turnover, in part due to the co-existence of defects in the so-called mitocheckpoints—mitochondrial biogenesis, fusion–fission, transport, and mitophagy (Figure 16.1). Consequently, these abnormalities result in an inefficient delivery of functional mitochondria into the synaptic terminals with the concomitant "synaptic starvation," ultimately leading to neuronal degeneration and demise. Within this scenario and having in mind the crucial role of these organelles for neuronal physiology, great expectation has been posed in mitochondrial medicine as a promising strategy to restore mitochondrial "health"

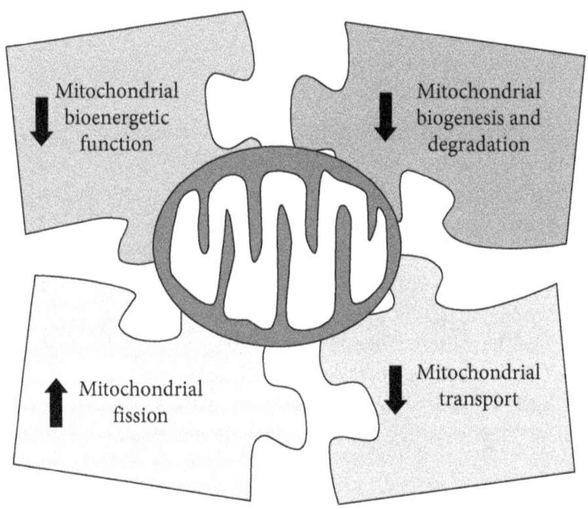

Figure 16.1. Mitochondrial pathobiology in Alzheimer's disease (AD). AD is characterized by an early decline in mitochondrial bioenergetic function as denoted by impaired cytochrome c oxidase (COX) activity even before the emergence of Aβ and tau pathologies. Hampered mitochondrial biogenesis and mitophagy are also two important pieces of this puzzle, contributing to defective mitochondrial turnover and reduced mitochondrial content in AD. Lastly, defects on mitochondrial trafficking and excessive mitochondrial fragmentation promotes mitochondrial mislocalization and ATP depletion in the presynaptic terminal, and ultimately synaptic and neuronal degeneration and loss.

and, thus, to tackle AD-related symptomatology and neuropathology in a timely manner. Despite the positive outcomes derived from preclinical studies, so far no efficacy of mitochondrial medicine was verified during clinical trials performed in AD subjects at moderate to severe stages of the disease. Under this perspective, we believe that the success of AD therapy may rely on future research aimed at describing and understanding in depth the temporal alterations in mitochondrial biology during the asymptomatic and prodromal stages of AD, where the hope resides, and the design of novel pharmacological interventions able to multitarget different aspects of these fascinating organelles, allowing a move away from the long-standing strategy of "one protein–one target–one drug."

Acknowledgments

Sónia C. Correia has a postdoctoral fellowship (SFRH/BPD/109822/2015 and SFRH/BPD/95770/2013, respectively) from the Fundação para a Ciência e a Tecnologia (FCT).

References

Angelova, P. R., & Abramov, A. Y. (2018). Role of mitochondrial ROS in the brain: from physiology to neurodegeneration. *FEBS Letters*, *92*(5), 692–702.

Archer, T. (2011). Physical exercise alleviates debilities of normal aging and Alzheimer's disease. *Acta Neurologica Scandinavica*, *123*(4), 221–238.

Atamna, H. (2006). Heme binding to Amyloid-beta peptide: Mechanistic role in Alzheimer's disease. *Journal of Alzheimer's Disease*, *10*(2–3), 255–266.

Atamna, H., & Frey, W. H., II. (2004). A role for heme in Alzheimer's disease: Heme binds amyloid beta and has altered metabolism. *Proceedings of the National Academy of Sciences of the United States of America*, *101*(30), 11153–1158.

Atlante, A., de Bari, L., Bobba, A., & Amadoro, G. (2017), A disease with a sweet tooth: Exploring the Warburg effect in Alzheimer's disease. *Biogerontology*, *18*(3), 301–319.

Baloyannis, S. J. (2006). Mitochondrial alterations in Alzheimer's disease. *Journal of Alzheimer's Disease*, *9*(2), 119–126.

Barnhart, E. L. (2016). Mechanics of mitochondrial motility in neurons. *Current Opinion in Cell Biology*, *38*, 90–9.

Bertholet, A. M., Delerue, T., Millet, A. M., Moulis, M. F., David, C., Daloyau, M., . . . Belenguer, P. (2016). Mitochondrial fusion/fission dynamics in neurodegeneration and neuronal plasticity. *Neurobiology of Disease*, *90*, 3–19.

Bosetti, F., Brizzi, F., Barogi, S., Mancuso, M., Siciliano, G., Tendi, E. A., . . . Solaini, G. (2002). Cytochrome c oxidase and mitochondrial F1F0-ATPase (ATP synthase) activities in platelets and brain from patients with Alzheimer's disease. *Neurobiology of Aging*, *23*(3), 371–376.

Braak, H., & Braak, E. (1995). Staging of Alzheimer's disease-related neurofibrillary changes. *Neurobiology of Aging, 16*(3), 271–278; discussion 78–84.

Brownlow, M. L., Joly-Amado, A., Azam, S., Elza, M., Selenica, M. L., Pappas, C., . . . Morgan, D. (2014). Partial rescue of memory deficits induced by calorie restriction in a mouse model of tau deposition. *Behavioural Brain Research, 271*, 79–88.

Bubber, P., Haroutunian, V., Fisch, G., Blass, J. P., & Gibson, G. E. (2005). Mitochondrial abnormalities in Alzheimer brain: Mechanistic implications. *Annals of Neurology, 57*(5), 695–703.

Burté, F., Carelli, V., Chinnery, P. F., & Yu-Wai-Man, P. (2015). Disturbed mitochondrial dynamics and neurodegenerative disorders. *Nature Reviews Neurology, 11*(1), 11–24.

Calkins, M. J., & Reddy, P. H. (2011). Amyloid beta impairs mitochondrial anterograde transport and degenerates synapses in Alzheimer's disease neurons. *Biochimica et Biophysica Acta, 1812*(4), 507–513.

Calkins, M. J., Manczak, M., Mao, P., Shirendeb, U., & Reddy, P. H. (2011). Impaired mitochondrial biogenesis, defective axonal transport of mitochondria, abnormal mitochondrial dynamics and synaptic degeneration in a mouse model of Alzheimer's disease. *Human Molecular Genetics, 20*(23), 4515–4529.

Calsolaro, V., & Edison, P. (2016). Alterations in glucose metabolism in Alzheimer's disease. *Recent Patents on Endocrine, Metabolic & Immune Drug Discovery, 10*(1), 31–39.

Cardoso, S., Carvalho, C., Correia, S. C., Seiça, R. M., & Moreira, P. I. (2016). Alzheimer's disease: From mitochondrial perturbations to mitochondrial medicine. *Brain Pathology, 26*(5), 632–647.

Caspersen, C., Wang, N., Yao, J., Sosunov, A., Chen, X., Lustbader, J.W., . . . Yan, S. D.(2005). Mitochondrial Abeta: A potential focal point for neuronal metabolic dysfunction in Alzheimer's disease. *FASEB Journal, 19*(14), 2040–2041.

Chen, H., & Chan, D. C. (2009). Mitochondrial dynamics—fusion, fission, movement, and mitophagy—in neurodegenerative diseases. *Human Molecular Genetics, 18*(R2), R169–R176.

Chetelat, G., Desgranges, B., de la Sayette, V., Viader, F., Eustache, F., & Baron, J.C. (2003). Mild cognitive impairment: Can FDG-PET predict who is to rapidly convert to Alzheimer's disease?. *Neurology, 60*(8), 1374–1377.

Cho, D. H., Nakamura, T., Fang, J., Cieplak, P., Godzik, A., Gu, Z., & Lipton, S. A. (2009). S-nitrosylation of Drp1 mediates beta-amyloid-related mitochondrial fission and neuronal injury. *Science, 324*(5923), 102–105.

Chou, J. L., Shenoy, D. V., Thomas, N., Choudhary, P. K., Laferla, F. M., Goodman, S. R., & Breen, G. A. (2011). Early dysregulation of the mitochondrial proteome in a mouse model of Alzheimer's disease. *Journal of Proteomics, 74*(4), 466–479.

Correia, S. C., Perry, G., & Moreira, P. I. (2016). Mitochondrial traffic jams in Alzheimer's disease - pinpointing the roadblocks. *Biochimica et Biophysica Acta, 1862*(10), 1909–1917.

Correia, S. C., Resende, R., Moreira, P. I., & Pereira, C. M. (2015). Alzheimer's disease-related misfolded proteins and dysfunctional organelles on autophagy menu. *DNA and Cell Biology, 34*(4), 261–273.

Correia, S. C., Santos, R. X., Carvalho, C., Cardoso, S., Candeias, E., Santos, M. S., . . . Moreira, P. I. (2012). Insulin signaling, glucose metabolism and mitochondria: Major players in Alzheimer's disease and diabetes interrelation. *Brain Research, 1441*, 64–78.

Correia, S. C., Santos, R. X., Santos, M. S., Casadesus, G., Lamanna, J. C., Perry, G., . . . Moreira, P. I. (2013). Mitochondrial abnormalities in a streptozotocin-induced rat model of sporadic Alzheimer's disease. *Current Alzheimer Research, 10*(4), 406–419.

Correia, S. C., Santos, R. X., Cardoso, S., Carvalho, C., Candeias, E., Duarte, A.I., . . . Moreira P. I. (2012). Alzheimer disease as a vascular disorder: Where do mitochondria fit? *Experimental Gerontology*, *47*(11), 878–886.

Cummins, N., & Götz, J. (2017). Shedding light on mitophagy in neurons: What is the evidence for PINK1/Parkin mitophagy in vivo? *Cellular and Molecular Life Sciences*, *75*(7), 115–1162

Devi, L., Prabhu, B. M., Galati, D. F., Avadhani, N. G., & Anandatheerthavarada, H. K. (2006). Accumulation of amyloid precursor protein in the mitochondrial import channels of human Alzheimer's disease brain is associated with mitochondrial dysfunction. *Journal of Neuroscience*, *26*(35), 9057–9068.

Drachman, D. A. (2014). The amyloid hypothesis, time to move on: Amyloid is the downstream result, not cause, of Alzheimer's disease. *Alzheimer's & Dementia*, *10*(3), 372–380.

Du, H., Guo, L., Yan, S., Sosunov, A. A., McKhann, G. M., & Yan, S. S. (2010). Early deficits in synaptic mitochondria in an Alzheimer's disease mouse model. *Proceedings of the National Academy of Sciences of the United States of America*, *107*(43), 18670–18675.

Du, L. L., Xie, J. Z., Cheng, X. S., Li, X. H., Kong, F. L., Jiang, X., . . . Zhou, X. W. (2014). Activation of sirtuin 1 attenuates cerebral ventricular streptozotocin-induced tau hyperphosphorylation and cognitive injuries in rat hippocampi. *Age (Dordr)*, *36*(2), 613–623.

Dumont, M., Kipiani, K., Yu, F., Wille, E., Katz, M., Calingasan, N. Y., . . . Beal M. F. (2011). Coenzyme Q10 decreases amyloid pathology and improves behavior in a transgenic mouse model of Alzheimer's disease. *Journal of Alzheimer's Disease*, *27*(1), 211–223.

Ebneth, A., Godemann, R., Stamer, K., Illenberger, S., Trinczek, B., & Mandelkow E. (1998). Overexpression of tau protein inhibits kinesin-dependent trafficking of vesicles, mitochondria, and endoplasmic reticulum: Implications for Alzheimer's disease. *Journal of Cell Biology*, *143*(3), 777–794.

Feldman, H. H., Godemann, R., Stamer, K., Illenberger, S., Trinczek, B., & Mandelkow, E. (2014). Alzheimer's disease research and development: A call for a new research roadmap. *Annals of the New York Academy of Sciences*, *1313*, 1–16.

Finkel, T., & Holbrook, N. J. (2000). Oxidants, oxidative stress and the biology of ageing. *Nature*, 408 (6809), 239–247.

Friedland, R. P., Jagust, W. J., Huesman, R. H., Koss, E., Knittel, B., Mathis, C. A., . . . Budinger T. F. (1989). Regional cerebral glucose transport and utilization in Alzheimer's disease. *Neurology*, *39*(11), 1427–1434.

Gan, X., Huang, S., Wu, L., Wang, Y., Hu, G., Li, G., . . . Yan, S. S. (2014). Inhibition of ERK-DLP1 signaling and mitochondrial division alleviates mitochondrial dysfunction in Alzheimer's disease cybrid cell. *Biochimica et Biophysica Acta*, *1842*(2), 220–231.

Gao, J., Wang, L., Liu, J., Xie, F., Su, B., & Wang, X. (2017). Abnormalities of Mitochondrial Dynamics in Neurodegenerative Diseases. *Antioxidants (Basel)*, *6*(2), E25.

Hansson Petersen, C. A., Alikhani, N., Behbahani, H., Wiehager, B., Pavlov, P. F., Alafuzoff, I., . . . Ankarcrona, M. (2008). The amyloid beta-peptide is imported into mitochondria via the TOM import machinery and localized to mitochondrial cristae. *Proceedings of the National Academy of Sciences of the United States of America*, *105*(35), 13145–13150.

Hardy, J. A., & Higgins, G. A. (1992). Alzheimer's disease: The amyloid cascade hypothesis. *Science*, *256*(5054), 184–185.

Harris, J. J., Jolivet, R., & Attwell, D. (2012). Synaptic energy use and supply. *Neuron*, *75*(5), 762–777.

Hirai, K., Aliev, G., Nunomura, A., Fujioka, H., Russell, R. L., Atwood, C. S., . . . Smith, M. A. (2001). Mitochondrial abnormalities in Alzheimer's disease. *Journal of Neuroscience, 21*(9), 3017–3023.

Iijima-Ando, K., Hearn, S. A., Shenton, C., Gatt, A., Zhao, L., & Iijima, K. (2009). Mitochondrial mislocalization underlies Abeta42-induced neuronal dysfunction in a Drosophila model of Alzheimer's disease. *PLoS One, 4*(12), e8310.

Jagust, W. J., Seab, J. P., Huesman, R. H., Valk, P. E., Mathis, C. A., Reed, B. R., . . . Budinger T. F. (1991). Diminished glucose transport in Alzheimer's disease: Dynamic PET studies. *Journal of Cerebral Blood Flow & Metabolism, 11*(2), 323–330.

Kane, L. A., Lazarou, M., Fogel, A. I., Li, Y., Yamano, K., Sarraf, S. A., . . . Youle, R. J. (2014). PINK1 phosphorylates ubiquitin to activate Parkin E3 ubiquitin ligase activity. *Journal of Cell Biology, 205*(2), 143–153.

Kann, O., & Kovacs, R. (2007). Mitochondria and neuronal activity. *Journal of Cerebral Blood Flow & Metabolism, 292*(2), C641–C657.

Karran, E., & De Strooper, B. (2016). The amyloid cascade hypothesis: Are we poised for success or failure? *Journal of Neurochemistry, 139*(Suppl 2), 237–252.

Karran, E., Mercken, M., & De Strooper, B. (2011). The amyloid cascade hypothesis for Alzheimer's disease: An appraisal for the development of therapeutics. *Nature Reviews Drug Discovery, 10*(9), 698–712.

Kim, G. H., Kim, J. E., Rhie, S. J., & Yoon, S. (2015). The Role of Oxidative Stress in Neurodegenerative Diseases. *Experimental Neurobiology, 24*(4), 325–340.

Kish, S. J., Bergeron, C., Rajput, A., Dozic, S., Mastrogiacomo, F., Chang, L. J., . . . Nobrega, J. N. (1992). Brain cytochrome oxidase in Alzheimer's disease. *Journal of Neurochemistry, 59*(2), 776–779.

Kopeikina, K. J., Carlson, G. A., Pitstick, R., Ludvigson, A .E., Peters, A., Luebke, J. I., . . . Spires-Jones, T. L. (2011). Tau accumulation causes mitochondrial distribution deficits in neurons in a mouse model of tauopathy and in human Alzheimer's disease brain. *American Journal of Pathology, 179*(4), 2071–2082.

Li, G., Zou, L. Y., Cao, C. M., & Yang, E. S. (2005). Coenzyme Q10 protects SHSY5Y neuronal cells from beta amyloid toxicity and oxygen-glucose deprivation by inhibiting the opening of the mitochondrial permeability transition pore. *Biofactors, 25*(1–4), 97–107.

Lin, M. Y., & Sheng, Z. H. (2015). Regulation of mitochondrial transport in neurons. *Experimental Cell Research, 334*(1), 35–44.

Manczak, M., & Reddy, P. H. (2012a). Abnormal interaction between the mitochondrial fission protein Drp1 and hyperphosphorylated tau in Alzheimer's disease neurons: Implications for mitochondrial dysfunction and neuronal damage. *Human Molecular Genetics, 21*(11), 2538–2547.

Manczak, M., & Reddy, P. H. (2012b). Abnormal interaction of VDAC1 with amyloid beta and phosphorylated tau causes mitochondrial dysfunction in Alzheimer's disease. *Human Molecular Genetics, 21*(23), 5131–5146.

Manczak, M., Calkins, M. J., & Reddy, P. H. (2011). Impaired mitochondrial dynamics and abnormal interaction of amyloid beta with mitochondrial protein Drp1 in neurons from patients with Alzheimer's disease: Implications for neuronal damage. *Human Molecular Genetics, 20*(13), 2495–2509.

Manczak, M., Anekonda, T. S., Henson, E., Park, B. S., Quinn, J., & Reddy, P. H. (2006). Mitochondria are a direct site of A beta accumulation in Alzheimer's disease neurons: Implications for free radical generation and oxidative damage in disease progression. *Human Molecular Genetics, 15*(9), 1437–1449.

Manczak, M., Mao, P., Calkins, M. J., Cornea, A., Reddy, A. P., Murphy, M. P., . . . Reddy, P. H. (2010). Mitochondria-targeted antioxidants protect against amyloid-beta toxicity in Alzheimer's disease neurons. *Journal of Alzheimer's Disease*, *20*(Suppl 2), S609–S631.

Marques-Aleixo, I., Santos-Alves, E., Balça, M. M., Rizo-Roca, D., Moreira, P. I., Oliveira, P. J., . . . Ascensão, A. (2015). Physical exercise improves brain cortex and cerebellum mitochondrial bioenergetics and alters apoptotic, dynamic and auto(mito)phagy markers. *Neuroscience*, *301*, 480–495.

Martin-Maestro, P., Gargini, R., Perry, G., Avila, J., & García-Escudero, V. (2016). PARK2 enhancement is able to compensate mitophagy alterations found in sporadic Alzheimer's disease. *Human Molecular Genetics*, *25*(4), 792–806.

Martin-Maestro, P., Gargini, R., A Sproul, A., García, E., Antón, L. C., Noggle, S., . . . García-Escudero, V. (2017). Mitophagy failure in fibroblasts and iPSC-derived neurons of Alzheimer's disease-associated presenilin 1 mutation. *Frontiers in Molecular Neuroscience*, *10*, 291.

Mastrogiacomo, F., Bergeron, C., & Kish, S. J. (1993), Brain alpha-ketoglutarate dehydrogenase complex activity in Alzheimer's disease. *Journal of Neurochemistry*, *61*(6), 2007–2014.

Matsubara, E., Bryant-Thomas, T., Pacheco Quinto, J., Henry, T. L., Poeggeler, B., Herbert, D., . . . Neria, E. (2003). Melatonin increases survival and inhibits oxidative and amyloid pathology in a transgenic model of Alzheimer's disease. *Journal of Neurochemistry*, *85*(5), 1101–1108.

McManus, M. J., Murphy, M. P., & Franklin, J. L. (2011). The mitochondria-targeted antioxidant MitoQ prevents loss of spatial memory retention and early neuropathology in a transgenic mouse model of Alzheimer's disease. *Journal of Neuroscience*, *31*(44), 15703–15715.

McWilliams, T. G., & Muqit, M. M. (2017)., PINK1 and Parkin: Emerging themes in mitochondrial homeostasis. *Current Opinion in Cell Biology*, *45*, 83–91.

Mielke, M. M., Vemuri, P., & Rocca, W. A. (2014). Clinical epidemiology of Alzheimer's disease: Assessing sex and gender differences. *Clinical Epidemiology*, *6*, 37–48.

Misgeld, T., & Schwarz, T. L. (2017). Mitostasis in neurons: Maintaining mitochondria in an extended cellular architecture. *Neuron*, *96*(3), 651–666.

Moreira, P. I., Santos, M. S., Sena, C., Nunes, E., Seiça, R., & Oliveira, C. R. (2005). CoQ10 therapy attenuates amyloid beta-peptide toxicity in brain mitochondria isolated from aged diabetic rats. *Experimental Neurology*, *196*(1), 112–119.

Moreira, P. I., Harris, P. L., Zhu, X., Santos, M. S., Oliveira, C. R., Smith, M. A., & Perry, G. (2007). Lipoic acid and N-acetyl cysteine decrease mitochondrial-related oxidative stress in Alzheimer disease patient fibroblasts. *Journal of Alzheimer's Disease*, *12*(2), 195–206.

Moreira, P. I., Siedlak, S. L., Wang, X., Santos, M. S., Oliveira, C. R., Tabaton, M., . . . Perry, G. (2007a). Autophagocytosis of mitochondria is prominent in Alzheimer disease. *Journal of Neuropathology & Experimental Neurology*, *66*(6), 525–532.

Moreira, P. I., Siedlak, S. L., Wang, X., Santos, M. S., Oliveira, C. R., Tabaton, M., . . . Perry, G. (2007b). Increased autophagic degradation of mitochondria in Alzheimer disease. *Autophagy*, *3*(6), 614–615.

Morris, M., Maeda, S., Vossel, K., & Mucke, L. (2011). The many faces of tau. *Neuron*, *70*(3), 410–426.

Morris, M. C., Maeda, S., Vossel, K., & Mucke, L. (2015). MIND diet associated with reduced incidence of Alzheimer's disease. *Alzheimer's & Dementia*, *11*(9), 1007–1014.

Mutisya, E. M., Bowling, A. C., & Beal, M. F. (1994). Cortical cytochrome oxidase activity is reduced in Alzheimer's disease. *Journal of Neurochemistry, 63*(6), 2179–2184.

Ni, H. M., Williams, J. A., & Ding, W. X. (2015). Mitochondrial dynamics and mitochondrial quality control. *Redox Biology, 4*, 6–13.

Nixon, R. A. (2007). Autophagy, amyloidogenesis and Alzheimer disease. *Journal of Cell Science, 120*(Pt 23), 4081–4091.

Nixon, R. A., Wegiel, J., Kumar, A., Yu, W. H., Peterhoff, C., Cataldo, A., & Cuervo, A. M. (2005). Extensive involvement of autophagy in Alzheimer disease: An immuno-electron microscopy study. *Journal of Neuropathology & Experimental Neurology, 64*(2), 113–122.

Nunomura, A., Perry, G., Aliev, G., Hirai, K., Takeda, A., Balraj, E. K., . . . Smith M. A. (2001). Oxidative damage is the earliest event in Alzheimer disease. *Journal of Neuropathology & Experimental Neurology, 60*(8), 759–767.

Palikaras, K., Lionaki, E., & Tavernarakis, N. (2015). Balancing mitochondrial biogenesis and mitophagy to maintain energy metabolism homeostasis. *Cell Death & Differentiation, 22*(9), 1399–1401.

Parker, W. D., Jr., Filley, C. M., & Parks, J. K. (1990). Cytochrome oxidase deficiency in Alzheimer's disease. *Neurology, 40*(8), 1302–1303.

Perez, M. J., Vergara-Pulgar, K., Jara, C., Cabezas-Opazo, F., & Quintanilla, R. A. (2018). Caspase-cleaved tau impairs mitochondrial dynamics in Alzheimer's disease. *Molecular Neurobiology, 55*(2), 1004–1018.

Persson, T., Popescu, B. O., & Cedazo-Minguez, A. (2014). Oxidative stress in Alzheimer's disease: Why did antioxidant therapy fail? *Oxidative Medicine and Cellular Longevity, 2014*, 427318.

Price, J. L., Davis, P. B., Morris, J. C., & White, D. L. (1991). The distribution of tangles, plaques and related immunohistochemical markers in healthy aging and Alzheimer's disease. *Neurobiology of Aging, 12*(4), 295–312.

Prince, M., Bryce, R., Albanese, E., Wimo, A., Ribeiro, W., & Ferri, C. P. (2013). The global prevalence of dementia: A systematic review and metaanalysis. *Alzheimer's & Dementia, 9*(1), 63–75 e2.

Princz, A., Kounakis, K., & Tavernarakis, N. (2018). Mitochondrial contributions to neuronal development and function. *Biological Chemistry, 399*(7), 723–739.

Qin, W., Haroutunian, V., Katsel, P., Cardozo, C. P., Ho, L., Buxbaum, J. D., & Pasinetti, G. M. (2009). PGC-1alpha expression decreases in the Alzheimer disease brain as a function of dementia. *Archives of Neurology, 66*(3), 352–361.

Querfurth, H. W., & LaFerla, F. M. (2010). Alzheimer's disease. *New England Journal of Medicine, 362*(4), 329–344.

Quintanilla, R. A., Dolan, P. J., Jin, Y. N., & Johnson, G. V. W. (2012). Truncated tau and Abeta cooperatively impair mitochondria in primary neurons. *Neurobiology of Aging, 33*(3), 619 e25–35.

Reddy, P. H., Manczak, M., & Yin, X. (2017). Mitochondria-Division Inhibitor 1 Protects Against Amyloid-beta induced Mitochondrial Fragmentation and Synaptic Damage in Alzheimer's Disease. *Journal of Alzheimer's Disease, 58*(1), 147–162.

Reddy, P. H., Manczak, M., Yin, X., & Reddy, A. P. (2018). Synergistic Protective Effects of Mitochondrial Division Inhibitor 1 and Mitochondria-Targeted Small Peptide SS31 in Alzheimer's Disease. *Journal of Alzheimer's Disease, 62*(4), 1549–1565.

Reddy, P. H., Tripathi, R., Troung, Q., Tirumala, K., Reddy, T. P., Anekonda, V., . . . Manczak, M. (2012). Abnormal mitochondrial dynamics and synaptic degeneration as early events in Alzheimer's disease: Implications to mitochondria-targeted antioxidant therapeutics. *Biochimica et Biophysica Acta, 1822*(5), 639–649.

Resende, R., Moreira, P. I., Proença, T., Deshpande, A., Busciglio, J., Pereira, C., & Oliveira C. R. (2008). Brain oxidative stress in a triple-transgenic mouse model of Alzheimer disease. *Free Radical Biology and Medicine, 44*(12), 2051–2057.

Rhein, V., Song, X., Wiesner, A., Ittner, L. M., Baysang, G., Meier, F., . . . Eckertm A. (2009). Amyloid-beta and tau synergistically impair the oxidative phosphorylation system in triple transgenic Alzheimer's disease mice. *Proceedings of the National Academy of Sciences of the United States of America, 106*(47), 20057–20062.

Rodolfo, C., Campello, S., & Cecconi, F. (2017). Mitophagy in neurodegenerative diseases. *Neurochemistry International, 117*, 156–166.

Rodriguez-Martin, T., Cuchillo-Ibáñez, I., Noble, W., Nyenya, F., Anderton, B. H., & Hanger, D. P. (2013). Tau phosphorylation affects its axonal transport and degradation. *Neurobiology of Aging, 34*(9), 2146–2157.

Rudnitskaya, E. A., Muraleva, N. A., Maksimova, K. Y., Kiseleva, E., Kolosova, N. G., & Stefanova, N.A. (2015). Melatonin Attenuates Memory Impairment, Amyloid-beta Accumulation, and Neurodegeneration in a Rat Model of Sporadic Alzheimer's Disease. *Journal of Alzheimer's Disease, 47*(1), 103–116.

Seo, A. Y., Joseph, A. M., Dutta, D., Hwang, J. C., Aris, J. P., & Leeuwenburgh, C. (2010). New insights into the role of mitochondria in aging: Mitochondrial dynamics and more. *Journal of Cell Science, 123*(Pt 15), 2533–2542.

Shaerzadeh, F., Motamedi, F., Minai-Tehrani, D., & Khodagholi, F. (2014). Monitoring of neuronal loss in the hippocampus of Abeta-injected rat: Autophagy, mitophagy, and mitochondrial biogenesis stand against apoptosis. *Neuromolecular Medicine, 16*(1), 175–190.

Shah, K., Desilva, S., & Abbruscato, T. (2012), The role of glucose transporters in brain disease: Diabetes and Alzheimer's disease. *International Journal of Molecular Sciences, 13*(10), 12629–12655.

Shahpasand, K., Uemura, I., Saito, T., Asano, T., Hata, K., Shibata, K., . . . Hisanaga. S. (2012). Regulation of mitochondrial transport and inter-microtubule spacing by tau phosphorylation at the sites hyperphosphorylated in Alzheimer's disease. *Journal of Neuroscience, 32*(7), 2430–2441.

Sharma, M., & Gupta, Y. K. (2002). Chronic treatment with trans resveratrol prevents intracerebroventricular streptozotocin induced cognitive impairment and oxidative stress in rats. *Life Sciences, 71*(21), 2489–2498.

Sheng, B., Wang, X., Su, B., Lee, H. G., Casadesus, G., Perry, G., & Zhu, X. (2012). Impaired mitochondrial biogenesis contributes to mitochondrial dysfunction in Alzheimer's disease. *Journal of Neurochemistry, 120*(3), 419–429.

Sheng, Z. H. (2014). Mitochondrial trafficking and anchoring in neurons: New insight and implications. *Journal of Cell Biology, 204*(7), 1087–1098.

Sheng, Z. H., & Cai, Q. (2012). Mitochondrial transport in neurons: Impact on synaptic homeostasis and neurodegeneration. *Nature Reviews Neuroscience, 13*(2), 77–93.

Stefanova, N. A., Maksimova, K. Y., Kiseleva, E., Rudnitskaya, E. A., Muraleva, N. A., & Kolosova, N. G. (2015). Melatonin attenuates impairments of structural hippocampal neuroplasticity in OXYS rats during active progression of Alzheimer's disease-like pathology. *Journal of Pineal Research, 59*(2), 163–177.

Steiner, J. L., Murphy, E. A., McClellan, J. L., Carmichael, M. D., & Davis, J. M. (2011). Exercise training increases mitochondrial biogenesis in the brain. *Journal of Applied* Physiology, *111*(4), 1066–1071.

Stokin, G. B., Lillo, C., Falzone, T. L., Brusch, R. G., Rockenstein, E., Mount, S. L. . . . Goldstein, L. S. (2005). Axonopathy and transport deficits early in the pathogenesis of Alzheimer's disease. *Science, 307*(5713), 1282–1288.

Sultana, R., & Butterfield, D. A. (2013). Oxidative modification of brain proteins in Alzheimer's disease: Perspective on future studies based on results of redox proteomics studies. *Journal of Alzheimer's Disease, 33*(Suppl 1), S243–S251.

Sung, S., Yao, Y., Uryu, K., Yang, H., Lee, V. M., Trojanowski, J. Q., & Praticò, D. (2004). Early vitamin E supplementation in young but not aged mice reduces Abeta levels and amyloid deposition in a transgenic model of Alzheimer's disease. *FASEB Journal, 18*(2), 323–325.

Swerdlow, R. H. (2009). Mitochondrial Medicine and the Neurodegenerative Mitochondriopathies. *Pharmaceuticals (Basel), 2*(3), 150–167.

Swerdlow, R. H., & Khan, S. M. (2004). A "mitochondrial cascade hypothesis" for sporadic Alzheimer's disease. *Medical Hypotheses, 63*(1), 8–20.

Swerdlow, R. H., Burns, J. M., & Khan, S. M. (2014). The Alzheimer's disease mitochondrial cascade hypothesis: Progress and perspectives. *Biochimica et Biophysica Acta, 1842*(8), 1219–1231.

Swerdlow, R. H., Koppel, S., Weidling, I., Hayley, C., Ji, Y., & Wilkins H. M. (2017). Mitochondria, cybrids, aging, and Alzheimer's disease. *Progress in Molecular Biology and Translational Science, 146*, 259–302.

Tretter, L., & Adam-Vizi, V. (2000). Inhibition of Krebs cycle enzymes by hydrogen peroxide: A key role of [alpha]-ketoglutarate dehydrogenase in limiting NADH production under oxidative stress. *Journal of Neuroscience, 20*(24), 8972–8979.

Turner, R. S., Thomas, R. G., Craft, S., van Dyck, C. H., Mintzer, J., Reynolds, B. A., . . . Aisen, P. S.; Alzheimer's Disease Cooperative Study. (2015). A randomized, double-blind, placebo-controlled trial of resveratrol for Alzheimer disease. *Neurology, 5*(16), 1383–1391.

Valla, J., Schneider, L., Niedzielko, T., Coon, K. D., Caselli, R., Sabbagh, M. N., . . . Reiman E. M. (2006). Impaired platelet mitochondrial activity in Alzheimer's disease and mild cognitive impairment. *Mitochondrion, 6*(6), 323–330.

Van Cauwenberghe, C., Schneider, L., Niedzielko, T., Coon, K. D., Caselli, R., Sabbagh, M. N., . . . Reiman, E. M. (2016). Caloric restriction: Beneficial effects on brain aging and Alzheimer's disease. *Mammalian Genome, 27*(7–8), 300–319.

Venturelli, M., Scarsini, R., & Schena, F. (2011). Six-month walking program changes cognitive and ADL performance in patients with Alzheimer. *American Journal of Alzheimer's Disease & Other Dementias, 26*(5), 381–388.

Vossel, K. A., Zhang, K., Brodbeck, J., Daub, A. C., Sharma, P., Finkbeiner, S., . . . Mucke L. (2010). Tau reduction prevents Abeta-induced defects in axonal transport. *Science, 330*(6001), 198.

Wang, J., Ho, L., Qin, W., Rocher, A. B., Seror, I., Humala, N., . . . Pasinetti, G. M. (2005). Caloric restriction attenuates beta-amyloid neuropathology in a mouse model of Alzheimer's disease. *FASEB Journal, 19*(6), 659–661.

Wang, X., Perry, G., Smith, M. A., & Zhu, X. (2010). Amyloid-beta-derived diffusible ligands cause impaired axonal transport of mitochondria in neurons. *Neurodegenerative Diseases, 7*(1–3), 56–59.

Wang, X., Wang, W., Li, L., Perry, G., Lee, H. G., & Zhu, X. (2014). Oxidative stress and mitochondrial dysfunction in Alzheimer's disease. *Biochimica et Biophysica Acta, 1842* (8), 1240–1247.

Wang, X., Su, B., Lee, H. G., Li, X., Perry, G., Smith, M. A., & Zhu, X. (2009). Impaired balance of mitochondrial fission and fusion in Alzheimer's disease. *Journal of Neuroscience*, *29*(28), 9090–9103.

Wang, X., Su, B., Siedlak, S. L., Moreira, P. I., Fujioka, H., Wang, Y., . . . Zhu, X. (2008). Amyloid-beta overproduction causes abnormal mitochondrial dynamics via differential modulation of mitochondrial fission/fusion proteins. *Proceedings of the National Academy of Sciences of the United States of America*, *105*(49), 19318–19323.

Westermann, B. (2010). Mitochondrial fusion and fission in cell life and death. *Nature Reviews Molecular Cell Biology*, *11*(12), 872–84.

Wild, P., & Dikic, I. (2010). Mitochondria get a Parkin' ticket. *Nature Cell Biology*, *12*(2), 104–106.

Winchester, J., Dick, M. B., Gillen, D., Reed, B., Miller, B., Tinklenberg, J., . . . Cotman, C. W. (2013). Walking stabilizes cognitive functioning in Alzheimer's disease (AD) across one year. *Archives of Gerontology and Geriatrics*, *56*(1), 96–103.

Wojsiat, J., Zoltowska, K. M., Laskowska-Kaszub, K., & Wojda, U. (2018). Oxidant/antioxidant imbalance in Alzheimer's disease: Therapeutic and diagnostic prospects. *Oxidative Medicine and Cellular Longevity*, *2018*, 6435861.

Wu, P., Shen, Q., Dong, S., Xu, Z., Tsien, J. Z., & Hu, Y. (2008). Calorie restriction ameliorates neurodegenerative phenotypes in forebrain-specific presenilin-1 and presenilin-2 double knockout mice. *Neurobiology of Aging*, *29*(10), 1502–1511.

Yamano, K., Matsuda, N., & Tanaka, K. (2016). The ubiquitin signal and autophagy: An orchestrated dance leading to mitochondrial degradation. *EMBO Reports*, *17*(3), 300–316.

Yang, X., Dai, G., Li, G., & Yang, E. S. (2010). Coenzyme Q10 reduces beta-amyloid plaque in an APP/PS1 transgenic mouse model of Alzheimer's disease. *Journal of Molecular Neuroscience*, *41*(1), 110–113.

Yang, X., Yang, Y., Li, G., Wang, J., & Yang, E. S. (2008). Coenzyme Q10 attenuates beta-amyloid pathology in the aged transgenic mice with Alzheimer presenilin 1 mutation. *Journal of Molecular Neuroscience*, *34*(2), 165–171.

Yao, J., Irwin, R. W., Zhao, L., Nilsen, J., Hamilton, R. T., & Brinton, R. D. (2009). Mitochondrial bioenergetic deficit precedes Alzheimer's pathology in female mouse model of Alzheimer's disease. *Proceedings of the National Academy of Sciences of the United States of America*, *106*(34), 14670–14675.

Ye, X., Sun, X., Starovoytov, V., & Cai, Q. (2015). Parkin-mediated mitophagy in mutant hAPP neurons and Alzheimer's disease patient brains. *Human Molecular Genetics*, *24*(10), 2938–2951.

Zhang, L., Trushin, S., Christensen, T. A., Bachmeier, B. V., Gateno, B., Schroeder, A., . . . Trushina, E. (2016). Altered brain energetics induces mitochondrial fission arrest in Alzheimer's disease. *Scientific Reports*, *6*, 18725.

Zhang, W., Gu, G. J., Shen, X., Zhang, Q., Wang, G. M., & Wang, P. J. (2015). Neural stem cell transplantation enhances mitochondrial biogenesis in a transgenic mouse model of Alzheimer's disease-like pathology. *Neurobiology of Aging*, *36*(3), 1282–1292.

Zhao, X. L., Wang, W. A., Tan, J. X., Huang, J. K., Zhang, X., Zhang, B. Z., . . . Huang, F. D. (2010). Expression of beta-amyloid induced age-dependent presynaptic and axonal changes in Drosophila. *Journal of Neuroscience*, *30*(4), 1512–1522.

PART 5

TREATMENT AND INTERVENTION

17

Cognitive Change and Elective Surgeries With Anesthesia

Considerations for Neuropsychologists and the Growing Field of Perioperative Cognitive Medicine

Margaret E. Wiggins, Carlos Hernaiz, Brenda G. Fahy, and Catherine C. Price

1. Case Examples

As a neuropsychologist, you may experience cases similar to the following:

- A 70-year-old patient reports having memory difficulties. After careful review of medical records and discussion of history onset, the patient reported that the problems developed after major back surgery that involved general anesthesia lasting at least 6 hours.
- An 80-year-old woman had a knee replacement surgery and a normal recovery until approximately 3 weeks postoperatively when she awoke one morning wondering why her leg was sore and painful. She had lost all memory for her surgical event and rehabilitation. She continues to have no recollection of any these events.
- An insurance company executive had a peripheral vascular operation and several months postoperatively found it impossible to perform required statistical calculations that were easy for him prior to surgery.
- A 67-year-old man now diagnosed with behavioral variant of frontotemporal dementia experienced an "unmasking" of his symptoms following surgical removal of a left temporal meningioma and delirium.

These cases demonstrate that surgery and accompanying anesthesia are not benign. There is increasing evidence to suggest significant cognitive vulnerability among patients with prodromal dementia or neurodegenerative diseases,

Margaret E. Wiggins, Carlos Hernaiz, Brenda G. Fahy, and Catherine C. Price, *Cognitive Change and Elective Surgeries With Anesthesia* In: *Vascular Disease, Alzheimer's Disease, and Mild Cognitive Impairment*. Edited by: David J. Libon, Melissa Lamar, Rodney A. Swenson, Kenneth M. Heilman, Oxford University Press (2020).
DOI: 10.1093/oso/9780190634230.003.0018

even in early stages when clinical symptoms are not yet present (Amini, Crowley, Hizel, Arias, Garvan et al., 2019; Culley et al., 2016; Evered et al., 2011). There is growing documentation that preoperative cognition and brain integrity are important risk factors for acute and long-term cognitive and neuronal change. For these reasons, neuropsychologists should be at the forefront of team-oriented approaches addressing perioperative cognitive medicine. Neuropsychologists and anesthesiologists are beginning to work together to appreciate interactions between preoperative brain integrity, intraoperative responses, and postoperative outcome.

To facilitate the future form of perioperative cognitive medicine, we designed this chapter to provide an overview of risk factors and relevant anesthesia considerations for dementia.

2. Background

Delirium and cognitive decline after surgery are two of the most frequently discussed domains within the geriatric anesthesia literature. Despite this, we currently have no clear answers about which anesthetics are most concerning or how neuroanatomical/physiological vulnerabilities interact with intraoperative factors. The underlying biological mechanisms of changes potentially due to anesthesia are unknown, and it is understudied whether individuals with early neurodegenerative pathologies respond differently to anesthesia or perioperative events. This is concerning as the World Health Organization reports an increase in older adults internationally. To date, one fourth to one third of older community dwelling individuals present with early signs of mild neurocognitive disorder (Luck et al., 2017) and are arriving to the preoperative environment relatively unaware of or denying the presence of their cognitive impairments (Amini, Crowley, Hizel, Arias, Garvan et al., 2019; Culley et al., 2016). Moreover, an increasing number of older adults are electing surgical procedures. We therefore need to remain alert to early indicators of potential neurodegenerative disorders and improve our understanding of appropriate perioperative care for such individuals. Failure to do so will hinder the development of intervention options. Identifying at-risk patients who may have nascent neurodegenerative disease is criterial as we learn how certain preoperative brain/cognitive profiles interact with anesthesia response (Giattino et al., 2017; Price et al., 2015) and predict acute (Huang et al., 2018) and long-term functional brain changes (Browndyke et al., 2017).

3. Risk Factors for Delirium or Cognitive Decline After Surgery With Anesthesia

3.1. Preoperative Risk Factors

Increased age is the most frequently cited risk for delirium and cognitive decline after noncardiac (Moller et al., 1998; Monk et al., 2008) and cardiac surgery (Frye, Kronmal, Schaff, Myers, & Gersh, 1992; Gardner et al., 1985; Tuman, McCarthy, Najafi, & Ivankovich, 1992). At least 15% of prospective study participants ≥65 years of age are experiencing memory and executive function declines postoperatively out to 3 months (Moller et al., 1998; Monk et al., 2008; Price et al., 2014). Aside from age, lower education is a well-known risk factor (e.g., Monk et al., 2008; Newman et al., 1995). Other published risk factors include lower performance on executive and memory tests before surgery (Greene et al., 2009; Price, Garvan, Hizel, Lopez, & Billings, 2017), elevated preoperative depression (Greene et al., 2009), greater medical co-morbidities, and preoperative evidence of nonsymptomatic stroke (Goto et al., 2001; Monk et al., 2008).

Aging has been shown to be associated with reductions in the function of large-scale, higher-order brain systems and networks, even in the absence of a pathological disease process (Andrews-Hanna et al., 2007). Furthermore, as individuals age there is an increased risk for cerebral white and gray matter loss, loss of cholinergic neurons (Schliebs & Arendt, 2011), reduced rates of neurogenesis (Galvan & Jin, 2007), and reduced brain reserve (Stern, 2009). These vulnerabilities may place the aged brain at greater risk for postoperative negative outcomes in response to perioperative stressors including intraoperative surgical stimuli.

3.2. Neurocognitive Status

A recent review conducted by Oresanya and colleagues (2014) found that in seven of nine studies examined preoperative cognitive impairment was independently associated with perioperative mortality (Bozic, Lau, Kurtz, Ong, & Berry, 2012; Bozic, Lau, Kurtz, Ong, Rubash, et al., 2012; Ho et al., 2005; Kim et al., 2012; Modini et al., 2012; Neuman et al., 2013; Schaller et al., 2012). However, they note that underdiagnosis of cognitive impairment can introduce considerable bias into these studies (Oresanya, Lyons, & Finlayson, 2014). Furthermore, a large study that included over 80,000 participants suggested that patients with cognitive impairment who were undergoing total knee arthroplasty had a 1.8×

higher risk of 9-day mortality when compared to cognitively well patients (Bozic, Lau, Kurtz, Ong, & Berry, 2012). In regard to delirium, publications that assessed delirium in orthopedic, urologic, vascular, cardiac, and abdominal patient populations were examined. Baseline cognitive impairment was associated with between a 2- and 17-fold increase in risk for acquiring postoperative delirium (Ansaloni et al., 2010; Bakker, Osse, Tulen, Kappetein, & Bogers, 2012; Chrispal, Mathews, & Surekha, 2010; Dai, Lou, Yip, & Huang, 2000; Freter, 2005; Furlaneto & Garcez-Leme, 2006; Juliebø et al., 2009; H. B. Lee et al., 2011; Otomo, Maekawa, Goto, Baba, & Yoshitake, 2013; Rudolph et al., 2007).

Cognitive impairment not only impacts postoperative outcomes, but it can also impact decision-making capacity regarding treatment options and potential preparation for surgical procedures. A review by Sessums and colleagues (2011) demonstrated that 2.8% of older adults without cognitive impairment, 20% of older adults with mild cognitive impairment (MCI), and 54% of older adults with Alzheimer's disease (AD) had limited decision-making capacity (Sessums, Zembrzuska, & Jackson, 2011). A novel and recent study by Arias and colleagues (2018) also shows that individuals with evidence of major neurocognitive disorder fail colonoscopy preparations. Colonoscopy is not considered a major surgical procedure, but it is routinely prescribed for older adults. Cognitive assessment for older adults appears relevant outside of the traditional parameters in which we are trained.

3.3. Genetics

After advanced age, carrying an apolipoprotein E4 (APOE4) allele is the second most influential risk factor for AD (Cunningham et al., 2017). The APOE4 allele is associated with amyloid accumulation, eventual emergence of dementia such as AD, and coronary artery disease. In relation to surgery outcome, patients with APOE4 are reported to have higher restenosis rates after coronary artery bypass grafting (CABG). Furthermore, while some suggest that APOE4 is associated with an increased risk of cognitive decline after CABG (Tardiff et al., 1997), others were unable to replicate this findings. In regard to delirium, a meta-analysis found an association between carrying the APOE4 allele and incidence of delirium (van Munster, Korevaar, Zwinderman, Leeflang, & de Rooij, 2009). However, recent studies have also been unable to replicate the conclusions of this meta-analysis in a postoperative population. Abelha and colleagues (2012) found APOE4 does not increase the risk of early postoperative delirium after surgery (Abelha et al., 2012). Other research also found no association between APOE genotype and postoperative delirium in 557 nondemented elderly patients undergoing major noncardiac surgery (Vasunilashorn et al., 2015) with no association found between APOE4 and delirium in the acute phase after stroke (Oldenbeuving, de Kort, Kappelle, van Dujin, & Roks, 2013). Despite the established associated with AD dementia and APOE4, the hypothesis that APOE4 predicts postoperative delirium has not generally been supported (Cunningham et al., 2017).

3.4. Mood Status

Research has found that depressive symptoms independently predict the development of postoperative delirium (Greene et al., 2009). Furthermore, depression has been found to impair cognition in patients with dementia and may predict early onset of age-related cognitive impairment. While preoperative depression can be treated with medications, there are reports that antidepressant medications such as tricyclic antidepressants are associated with the development of postoperative delirium. The mechanisms by which tricyclics and other anticholinergic mediations interact with surgery variables such as type of anesthesia (general vs. regional) to induce delirium is speculative and requires further investigation.

3.5. Frailty

Between 25% and 50% of adults over the age of 85 are estimated to be frail (L. P. Fried et al., 2001; Song, Mitnitski, & Rockwood, 2010). Frailty in older adults develops as a result of age-related decline in physiological functioning. Collectively, this decline increases vulnerability to sudden changes in health status (even from independent living to dependent living) as triggered by minor stressors (Clegg, Young, Iliffe, Rikkert, & Rockwood, 2013). Research on community-dwelling older adults has demonstrated that frailty has a stronger association with death than either advanced age or comorbidity status (Song et al., 2010).

Frailty has both risks and consequences that overlap with delirium. For example, increased age and increased disease status are both common risks for frailty and delirium, and functional dependence is a common outcome for frailty and delirium (Leung, Tsai, & Sands, 2011). There is also overlap in the etiology for both frailty and changes in cognition. For example, cerebrovascular disease is related to both delirium (Leung et al., 2007) and frailty (Newman et al., 2001) after surgery.

Frailty status interacts with the perioperative environment as higher frailty scores are associated with higher risk for delirium in older adults undergoing noncardiac surgery (Leung et al., 2011). Furthermore, in a sample of older adults undergoing cardiac surgery, frailty status independently resulted in a threefold to eightfold increase in the risk of delirium after surgery (Jung et al., 2015). The addition of frailty in standard preoperative risk prediction models (such as the European System for Cardiac Operative Risk Evaluation II [EUROSCORE II]; Nashef et al., 2012) significantly improved the ability to predict delirium, which has implications for opportunities regarding improved delirium intervention and optimal patient care (Jung et al., 2015). Additionally, survival following delirium is poor, but the combination of delirium and frailty leads to a particularly poor prognosis (Eeles, White, O'Mahony, Bayer, & Hubbard, 2012).

3.6. Anticholinergic Medication and Polypharmacy

Neurodegenerative brain diseases can be associated with changes in the cholinergic system. Moreover, acetylcholine (ACh) is a neurotransmitter that is known to regulate higher-order cognition including learning and memory. Anticholinergic medications act in opposition to acetylcholine and inhibit the transmission of nerve impulses in the parasympathetic nervous system. Anticholinergic medications have been identified by the American Geriatrics Society Beers Criteria (AGS Beers Criteria®) for Potentially Inappropriate Medications Use in Older Adults as a class of medications that should be avoided by older adults if possible (Ness, Hoth, Barnett, Shorr, & Kaboli, 2006). In adults older than 65, anticholinergic medications have been associated with adverse outcomes including symptoms of delirium, dementia, or cognitive impairment (Ness et al., 2006).

Neuropsychologists and other medical care providers should be keenly aware of their patients' medication regiment prior to surgery, especially in the context of anticholinergics. Acetylcholine production decreases with aging and to a greater degree in older adults with AD or other dementia pathologies (Tune, 2001). Peripheral effects of anticholinergic medications may impact vision, the oral cavity, gastrointestinal functioning, cardiovascular functioning, the urinary tract, and the central nervous system (Feinberg, 1993; Tune, 2001), all potentially leading to impaired activities of daily living, falls, increased risk of infection, decreased nutritional status, anxiety, pain, incontinence, and loss of independence (Tune, 2001). However, central effects of anticholinergic medications in older adults may be of even greater clinical significance and include confusion, delirium, and cognitive and functional decline (Brombo et al., 2018; Ness et al., 2006; Tune, 2001). Furthermore, cognitive decline potentially associated with anticholinergic medications persists in the year after hospital discharge (Brombo et al., 2018). Not only should the medical team be aware of anticholinergic medications, but they should also consider the effects of polypharmacy. Polypharmacy may be present in up to 18% of older adults (Rawle, Cooper, Kuh, & Richards, 2018) and is associated with an increased fall risk, hospitalization, premature mortality, adverse reactions to drugs, and cognitive impairment (T. R. Fried et al., 2014). By being aware of potential risk factors for delirium and cognitive impairment after surgery such as medication regiment, the care team can intervene earlier and make necessary modifications prior to the patient undergoing surgery.

4. Operative Risk Factors

4.1. Anesthesia and Dementia

There has been relatively little research regarding the impact of anesthetics on patients who meet criteria for MCI or dementia. However, numerous studies have attempted to understand this question using basic science models. Due to the extensive literature on this topic, only a few additional key points concerning anesthesia will be covered in this chapter.

One of the difficulties in assessing the effects of anesthetics on patients with dementia is the fact that an anesthetic, whether regional or general, is rarely (if ever) delivered without a concomitant surgical procedure. Surgery causes a stress response via the activation of endocrine, metabolic, and inflammatory responses. The inflammatory response is activated not only locally at the wound site can trigger an systemic inflammatory response which has the potential to be harmful to the brain (Angele & Chaudry, 2005; Lenz, Franklin, & Cheadle, 2007). A major challenge conducting this research revolves the need for an appropriate control group that does not require surgery. In one retrospective study that attempted to control for surgical procedure, patients undergoing CABG were compared to patients with other known cardiovascular diseases requiring a percutaneous transluminal coronary angioplasty intervention (T. A. Lee, Wolozin, Weiss, & Bednar, 2005). In this study, the patients who underwent CABG had an adjusted risk of dementia of 1.7 for up to 6 years postoperatively compared to those who underwent the percutaneous procedure. Therefore, while the mechanisms for anesthesia leading to an increased risk for dementia are unclear, future research should further investigate this topic.

4.2. Anesthetic Effects: Brain–Behavior Models

Agents that are used to produce the desired effects of general anesthesia have both benefits and risks. While general anesthetic agents lead to loss of consciousness and memory function and prevent pain and movement during the procedure, they also decrease the release of ACh and cholinergic transmission (Fodale, Quattrone, Trecroci, Caminiti, & Santamaria, 2006). Although some reports on anesthetic agents such as the volatile agent isoflurane have suggested that it may have properties that protect against neurotoxicity, other reports have concerns about its potential neurotoxicity. One study showed that in mouse models, isoflurane reduces cell death (Zhan, Fahlman, & Bickler, 2006). However, this was only seen in young mice and therefore the neuroprotective effect appears to be age dependent (Zhan et al., 2006). On the contrary, other studies of mouse models with AD have found that isoflurane increases amyloid pathology (Eckenhoff et al., 2004; Perucho et al., 2010). In addition to increases in amyloid-beta (Aβ) protein level, an additional study found that isoflurane also induced caspase activation in mice (Xie et al., 2008). In human neuroglioma cells, isoflurane produced neurotoxic effects including inducing caspase activation, extracellular accumulation of Aβ, and cell death (Xie et al., 2006).

A newer volatile anesthetic, desflurane, which differs from isoflurane and sevoflurane, has been shown in human neuroglioma cells to not activate caspase-3 or impact amyloid precursor protein processing or Aβ accumulation (Y. Zhang et al., 2012). Comparing spinal anesthesia to general anesthesia with isoflurane or desflurane, isoflurane but not desflurane increased cerebrospinal levels of Aβ proteins in humans (B. Zhang et al., 2013). While the literature regarding anesthesia and brain-behavior models is mixed, it appears as if the majority of research suggests that isoflurane has neurotoxic effects of the brain. This should be monitored closely in the perioperative environment.

4.3. Deep of Anesthesia

It is frequently discussed whether depth of anesthesia during surgery can have negative postoperative cognitive and functional outcomes such as delirium. One study conducted in a sample of older adults undergoing hip fracture with spinal anesthesia found that the use of light sedation decreased the prevalence of delirium by 50% compared with deep sedation (Sieber et al., 2010). Additional research suggests that depth of sedation, as measured by two-channel derived electroencephalography (EEG) monitors, is a risk factor for delirium and even potentially mortality in the elderly (Monk et al., 2008). Another means to assess for depth of sedation is the Bispectral Index Monitor (BIS; Rampil, 1998). The BIS converts EEG readings into a simplified number that represents hypnotic depth. Despite literature demonstrating that anesthetic depth can impact postoperative outcome, some anesthesiologists disregard BIS readings or consider EEG metrics to be unreliable. This is because rapid fluctuations can occur in EEG-derived BIS values for the same patient throughout surgery, even during stable periods of monitoring. However, it can be hypothesized that fluctuations should be anticipated or even expected, particularly in older adults. It has been shown that EEG variability is more prominent in adults with lower levels of intelligence (Barrett & Eysenck, 1994), schizophrenia (Shin et al., 2015), AD, and Lewy body disease (Andersson, Hansson, Minthon, Rosen, & Londos, 2008). Furthermore, neurophysiological variability has been known to associate with cortical thinning, brain shrinkage, and atrophy of the frontoparietal region of the brain (Moretti, 2015a, 2015b; Rossini et al., 2008). Therefore, variability in anesthetic depth during surgery may provide important insight into the brain's response to anesthesia that could impact postoperative outcomes. An exploratory substudy of a larger National Institutes of Health–funded investigation, with primary outcomes of postoperative decline in memory and executive function after total knee arthroplasty, assessed the contribution of preoperative cognition and brain markers on intraoperative neurophysiological variability during general anesthesia as measured from the BIS. This study posited a theoretical framework of premorbid cognitive reserve, brain integrity (gray and white matter markers of neurodegenerative disease), and current cognition (specifically processing speed/working memory, episodic memory). First, premorbid cognitive reserve represents psychosocial, experiential factors (e.g., greater educational attainment), and genetic factors (e.g., childhood intelligence) that enable the brain to withstand injury. Cognitive reserve represents foundational synaptic density distinct from neurodegenerative brain pathologies; individuals with significant amounts of reserve can have substantial neurodegenerative disease markers without clinical manifestation. Second, current brain integrity represents the status of an individuals' gray and white matter as seen on brain magnetic resonance. Entorhinal cortical thickness, leukoaraiosis (i.e., white matter disease), and lateral ventricular volume are three well-established neuroimaging markers of early neurodegenerative pathology. Lastly, cognitive domains of the frontal-subcortical/thalamocortical system (i.e., processing speed and working memory) and medial/lateral temporal systems (i.e., episodic memory encoding and retrieval) are most vulnerable to aging vascular pathologies. Research has yet to examine the effects of intraindividual variability during anesthesia on postoperative cognitive outcome.

4.4. General Versus Spinal Anesthesia

Research assessing cognition in older adults with general versus spinal anesthesia has been conducted, and overall these studies found minimal or no significant differences in postoperative cognition between anesthetic groups (Bigler et al., 1985; Ghoneim et al., 1988; Jones et al., 1990; Mazul-Sunko et al., 2010; Nielson et al., 1990; Rasmussen et al., 2003; Xu et al., 2016). Of the studies that found differences in cognitive performance across groups after surgery, one study found that individuals who received general anesthesia improved in processing speed when compared to those who received local anesthesia (Jones et al., 1990). However, other researchers found that those who received local anesthesia performed better on measures of orientation than those who received general anesthesia (Mazul-Sunko et al., 2010; Xu et al., 2016). In a classic paper assessing postoperative changes in cognition, there was no causative relationship between general anesthesia and long-term cognitive changes (Rasmussen et al., 2003). However, there are several critical limitations of the previous studies to consider. Cognitive cut-points for inclusion were unclear (Bigler et al., 1985; Ghoneim et al., 1988; Jones et al., 1990; Mazul-Sunko et al., 2010; Nielson et al., 1990; Rasmussen et al., 2003). The inclusion of memory measures was negligible, yet we know memory is one of the cognitive domains most susceptible to decline after surgery. Furthermore, the majority of research was conducted in the 1980s and 1990s. Since that time, spinal and general anesthetic techniques have been updated and refined. For all of these reasons, there is no clear indication that spinal anesthesia results in improved outcome relative to general anesthesia.

4.5. Rewarming Rate in the Context of Cardiac Surgery

In 1958, hypothermia was first introduced as a method for controlling oxygen circulation during cardiac surgery (Sealy, Brown, & Young, 1958) and has since been used frequently in perioperative settings. Hypothermia has been shown to improve both myocardial and cerebral tolerance to the impacts of ischemia during the perioperative process (Buckberg et al., 1977; Busto, Dietrich, Globus, & Ginsberg, 1989; Govier et al., 1984; Marion, Obrist, Carlier, Penrod, & Darby, 1993). However, hypothermia requires rewarming the body to a normal temperature. Rapid rewarming is associated with reaching temperatures beyond the desired rewarmed temperature. This can result in exposure to hyperthermic temperatures and increase potential for negative outcomes (Grigore, Murray, Ramakrishna, & Djaiani, 2009), perhaps due in part to higher cerebral blood flow and the location of carotid origins being nearby the aortic cannulation site in cardiac surgeries (Cook, Orszulak, Daly, & Buda, 1996).

In human studies, research has shown that a slower rewarming rate with lower peak temperatures leads to better cognitive performance after cardiac surgery (Grigore et al., 2002). Similarly, a prospective, randomized, clinical trial demonstrated that patients undergoing CABG who were rewarmed to 37°C, compared with a group who experienced limited rewarming, had significant declines in neurocognitive testing performance (Sahu et al., 2009). Similar findings have been seen in mouse models, such that hypothermic neuroprotection was maximized when paired with limited rewarming and extended postoperative hypothermia programs (de Lange, Jones, Mackensen, & Grocott, 2008).

4.6. Emboli

Emboli as a potential cause for cognitive complications has been studied in both noncardiac and cardiac surgery populations. In orthopedic surgery, one potential cause for the development of delirium is cerebral fat embolism (Cox et al., 2011; Barak et al., 2008; Forteza et al., 1999; Koessler & Pitto, 2002; Rodriguez et al., 2005). Cerebral fat embolism occurs when lipid microemboli are sent to the brain via the blood stream (Cox et al., 2011). There are two theories as to how fat emboli occur: the mechanical theory and the biochemical theory. The mechanical theory suggests that emboli can occur when intramedullary pressure is increased during processes such as nailing of long bones (Christie, Robinson, Pell, McBirnie, & Burnett, 1995; Giannoudis, Tzioupis, & Pape, 2006; Talucci, Manning, Lampard, Bach, & Carrico, 1983). The biochemical theory suggests that free fatty acids are released via lipases (Fabian, 1993). In either theory, fat is passed through the heart where it is sent to organs, including the brain (Brondén, Dencker, Allers, Plaza, & Jönsson, 2006; Glover & Worthley, 1999), leading to postoperative complications such as delirium.

Research regarding emboli in relation to cardiac surgery has found a significant relationship between the number of emboli and negative postoperative cognitive outcomes (Pugsley et al., 1990). Furthermore, research on patients undergoing cardiac procedures has demonstrated an association between increasing age and number of emboli present (Stump, Tegeler, Newman, Wallenhaupt, & Roy, 1992). However, conclusions based on such studies are limited as there is difficulty in differentiating whether the emboli are from the air (derived from the surgical field) or particulate in nature (derived from fat, muscle fragments, platelet aggregates, calcium particles, lipid droplets, etc.; Stump, Rogers, Hammon, & Newman, 1996). Regardless of the cause of emboli, patients should be monitored both intraoperatively and postoperatively for signs of complications.

5. Postoperative Factors

5.1. Blood Levels

Not only do surgical factors potentially impact the brain, but physical factors such as abnormal blood values and blood loss may impact brain functioning in the perioperative environment. The association of blood loss and hematocrit levels on postoperative outcomes have been studied following both cardiac and noncardiac surgery, but findings have been mixed. Research has shown that arterial oxygenation factors such as blood hemoglobin (the oxygen transport protein within blood cells) and partial pressure of oxygen (PaO_2) were reduced among patients with delirium onset (Axèll, Malmros, Bergbom, & Lundberg, 2002). Specifically, it was found that patients with severe delirium had significantly lower hemoglobin concentrations than patients with moderate delirium and patients without delirium (Axèll et al., 2002). This is in line with findings from other research suggesting that intraoperative blood loss, postoperative blood transfusions, and the lowest postoperative hematocrit value were associated with delirium onset such that patients who developed delirium experienced greater intraoperative blood loss and received more postoperative blood transfusions (Marcantonio, Goldman, Orav, Cook, & Lee, 1998). Other research has shown that postoperative oxygen saturation is associated with delirium (Moller et al., 1993), however the same authors did not find an association with cognitive functioning (Moller et al., 1998). Taken together, if there is indeed an association between blood content or levels and delirium, it is critical that physicians and anesthesiologists monitor blood levels both during and after surgery and potentially decrease the risk of delirium with prompt administration of oxygen therapy.

5.2. Oxygenation

While delirium is sometimes treated with sedatives, leading to potentially serious negative side effects, it can also be treated with supplementary oxygen. Early research on the effects of treatments with supplementary oxygen found that after operation, there was a trend toward individuals with delirium experiencing more hypoxemic episodes than individuals without delirium (Aakerlund & Rosenberg, 1994). It was also found that mean oxygen saturation was lower and the time spent with oxygen saturation under 85% was greater in the individuals with delirium than in individuals without delirium on the second night after operation (Aakerlund & Rosenberg, 1994), which is when the risk of hypoxemia has been shown to be highest (Entwistle, Roe, Sapsford, Berrisford,

& Jones, 1991). All patients with delirium were successfully treated with supplementary oxygen, therefore suggesting that delirium is related to inadequate oxygenation after surgery (Entwistle, Roe, Sapsford, Berrisford, & Jones, 1991). However, research on the efficacy of monitoring oxygen levels has been mixed. Research conducted by Moller and colleagues (1993) did not find any differences in postoperative cognitive impairment between individuals who did or did not receive pulse oximetry monitoring in the perioperative environment (Moller et al., 1993). However, extensive research has not been conducted on the effects of oxygen therapy after surgery and should be considered in the future.

6. Should We Label Perioperative Cognitive Change?

Evered and colleagues (2018) point out that the majority of the literature regarding cognitive changes in the perioperative period has been in isolation from the general population of older adults not undergoing surgical procedures. In fact, postoperative cognitive dysfunction (POCD) has become an area of research rather than a clinical diagnosis which limits its utility. A formal clinical classification regarding POCD may be necessary for several reasons. For one, the number of patients over the age of 60 undergoing surgery has significantly increased. Second, the diagnostic criteria for cognitive changes related to the perioperative environment should not be differentiated from neurocognitive disorders in the general population. Third, the terminology of neurocognitive changes associated with the perioperative environment should be aligned with other neurocognitive disorders to promote cross-specialty communication and aid clinical management of patients as neurocognitive disorders occur frequently in the community (Evered et al., 2018). Therefore, Evered and colleagues (2018) aimed to develop terminology that can be used in the classification of neurocognitive status in the general population for studies examining changes postsurgically. They discussed that the fifth edition of the *Diagnostic and Statistical Manual for Mental Disorders* (DSM-5) and the National Institute for Aging and the Alzheimer Association (NIA-AA) are the two diagnostic guidelines currently recognized in clinical procedures. They recommended an umbrella term of "perioperative neurocognitive disorders" be used to identify cognitive changes or impairments observed or reported during the preoperative or postoperative period (Evered et al., 2018). For pre-existing cognitive impairment, terminology should be considered in terms of cognitive impairment that might be identified in the general community, such as mild neurocognitive disorder (MCI) or major neurocognitive disorder (dementia; Evered et al., 2018). In regard to delirium, "postoperative delirium" should be recognized as a specific category that is consistent with current DSM-5 terminology and that has appropriate specifiers. It is suggested that "postoperative delirium" be defined as occurring in the hospital up to 1 week after surgery or until discharge (whichever is first) and meets DSM-5 diagnostic criteria (Evered et al., 2018). This group also pointed out that the criteria for POCD have been confined to research settings. As such there us variability regarding diagnostic criteria that have been employed to classify an individual as experiencing POCD (Evered et al., 2018). These researchers recommended that terminology designating impairment or change in cognition associated with surgery be changed from POCD to "delayed neurocognitive recovery" and mild or major neurocognitive disorder, depending on timeline and severity (Evered et al., 2018).

The current chapter uses the terminology "POCD" to refer to cognitive changes in the context of surgery. Moving forward, it is critical that neuropsychologists and the perioperative care team adopt a nomenclature for postoperative cognitive changes that is in line with clinical practice. This would allow for both better research opportunities and enhanced clinical diagnostic abilities.

7. Neuropsychologists as Team Builders for Perioperative Cognitive Medicine

The American Society of Anesthesiology, International Anesthesia Research Society, and the Society for Perioperative Anesthesia (SPAQUI) have published papers addressing the need for cognitive screening measures in the preoperative environment. Studies show that these screenings identify symptoms of mild to major neurocognitive disorder in 19% to 33% of older adults scheduled for elective surgical procedures (Amini, Crowley, Hizel, Arias, Libon, et al., 2019; Culley et al., 2016) and predict cognitive and noncognitive complications after surgery and anesthesia (Price et al., 2017). Most screening instruments include variants of short traditional neuropsychological/neurological tools, such as the three-word memory test, counting backwards from 100 by 7, or spelling the word "WORLD" backwards such as in the Mini-Cog (Borson, Scanlan, Chen, & Ganguli, 2003), the Mini-Mental State Examination (Folstein, Robins, & Helzer, 1983), and clock drawing to command and copy (Libon, Malamut, Swenson, Sands, & Cloud, 1996). Yet, routine inclusion of preoperative cognitive screening for dementia or delirium is in its infancy. We are only beginning to learn how to integrate educational and cognitive screenings into busy clinical settings and to appropriately report and implement cognitive/memory screening data for perioperative management. Very few hospitals include cognitive screening of older adults as a routine component of their preoperative evaluation. Even fewer hospitals collaborate with neuropsychologists and geriatricians for more integrated preoperative and postoperative care.

The University of Florida Health System has established a screening program where patients who "fail" a preadmission cognitive/memory screen are referred to neuropsychologists and/or geriatric medicine physicians (Amini, Crowley, Hizel, Arias, Libon, et al., 2019; Arias, Bursian, Sappenfield, & Price, 2018). These assessments identify modifiable risk factors such as anticholinergic burden or polypharmacy, provide the anesthesia–surgical team with considerations about the type of cognitive impairment, and provide recommendations for inpatient geriatric medicine follow-up and closer in-patient and home-based delirium monitoring. Patients at-risk for developing delirium are then educated (with their families) on perioperative risks, thus enhancing patient-centered care (for an example, see Arias et al., 2018). With perioperative follow-up, teams monitor for delirium and inform patients and family about the possibility of a longer hospitalization and discharge to a nursing facility rather than home. Patient reports are available to the anesthesiology and surgery team prior to the surgical procedure so that anesthesiologists and surgeons can tailor their care based on their preoperative profile, when possible.

This form of integrated care, however, requires close collaboration between anesthesiology, neuropsychology, and geriatric medicine. Prospective studies are needed to address the relationships between preoperative cognitive impairment and type/depth of anesthesia, invasiveness of the surgical procedure, biomarker changes, and patient outcomes to identify best practices for the care of our older patients. Addressing cognition within the preoperative environment is relevant to identify risk for neurocognitive decline.

8. Future Directions

We need more collaborative and prospective investigations addressing interactions between anesthesia, brain structure, and brain function. Results from a prospective longitudinal study (Huang et al., 2018) show significant reductions in resting state functional MRI connectivity for three major networks of interest (default mode network [DMN], salience network, salience network, central executive network) in nondemented older adults electing unilateral total knee arthroplasty under general anesthesia. By using a novel application of reliable change statistics to functional MRI data, they show that 15% of surgery participants significantly declined across all three functional networks and an additional 8% declined in at least one network for a total of 23% of the sample showing declined in one or more networks (Huang et al., 2018). Pain, opioid medication dose at the time of the postoperative MRI, estimates of premorbid cognitive function (vocabulary, reading ability, education), an estimate of brain reserve (total intracranial volume), and group differences in baseline global cognition did not significantly contribute to or explain network connectivity decline (Huang et al., 2018). Rather, an estimate of preoperative brain integrity (ventricular volume) and current cognitive function explained functional connectivity decline with this specific to the DMN (Huang et al., 2018). A follow-up study with a larger sample showed that individuals meeting MCI were the most vulnerable to this change (Hardcastle et al., 2019). Changes in the DMN is also reported after cardiothoracic surgery, with evidence suggesting this change predicts later cognitive change (Browndyke et al., 2017). These findings in combination with recent studies showing that cognition and brain integrity prior to surgery predict basic two-channel EEG anesthesia response (Hernaiz et al., 2019), suggesting that neuropsychologists can play a pivotal role in improving brain–anesthesia interactions. Future research should assess whether types of preoperative cognitive abilities predict greater changes in functional connectivity and why brains are vulnerable to change after surgery. Neuropsychologists have the knowledge, patient skills, and research skills necessary to conduct this research with a collaborative team of anesthesiologists, surgeons, and geriatricians. Furthermore, neuropsychologists need to remain aware of this research so that we are not taken by surprise when our patients report abrupt cognitive change or neurological symptoms following minor or major surgical procedures.

References

Aakerlund, L. P., & Rosenberg, J. (1994). Postoperative delirium: Treatment with supplementary oxygen. *British Journal of Anaesthesia, 72*(3), 286–290. https://doi.org/10.1093/bja/72.3.286

Abelha, F. J., Fernandes, V., Botelho, M., Santos, P., Santos, A., Machado, J. C., & Barros, H. (2012). Apolipoprotein E e4 allele does not increase the risk of early postoperative delirium after major surgery. *Journal of Anesthesia, 26*(3), 412–421. https://doi.org/10.1007/s00540-012-1326-5

Amini, S., Crowley, S., Hizel, L., Arias, F., Libon, D. J., Tighe, P., Giordano, C., Garvan, C., Enneking, F. K., & Price, C. (2019). Feasibility and rationale for incorporating frailty and cognitive screening protocols in a preoperative anesthesia clinic. *Anesthesia & Analgesia, 129*, 830–838.

Amini, S., Crowley, S. J., Hizel, L. P., Arias, F., Libon, D. J., Tighe, P., . . . Price, C. C. (2019). Feasibility and rationale for incorporating frailty and cognitive screening protocols in a preoperative anesthesia clinic. *Anesthesia & Analgesia*, 129(3), 830–838.

Ansaloni, L., Catena, F., Chattat, R., Fortuna, D., Franceschi, C., Mascitti, P., & Melotti, R. M. (2010). Risk factors and incidence of postoperative delirium in elderly patients after elective and emergency surgery. *BJS, 97*(2), 273–280. https://doi.org/10.1002/bjs.6843

Andersson, M., Hansson, O., Minthon, L., Rosen, I., & Londos, E. (2008). Electroencephalogram variability in dementia with lewy bodies, Alzheimer's disease and controls. *Dementia and Geriatric Cognitive Disorders, 26*(3), 284–290.

Andrews-Hanna, J. R., Snyder, A. Z., Vincent, J. L., Lustig, C., Head, D., Raichle, M. E., & Buckner, R. L. (2007). Disruption of large-scale brain systems in advanced aging. *Neuron, 56*(5), 924–935. https://doi.org/10.1016/j.neuron.2007.10.038

Angele, M. K., & Chaudry, I. H. (2005). Surgical trauma and immunosuppression: Pathophysiology and potential immunomodulatory approaches. *Langenbeck's Archives of Surgery, 390*(4), 333–341. https://doi.org/10.1007/s00423-005-0557-4

Arias, F., Bursian, A. C., Sappenfield, J. W., & Price, C. C. (2018). Delirium history and preoperative mild neurocognitive disorder: An opportunity for multidisciplinary patient-centered care. *The American Journal of Case Reports, 19*, 1324–1328. https://doi.org/10.12659/AJCR.911437

Axèll, A. I. R. G., Malmros, C. W., Bergbom, I. L., & Lundberg, D. B. A. (2002). Intensive care unit syndrome/delirium is associated with anemia, drug therapy and duration of ventilation treatment. *Acta Anaesthesiologica Scandinavica, 46*(6), 726–731. https://doi.org/10.1034/j.1399-6576.2002.460616.x

Bakker, R. C., Osse, R. J., Tulen, J. H. M., Kappetein, A. P., & Bogers, A. J. J. C. (2012). Preoperative and operative predictors of delirium after cardiac surgery in elderly patients. *European Journal of Cardio-Thoracic Surgery, 41*(3), 544–549. https://doi.org/10.1093/ejcts/ezr031

Barak, M., Kabha, M., Norman, D., Soudry, M., Kats, Y., & Milo, S. (2008). Cerebral microemboli during hip fracture fixation: A prospective study. *Anesthesia & Analgesia, 107*(1), 221–225. https://doi.org/10.1213/ane.0b013e3181770abb

Barrett, P. T., & Eysenck, H. J. (1994). The relationship between evoked potential component amplitude, latency, contour length, variability, zero-crossings, and psychometric intelligence. *Personality and Individual Differences, 16*(1), 3–32.

Bigler, D., Adelhøj, B., Petring, O. U., Pederson, N. O., Busch, P., & Kalhke, P. (1985). Mental function and morbidity after acute hip surgery during spinal and general anaesthesia. *Anaesthesia, 40*(7), 672–676. https://doi.org/10.1111/j.1365-2044.1985.tb10949.x

Borson, S., Scanlan, J. M., Chen, P., & Ganguli, M. (2003). The Mini-Cog as a screen for dementia: validation in a population-based sample. *Journal of the American Geriatrics Society, 51*(10), 1451–1454.

Bozic, K. J., Lau, E., Kurtz, S., Ong, K., & Berry, D. J. (2012). Patient-related risk factors for postoperative mortality and periprosthetic joint infection in Medicare patients undergoing TKA. *Clinical Orthopaedics and Related Research®, 470*(1), 130–137. https://doi.org/10.1007/s11999-011-2043-3

Bozic, K. J., Lau, E., Kurtz, S., Ong, K., Rubash, H., Vail, T. P., & Berry, D. J. (2012). Patient-related risk factors for periprosthetic joint infection and postoperative mortality following total hip arthroplasty in Medicare patients. *The Journal of Bone and Joint Surgery-American Volume, 94*(9), 794–800. https://doi.org/10.2106/JBJS.K.00072

Brombo, G., Bianchi, L., Maietti, E., Malacarne, F., Corsonello, A., Cherubini, A., . . . Volpato, S. (2018). Association of anticholinergic drug burden with cognitive and functional decline over time in older inpatients: Results from the CRIME Project. *Drugs & Aging, 35*(10), 917–924. https://doi.org/10.1007/s40266-018-0584-9

Brondén, B., Dencker, M., Allers, M., Plaza, I., & Jönsson, H. (2006). Differential distribution of lipid microemboli after cardiac surgery. *The Annals of Thoracic Surgery, 81*(2), 643–648. https://doi.org/10.1016/j.athoracsur.2005.08.006

Browndyke, J. N., Berger, M., Harshbarger, T. B., Smith, P. J., White, W., Bisanar, T. L., . . . Mathew, J. P. (2017). Resting-state functional connectivity and cognition after major cardiac surgery in older adults without preoperative cognitive impairment: Preliminary findings. *Journal of the American Geriatrics Society*, *65*(1), e6–e12. https://doi.org/10.1111/jgs.14534

Buckberg, G. D., Brazier, J. R., Nelson, R. L., Goldstein, S. M., McConnell, D. H., & Cooper, N. (1977). Studies of the effects of hypothermia on regional myocardial blood flow and metabolism during cardiopulmonary bypass. I. The adequately perfused beating, fibrillating, and arrested heart. *The Journal of Thoracic and Cardiovascular Surgery*, *73*(1), 87–94.

Busto, R., Dietrich, W. D., Globus, M. Y., & Ginsberg, M. D. (1989). The importance of brain temperature in cerebral ischemic injury. *Stroke*, *20*(8), 1113–1114.

Chrispal, A., Mathews, K. P., & Surekha, V. (2010). The clinical profile and association of delirium in geriatric patients with hip fractures in a tertiary care hospital in India, *58*, 5.

Christie, J., Robinson, C. M., Pell, A. C., McBirnie, J., & Burnett, R. (1995). Transcardiac echocardiography during invasive intramedullary procedures. *Journal of Bone and Joint Surgery (British Volume)*, *77*(3), 450–455.

Clegg, A., Young, J., Iliffe, S., Rikkert, M. O., & Rockwood, K. (2013). Frailty in elderly people. *Lancet*, *381*(9868), 752–762. https://doi.org/10.1016/S0140-6736(12)62167-9

Cook, D. J., Orszulak, T. A., Daly, R. C., & Buda, D. A. (1996). Cerebral hyperthermia during cardiopulmonary bypass in adults. *Journal of Thoracic and Cardiovascular Surgery*, *111*(1), 268–269. https://doi.org/10.1016/S0022-5223(96)70425-7

Cox, G., Tzioupis, C., Calori, G. M., Green, J., Seligson, D., & Giannoudis, P. V. (2011). Cerebral fat emboli: A trigger of post-operative delirium. *Injury*, *42*, S6–S10. https://doi.org/10.1016/S0020-1383(11)70005-5

Culley, D. J., Flaherty, D., Reddy, S., Fahey, M. C., Rudolph, J., Huang, C. C., . . . Crosby, G. (2016). Preoperative cognitive stratification of older elective surgical patients: A cross-sectional study. *Anesthesia and Analgesia*, *123*(1), 186–192. https://doi.org/10.1213/ANE.0000000000001277

Cunningham, E. L., Mawhinney, T., Beverland, D., O'Brien, S., McAuley, D. F., Cairns, R., . . . McGuinness, B. (2017). Observational cohort study examining apolipoprotein E status and preoperative neuropsychological performance as predictors of post-operative delirium in an older elective arthroplasty population. *Age & Ageing*, *46*(5), 779–786. https://doi.org/10.1093/ageing/afx042

Dai, Y.-T., Lou, M.-F., Yip, P.-K., & Huang, G.-S. (2000). Risk factors and incidence of postoperative delirium in elderly Chinese patients. *Gerontology*, *46*(1), 28–35. https://doi.org/10.1159/000022130

de Lange, F., Jones, W. L., Mackensen, G. B., & Grocott, H. P. (2008). The effect of limited rewarming and postoperative hypothermia on cognitive function in a rat cardiopulmonary bypass model. *Anesthesia & Analgesia*, *106*(3), 739. https://doi.org/10.1213/ane.0b013e318162d026

Eckenhoff, R. G., Johansson, J. S., Wei, H., Carnini, A., Kang, B., Wei, W., . . . Eckenhoff, M. F. (2004). Inhaled anesthetic enhancement of amyloid-β oligomerization and cytotoxicity. *Anesthesiology*, *101*(3), 703–709.

Eeles, E. M. P., White, S. V., O'Mahony, S. M., Bayer, A. J., & Hubbard, R. E. (2012). The impact of frailty and delirium on mortality in older inpatients. *Age & Ageing*, *41*(3), 412–416. https://doi.org/10.1093/ageing/afs021

Entwistle, M. D., Roe, P. G., Sapsford, D. J., Berrisford, R. G., & Jones, J. G. (1991). Patterns of oxygenation after thoracotomy. *British Journal of Anaesthesia*, *67*(6), 704–711. https://doi.org/10.1093/bja/67.6.704

Evered, L. A., Silbert, B. S., Scott, D. A., Maruff, P., Ames, D., & Choong, P. F. (2011). Preexisting cognitive impairment and mild cognitive impairment in subjects presenting for total hip joint replacement. *Anesthesiology: The Journal of the American Society of Anesthesiologists, 114*(6), 1297–1304. https://doi.org/10.1097/ALN.0b013e31821b1aab

Evered, L., Silbert, B., Knopman, D. S., Scott, D. A., DeKosky, S. T., Rasmussen, L. S., . . . Xie, Z. (2018). Recommendations for the nomenclature of cognitive change associated with anaesthesia and surgery—2018. *British Journal of Anaesthesia, 121*(5), 1005–1012. https://doi.org/10.1016/j.bja.2017.11.087

Fabian, T. C. (1993). Unraveling the fat embolism syndrome. *New England Journal of Medicine, 329*(13), 961–963. https://doi.org/10.1056/NEJM199309233291313

Feinberg, M. (1993). The problems of anticholinergic adverse effects in older patients. *Drugs & Aging, 3*(4), 335–348. https://doi.org/10.2165/00002512-199303040-00004

Fodale, V., Quattrone, D., Trecroci, C., Caminiti, V., & Santamaria, L. B. (2006). Alzheimer's disease and anaesthesia: implications for the central cholinergic system. *BJA: British Journal of Anaesthesia, 97*(4), 445–452.

Folstein, M. F., Robins, L. N., & Helzer, J. E. (1983). The mini-mental state examination. *Archives of general psychiatry, 40*(7), 812–812.

Forteza, A. M., Koch, S., Romano, J. G., Zych, G., Bustillo, I. C., Duncan, R. C., & Babikian, V. L. (1999). Transcranial doppler detection of fat emboli. *Stroke, 30*(12), 2687–2691.

Freter, S. H. (2005). Predicting post-operative delirium in elective orthopaedic patients: The Delirium Elderly At-Risk (DEAR) instrument. *Age & Ageing, 34*(2), 169–171. https://doi.org/10.1093/ageing/afh245

Fried, L. P., Tangen, C. M., Walston, J., Newman, A. B., Hirsch, C., Gottdiener, J., . . . McBurnie, M. A. (2001). Frailty in older adults: Evidence for a phenotype. *Journals of Gerontology Series A: Biological Sciences and Medical Sciences, 56*(3), M146–M157. https://doi.org/10.1093/gerona/56.3.M146

Fried, T. R., O'Leary, J., Towle, V., Goldstein, M. K., Trentalange, M., & Martin, D. K. (2014). Health outcomes associated with polypharmacy in community-dwelling older adults: A systematic review. *Journal of the American Geriatrics Society, 62*(12), 2261–2272. https://doi.org/10.1111/jgs.13153

Frye, R. L., Kronmal, R., Schaff, H. V., Myers, W. O., & Gersh, B. J. (1992). Stroke in coronary artery bypass graft surgery: an analysis of the CASS experience. *International Journal of Cardiology, 36*(2), 213–221. https://doi.org/10.1016/0167-5273(92)90009-R

Furlaneto, M. E., & Garcez-Leme, L. E. (2006). Delirium in elderly individuals with hip fracture: Causes, incidence, prevalence, and risk factors. *Clinics, 61*(1), 35–40. https://doi.org/10.1590/S1807-59322006000100007

Galvan, V., & Jin, K. (2007). Neurogenesis in the aging brain. *Clinical Interventions in Aging, 2*(4), 605–610.

Gardner, T. J., Horneffer, P. J., Manolio, T. A., Pearson, T. A., Gott, V. L., Baumgartner, W. A., . . . Reitz, B. A. (1985). Stroke following coronary artery bypass grafting: a ten-year study. *The Annals of Thoracic Surgery, 40*(6), 574–581.

Ghoneim, M. M., Hinrichs, J. V., O'Hara, M. W., Mehta, M. P., Pathak, D., Kumar, V., & Clark, C. R. (1988). Comparison of psychologic and cognitive functions after general or regional anesthesia. *Anesthesiology, 69*(4), 507–515.

Giannoudis, P. V., Tzioupis, C., & Pape, H.-C. (2006). Fat embolism: The reaming controversy. *Injury, 37*(4), S50–S58. https://doi.org/10.1016/j.injury.2006.08.040

Giattino, C. M., Gardner, J. E., Sbahi, F. M., Roberts, K. C., Cooter, M., Moretti, E., . . . Brigman, B. E. (2017). Intraoperative frontal alpha-band power correlates with preoperative neurocognitive function in older adults. *Frontiers in systems neuroscience, 11*, 24. https://doi.org/10.3389/fnsys.2017.00024

Glover, P., & Worthley, L. I. (1999). Fat embolism. *Critical Care and Resuscitation, 1*(3), 276–284.

Goto, T., Baba, T., Honma, K., Shibata, Y., Arai, Y., Uozumi, H., & Okuda, T. (2001). Magnetic resonance imaging findings and postoperative neurologic dysfunction in elderly patients undergoing coronary artery bypass grafting. *The Annals of Thoracic Surgery, 72*(1), 137–142.

Govier, A. V., Reves, J. G., McKay, R. D., Karp, R. B., Zorn, G. L., Morawetz, R. B., . . . Freeman, A. M. (1984). Factors and their influence on regional cerebral blood flow during nonpulsatile cardiopulmonary bypass. *Annals of Thoracic Surgery, 38*(6), 592–600.

Greene, N. H., Attix, D. K., Weldon, B. C., Smith, P. J., McDonagh, D. L., & Monk, T. G. (2009). Measures of executive function and depression identify patients at risk for postoperative delirium. *Anesthesiology, 110*(4), 788–795. https://doi.org/10.1097/ALN.0b013e31819b5ba6

Grigore, A. M., Grocott, H. P., Mathew, J. P., Phillips-Bute, B., Stanley, T. O., Butler, A., . . . Newman, M. F. (2002). The rewarming rate and increased peak temperature alter neurocognitive outcome after cardiac surgery. *Anesthesia & Analgesia, 94*(1), 4. https://doi.org/10.1213/00000539-200201000-00002

Grigore, A. M., Murray, C. F., Ramakrishna, H., & Djaiani, G. (2009). A core review of temperature regimens and neuroprotection during cardiopulmonary bypass: Does rewarming rate matter? *Anesthesia & Analgesia, 109*(6), 1741. https://doi.org/10.1213/ANE.0b013e3181c04fea

Hardcastle, C., Huang, H., Crowley, S. J., Tanner, J. J., Hernaiz, C., Rice, M., . . . Price, C. C. (2019). Mild cognitive impairment and decline in resting state functional connectivity after total knee arthroplasty with general anesthesia. *Journal of Alzheimer's Disease, 69*(4), 1003–1018.

Hernaiz, C., Tanner, J. J., Wiggins, M. E., Sinha, P., Parvataneni, H., Seubert, C., . . . Price, C. C. (2019). Preoperative cognitive reserve and brain integrity predict two-channel EEG intraindividual variability from time of tourniquet up to tourniquet down during total knee arthroplasty. *PLoS One, 14*(5), e0216209.

Ho, P. M., Masoudi, F. A., Peterson, P. N., Shroyer, A. L., McCarthy, M., Grover, F. L., . . . Rumsfeld, J. S. (2005). Health-related quality of life predicts mortality in older but not younger patients following cardiac surgery. *American Journal of Geriatric Cardiology, 14*(4), 176–182.

Huang, H., Tanner, J. J., Parvataneni, H., Rice, M., Horgas, A., Ding, M., & Price, C. (2018). Impact of total knee arthroplasty with general anesthesia on brain networks: Cognitive efficiency and ventricular volume predict functional connectivity decline in older adults. *Journal of Alzheimer's Disease, 62*(1), 319–333. https://doi.org/10.3233/JAD-170496

Jones, M. J., Piggott, S. E., Vaughan, R. S., Bayer, A. J., Newcombe, R. G., Twining, T. C., . . . Rosen, M. (1990). Cognitive and functional competence after anaesthesia in patients aged over 60: Controlled trial of general and regional anaesthesia for elective hip or knee replacement. *BMJ, 300*(6741), 1683–1687.

Juliebø, V., Bjøro, K., Krogseth, M., Skovlund, E., Ranhoff, A. H., & Wyller, T. B. (2009). Risk factors for preoperative and postoperative delirium in elderly patients with hip fracture. *Journal of the American Geriatrics Society*, *57*(8), 1354–1361. https://doi.org/10.1111/j.1532-5415.2009.02377.x

Jung, P., Pereira, M. A., Hiebert, B., Song, X., Rockwood, K., Tangri, N., & Arora, R. C. (2015). The impact of frailty on postoperative delirium in cardiac surgery patients. *Journal of Thoracic and Cardiovascular Surgery*, *149*(3), 869–875.e2. https://doi.org/10.1016/j.jtcvs.2014.10.118

Kim, S.-M., Moon, Y.-W., Lim, S.-J., Yoon, B.-K., Min, Y.-K., Lee, D.-Y., & Park, Y.-S. (2012). Prediction of survival, second fracture, and functional recovery following the first hip fracture surgery in elderly patients. *Bone*, *50*(6), 1343–1350. https://doi.org/10.1016/j.bone.2012.02.633

Koessler, M., & Pitto, R. (2002). Fat embolism and cerebral function in total hip arthroplasty. *International Orthopaedics*, *26*(5), 259–262. https://doi.org/10.1007/s00264-002-0380-2

Lee, H. B., Mears, S. C., Rosenberg, P. B., Leoutsakos, J.-M. S., Gottschalk, A., & Sieber, F. E. (2011). Predisposing factors for postoperative delirium after hip fracture repair in individuals with and without dementia. *Journal of the American Geriatrics Society*, *59*(12), 2306–2313. https://doi.org/10.1111/j.1532-5415.2011.03725.x

Lee, T. A., Wolozin, B., Weiss, K. B., & Bednar, M. M. (2005). Assessment of the emergence of Alzheimer's disease following coronary artery bypass graft surgery or percutaneous transluminal coronary angioplasty. *Journal of Alzheimer's Disease*, *7*(4), 319–324.

Lenz, A., Franklin, G. A., & Cheadle, W. G. (2007). Systemic inflammation after trauma. *Injury*, *38*(12), 1336–1345. https://doi.org/10.1016/j.injury.2007.10.003

Leung, J. M., Sands, L. P., Wang, Y., Poon, A., Kwok, P., Kane, J., & Pullinger, C. (2007). Apolipoprotein E e4 allele increases the risk of early postoperative delirium in older patients undergoing noncardiac surgery. *Anesthesiology*, *107*(3), 406–411.

Leung, J. M., Tsai, T. L., & Sands, L. P. (2011). Preoperative frailty in older surgical patients is associated with early postoperative delirium. *Anesthesia and Analgesia*, *112*(5), 1199–1201. https://doi.org/10.1213/ANE.0b013e31820c7c06

Libon, D. J., Malamut, B. L., Swenson, R., Sands, L. P., & Cloud, B. S. (1996). Further analyses of clock drawings among demented and nondemented older subjects. *Archives of Clinical Neuropsychology*, *11*(3), 193–205.

Luck, T., Then, F. S., Schroeter, M. L., Witte, V., Engel, C., Loeffler, M., . . . Riedel-Heller, S. G. (2017). Prevalence of DSM-5 mild neurocognitive disorder in dementia-free older adults: results of the population-based LIFE-adult-study. *The American Journal of Geriatric Psychiatry*, *25*(4), 328–339. https://doi.org/10.1016/j.jagp.2016.07.001

Marcantonio, E. R., Goldman, L., Orav, E. J., Cook, E. F., & Lee, T. H. (1998). The association of intraoperative factors with the development of postoperative delirium. *American Journal of Medicine*, *105*, 380–384.

Marion, D. W., Obrist, W. D., Carlier, P. M., Penrod, L. E., & Darby, J. M. (1993). The use of moderate therapeutic hypothermia for patients with severe head injuries: A preliminary report. *Journal of Neurosurgery*, *79*(3), 354–362.

Mazul-Sunko, B., Hromatko, I., Tadinac, M., Sekulić, A., Ivanec, Z., Gvozdenović, A., . . . Lovricević, I. (2010). Subclinical neurocognitive dysfunction after carotid endarterectomy-the impact of shunting. *Journal of Neurosurgical Anesthesiology*, *22*(3), 195–201. https://doi.org/10.1097/ANA.0b013e3181d5e421

Modini, C., Romagnoli, F., Milito, R. D., Romeo, V., Petroni, R., Torre, F. L., & Catani, M. (2012). Octogenarians: An increasing challenge for acute care and colorectal surgeons.

An outcomes analysis of emergency colorectal surgery in the elderly. *Colorectal Disease, 14*(6), e312–e318. https://doi.org/10.1111/j.1463-1318.2012.02934.x

Moller, J., Cluitmans, P., Rasmussen, L., Houx, P., Rasmussen, H., Canet, J., . . . Gravenstein, J. (1998). Long-term postoperative cognitive dysfunction in the elderly: ISPOCD1 study. *Lancet, 351*(9106), 857–861. https://doi.org/10.1016/S0140-6736(97)07382-0

Moller, J. T., Svennild, I., Johannessen, N. W., Jensen, P. F., Espersen, K., Gravenstein, J. S., . . . Johansen, S. H. (1993). Perioperative monitoring with pulse oximetry and late postoperative cognitive dysfunction. *British Journal of Anaesthesia, 71*(3), 340–347. https://doi.org/10.1093/bja/71.3.340

Monk, T. G., Weldon, B. C., Garvan, C. W., Dede, D. E., Aa, M. T. van der, Heilman, K. M., & Gravenstein, J. S. (2008). Predictors of cognitive dysfunction after major noncardiac surgery. *Anesthesiology, 108*(1), 18–30. https://doi.org/10.1097/01.anes.0000296071.19434.1e

Moretti, D. V. (2015a). Conversion of mild cognitive impairment patients in Alzheimer's disease: Prognostic value of Alpha3/Alpha2 electroencephalographic rhythms power ratio. *Alzheimer's Research & Therapy, 7*(1). https://doi.org/10.1186/s13195-015-0162-x

Moretti, D. V. (2015b). Theta and alpha EEG frequency interplay in subjects with mild cognitive impairment: Evidence from EEG, MRI, and SPECT brain modifications. *Frontiers in Aging Neuroscience, 20*(7).

Nashef, S. A. M., Roques, F., Sharples, L. D., Nilsson, J., Smith, C., Goldstone, A. R., & Lockowandt, U. (2012). EuroSCORE II. *European Journal of Cardio-Thoracic Surgery, 41*(4), 734–745. https://doi.org/10.1093/ejcts/ezs043

Ness, J., Hoth, A., Barnett, M. J., Shorr, R. I., & Kaboli, P. J. (2006). Anticholinergic medications in community-dwelling older veterans: Prevalence of anticholinergic symptoms, symptom burden, and adverse drug events. *American Journal of Geriatric Pharmacotherapy, 4*(1), 42–51. https://doi.org/10.1016/j.amjopharm.2006.03.008

Neuman, H. B., O'Connor, E. S., Weiss, J., LoConte, N. K., Greenblatt, D. Y., Greenberg, C. C., & Smith, M. A. (2013). Surgical treatment of colon cancer in patients aged 80 years and older. *Cancer, 119*(3), 639–647. https://doi.org/10.1002/cncr.27765

Newman, M. F., Croughwell, N. D., Blumenthal, J. A., Lowry, E., White, W. D., Spillane, W., . . . Reves, J. G. (1995). Predictors of cognitive decline after cardiac operation. *The Annals of Thoracic Surgery, 59*(5), 1326–1330.

Newman, A. B., Gottdiener, J. S., McBurnie, M. A., Hirsch, C. H., Kop, W. J., Tracy, R., . . . Fried, L. P. (2001). Associations of subclinical cardiovascular disease with frailty. *The Journals of Gerontology Series A: Biological Sciences and Medical Sciences, 56*(3), M158–M166.

Nielson, W. R., Gelb, A. W., Casey, J. E., Penny, F. J., Merchant, R. N., & Manninen, P. H. (1990). Long-term cognitive and social sequelae of general versus regional anesthesia during arthroplasty in the elderly. *Anesthesiology, 73*(6), 1103–1109.

Oldenbeuving, A. W., de Kort, P. L. M., Kappelle, L. J., van Dujin, C. M., & Roks, G. (2013). Delirium in the acute phase after stroke and the role of the apolipoprotein E gene. *The American Journal of Geriatric Psychiatry, 21*(10), 935–937.

Oresanya, L. B., Lyons, W. L., & Finlayson, E. (2014). Preoperative assessment of the older patient: A narrative review. *JAMA, 311*(20), 2110–2120. https://doi.org/10.1001/jama.2014.4573

Otomo, S., Maekawa, K., Goto, T., Baba, T., & Yoshitake, A. (2013). Pre-existing cerebral infarcts as a risk factor for delirium after coronary artery bypass graft surgery.

Interactive CardioVascular and Thoracic Surgery, 17(5), 799–804. https://doi.org/10.1093/icvts/ivt304

Perucho, J., Rubio, I., Casarejos, M. J., Gomez, A., Rodriguez-Navarro, J. A., Solano, R. M., . . . Mena, M. A. (2010). Anesthesia with isoflurane increases amyloid pathology in mice models of Alzheimer's disease. *Journal of Alzheimer's Disease, 19*(4), 1245–1257. https://doi.org/10.3233/JAD-2010-1318

Price, C. C., Tanner, J. J., Schmalfuss, I., Garvan, C. W., Gearen, P., Dickey, D., . . . Bowers, D. (2014). A pilot study evaluating presurgery neuroanatomical biomarkers for postoperative cognitive decline after total knee arthroplasty in older adults. *Anesthesiology: The Journal of the American Society of Anesthesiologists, 120*(3), 601–613.

Price, C. C., Garvan, C., Hizel, L. P., Lopez, M. G., & Billings, F. T. (2017). Delayed recall and working memory MMSE domains predict delirium following cardiac surgery. *Journal of Alzheimer's Disease, 59*(3), 1027–1035. https://doi.org/10.3233/JAD-170380

Pugsley, W., Treasure, T., Klinger, L., Newman, S., Pascalis, C., & Harrison, M. (1990). Microemboli and cerebral impairment during cardiac surgery. *Journal of Vascular Surgery, 24*, 34–43.

Rampil, I. J. (1998). A primer for EEG signal processing in anesthesia. *Anesthesiology, 89*(4), 980–1002.

Rasmussen, L. S., Johnson, T., Kuipers, H. M., Kristensen, D., Siersma, V. D., Vila, P., . . . Moller, J. T. (2003). Does anaesthesia cause postoperative cognitive dysfunction? A randomised study of regional versus general anaesthesia in 438 elderly patients. *Acta Anaesthesiologica Scandinavica, 47*(3), 260–266. https://doi.org/10.1034/j.1399-6576.2003.00057.x

Rawle, M. J., Cooper, R., Kuh, D., & Richards, M. (2018). Associations between polypharmacy and cognitive and physical capability: A British birth cohort study. *Journal of the American Geriatrics Society, 66*(5), 916–923. https://doi.org/10.1111/jgs.15317

Rodriguez, R. A., Tellier, A., Grabowski, J., Fazekas, A., Turek, M., Miller, D., . . . Giachino, A. (2005). Cognitive dysfunction after total knee arthroplasty. *Journal of Arthroplasty, 20*(6), 763–771. https://doi.org/10.1016/j.arth.2005.05.004

Rossini, P. M., Buscema, M., Capriotti, M., Grossi, E., Rodriguez, G., Del Percio, C., & Babiloni, C. (2008). Is it possible to automatically distinguish resting EEG data of normal elderly vs. mild cognitive impairment subjects with high degree of accuracy? *Clinical Neurophysiology, 119*(7), 1534–1545. https://doi.org/10.1016/j.clinph.2008.03.026

Rudolph, J. L., Jones, R. N., Rasmussen, L. S., Silverstein, J. H., Inouye, S. K., & Marcantonio, E. R. (2007). Independent vascular and cognitive risk factors for postoperative delirium. *American Journal of Medicine, 120*(9), 807–813. https://doi.org/10.1016/j.amjmed.2007.02.026

Sahu, B., Chauhan, S., Kiran, U., Bisoi, A., Lakshmy, R., Selvaraj, T., & Nehra, A. (2009). Neurocognitive function in patients undergoing coronary artery bypass graft surgery with cardiopulmonary bypass: The effect of two different rewarming strategies. *Journal of Cardiothoracic and Vascular Anesthesia, 23*(1), 14–21. https://doi.org/10.1053/j.jvca.2008.07.010

Schaller, F., Sidelnikov, E., Theiler, R., Egli, A., Staehelin, H. B., Dick, W., . . . Bischoff-Ferrari, H. A. (2012). Mild to moderate cognitive impairment is a major risk factor for mortality and nursing home admission in the first year after hip fracture. *Bone, 51*(3), 347–352. https://doi.org/10.1016/j.bone.2012.06.004

Schliebs, R., & Arendt, T. (2011). The cholinergic system in aging and neuronal degeneration. *Behavioural Brain Research*, *221*(2), 555–563. https://doi.org/10.1016/j.bbr.2010.11.058

Sealy, W. C., Brown, I. W., & Young, W. G. (1958). A report on the use of both extracorporeal circulation and hypothermia for open heart surgery. *Annals of Surgery*, *147*(5), 603–613.

Sessums, L. L., Zembrzuska, H., & Jackson, J. L. (2011). Does this patient have medical decision-making capacity? *JAMA*, *306*(4), 420–427. https://doi.org/10.1001/jama.2011.1023

Shin, K. S., Kim, J. S., Kim, S. N., Hong, K. S., O'Donnell, B. F., Chung, C. K., & Kwon, J. S. (2015). Intraindividual neurophysiological variability in ultra-high-risk for psychosis and schizophrenia patients: Single-trial analysis. *Npj Schizophrenia*, *1*(1). https://doi.org/10.1038/npjschz.2015.31

Sieber, F. E., Zakriya, K. J., Gottschalk, A., Blute, M.-R., Lee, H. B., Rosenberg, P. B., & Mears, S. C. (2010). Sedation depth during spinal anesthesia and the development of postoperative delirium in elderly patients undergoing hip fracture repair. *Mayo Clinic Proceedings*, *85*(1), 18–26. https://doi.org/10.4065/mcp.2009.0469

Song, X., Mitnitski, A., & Rockwood, K. (2010). Prevalence and 10-year outcomes of frailty in older adults in relation to deficit accumulation. *Journal of the American Geriatrics Society*, *58*(4), 681–687. https://doi.org/10.1111/j.1532-5415.2010.02764.x

Stern, Y. (2009). Cognitive reserve. *Neuropsychologia*, *47*(10), 2015–2028. https://doi.org/10.1016/j.neuropsychologia.2009.03.004

Stump, D.A., Tegeler, C. H., Newman, S. P., Wallenhaupt, S., & Roy, R. C. (1992). Older patients have more emboli during coronary artery bypass graft surgery. *Anesthesiology*, *77*, A52.

Stump, D. A., Rogers, A. T., Hammon, J. W., & Newman, S. P. (1996). Cerebral emboli and cognitive outcome after cardiac surgery. *Journal of Cardiothoracic and Vascular Anesthesia*, *10*(1), 113–119. https://doi.org/10.1016/S1053-0770(96)80186-8

Talucci, R. C., Manning, J., Lampard, S., Bach, A., & Carrico, C. J. (1983). Early intramedullary nailing of femoral shaft fractures: A cause of fat embolism syndrome. *American Journal of Surgery*, *146*(1), 107–111.

Tardiff, B. E., Newman, M. F., Saunders, A. M., Strittmatter, W. J., Blumenthal, J. A., White, W. D., . . . Reves, J. G. (1997). Preliminary report of a genetic basis for cognitive decline after cardiac operations. *Annals of Thoracic Surgery*, *64*, 715–720.

Tuman, K. J., McCarthy, R. J., Najafi, H., & Ivankovich, A. D. (1992). Differential effects of advanced age on neurologic and cardiac risks of coronary artery operations. *The Journal of Thoracic and Cardiovascular Surgery*, *104*(6), 1510–1517.

Tune, L. E. (2001). Anticholinergic effects of medication in elderly patients. *Journal of Clinical Psychiatry*, *62*(Suppl 21), 11–14.

van Munster, B. C., Korevaar, J. C., Zwinderman, A. H., Leeflang, M. M., & de Rooij, S. E. J. A. (2009). The association between delirium and the apolipoprotein e epsilon 4 allele: New study results and a meta-analysis. *American Journal of Geriatric Psychiatry*, *17*(10), 856–862.

Vasunilashorn, S., Ngo, L., Kosar, C. M., Fong, T. G., Jones, R. N., Inouye, S. K., & Marcantonio, E. R. (2015). Does apolipoprotein E genotype increase risk of postoperative delirium? *American Journal of Geriatric Psychiatry*, *23*(10), 1029–1037. https://doi.org/10.1016/j.jagp.2014.12.192

Xie, Z., Culley, D. J., Dong, Y., Zhang, G., Zhang, B., Moir, R. D., . . . Tanzi, R. E. (2008). The common inhalation anesthetic isoflurane induces caspase activation and increases amyloid β-protein level in vivo. *Annals of Neurology*, *64*(6), 618–627. https://doi.org/10.1002/ana.21548

Xie, Z., Dong, Y., Maeda, U., Alfille, P., Culley, D. J., Crosby, G., & Tanzi, R. E. (2006). The common inhalation anesthetic isoflurane induces apoptosis and increases amyloid β protein levels. *Anesthesiology*, *104*(5), 988–994.

Xu, G.-H., Zhang, Q.-M., Chen, C., Shen, Q.-Y., Liu, X.-S., Shi, J.-F., . . . Wang, K. (2016). Comparison of the type and severity of early attentional network decline after total intravenous or epidural anesthesia in middle-aged women after gynecological surgery. *International Clinical Psychopharmacology*, *31*(5), 293–299. https://doi.org/10.1097/YIC.0000000000000129

Zhan, X., Fahlman, C. S., & Bickler, P. (2006). Isoflurane neuroprotection in rat hippocampal slices decreases with aging: Changes in intracellular Ca2+ regulation and *N*-methyl-d-aspartate receptor–mediated Ca2+ influx. *Anesthesiology*, *104*, 995–1003.

Zhang, B., Tian, M., Zheng, H., Zhen, Y., Yue, Y., Li, T., . . . Xie, Z. (2013). Effects of anesthetic isoflurane and desflurane on human cerebrospinal fluid Aβ and τ level. *Anesthesiology*, *119*(1), 52–60. https://doi.org/10.1097/ALN.0b013e31828ce55d

Zhang, Y., Xu, Z., Wang, H., Dong, Y., Shi, H. N., Culley, D. J., . . . Xie, Z. (2012). Anesthetics isoflurane and desflurane differently affect mitochondrial function, learning, and memory. *Annals of Neurology*, *71*(5), 687–698. https://doi.org/10.1002/ana.23536

18
Management of Mild Cognitive Impairment

Ramit Ravona-Springer and Amos D. Korczyn

1. Introduction

Mild cognitive impairment (MCI) is considered an intermediate state between normal aging and dementia. In light of increasing awareness of the need for preventive treatment strategies in patients that are not yet clinically demented, patients diagnosed with MCI may be an important population to target for treatment. However, MCI is a heterogeneous entity with multiple etiologies (see Chapter 2 of this volume), different clinical presentations (e.g., amnestic, executive, mixed), and varying diagnostic criteria (Ash & Korczyn, 2011). There is also variability in clinical outcomes over time regarding rates of progression. An MCI diagnosis generally means that the patient, while not demented, has some recently acquired neurocognitive deficits that may be predictive of further neurocognitive and functional decline and dementia. Diagnosing patients with MCI may have a detrimental effect as the patient may interpret this as meaning that he or she is on an accelerated downhill slope while, in fact, a significant number of people who are diagnosed as having MCI may maintain stability or revert to normality (Canevelli et al., 2016). However, patients and their family's awareness of this diagnosis may benefit from detailed diagnostic work-up, ongoing monitoring, support, and treatment, if available, to help with significant functional and health-care–related decisions.

2. Possible Interventions

Mixed results have been reported regarding the efficacy of pharmacological treatment or food supplements aimed at improving neurocognitive function in MCI or preventing conversion to dementia (Farina, Llewellyn, Isaac, & Tabet, 2017; Fitzpatrick-Lewis, Warren, Ali, Sherifali, & Raina, 2015; M.-M. Li et al., 2014; Yang, Wang, Sun, Zhang, & Liu, 2016). As will be discussed later, this literature is likely complex due to the heterogeneity of presentation in various types

Ramit Ravona-Springer and Amos D. Korczyn, *Management of Mild Cognitive Impairment* In: *Vascular Disease, Alzheimer's Disease, and Mild Cognitive Impairment*. Edited by: David J. Libon, Melissa Lamar, Rodney A. Swenson, Kenneth M. Heilman, Oxford University Press (2020).
DOI: 10.1093/oso/9780190634230.003.0019

of MCI and dementia. In addition, there is evidence to support the efficacy of nonpharmacological interventions in patients with MCI such as mental activity, aerobic exercise, and better management of cardiovascular risk factors (Hong, Jang, Hwang, Roh, & Lee, 2015; Langa & Levine, 2014; Ströhle et al., 2015; Wang et al., 2014).

3. Heterogeneity of Clinical Phenotype

Some clinical phenotypes of MCI may be at higher risk for future conversion to dementia than others. For example, presence of neuropsychiatric symptoms, specifically depression and apathy (Teng, Lu, & Cummings, 2007), lack of insight (Roberts, Clare, & Woods, 2009), subtle gait abnormalities including falls, and brain alterations as seen on computed tomography (CT) or magnetic resonance imaging (MRI) studies (Serra et al., 2016) have all been associated with higher risk for conversion to dementia.

In addition to AD-related neuropathology, many other processes affecting the brain may cause neurocognitive impairment, each with its own prognosis (Abner et al., 2017; Brenowitz et al., 2017). The situation is even more complicated in that significant number of patients show mixed pathology, including amyloid and neurofibrillary deposits, vascular changes, synucleinopathy, and other neuropathological changes. In one clinical-pathological study, only 41% of the variability in cognitive decline was explained by these neuropathologies (Wilson et al., 2013). Thus, it cannot be expected that any single intervention would necessarily stop decline in all cases.

4. Clinical Evaluation

Patients with MCI need to be evaluated for the presence of treatable causes that could account for neurocognitive decline, such as vitamin deficiency, including thiamine, B-12, and vitamin D, folic acid; thyroid dysfunction; infection; and other systemic/metabolic organ system that may affect neurocognitive abilities. Brain imaging with MRI or CT should always be considered to rule out structural disease and/or assess the form of atrophic changes. Positron emission tomography studies for amyloid and tau, as well as a lumbar puncture with analysis of the cerebral spinal fluid, can help determine the probability of developing dementia such as AD. In addition, there are many treatable diseases that can also cause MCI (e.g., organ failure, chronic meningitis, autoimmune diseases, etc.). Therefore, a careful medical evaluation is a necessary component for any patient who presents with suspected neurocognitive alterations.

5. Importance of Neuropsychiatric Assessment

Consideration should also be given to the patients' psychosocial status (e.g., a person living by himself or herself should be evaluated for possible dietary insufficiency, alcoholism, social isolation and depression, each of which are potentially treatable conditions). A neuropsychiatric evaluation may identify depression, apathy, or anxiety. All of these problems are amenable to treatment and may also serve as markers for future neurocognitive decline. Both patient and informant interview should be part of any neuropsychiatric evaluation. The clinician should learn if the patient's complaints (or lack of) are disproportionate to the actual objective abnormalities and/or caregiver's report. Patient complaints that are mild in comparison to objective abnormalities (anosodiaphoria) or denial (anosognosia) may suggest that the patient lacks insight, a common phenomenon in dementia and MCI (Roberts et al., 2009). The presence of these disorders may reflect the extent of neurocognitive decline and may be associated with higher risk for incipient dementia or, alternatively, may reflect psychological denial. Conversely, subjective complaints that are worse than performance on objective tests may reflect the presence of anxiety or depression, leading to a different therapeutic strategy.

6. Interventions

A common approach to develop drug intervention is to create an animal model of MCI-AD (i.e., MCI that will progress to dementia). Unfortunately, animal models are often based on a narrow conceptualization of underlying disease mechanisms (Y. Li, 2013), mainly the amyloid cascade hypothesis, and do not take into consideration the increasing evidence of neuropathological heterogeneity. As previously stated, many patients with MCI likely present with mixed underlying neuropathology (Korczyn, 2006; Schneider, Aggarwal, Barnes, Boyle, & Bennett, 2009). A question that has been addressed is how different underlying neuropathological and other medical processes interact and how this modifies putative treatment.

6.1. Medications

The U.S. Food and Drug Administration registers studies done for various purposes (https://clinicaltrials.gov/). Among them are over 100 formal studies aimed at treating MCI patients. These studies employ drugs of various chemical structures, including antiamyloid antibodies, γ and β secretase inhibitors, cholinesterase inhibitors such as donepezil, rivastigmine, galantamine, and ladostigil. *N*-methyl-D-aspartate receptor antagonists such as memantine, monoamine oxidase-B inhibitors, stimulants (methylphenidate, atomoxetine), melatonin, cilostazol, the iron chelator deferiprone, the antidiabetic pioglitazone, and more. Although there have been many negative findings, several papers exploring this area offer some clues for potential improvement in demonstrating benefit from medication attempts.

Studies have revealed some effectiveness in treatment with donezepil alone or when combined with memantine in reducing the level of neurocognitive decline when compared to untreated patients, with additional benefit in reducing caregiver burden in patient groups with mild/moderate AD (Fillit, Gutterman, & Brooks, 2000; Hashimoto, Yatabe, Kaneda, Honda, & Ikeda, 2009) as well is in patients with vascular dementia (Black et al., 2003). A systematic review and meta-analysis of combination treatment for AD with donepezil and memantine revealed only small, but significant, effect sizes were found favoring combination therapy for patients with moderate to severe AD (Knapp et al., 2016).

These data suggest that if some beneficial effects have been noted in patients with dementia, earlier intervention with using these agents in MCI might also prove efficacious. A meta-analysis addressing whether medications like donepezil would delay conversion from MCI to AD found that long-term use may attenuate the risk of progression to AD/dementia (Lee et al., 2015). Nonetheless results have not been overly dramatic.

An intriguing study by Edmonds et al. (2018) underscores the presence of diagnostic error in the original donepezil/vitamin E drug trial. By using actuarial based neuropsychological criteria to eliminate patient classification approximately one third of patients diagnosed with MCI were actually determined to be false positives. Once these patients were removed from an original sample, it was determined that treatment with donepezil was associated with a significantly lower rate of progression to AD dementia over a 3-year period. In addition, Jak et al. (2009) have done pioneering work showing that utilizing precision-based neuropsychological criteria for determining MCI diagnostic groups (as compared to conventional Petersen/Winblad criteria as operationalized by the Alzheimer's Disease Neuroimaging Initiative) not only greatly improves accurate diagnosis of MCI groups but also results in better determinations of biomarker associations and progression/conversion rates (see Chapter 3 of this volume).

6.2. Cognitive Interventions

The rationale for cognitive intervention as a means to treat or slow the progression of related to neurocognitive decline is associated with higher education and engagement in cognitive activities throughout life (Martin, Clare, Altgassen, Cameron, & Zehnder, 2011). Animal models demonstrate better neurocognitive performance after exposure to richer environments (Gonçalves et al., 2018). However, the exact type of training versus rehabilitation and optimal timing and duration, as well as generalizability of neurocognitive interventions to real life, are yet to be demonstrated. Suggested interventions should likely be personalized to age, pattern of neurocognitive performance, fields of interest, etc. High-level studies are difficult to conduct, and double-blind studies are almost impossible. Nonetheless, patient should be encouraged to be involved in such activities as long as possible. Computer-based methods have been suggested but have not been validated (Klimova, 2016). A potentially prophylactic activity against neurocognitive decline is writing an autobiography (Subramaniam, Woods, & Whitaker, 2014). This is an activity that can involve offspring who are often grateful for this experience.

6.3. Physical Activity

Epidemiological studies suggest that individuals who are involved in recreational physical activity are less likely to develop dementia (Ströhle et al., 2015). Several mechanisms of how recreational physical activity protect against dementia have been suggested like reducing vascular pathology, increasing vertebral blood flow, and, reducing cardiovascular risk (Gallaway et al., 2017).

6.4. Dietary Management

Several epidemiological studies suggest that diet both potentiates and can be used to help manage emergence of neurocognitive decline. The beneficial role of the Mediterranean diet, characterized by high content of olive oil, nuts, vegetables and fruits, legumes, and fish and low content of animal has been shown to be associated with lower risk for dementia, lower MRI white matter hyperintensities, and better neurocognitive functioning (Gu et al., 2015; Lourida et al., 2013; Scarmeas et al., 2011). Regarding the use of alcohol, data suggest that low to moderate use of alcohol may be beneficial. However, exact constituents of food and wine as may be potentially neuroprotective is unknown (Panza et al., 2012). Some food additives, particularly omega-3 have been suggested, but, as reported by Yassine and colleagues (2017), results in clinical trials are inconsistent and probably differ by age and neurocognitive status of participants, duration, and type of intervention and level of consumption of omega-3 prior to intervention. In a recent review, these authors suggested that nondemented apolipoprotein E carriers, but not noncarriers, may benefit from high doses of docosahexaenoic acid, an essential omega-3 fatty acid, for prevention of dementia (Yassine et al., 2017).

6.5. Risk Factor Management

Obesity and diabetes mellitus are known risk factors for MCI and dementia, and therefore weight reduction by calorie restriction and low carbohydrate diets are logical interventions in some cases. Nevertheless, acute weight loss and change in caloric intake in old age may also be harmful. Additional studies are required to understand the exact role of diet, optimal timing and intensity of dietary interventions, and the type of MCI for which these interventions are most expected to be beneficial (Areosa Sastre, Vernooij, González-Colaço Harmand, & Martínez, 2017; Mendiola-Precoma, Berumen, Padilla, & Garcia-Alcocer, 2016; Simó, Ciudin, Simó-Servat, & Hernández, 2017). Hypertension, dyslipidemia, smoking, physical inactivity, depression, and limited social interaction have repeatedly and convincingly been shown to be associated with cognitive decline in old age (Anstey, Eramudugolla, & Dixon, 2014; Norton, Matthews, Barnes, Yaffe, & Brayne, 2014). Similarly, increased risk for incident dementia has been demonstrated in subjects with sleep abnormalities such as obstructive sleep apnea and short sleep duration (Lutsey et al., 2018).

6.6. Brain Stimulation

Attempts to stimulate brain activity using transcranial magnetic stimulation, direct current electrical stimulation, or intracranial electrical stimuli to various brain targets are being tested, but none has been advanced beyond the experimental stage (Birba et al., 2017).

7. Recommendations

At the present time, the clinician working with patients who present with MCI should make efforts to identify an underlying process and consider appropriate treatment, if possible. An excellent summary of evidence-based interventions on modifiable risk factors for neurocognitive decline and dementia has been provided by World Dementia Council (Baumgart et al., 2015). Optimal management of diet and exercise, treating neuropsychiatric problems, and encouraging appropriate psychosocial relationships are likely the best available tools to forestall and/or mitigate neurocognitive decline associated with MCI and dementia.

References

Abner, E. L., Kryscio, R. J., Schmitt, F. A., Fardo, D. W., Moga, D. C., Ighodaro, E. T., . . . Nelson, P. T. (2017). Outcomes after diagnosis of mild cognitive impairment in a large autopsy series. *Annals of Neurology*, *81*(4), 549–559. http://doi.org/10.1002/ana.24903

Anstey, K. J., Eramudugolla, R., & Dixon, R. A. (2014). Contributions of a risk assessment approach to the prevention of Alzheimer's disease and dementia. *Journal of Alzheimer's Disease*, *42*(Suppl 4), S463–S473. http://doi.org/10.3233/JAD-141248

Areosa Sastre, A., Vernooij, R. W., González-Colaço Harmand, M., & Martínez, G. (2017). Effect of the treatment of Type 2 diabetes mellitus on the development of cognitive impairment and dementia. *Cochrane Database of Systematic Reviews*, 6. http://doi.org/10.1002/14651858.CD003804.pub2

Ash, E, & Korczyn, A. D. (2011). Is amnestic mild cognitive impairment a useful concept? *Future Medicine*, *7*(1), 107–122.

Baumgart, M., Snyder, H. M., Carrillo, M. C., Fazio, S., Kim, H., & Johns, H. (2015). Summary of the evidence on modifiable risk factors for cognitive decline and dementia: A population-based perspective. *Alzheimer's & Dementia*, *11*(6), 718–726. http://doi.org/10.1016/j.jalz.2015.05.016

Birba, A., Ibáñez, A., Sedeño, L., Ferrari, J., García, A. M., & Zimerman, M. (2017). Non-invasive brain stimulation: A new strategy in mild cognitive impairment? *Frontiers in Aging Neuroscience*, *9*. http://doi.org/10.3389/fnagi.2017.00016

Black, S., Román, G. C., Geldmacher, D. S., Salloway, S., Hecker, J., Burns, A., . . . Pratt, R. (2003). Efficacy and tolerability of donepezil in vascular dementia: Positive results of a 24-week, multicenter, international, randomized, placebo-controlled clinical trial. *Stroke*, *34*(10), 2323–2330. http://doi.org/10.1161/01.STR.0000091396.95360.E1

Brenowitz, W. D., Hubbard, R. A., Keene, C. D., Hawes, S. E., Longstreth, W. T., Woltjer, R. L., & Kukull, W. A. (2017). Mixed neuropathologies and estimated rates of clinical progression in a large autopsy sample. *Alzheimer's & Dementia*, *13*(6), 654–662. http://doi.org/10.1016/j.jalz.2016.09.015

Canevelli, M., Grande, G., Lacorte, E., Quarchioni, E., Cesari, M., Mariani, C., . . . Vanacore, N. (2016). Spontaneous reversion of mild cognitive impairment to normal cognition: A systematic review of literature and meta-analysis. *Journal of the American Medical Directors Association*, *17*(10), 943–948. http://doi.org/10.1016/j.jamda.2016.06.020

Edmonds, E. C., Ard, M. C., Edland, S. D., Galasko, D. R., Salmon, D. P., & Bondi, M. W. (2018). Unmasking the benefits of donepezil via psychometrically precise identification of mild cognitive impairment: A secondary analysis of the ADCS vitamin E and donepezil in MCI study. *Alzheimer's & Dementia*, *4*, 11–18. http://doi.org/10.1016/j.trci.2017.11.001

Farina, N., Llewellyn, D., Isaac, M. G. E. K. N., & Tabet, N. (2017). Vitamin E for Alzheimer's dementia and mild cognitive impairment. *Cochrane Database of Systematic Reviews, 4*. http://doi.org/10.1002/14651858.CD002854.pub5

Fillit, H. M., Gutterman, E. M., & Brooks, R. L. (2000). Impact of donepezil on caregiving burden for patients with Alzheimer's disease. *International Psychogeriatrics, 12*(3), 389–401. http://doi.org/10.1017/S1041610200006499

Fitzpatrick-Lewis, D., Warren, R., Ali, M. U., Sherifali, D., & Raina, P. (2015). Treatment for mild cognitive impairment: A systematic review and meta-analysis. *CMAJ Open, 3*(4), E419–E427. http://doi.org/10.9778/cmajo.20150057

Gallaway, P., Miyake, H., Buchowski, M., Shimada, M., Yoshitake, Y., Kim, A., & Hongu, N. (2017). Physical activity: A viable way to reduce the risks of mild cognitive impairment, Alzheimer's disease, and vascular dementia in older adults. *Brain Sciences, 7*(12), 22. http://doi.org/10.3390/brainsci7020022

Gonçalves, L. V., Herlinger, A. L., Ferreira, T. A. A., Coitinho, J. B., Pires, R. G. W., & Martins-Silva, C. (2018). Environmental enrichment cognitive neuroprotection in an experimental model of cerebral ischemia: Biochemical and molecular aspects. *Behavioural Brain Research, 348*, 171–183. http://doi.org/10.1016/j.bbr.2018.04.023

Gu, Y., Brickman, A. M., Stern, Y., Habeck, C. G., Razlighi, Q. R., Luchsinger, J. A., . . . Scarmeas, N. (2015). Mediterranean diet and brain structure in a multiethnic elderly cohort. *Neurology, 85*(20), 1744–1751. http://doi.org/10.1212/WNL.0000000000002121

Hashimoto, M., Yatabe, Y., Kaneda, K., Honda, K., & Ikeda, M. (2009). Impact of donepezil hydrochloride on the care burden of family caregivers of patients with Alzheimer's disease. *Psychogeriatrics, 9*(4), 196–203. http://doi.org/10.1111/j.1479-8301.2009.00302.x

Hong, Y. J., Jang, E. H., Hwang, J., Roh, J. H., & Lee, J.-H. (2015). The efficacy of cognitive intervention programs for mild cognitive impairment: A systematic review. *Current Alzheimer Research, 12*(6), 527–542.

Jak, A. J., Bondi, M. W., Delano-Wood, L., Wierenga, C., Corey-Bloom, J., Salmon, D. P., & Delis, D. C. (2009). Quantification of five neuropsychological approaches to defining mild cognitive impairment. *American Journal of Geriatric Psychiatry, 17*(5), 368–375. http://doi.org/10.1097/JGP.0b013e31819431d5

Klimova, B. (2016). Computer-based cognitive training in aging. *Frontiers in Aging Neuroscience, 8*. http://doi.org/10.3389/fnagi.2016.00313

Knapp, M., King, D., Romeo, R., Adams, J., Baldwin, A., Ballard., . . . Howard, R. (2016). Cost-effectiveness of donepezil and memantine in moderate to severe Alzheimer's disease (the DOMINO-AD trial). *Internal Journal of Geriatric Psychiatry, 12*, 1205–1216. http://doi.org/10.1002/gps.4583

Korczyn, A. D. (2006). Mixed dementia: The most common cause of dementia. *Annals of the New York Academy of Sciences, 977*, 129–134.

Langa, K. M., & Levine, D. A. (2014). The diagnosis and management of mild cognitive impairment. *JAMA, 312*(23), 2551. http://doi.org/10.1001/jama.2014.13806

Lee, J. H., Jeong, S. K., Kim, B. C., Park, K. W., & Dash A. (2015). Donepezil across the spectrum of Alzheimer's disease: Dose optimization and clinical relevance. *Acta Neurologica Scandavavia, 131,* 259–67. http://doi.org/10.1111/ane.12386

Li, M.-M., Yu, J.-T., Wang, H.-F., Jiang, T., Wang, J., Meng, X.-F., . . . Tan, L. (2014). Efficacy of vitamins B supplementation on mild cognitive impairment and Alzheimer's disease: A systematic review and meta-analysis. *Current Alzheimer Research, 11*(9), 844–852.

Li, Y. (2013). Establishment of experimental models for Alzheimer's disease research. *International Journal of Neuroscience, 123*(12), 823–831. http://doi.org/10.3109/00207454.2013.804821

Lourida, I., Soni, M., Thompson-Coon, J., Purandare, N., Lang, I. A., Ukoumunne, O. C., & Llewellyn, D. J. (2013). Mediterranean diet, cognitive function, and dementia: A systematic review. *Epidemiology, 24*(4), 479–489. http://doi.org/10.1097/EDE.0b013e3182944410

Lutsey, P. L., Misialek, J. R., Mosley, T. H., Gottesman, R. F., Punjabi, N. M., Shahar, E., . . . Alonso, A. (2018). Sleep characteristics and risk of dementia and Alzheimer's disease: The Atherosclerosis Risk in Communities Study. *Alzheimer's & Dementia, 14*(2), 157–166. http://doi.org/10.1016/j.jalz.2017.06.2269

Martin, M., Clare, L., Altgassen, A. M., Cameron, M. H., & Zehnder, F. (2011). Cognition-based interventions for healthy older people and people with mild cognitive impairment. *Cochrane Database of Systematic Reviews*, 1. http://doi.org/10.1002/14651858.CD006220.pub2

Mendiola-Precoma, J., Berumen, L. C., Padilla, K., & Garcia-Alcocer, G. (2016). Therapies for prevention and treatment of Alzheimer's disease. *BioMed Research International, 2016*(2), 1–17. http://doi.org/10.1155/2016/2589276

Norton, S., Matthews, F. E., Barnes, D. E., Yaffe, K., & Brayne, C. (2014). Potential for primary prevention of Alzheimer's disease: An analysis of population-based data. *Lancet Neurology, 13*(8), 788–794. http://doi.org/10.1016/S1474-4422(14)70136-X

Panza, F., Frisardi, V., Seripa, D., Logroscino, G., Santamato, A., Imbimbo, B. P., . . . Solfrizzi, V. (2012). Alcohol consumption in mild cognitive impairment and dementia: Harmful or neuroprotective? *International Journal of Geriatric Psychiatry, 27*(12), 1218–1238. http://doi.org/10.1002/gps.3772

Roberts, J. L., Clare, L., & Woods, R. T. (2009). Subjective memory complaints and awareness of memory functioning in mild cognitive impairment: A systematic review. *Dementia and Geriatric Cognitive Disorders, 28*(2), 95–109. http://doi.org/10.1159/000234911

Scarmeas, N., Luchsinger, J. A., Stern, Y., Gu, Y., He, J., DeCarli, C., . . . Brickman, A. M. (2011). Mediterranean diet and magnetic resonance imaging-assessed cerebrovascular disease. *Annals of Neurology, 69*(2), 257–268. http://doi.org/10.1002/ana.22317

Schneider, J. A., Aggarwal, N. T., Barnes, L., Boyle, P., & Bennett, D. A. (2009). The neuropathology of older persons with and without dementia from community versus clinic cohorts. *Journal of Alzheimer's Disease, 18*(3), 691–701. http://doi.org/10.3233/JAD-2009-1227

Serra, L., Cercignani, M., Mastropasqua, C., Torso, M., Spano, B., Makovac, E., . . . Bozzali, M. (2016). Longitudinal changes in functional brain connectivity predicts conversion to Alzheimer's disease. *Journal of Alzheimer's Disease, 51*(2), 377–389. http://doi.org/10.3233/JAD-150961

Simó, R., Ciudin, A., Simó-Servat, O., & Hernández, C. (2017). Cognitive impairment and dementia: A new emerging complication of type 2 diabetes—The diabetologist's perspective. *Acta Diabetologica, 54*(5), 417–424. http://doi.org/10.1007/s00592-017-0970-5

Ströhle, A., Schmidt, D. K., Schultz, F., Fricke, N., Staden, T., Hellweg, R., . . . Rieckmann, N. (2015). Drug and exercise treatment of Alzheimer disease and mild cognitive impairment: A systematic review and meta-analysis of effects on cognition in randomized controlled trials. *American Journal of Geriatric Psychiatry*, *23*(12), 1234–1249. http://doi.org/10.1016/j.jagp.2015.07.007

Subramaniam, P., Woods, B., & Whitaker, C. (2014). Life review and life story books for people with mild to moderate dementia: A randomised controlled trial. *Aging & Mental Health*, *18*(3), 363–375. http://doi.org/10.1080/13607863.2013.837144

Teng, E., Lu, P. H., & Cummings, J. L. (2007). Neuropsychiatric symptoms are associated with progression from mild cognitive impairment to Alzheimer's disease. *Dementia and Geriatric Cognitive Disorders*, *24*(4), 253–259. http://doi.org/10.1159/000107100

Wang, C., Yu, J.-T., Wang, H.-F., Tan, C.-C., Meng, X.-F., & Tan, L. (2014). Non-pharmacological interventions for patients with mild cognitive impairment: A meta-analysis of randomized controlled trials of cognition-based and exercise interventions. *Journal of Alzheimer's Disease*, *42*(2), 663–678. http://doi.org/10.3233/JAD-140660

Wilson, R. S., Boyle, P. A., Yu, L., Barnes, L. L., Schneider, J. A., & Bennett, D. A. (2013). Life-span cognitive activity, neuropathologic burden, and cognitive aging. *Neurology*, *81*(4), 314–321. http://doi.org/10.1212/WNL.0b013e31829c5e8a

Yang, G., Wang, Y., Sun, J., Zhang, K., & Liu, J. (2016). Ginkgo biloba for mild cognitive impairment and Alzheimer's disease: A systematic review and meta-analysis of randomized controlled trials. *Current Topics in Medicinal Chemistry*, *16*(5), 520–528.

Yassine, H. N., Braskie, M. N., Mack, W. J., Castor, K. J., Fonteh, A. N., Schneider, L. S., . . . Chui, H. C. (2017). Association of docosahexaenoic acid supplementation with alzheimer disease stage in apolipoprotein E ε4 carriers. *JAMA Neurology*, *74*(3), 339. http://doi.org/10.1001/jamaneurol.2016.4899

Index

Tables, figures and boxes are indicated by *t*, *f* and *b* following the page number

For the benefit of digital users, indexed terms that span two pages (e.g., 52–53) may, on occasion, appear on only one of those pages.

abulia, 166–67
acetylcholinesterase inhibitors, 62
Acosta, L. M., 161–62
action disorganization syndrome. *See* ideational apraxia
action-intentional disorders
  characterization, 164–66
  defective response inhibition, 169
  diseases associated with, 172
  motor impersistence, 169
  motor preservation, 171
  pathophysiology, 173
  stroke and, 172–73
  sub types of, 166–77
activities of daily living (ADL), 103
ADAM-10, 268–69
aging
  age-related neuropathology, 348–50, 349*f*
  cerebrovascular tissue injury neuropathology, 341–45
  hemodynamic impairment patterns in, 307–9
  minority populations, neuropathological assessment, 357
  as surgical risk factor, 435
  vessel pathologies, 336–40, 337*f*
AGS Beers Criteria, 438
akinesia/hypokinesia
  body-centered hemispatial, 166
  clinical signs, 166
  directional/hemispatial, of arm, 168
  endogenously (endo-evoked), 166–68
  exogenously evoked (exo-evoked), 166–68
  hypokinesia, 167, 173
  sub types of, 166
  testing, 167
Albert, M. L., 173
Albert, M. S., 55–56
alcohol consumption
  as CVD risk factor, 10, 13*t*, 18*t*
  gender differences in, 10–11
  MRI studies, 16
Alexander, G. E., 176
Alexander, M. P., 176–77
Alzheimer's disease
  action-intentional disorder-associated, 172–73
  amyloid cascade hypothesis, xv, 31, 275–76, 408
  animal models, 221
  arterial stiffness (*see* arterial stiffness)
  brain structural alterations in, 241–42
  brain volumetry imaging, 209, 211*f*
  cerebral blood flow in, 282–83
  cerebrovascular resistance imaging studies, 287–88
  cerebrovascular resistance in, 284–91, 285*b*, 286*f*, 308–9
  characterization, 274–76, 375–77, 407–8
  conceptual knowledge impairment in, 116
  connectomics, multimodal imaging, 250–52
  context independent *vs.* dependent profiles, 40–41
  cortical signature, 212–13, 214*f*
  cortical thickness studies, 212
  CVD contribution, 213–17
  CVD risk congruence, 247*f*, 247
  CVD risk imaging, 242, 244*t*
  diagnosis *vs.* classification, 45–46
  epidemiology, 3
  genetic forms of, 275–76, 316, 408

Alzheimer's disease (*cont.*)
graphomotor preservation in, 41
gray matter/subcortical structures imaging, 242–47
hemodynamic changes in (*see* hemodynamic impairment)
heterogeneity of, 30
ideational apraxia-associated, 164
ideomotor apraxia-associated, 158
impaired temporal gradients in, 44–45
impairment level in everyday function, 108, 118
lifestyle patterns factors, statistical analyses, 137
memory impairment, statistical analyses, 138–39
microbleeds as predictive, 215–17, 216*f*, 222–23
mitochondrial bioenergetics/oxidative stress in, 410–11
mitochondrial dynamics in, 412–16
mixed, 348–52, 349*f*
neuropathology heterogeneity in, 33–34
neuropathology of, 335–36
neuropsychological heterogeneity in, 38–40
pathological studies, 210–11
pathophysiology, 130, 315–16
phenotypes, latent class analysis, 39
phenotypes, mixed pathology impacts on, 352–54
phenotypes, statistical modeling of, 38
phenotypes statistical modeling, in treatment, 39
profiles, statistical analyses, 134–36, 137, 138–40
protein pathology in MCI, 72
risk/development, 243, 245*t*
service utilization patterns, statistical analyses, 134
sleep patterns, statistical analyses, 134
small subcortical infarcts as predictors, 217*f*, 217, 218*f*, 219*f*
staging criteria, 55
stroke and, 8–9, 223–24
structural MRI applications, 208–9
subgroups, statistical analyses, 134
vascular disease and, 32
vascular dysfunction in regulation of, 34–38
vascular hypothesis, 261–63
vascular risk factors studies, 20–22
verbal concept formation in, 42
visuospatial impairment, statistical analyses, 138
white matter imaging, 248–50, 250*f*
white matter microstructure in, 225
WMHs as predictive, 190, 215*f*, 215, 218–21
Alzheimer's Disease Cooperative Study (ADCS), 62–63
Alzheimer's Disease Neuroimaging Initiative (ADNI), 243–47, 262–63, 281–82, 386–87, 461
amygdala volume studies
AD prediction, 243–47
cerebral blood flow, 282–83
mixed AD neuropathology, 349*f*
MRI, 71
amyloid cascade hypothesis, xv, 31, 275–76, 408
An, X., 88–89
anesthesia. *See also* perioperative cognitive medicine
background, 434
brain–behavior models, 440
case studies, 433–34
dementia and, 439
depth of, 440
emboli, 443
general *vs.* spinal, 442
rewarming rate, 442
animal studies
Alzheimer's disease, 221
ApoE4, 269
cerebral perfusion, 286–87
dementia, 32–33
anterior cingulate cortex volume studies, 114
anterior cingulate gyrus in brain connectivity, 176
anticholinergics as surgical risk factor, 438
antioxidant therapy, 418–19
apolipoprotein ε4 (ApoE4)
animal studies, 269
arterial stiffening relationships, 281

in BBB integrity, 269
cardiovascular risk factors and, 20, 21*t*
cerebrovascular lesions and, 37
CSF albumin index, 263–65
genotype in MCI, 75, 134–35
isoforms in dementia risk, 340
LPA analysis, 61–62
PET imaging, 72–73
as risk factor, 7, 130, 275–76
statistical analyses, 137
as surgical risk factor, 436
APP, 275–76
APP biomarkers, 387
applause test, 171–72
apraxia. *See also specific forms of apraxia by name*
characterization, 147
limb apraxia, task-specific forms of, 148
praxic-movement programs, 146–47
terminology, 103
upper limb apraxia, forms of, 148–49
ARIA/ARIA-E/ARIA-H, 223
ARIC study, 8
arterial spin labeling
AD, cerebral blood flow in, 283
cerebrovascular resistance, 288
hemodynamic impairment, 307
arterial stiffness. *See also* pressure pulsatility
AD, cerebral blood flow in, 282–83
AD pathology and, 281–82
brain, impacts on, 277
cerebrovascular resistance and, 284–90, 285*b*, 286*f*
cerebrovascular resistance imaging studies, 287–88
cognitive decline and, 278–81
as CVD risk factor, 11, 13*t*, 89–90
markers of, 277–78
MRI studies, 16
pathophysiology of, 276–77
arteriosclerosis, 338
atherosclerosis, 351
autoantibody biomarkers, 389–91
autopsy studies, 34
Azarpazhooh, M. R., 34
$A\beta_{42}$, 378–80, 385, 386–87
BACE1 biomarkers, 387
Bailey, H. R., 114
Bangen, K. J., 8–9, 115–16
Barber, R., 386–87
Barrett, A. M., 156–57
basal ganglia networks in brain connectivity, 176
Basso, A., 156–57
BDNF as biomarker, 20–22, 21*t*
Beeber, A. S., 134
Bell-McGinty, S., 71
Benetos, A., 280–81
Bennett, J. A., 161–62
Binswanger's disease, 266–67
biomarkers
ADAM-10, 268–69
in AD staging, 55–56
APOE (*see* apolipoprotein ε4 [ApoE4])
apolipoproteins, 381
arterial integrity, 92
autoantibodies, 389–91
$A\beta_{42}$, 378, 385, 386–87
$A\beta_{42}$/tau combined, 380
BDNF, 381
blood, in VCI, 93
blood-based, 384–89
blood–brain barrier, 382
cell signaling/inflammation associated proteins, 386
cortical atrophy studies, 70
CSF-based, 377–85
diagnostic value of, 375–77
disease progression studies, 69
endosome-lysosome system, 382
exosomes, 388
goals/obstacles, 377–78
hippocampal atrophy studies, 70
MCA-PI, 93
microRNAs, 383, 388–89
neurogranin, 381
platelets, 387
S100B, 382–83
stroke, 20–22, 93–94
tau, 72, 379, 385, 386–87
ubiquitin, 381
vascular risk factors studies, 20–22, 21*t*
for VCI, 92–93
VILIP-1, 381
α-synuclein, 382

Bispectral Index Monitor (BIS), 440–41
Blennow, K., 264
blood–brain barrier
  alterations in neuropathology, 35
  ApoE4 in damage to, 37
  APOE-ε4, 269
  Aβ clearance, 312–13
  Aβ peptides modulation by, 32–33
  biomarkers, 382
  CSF albumin index (Q_{alb}), 263–65, 266
  DCE-MRI, 265–68
  dysfunction of, neuropathology, 355
  hemodynamic impairment effects, 311
  longitudinal studies of, 263–64
  plasma triglycerides in variance, 264–65
  sPDGFRβ, 268–69
  vascular hypothesis of AD, 261–63
Bombois, S., 191
Bondi, M. W., 66, 67–68, 67*t*, 69, 110
bootstrap likelihood ratio test, 132
Bowman, G. L., 263–65
Boyle, P. A., 33–34, 112
Braak, E., 315–16, 335
Braak, H., 315–16, 335
brachial-ankle PWV (baPWV), 277–78
brain connectivity, 175–77
brain infarcts, 341, 342*f*, 350–52
brain volumetry imaging, 209, 211*f*
Broca, P., 174–75
Burgmans, S., 266

CAA. *See* cerebral amyloid angiopathy
CADASIL, 339
Cahn-Weiner, D. A., 112–13
Cairns, H., 172
caloric restriction interventions, 420
cancellation test, 172
CARASIL, 339
Cardiovascular Health Study, 190–91
Cardiovascular Health Study Cognition Study, 93
cardiovascular risk factors
  alcohol consumption, 10, 13*t*, 18*t*
  arterial stiffness, 11, 13*t*, 89–90
  brain area congruence, 247*f*, 247
  cumulative, 12, 13*t*, 17
  diabetes, 8, 13*t*, 18*t*, 21*t*, 36, 242
  FSRP, 12, 13*t*, 17
  hypercholesterolemia, 18*t*
  hyperlipidemia, 37
  hypertension, 6, 10, 13*t*, 18*t*, 36, 89–90, 242
  imaging, 242
  midlife, 21*t*
  neuropathological correlates, 355
  obesity, 9, 13*t*, 18*t*
  overview, 5–6
  pressure pulsatility, 11, 13*t*, 89–90
  prevalence, 314
  serum cholesterol, 9, 13*t*, 37
  smoking, 9, 13*t*, 18*t*
carotid-femoral pulse wave velocity (CFPWV) studies, 11, 16–17
carotid-femoral PWV (cfPWV), 277–78
CERAD, 333–34, 335–36
cereboretinal vasculopathy, 339
cerebral amyloid angiopathy
  APOE association with, 340
  lobar intracerebral hemorrhage and, 340, 345
  microbleed association with, 222, 310–11, 345, 352
  microinfarct association with, 350–52
  neuropathology, 336, 337*f*, 338, 340, 343
cerebral amyloidosis, 11–12, 275–76, 281, 290–91
cerebral hemorrhages neuropathology, 343, 344*f*
cerebral microbleeds. *See* microbleeds
cerebral SVD
  cerebral microbleeds (*see* microbleeds)
  characterization, 187
  in cognitive decline, 188–89
  cortical superficial siderosis, 188
  cortical thinning in, 197
  frontoparietal network disruption in, 197
  hereditary, 339
  lacunes/presumed vascular origin, 188
  longitudinal studies, 193–94, 199–200
  methodology, 188–89
  neuroimaging nomenclature, 187–88
  neuropathology, 351
  perivascular spaces, 188, 199–201, 200*t*, 310–11

small subcortical infarcts (*see* small subcortical infarcts)
small subcortical infarcts as predictors of AD, 217*f*
vascular injury/ neurodegeneration, 309–11
vessel pathologies, 336–40, 337*f*
WMHs as predictive in diagnosis, 190
WMHs as predictive of cognitive decline, 192, 200*t*
WMHs in, 187, 189–94, 310–11
cerebrovascular reactivity (CVR), 305–6
cerebrovasculature, 303–4
cholesterol as CVD risk factor, 9
Clark, L. R., 32, 57–59, 64*t*
Clerici, F., 190
clinical amnesia, 84
Clinical Dementia Rating (CDR), 53
clinic-based neuropathological assessment, 356
cognitive decline
age-related neuropathology, 348–50, 349*f*
conceptual knowledge, 116
episodic memory impairment, 112, 117–18
everyday functioning assessment, 119
everyday function multidimensionality, 113
executive function impairment, 112, 117–18
financial abilities, 109–10
impairment level in everyday function, 108
methodology, 103
microerrors/microslips, 106, 117
omission–commission model, 113
phenotypes, mixed pathology impacts on, 352–54
resource theory, 111
self-report *vs.* informant-report, 110
as surgical risk factor, 435
terminology, 103
Cohen, M. L., 171
Cohen, R. A., 112
coin rotation task, 160–61
collagen type IV mutations, 339
Combarros, O., 176–77
community-based neuropathological assessment, 356–58
conceptual apraxia
clinical signs, 108
etiologies, 113
pathophysiology, 112
terminology, 103, 148–49, 162–63
Constantine, G. L., 136
construction apraxia, 148
context independent *vs.* dependent profiles, 40–41
cortical superficial siderosis, 188
cortical thickness studies
in cerebral SVD, 197
longitudinal studies in AD, 212–13
structural MRI, 212
corticobasal degeneration, action-intentional disorder-associated, 172–73
COX activity impairment, 410–11
crossed-response inhibition task, 170
Crutch, S. J., 164
CSF albumin index (Q_{alb}), 263–65, 266
Cullum, C. M., 386–87

DASH diet, 94–95
Davidson, J. E., 134–35, 138–39
day-out task, 106
Debette, S., 9–10, 15, 16
default mode network (DMN), 447–48
defective response inhibition, 165, 169
De Groot, J. C., 192–93
Delano-Wood, L., 57, 64*t*, 73–74, 110
Delon, S., 304
DeLong, M. R., 176
dementia
age-related neuropathology, 348–50, 349*f*
anesthesia and, 439
animal models, 32–33
autoantibody biomarkers, 389–91
hemodynamic impairment patterns in, 307–9
neuropathological basis of, 333–35
phenotypes, mixed pathology impacts on, 352–54
post stroke, neuropathology, 348
profile similarities, statistical analyses, 138–39

dementia (*cont.*)
service utilization patterns, statistical analyses, 134
vascular disease and, 32
vascular risk factors studies, 20–22
vessel pathologies, 336–40, 337*f*
WMHs as predictive, 190
depression, 437
De Renzi, E., 162–63, 168
desflurane, 440
Devi, L., 411
diabetes
BBB permeability in, 267
as CVD risk factor, 8, 13*t*, 18*t*, 21*t*, 36, 242
management, 463
MRI studies, 16
neuropathological correlates, 355–56
Diaz-Arrastia, R., 386–87
diffusion tensor imaging (DTI)
cerebral SVD, 189
MCI, 74
small subcortical infarcts, 217, 218*f*, 219*f*
white matter, in AD, 248–49, 250*f*
white matter microstructure in AD, 225
dissociation apraxia
clinical signs, 162
terminology, 148–49
verbal, 162–63
Dolan, P. J., 417–18
Dominantly Inherited Alzheimer's Network, 220
donepezil, 62, 460–61
dorsal PFC volume studies, 114
Douiri, A., 94–95
Down's syndrome, 275–76
dressing apraxia, 148
Drosophila melanogaster studies, 417–18
DRP-1 impairment, 412–14, 419–20
DSM-5 guidelines, 85, 86*t*, 445–46
DTI tractography, 225
Dubois, B., 171–72
Duvernoy, H. M., 304

Edland, S. D., 281–82
Edmonds, E. C., 39–40, 46, 58, 61, 62–63, 64*t*, 71–72, 110, 461
Elias, M. F., 7, 10–11
Elias, P. K., 8
Eliassen, C. F., 70
entropy, 132
Epidemiology of Dementia Study, 20
episodic memory. *See also* memory
alcohol consumption studies, 10–11
assessment of, 107–8
brain infarcts effects on, 350–51
impairment in cognitive decline, 112, 117–18
PrVLT studies, 43
WMAs, MRI studies, 38–39
Eppig, J. S., 61, 64*t*, 133
Erkinjuntti, T., 84–85
Evered, L., 445–46
Everyday Cognition (ECog) Scale, 104–5
executive function
aerobic training in treatment of, 94
anesthesia depth and, 440
cerebral microbleeds as predictors of cognitive decline without dementia, 199
diabetes effects on, 8–9
dysregulation/preservation, 41
impairment in cognitive decline, 112, 117–18
pressure pulsatility and, 279
serum cholesterol effects on, 10
small subcortical infarcts as predictors of cognitive decline, 196
smoking effects on, 9
subcortical lacunes impairments, 90
vascular cognitive impairment, 91
exosome biomarkers, 388

Fabry disorder, 339
Faglioni, P., 156–57
Farias, S. T., 109
Farmer, M. E., 6–7, 10–11
Ferriera, D., 135
Fogassi, L., 161
Forrester, S. N., 133, 136, 138–39
fractional anisotropy, 225, 248–49
frailty as surgical risk factor, 437
Framingham Heart Study
cardiovascular risk factors (*see* cardiovascular risk factors)
conventional *vs.* comprehensive criteria/MCI, 68–69

described, 4–5
MRI (*see* MRI studies)
neuropsychological testing, 5, 6–12
WMHs as predictive, 190
Framingham Offspring Study, 192–93
Framingham Risk Score (FRS), 12
Freund, H. J., 156–57, 161
frontal aging hypothesis, 209–10
frontal lobes in brain connectivity, 175–76
frontal pole, MRI studies, 71
FSRP score studies, 8–10
functional hyperemia, 305–6
Fuster, J., 44

Galasko, D. R., 110
Gall, F. J., 174–75
Gallo, J. L., 113–14
Garrett, K. D., 91–92
Gasparovic, C., 91–92
Geschwind, N., 154, 174–75
Ghacibeh, G. A., 161–62
Giovannetti, T., 42–43, 110–11, 113–14, 164
glabella reflex testing, 169–70
glia limitans, 262
Global Deterioration Scale (GDS), 53
Golob, E. J., 265–66
go/no-go test, 170
Goodglass, H., 151–52
Grau-Olivares, M., 91
Guoping, P., 93–94
Gupta, A., 9–10

Haaland, K. Y., 156–57
Hachinski, V. C., 84
Hachinski Ischemic Scale, 84
Hall, J., 386–87
Halsband, U., 155
Hanfelt, J. J., 59–60, 64*t*, 137–38
Hanna-Pladdy, B., 157–58, 161–62
Hansson Petersen, C. A., 411
Hayden, K. M., 135, 139
Heilman, K. M., 155, 161–62, 167
hemodynamic impairment
AD pathology interactions, 311–13
cardiac dysfunction in, 314–16
cerebrovasculature, 303–4
clinical impact of, 302–3
patterns in dementia/aging, 307–9
regulation mechanisms, 304–6
vascular injury/ neurodegeneration, 309–11
hereditary cerebral hemorrhage with amyloidosis, 339
high blood pressure. *See* hypertension
high-risk populations studies
cerebral SVD, 192
MCI to dementia conversion, prediction of, 193–94
minority populations, neuropathological assessment, 357
hippocampal sclerosis, 333–34, 348–50, 353–54
hippocampal volume studies
Alzheimer's disease, structural MRI, 210–12, 211*f*
BBB integrity, 266
cerebral blood flow, 282–83
cerebral SVD, 190–91
diabetes, 242
hypertension, 242
MCI status, 69
in MCI sub types, 70
mixed AD neuropathology, 349*f*
omission–commission model, 114
small subcortical infarcts, 197–98
vascular dementia, 347–48
Hirai, K., 413
HOMA-IR model, 8–9
home/action monitoring, 107
homocysteine concentration as biomarker, 20–22
Honolulu Aging Study, 33–34
Honolulu-Asia Aging Study, 193
Hsu, C. L., 94
Hu, W. T., 386–87
Hummelsheim, H., 156–57, 161
Huntington's disease, 172–73
hyperlipidemia, 37
hypertension
cerebrovascular resistance and, 285–86
as CVD risk factor, 6, 10, 13*t*, 18*t*, 36, 89–90, 242
MRI studies, 15
neuropathological correlates, 356

hypertensive arteriopathy, 338
hypokinesia, 167

ideational apraxia
clinical signs, 162
diseases associated with, 164
pathophysiology, 163
terminology, 103, 148
ideomotor apraxia
Alzheimer's disease associated with, 158
basal ganglia/thalamus, 157
clinical signs, 151
convexity premotor cortex, 156
Parkinson plus syndromes associated with, 159
Parkinson's disease associated with, 159
pathophysiology, 153
stroke and, 158
superior longitudinal fasciculus, 155
supplementary motor area, 156, 157
terminology, 148
vascular diseases associated with, 158
IgG biomarkers, 389–91
inflammation, 354–56
innervatory apraxia. *See* limb-kinetic apraxia
instrumental activities of daily living (IADL), 103
insulin resistance, 20–22, 21*t*, 36
internal configuration errors, 151–52
Iqbal, K., 137
isoflurane, 440
Iturria-Medina, Y., 32

Jak, A. J., 66, 67–68, 67*t*, 69, 461
Jansen, J. F., 266
Jarvie, G., 280
Jefferson, A. L., 20, 113
Jin, Y. N., 417–18
Johnson, G. V. W., 417–18
Johnston, S. A., 390
Jokinen, H., 91
Jorge, R. E., 176–77

Kaplan, E., 151–52
Kaye, J. A., 264–65
Kertesz, A., 173
Khodagholi, F., 414–15
Kim, E. J., 173
Kim, M. J., 70–71
Kim, S., 190
Kinsbourne, M., 174
Kirchberg, B. C., 116–17
Kittner, S. J., 10–11
Knopman, D., 8
Kodadek, T., 390
Köhler, S., 137, 139
Kopeikina, K. J., 416–17
Kramer, J. H., 90
Krebs cycle impairment, 410–11
Kuypers, H. G., 161

lacunar infarcts, 342*f*
LADIS Study, 195, 196
Lam, L. C. W., 138–39
Lamar, M., 41–42, 44–45
large vessel atherosclerosis, 336
latent class analysis (LCA)
applications of, 131–32, 140–41
described, 131–32
mild cognitive impairment, 59, 64*t*
research examples, 132–40
latent profile analysis (LPA)
applications of, 131–32, 140–41
described, 131–32
mild cognitive impairment, 59, 64*t*
research examples, 132–40
Lawrence, D. G., 161
Leiguarda, R. C., 159–60, 164
Leoutsakos, J- M. S., 136, 138–39
letters FAS studies, 7, 44–45
leukoaraiosis. *See* white matter hyperintensities
Levitsky, W., 174–75
Lewy body dementia, 348, 349*f*, 352–53, 357–59, 440–41
Li, C., 88–89
Li, X., 92–93
Libon, D. J., 39, 57, 64*t*, 84, 113–14, 135–36
Liepmann, H., 148, 153–54, 160, 161, 162–64
lifestyle interventions, 420
limb-kinetic apraxia
clinical signs, 160
etiologies, 162
pathophysiology, 161
terminology, 148

lipohyalinosis, 310, 338
Liu, Q., 92
Lopez, O. L., 191
López-Olóriz, J., 93
Loring, D. W., 161–62
loss of volition, 166–67
Luria, A. R., 40–41, 170
Lyketsos, C. G., 136, 138–39

Magee, D. M., 390
Maillard, P., 15
Marquine, M. J., 194
Marsden, C. D., 157–58
McFall, G. P., 279
McGuinness, B., 60–61, 64*t*, 138–39
MCI. *See* mild cognitive impairment
McManus, M. J., 419
mdivi-1 therapy, 419–20
Meador, K. J., 161–62, 166
Mecocci, P., 264
medial temporal lobes. *See* MTL atrophy studies
Mediterranean–DASH MIND diet, 94–95
Mediterranean diet, 94–95, 462–63
melatonin therapy, 418–19
melokinetic apraxia. *See* limb-kinetic apraxia
memory. *See also* episodic memory
  anesthesia depth and, 440
  impairment *vs.* clinical amnesia, 84
  small subcortical infarcts as predictors of cognitive decline, 196
  subcortical lacunes impairments, 90
microarray studies, 390–91
microbleeds
  in cerebral SVD, 309–11
  MRI studies, 345
  neuropathology, 343, 344*f*
  PiB PET studies, 345
  as predictors of AD, 215–17, 216*f*, 222–23
  as predictors of cognitive decline, 199, 200*t*
  as predictors of diagnosis, 198
  stroke and, 199
microerrors/microslips, 106, 117
microinfarcts, 342–43
microRNA biomarkers, 383, 388–89
middle cerebral artery-pulsatility index (MCA-PI), 93
mild cognitive impairment
  acetylcholinesterase inhibitors in, 62
  AD protein pathology in, 72
  AD staging criteria, 55
  amnestic, 59–60, 63, 69, 70–71
  APOE genotype in, 75
  autoantibody biomarkers, 389–91
  blood pressure studies, 6–7
  brain stimulation, 463
  characterization, 3, 52–53, 129–30, 458
  clinical evaluation, 459
  clinical phenotype heterogeneity, 459
  cluster analytic models of, 57, 64*t*
  cognitive interventions, 462
  comprehensive diagnostic criteria, 66–68, 67*t*
  conventional diagnostic criteria, 53, 63
  core clinical criteria, 55
  cortical atrophy studies, 70
  DCE-MRI, 265–68
  dietary management, 462
  differential functional profiles in, 115–16
  donepezil/vitamin E trial, 39–40
  DTI studies, 74
  everyday functioning declines, 109
  executive function/language impairments, 59–60
  functional difficulties detection, 118
  functional impairments/ neuropsychiatric features, 59–60
  hippocampal atrophy studies, 70
  interventions, 458–59, 460–63
  latent mixture models of, 59, 64*t*
  MCI to dementia conversion, 88, 190–91, 308–9
  MCI to dementia conversion, prediction of, 89, 192–93, 198, 212, 218–21
  MCI to VaD conversion, 137–38
  medications, 460
  memory impairment, statistical analyses, 139
  minimally impaired subtype, 59–60
  mixed multidomain, 59–60, 63, 70
  neuropsychiatric assessment, 460

mild cognitive impairment (*cont.*)
neuropsychological subtypes, 56–63
omission–commission model in, 115
physical activity, 462
prodromal dementia identification, 53
profiles, statistical analyses, 134–36, 137, 139–40
profile similarities, statistical analyses, 138–39
pure amnestic, 59–60
risk factor management, 463
risk profiles, statistical analyses, 136, 137–38
small/ lacunar infarcts studies, 197
statistical techniques summary, 63
symptom profiles, statistical analyses, 133
vascular risk factors, 88 (*see also* cardiovascular risk factors)
vascular risk factors studies, 20–22
white matter pathology in, 73
Miles, W. R., 8
Miller, B. D., 167
Minai-Tehrani, D., 414–15
minority populations, neuropathological assessment, 357
Mishkin, M., 154
mitochondria
bioenergetics/oxidative stress in AD, 410–11
dynamics in AD, 412–18
fusion–fission dynamics, 412
neuronal populations role, 408–10
pathobiology in AD, 421*f*, 421–22
as therapeutic targets, 418–20
transport in AD, 416
turnover in AD, 414
mitofusins impairment, 412–14
MitoQ therapy, 419
MOAS phenotype, 413
modularity hypotheses, 174–75
Montagne, A., 266
Monte Carlo simulation studies, 132
Monza, D., 159–60
Moran, M., 139
Morris, J. C., 57, 60–61, 67*t*
Moser, D. J., 112
Motamedi, F., 414–15
motor impersistence, 165, 169
motor preservation, 171
Mountcastle, V. B., 175
mouse models
AD vascular dysfunction, 311–12
Aβ homeostasis, 32–33
mitochondrial dysfunction/cognitive deficits, 419–20
MRI studies
alcohol consumption, 16
amnestic MCI, 88–89
arterial stiffness, 16
atrial fibrillation, 15
blood pressure, 15
BMI, 16
cerebral blood flow, 283
cerebral SVD, 191, 197–98
cholesterol, 16
cortical atrophy, 70
diabetes, 16
diet, 16
FHS, 12–17
hypertension, 15
microbleeds, 198, 345
obesity, 16
pressure pulsatility, 16
SCIs, 15
small subcortical infarcts, 195–96, 197–98
smoking, 16
MTL atrophy studies
AD prediction, 243–47
Alzheimer's disease, structural MRI, 210–11
BBB integrity, 266
CBF patterns, 308–9
cerebral blood flow, 284
cerebral SVD, 191–92
omission–commission model, 114
multi-infect dementia, 84
multiple sclerosis, 353
multisystem atrophy, ideomotor apraxia and, 159–60
Mungas, D., 196–97
Myerson's sign testing, 169–70

Nakaoku, Y., 91
Nation, D. A., 267–69, 281–82

National Heart, Lung, and Blood Institute Twin Study, 193
Naturalistic Action Test (NAT), 105–7, 113–14
neural stem cell transplantation, 419–20
neuropathology assessments, 358–59
neurovascular coupling, 305–6
NIA-AA guidelines, 333–34, 359, 445–46
NIA Reagan, 335–36
NIH EXAMINER, 119
Niki, C., 163–64
Nilsson, E. D., 280
Nirkko, A. C., 161
Nishtala, A., 7, 8–10
n–m test, 171–72
nonamyloid SVD. *See* cerebral SVD
Norton, M. C., 137
novel-concept formation impairments, 90
Nyenhuis, D. L., 91, 94

obesity
  as CVD risk factor, 9, 13*t*, 18*t*
  dietary management, 462
  management, 463
  MRI studies, 16
O'Bryant, S. E., 386–87
Ohara, T., 88
olivopontocerebellar atrophy, 172–73
omission–commission model, 113
OPA-1 impairment, 412–14
Oregon Brain Aging Study, 192–93
Oresanya, L. B., 435–36

pantomimes, 151–52, 155, 158–59
parallel processing, 174
Parkinson plus syndromes, 159, 172–73
Parkinson's disease
  action-intentional disorder-associated, 172–73
  autoantibody biomarkers, 389–91
  defective response inhibition in, 171
  functional impairments in, 114–15
  ideational apraxia-associated, 164
  ideomotor apraxia-associated, 159
  letters FAS studies, 44–45
  preservation disorders treatment, 176–77
  α-synuclein as biomarker, 382
Pase, M. P., 20
pathological inertia construct, 40–41
Paul, R. H., 108–9, 112
Pavlovic, A. M., 197
PC DHA as biomarker, 20–22
Pedelty, L., 94
pegboard task, 160–61
performance-based measures, 105–8
perioperative cognitive medicine. *See also* anesthesia
  anesthesia, dementia and, 439
  anesthesia rewarming rate, 442
  background, 434
  blood levels, 444
  case studies, 433–34
  change, labeling, 445–46
  emboli, 443
  neuropsychologists as team builders, 446–47
  operative risk factors, 439–43
  oxygenation, 444
  postoperative risk factors, 444–45
  risk factors, 435–38
perivascular spaces, 188, 199–201, 200*t*, 310–11
Perry, G., 417–18
Petersen, R. C., 53–54, 57, 60–61, 67*t*
PET imaging
  AD protein pathology, 72–73
  amyloid levels/WMH in AD, 220–21
  glucose metabolism in AD, 410–11
Pharr, V., 159–60
phenotypes
  latent class analysis, 39
  mixed pathology impacts on, 352–54
  statistical modeling of, 38
  statistical modeling of, in treatment, 39
PiB PET studies, 345
plasma homocysteine concentration as biomarker, 20–22
Poeck, K., 162–63
Poizner, H., 153
polypharmacy as surgical risk factor, 438
posterior cortex volume studies, 114
post mortem examinations, 34
postoperative cognitive dysfunction, 445–46
postural errors, 151–52, 157–58

Pramstaller, P. P., 157–58
praxicons, 154–55
praxis recognition disorders, 153
pressure pulsatility. *See also* arterial stiffness
  cognitive decline and, 278–79
  as CVD risk factor, 11, 13*t*, 89–90
  executive function and, 279
  MRI studies, 16
Price, C. C/, 38, 43
prodromal dementia identification, 53
progressive nuclear palsy, 172–73
PSEN1/PSEN2, 275–76
pulse pressure. *See* pressure pulsatility
PVS. *See* perivascular spaces

Qin, W., 415–16
questionnaires, 103–5
Quinn, J. F., 264–65
Quintanilla, R. A., 417–18
Qureshi, M., 162–63

Rabkin, S. W., 280
Raymer, A. M., 151–52
Razani, J., 9–10
reactive oxygen species, 408–9, 418–19
Reddy, M. M., 390
Religious Orders Study, 347
resource theory, 111
Restrepo, L., 390
Rockwood, K., 84–85
Román, G. C., 84–85
Root, H. F., 8
Rossor, M. N., 164
Rothi, L. J. G., 155
Rotterdam Study, 94–95, 192–93, 198
Royall, D. R., 112–13
Rush Alzheimer's Disease Center MAP, 248
Rush Memory and Aging Project, 347

Sachdev, P. S., 91–92
Sadowski, M., 32–33
Salmon, D. P., 110
Sandson, J., 173
Schaefer, E. J., 20–22
Scheltens, N. M., 138
Schmidt, K. S., 113–14
Schneider, J. A., 33–34
Seidel, G. A., 114
semantic dementia, 116–17, 150
serial list-learning test studies, 32
serum cholesterol as CVD risk factor, 9, 13*t*, 37
Seshadri, S., 17
Sestito, N., 113–14
Shaerzadeh, F., 414–15
Silbert, L. C., 192–93
Skoog, I., 263–64
small subcortical infarcts
  characterization, 194–99
  lacunar, 342*f*, 342
  as predictors of AD, 217
  as predictors of cognitive decline, 196, 200*t*
  as predictors of diagnosis, 195
  terminology, 188–89
small vessel disease. *See* cerebral SVD
Smith, E. E., 88–89
Smith, G. W., 136
Smith, M. A., 417–18
smoking, 9, 13*t*, 16, 18*t*
sporadic nonamyloid microangiopathy. *See* cerebral SVD
SS-31 therapy, 419–20
Staekenborg, S. S., 191
Stafford, P., 390
Starr, J. M., 267
statistical modeling
  latent class/latent profile analyses, 131–32
  in MCI, summary, 63
  person-centered techniques, examples, 132–40
  phenotypes, in treatment, 39
  of phenotypes, 38
  variable- /person-centered techniques, 130–31, 140–41
Stephan, B. C. M., 89–90
striatonigral degeneration, 172–73
Strick, P. L., 176
stroke
  action intentional deficits and, 172–73
  Alzheimer's disease and, 8–9, 223–24
  arterial integrity, post stroke, 92
  biomarkers, 20–22, 93–94

brain connectivity and, 175
cholinesterase inhibitors treatment, 176–77
cognitive disabilities, post stroke, 90
cortical/subcortical, studies, 157–58
dementia evolution and, 88–90, 130, 137–38, 224
FSRP as predictive, 5–6, 12, 13*t*, 17
hemispheric, studies, 150, 153
ideomotor apraxia and, 158
ischemic, 84, 88–89, 94–95, 199
microbleeds and, 199
prevention of, 94–95
resource theory, 111
as risk factor, 4
SCIs as risk factor, 15
small/lacunar infarcts, 195–97
strategic, 83
structural MRI, 195–97
terminology, 223–24
WMHs as predictive of, 190–92
structural MRI
brain volumetry imaging, 209, 211*f*
cerebral microbleeds as predictors of AD, 222–23
cortical thickness studies, 212
CVD contribution to AD, 213–17
stroke, 195–97
white matter hyperintensities, 218–21
Su, M. Y., 265–66
subcortical infarcts. *See* small subcortical infarcts
subcortical white matter disease, 91
systolic blood pressure, interarm differences, 21*t*
Szeto-Schiller therapy, 419

Takahashi, Y., 88–89
Tan, Z. S., 8–9, 16
tau biomarkers, 72, 379–80, 385, 386–87
TDP-43, 333–34, 348, 353–54
temporal gradients, impaired studies, 44–45
temporal lobe epilepsy, 353
Texas Alzheimer's Research Consortium, 386–87
3-City Dijon MRI study, 192–93
tissue injury neuropathology, 341–45
transcranial Doppler
AD, cerebral blood flow in, 282
cerebrovascular resistance, 287
Tsao, C. W., 11, 16–17
two-hit hypothesis, 35

Uluduz, D., 159–60
Ungerleider, L. G., 154
Urban, S., 69

van de Haar, H. J., 266
van den Heuvel, D. M., 194
van der Flier, W. M., 193
Vannson, J. L., 304
Van Straaten, E. C., 191
vascular cognitive impairment, 84
arterial integrity, 92
background, 84–85
biomarkers for, 92–93
blood biomarkers, 93
cerebrovascular resistance in, 308
characterization, 83–84, 274–76
classification, 85, 86*t*
cognitive disabilities, post stroke, 90
empirical support for, 85–90
hemodynamic changes in (*see* hemodynamic impairment)
MCI to dementia conversion, 88
MCI to dementia conversion, prediction of, 89
neuropsychology of, 90–91
public health issues, 94–95
risk factors, 88 (*see also* cardiovascular risk factors)
subcortical white matter disease, 91
treatment, 94–95
vascular dementia
BBB disruption in, 264–65
BBB permeability in, 266–67
context independent *vs.* dependent profiles, 40–41
CSF albumin index, 263–65
diagnosis *vs.* classification, 45–46
episodic memory impairment, 112
executive function impairment, 112, 118
graphomotor preservation in, 41
heterogeneity of, 30

vascular dementia (*cont.*)
impaired temporal gradients in, 44–45
impairment level in everyday function, 108
neuropathology, 346–48
neuropathology heterogeneity in, 33–34
neuropsychological heterogeneity in, 38–40
pathophysiology, 130
phenotypes, latent class analysis, 39
phenotypes, statistical modeling of, 38
phenotypes statistical modeling, in treatment, 39
profiles, statistical analyses, 139–40
service utilization patterns, statistical analyses, 134
vascular dysfunction in regulation of, 34–38
verbal concept formation in, 42
WMHs as predictive, 190
vascular hypothesis of AD, 261–63
VCI. *See* vascular cognitive impairment
venous collagenosis, 339
Verdelho, A., 192
Villeneuve, S., 88–89
Virchow-Robin spaces. *See* perivascular spaces
Virtual Kitchen Challenge, 106–7
virtual reality tasks, 106–7
visual processing networks, 154
vitamin antioxidants in VCI treatment, 94
volition, loss of, 166–67
Vuong-Lo-Mendell-Rubin likelihood ratio test, 132

Waldstein, S. R., 279
Wang, B. W., 34
Wang, H., 265–66
Wang, X., 413–14, 417–18
Warrington, E. K., 164
Washington Heights/Inwood Columbia Aging Project (WHICAP), 190–91
Watson, R. T., 156, 167
Weiner, M., 386–87
Wharton, S. B., 33–34
White, L. R., 10–11
white matter hyperintensities
in cerebral SVD, 187, 189–94, 310–11
executive function impairment, 112
FLAIR MRI studies, 91–92, 266–67
imaging in AD, 248–50, 250*f*
inflammation in, 354–56
interactive hypotheses, 189–90
longitudinal studies, 193–94
MRI studies, 38, 41–42, 43, 89–90
MR spectroscopy studies, 91–92
neuropathology, 345
as predictive in AD, 190, 215*f*, 215, 216*f*, 218–21
as predictive of cerebral SVD, 190
as predictive of cognitive decline, 192, 200*t*
as predictive of stroke, 190–92
PVS dilatation as predictive, 199–200, 200*t*
as risk factor, 21*t*
structural MRI, 218–21
subcortical lacunes impairments, 90
subcortical white matter disease, 91
Winblad, B., 54
Windkessel effect, 277
WMH. *See* white matter hyperintensities
Wolf, P. A., 10, 20
Wolfson, L., 193–94

Xiao, G., 386–87

Yan, L., 288
Yao, M., 199–200
Yassine, H. N., 462–63
Yip, A. G., 37

Zanetti, M., 88
Zhang, W., 419–20
Zhang, Y., 88
Zhu, X., 417–18
Zhu, Y. C., 199–200

Printed in the USA
CPSIA information can be obtained
at www.ICGtesting.com
CBHW081744190724
11856CB00005B/339

9 780190 634230